HANDBOOK OF HEALTH RESEARCH METHODS

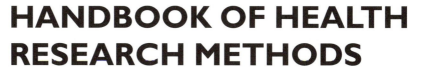

HANDBOOK OF HEALTH RESEARCH METHODS

Investigation, measurement and analysis

Edited by Ann Bowling and Shah Ebrahim

Open University Press

Open University Press
McGraw-Hill Education
McGraw-Hill House
Shoppenhangers Road
Maidenhead
Berkshire
England
SL6 2QL

email: enquiries@openup.co.uk
world wide web: www.openup.co.uk

and Two Penn Plaza, New York, NY 10121-2289, USA

First published 2005
Reprinted 2006, 2007

A catalogue record of this book is available from the British Library

ISBN–10: 0 335 21460 6 (pb)   0 335 21461 4 (hb)
ISBN–13: 978 0335 214600 (pb)   978 0335 2146 1 7 (hb)

Library of Congress Cataloging-in-Publication Data
CIP data applied for

Typeset by RefineCatch Limited, Bungay, Suffolk
Printed in the UK by Bell and Bain Ltd, Glasgow

Contents

List of contributors

Dr Joy Adamson, Department of Health Sciences, University of York, UK.

Dr Geraldine Barrett, Department of Health and Social Care, Brunel University, UK.

Dr Jane P. Biddulph, Department of Primary Care and Population Sciences, University College London, University of London, UK.

Professor Ann Bowling, Department of Primary Care and Population Sciences, University College London, University of London, UK.

Ms Sara Brookes, Department of Social Medicine, University of Bristol, UK.

Dr Jackie Brown, MRC Health Services Research Collaboration, Department of Social Medicine, University of Bristol, UK.

Dr Simon Carter, Sociology Group, Department of Public Health and Policy, London School of Hygiene and Tropical Medicine, University of London, UK.

Professor Michel P. Coleman, Non-Communicable Disease Epidemiology Unit, London School of Hygiene and Tropical Medicine, University of London, UK.

Dr Paul Cullinan, Department of Occupational and Environmental Medicine, National Heart and Lung Institute, Imperial College London, University of London, UK.

Professor George Davey Smith, Department of Social Medicine, University of Bristol, UK.

Professor Paul Dieppe, MRC Health Services Research Collaboration, Department of Social Medicine, University of Bristol, UK.

Professor Jenny Donovan, Department of Social Medicine, University of Bristol, UK.

Dr Craig Duncan, Institute for the Geography of Health, University of Portsmouth, UK.

Professor Shah Ebrahim, Department of Social Medicine, University of Bristol, UK.

Dr Vikki Entwistle, Health Services Research Unit, Department of Public Health, University of Aberdeen, UK.

Dr Clare Harries, Department of Psychology, University College London, University of London, UK.

Dr Lesley Henderson, Department of Human Sciences, Brunel University, UK.

Professor Kelvyn Jones, School of Geographical Sciences, University of Bristol, UK.

Dr Olga Kostopoulou, Department of Primary Care and General Practice, University of Birmingham, UK.

Dr Sarah J. Lewis, Department of Social Medicine, University of Bristol, UK.

Dr Richard Martin, Department of Social Medicine, University of Bristol, UK.

Professor Martin McKee, European Centre on Health of Societies in Transition, London School of Hygiene and Tropical Medicine, University of London, UK.

Professor Graham Moon, Institute for the Geography of Health, University of Portsmouth, UK.

Dr Ellen Nolte, European Centre on Health of Societies in Transition, London School of Hygiene and Tropical Medicine, University of London, UK.

Dr Alan O'Rourke, Institute of General Practice, School of Health and Related Research (ScHARR), University of Sheffield, UK.

Professor Ann Oakley, Social Science Research Unit, Institute of Education, University of London, UK.

Professor Tim Peters, Academic Unit of Primary Health Care, Department of Community Based Medicine, University of Bristol, UK.

Dr Tina Ramkalawan, MRC Health Services Research Collaboration, Department of Social Medicine, University of Bristol, UK.

Ms Caroline Sanders, Department of Social Medicine, University of Bristol, UK.

Dr Mary Shaw, Department of Social Medicine, University of Bristol, UK.

Dr Andrew Steptoe, Psychobiology Group, Department of Epidemiology and Public Health, University College London, University of London, UK.

Dr Jonathan Sterne, Department of Social Medicine, University of Bristol, UK.

Dr Anne Stiggelbout, Department of Medical Decision Making, Leiden University, The Netherlands.

Dr S. V. Subramanian, Harvard School of Public Health, Harvard University, USA.

Dr Kate Tilling, Department of Social Medicine, University of Bristol, UK.

Dr Liz Twigg, Institute for the Geography of Health, University of Portsmouth, UK.

Dr Suzanne Wait, Judge Institute of Management Studies, University of Cambridge, UK.

Preface

This book aims to assist researchers from clinical and non-clinical disciplines to plan, carry out, analyse and evaluate research on population health, health outcomes and health care delivery. A sound knowledge of research methods is important to all professionals involved in health policy and the delivery of health care. It is increasingly common for researchers from different disciplines to work together, and this book also aims to provide insight into their different research perspectives and methods. The focus of the book therefore reflects a multidisciplinary approach to research that is relevant to a wide range of students and researchers.

The book includes an impressive number of authors, all of whom are active and experienced investigators, with international reputations in their area of expertise. While the length of each chapter varies, depending on its aims and subject matter, the authors have each provided a comprehensive guide to their specialist topics, pitched at a level suitable for a multidisciplinary readership. Where appropriate, authors have included a list of further reading and resources to point the reader towards more detailed material. It is hoped that this book will introduce readers to research methodology across disciplines, and increase awareness of some of the critical issues involved in investigating health and health services.

Ann Bowling and Shah Ebrahim

Part I
Introduction

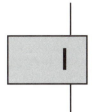

Research on health and health care

Paul Dieppe

He who has choice has trouble.
(Dutch proverb)

Doubt is not a pleasant condition, but certainty is absurd.
(Voltaire)

All democratic governments are rightly concerned with the education and health of the populations they serve. But modern democracies are finding it increasingly difficult to maintain the health of their people in equitable and cost-effective ways. They need research on the effectiveness, outcomes, access to and costs of the varying options available to us to improve the health of individuals and populations. This book is about the methods needed to do that research. In this introductory chapter, one of the principles behind all health problems, as well as health care research – uncertainty – is explored.

Health, disease and illness

Health is difficult to define. Literally it means 'wholeness' and it can be thought of as the ability of an individual to fulfil their potential. In practice, health has often been used to denote the absence of disease and, as outlined below, modern health services and health research have concentrated on the prevention or treatment of disease rather than on health. But this may not be sufficient for our increasingly demanding and wealthy western populations. They may prefer the World Health Organization's definition of health as 'A state of complete physical, mental and social wellbeing' (WHO 1948). But this utopian state is difficult to achieve, except perhaps fleetingly (Skrabanek and McCormick 1998).

Disease can be defined as an abnormality of the structure or function of the body (a definition that raises the difficult question of what we think of as normal, and how much diversity we are willing to accept). An illness is a symptom experience, which can include features such as pain or distress, restriction of normal activities (disability), or reduced ability to participate in life in the ways in which an individual would like. It is now customary to consider disease and illness within a 'biopsychosocial model', which stresses the importance of environmental and personal factors, and their interactions with a disease on health. Disease and illness can lead to sickness – which is the role played by people with illness in our society. But the illness experience and sickness are not always caused by disease; they depend on psychosocial factors as well. Health care professionals spend a lot of their time with people with illness but not disease.

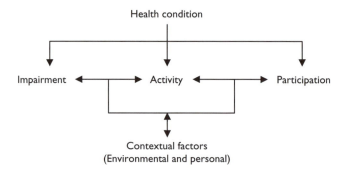

Figure 1.1

Source: Adapted, with permission from The International Classification of Impairment, Disability and Handicap (WHO 1999).

    Therefore, health problems are about sensations that we consider to be less than ideal, and/or about what our society regards as abnormalities of body or mind. They also embody things that we see as an internal threat to our identity and ourselves. An external threat can come from something like the perceived risk of a terrorist attack, and can engender symptoms associated with disease, such a pain and anxiety. An internal threat occurs when our body or mind appears to let us down or malfunction, resulting in uncertainty about who or what we are and about our future.
    The WHO (1999) model (see Figure 1.1) suggests that a health condition (any disease or illness) is one of the factors that dictates what one is able to do (activities) and how much one is able to take part in society (participation). A key health-related variable is impairment (loss of a certain bodily function). Other contextual factors also affect activities and participation; they include external (environmental) factors, such as culture, housing and income, and internal (personal) factors such as psychological status, motivation and educational attainments. All factors interact.

Health care

    As Horacio Fabrega (1997) and others have said, illness can be regarded as embodying an increase in uncertainty among individuals and societies. Members of the society try to reduce or eliminate that uncertainty through knowledge structures related to disease, illness and healing. Two main systems emerge in most societies – the informal, lay or folk systems of healing, and the formal or professional structures. Most health care, in every country in the world, takes place within the informal sector.
    Societies are diverse, and often seem to need more than one type of professional health care system to accommodate the varying views, priorities and approaches of the different individuals within them. This has been termed 'medical pluralism' and leads to a situation in which a sick individual can choose help from a system that fits best with their own perceptions of the problem. However, over the last two centuries, the biomedical model has become hugely dominant in western society, eclipsing most other concepts of health and health care. This dominance has been aided by regulation and research. Alternatives are available through what we pejoratively call 'complementary and alternative medicine' – but we now appear to be doing

our best to incorporate them into the biomedical model by carrying out scientific research on them and rejecting those that do not seem to work in ways that biomedicine understands. The result is three main systems of health care:

1 lay advice and folk remedies;
2 biomedicine, working within state-funded, regulated systems;
3 complementary and alternative traditions and healers, who tend to be marginalized by the biomedical movement.

The biomedical revolution has been enormously successful. Many conditions that would have been fatal in the past can now be treated successfully with modern drugs and surgery. However, within this success story there appear to be two significant problems:

1 our society remains uncertain about its health and health care;
2 the systems that we have built up around the biomedical model of health care are not well equipped to deal with chronic illness.

The persisting uncertainty about health in our population is apparent from the extent of the utilization of complementary and alternative practices; this often takes place in conjunction with the utilization of modern biomedicine. We go to alternative practitioners, who work outside the biomedical model even though we do not always think that they can 'cure' us in the conventional sense. We are looking for something else in relation to our uncertainty about our health.

During a time of enormous advances in biomedicine and biomedical research, and in the number and complexity of the interventions available to help people with disease and illness, two major new trends have put increasing pressure on western health systems:

1 the development of expensive technologies for health care delivery in place of simple, cheaper options;
2 the rise in the prevalence of chronic disease.

The two issues are interrelated.

Take, for example, the case of kidney failure. Until the 1960s all you could offer someone whose kidneys were failing was supportive care until they died. Then along came dialysis, followed by kidney transplantation. These are great success stories, allowing huge numbers of people to be kept alive for much longer. But they are expensive, and they do not always 'cure' the individual with the kidney problem, who may remain ill for years, and in need of human caring and expensive drugs, in spite of the 'successful' renal transplantation.

Scientific research often results in more expensive options in health care, for diagnosis as well as treatment. For example, we have replaced the humble, cheap X-ray machine, housed in a van or shed and operated by a single radiographer, with the expensive and complex magnetic resonance imaging suite in which you can find an army of physicists, radiographers and radiologists.

Disease and illness varies in different cultures and continents, and changes over time. In many parts of the world malnutrition, infection and injury are still the dominant health problems. However, in the rich western countries chronic disease is becoming the major issue. There are several reasons for this:

1 diminishing importance of malnutrition and infection;
2 increasing age of the population;
3 increasing prevalence of chronic disease risk factors such as obesity;
4 partial treatment of acute conditions (the ability to keep more people with diseases alive for longer, but without completely 'curing' them);

5 the creation of chronic diseases without illness (hypertension for example – the diagnosis of which can lead to great anxiety);

6 the invention of chronic illness without disease (e.g. awareness of environmental hazards and the cultural belief that they are making you 'ill').

We are adapting quickly to the influx of modern new technologies in health care, in part because of the love affair that health care professionals have developed for expensive bits of equipment that they can use to try and help their patients. But we are not adapting so well to the rise in chronic health problems, and health care professionals are still taught more about the management of acute crises than they are about chronic health care.

Our systems of hospitals and clinics was designed and set up to deal with acute crises. They remain excellent at dealing with people who have a myocardial infarction, or get knocked down and fracture a leg. Triage takes place in a well-equipped accident and emergency department, followed by referral to the specialist cardiologist or orthopaedic surgeon respectively, who then administers the necessary technology, according to current, evidence-based protocols. But these systems are not so good at dealing with the person with chronic disease, or the individual who is ill, but not diseased. Indeed, super-specialization and increasing fragmentation of health care into 'cells' built around systems or diseases may be acting to the direct disadvantage of such people. Although primary care remains strong in the UK and many other countries, it is increasingly difficult to find a 'general physician' who can look at all aspects of the health and care of someone with multiple, difficult problems.

Health care research

In the previous sections the concept of illness as 'uncertainty' (about your body, your mind, your identity and your future) was introduced. Uncertainty is also the underlying principle behind all research.

Although physicists may be able to predict the next eclipse of the sun with astounding accuracy and very little uncertainty, in the biological and social sciences uncertainty always remains high, however much evidence is brought to bear on the problem. We do research to reduce the degree of uncertainty, but we cannot abolish it. We do not 'know' anything for certain (sadly this concept seems lost on the general public, who are encouraged to believe that medical scientists can come up with definitive answers to their problems).

As Kerlinger (1986) pointed out, we get to know things in one of three main ways:

1 by authority (we are told the 'truth' by someone we believe in);
2 by intuition (it is our judgement that, or it seems to stand to reason that, something is true);
3 by scientific methods (which involve the key principle of self-correction).

The scientific method finds things out by research that is characterized by control and replication:

• *control* means that the central observations or experiments take place in a known framework, so that the causes of the results can be identified;
• *replication* means that if the work was repeated the answer should be the same.

In the physical sciences quantitative methods are pre-eminent: hypotheses are constructed and tested in experiments that take place in tightly controlled conditions, outcomes are measured with high precision, and the findings are always carefully replicated. The same positivist methodology is valuable in the biological and social sciences, although a wide range of different quantitative methods and approaches are needed to help acquire reliable, replicable data on complex biological or health care systems. But the great complexity of these systems, the huge variations in individual human behaviour and outcomes, and the positivist belief in a single truth for all, can limit the value and applicability of classical quantitative methods if used in isolation. For these reasons qualitative as well as quantitative research methods have to be used in biological and social sciences, including health research.

Qualitative methods, such as the collection of narratives, interviews, focus groups and ethnographic work, can provide rich insights into the experience of individuals, the meaning and interpretation of those experiences, and the likely relationships between different factors. Although often working in a hypothesis-free environment they can also be very helpful in the formation of new hypotheses to be tested by quantitative methods. Qualitative research methods uncover a different type of truth, but one that is no less important. Its limitations stem largely from problems of replication and in the time taken to acquire and interpret the data.

The methods used to undertake health and health care research are diverse. But all lead to the acquisition of new data, and share the need for storage, analysis and interpretation of those data. Computers have revolutionized our ability to deal with the vast quantities and diverse types of data obtained within health research, and to increase output. The massive rise in research outputs over recent years has led to a further division of health research into 'primary' and 'secondary' types. Primary research involves observation and experiment to gain new data. Secondary research involves finding and analysing research done by others.

Health and health care research are needed in order to reduce the uncertainty associated with the diagnosis, treatment and delivery of health care to all of those people in our society who are in need of it. There is a massive spectrum of such research, ranging from laboratory investigations on single molecules in tightly-controlled conditions, to observations on the complex behaviours within populations or systems of health care delivery.

This book is concerned with applied research on health and health services, rather than basic biological investigations. This spans a continuum from studies on individuals to those on groups of subjects and finally on populations and systems. It should be seen as a broad range of research techniques rather than a speciality or discipline. It covers all aspects of health care, including prevention, diagnosis and treatment and includes research on patients as well as healthy volunteers.

Health services research

The term 'health services research' (HSR) has been used to cover most of the methods and approaches to research described in this book. In general terms, HSR seeks knowledge and evidence that will lead to improvements in the delivery of health care; it is not a distinct discipline or profession, rather it is a set of techniques used in applied health research with the aim of improving health, health care and its delivery – it covers a huge range of activities.

As part of an attempt to provide a framework for HSR, and help delineate its borders with clinical research, audit and quality assurance (see below), the Medical Research Council's Health Services Research Collaboration and others have suggested that the main purpose of HSR should be to attempt to integrate the four main requirements of a good health service – i.e. that it should be *effective*, *efficient*, *equitable* and *acceptable* – and to research methods of implementing such services.

Effectiveness

It is obvious that anything we try to do to improve health and health care should work. And yet, many of the things we do probably have no effect. In medical literature two different aspects of whether something 'works' or not are distinguished – efficacy, which is whether an intervention helps a clearly defined group of people on whom it is tested, and effectiveness, which denotes the ability of that intervention to work for everyone who might need it. This raises the issue of whether the results of a trial (carried out using the scientific method, in carefully controlled conditions) is generalizible to the whole population, as discussed later in this book (see Chapter 5).

Efficiency

Efficiency means value for money. As interventions become increasingly expensive, efficiency becomes increasingly important. Health economists have developed a variety of ways of comparing the cost-effectiveness of different interventions and strategies. One of HSR's major challenges is to find out what strategies are likely to have the greatest pay-off to society as a whole, as well as to sick individuals. For example, it may be that we would be better off spending most of a country's health budget on the prevention of smoking and obesity, rather than on the provision of services for people who have developed diseases that result from these problems. But it is clear that we have not yet learnt how to control smoking and obesity, and another aspect of HSR is research into how behavioural change might be achieved.

Equity

Although not a central issue in health care for all advanced nations, the concept that health care should be available to everyone who needs it was one of the founding principles behind the establishment of the UK National Health Service. But equity of health services could mean a variety of different things: it could mean equity of access, equity of opportunity or equity of outcome. In the UK, equity of access, rather than equity of opportunity, has come to dominate the political debate. Concerns about equity are growing, with increasing awareness of the problems of diversity in society and the strong link between disadvantage and health problems.

Acceptability

Over the last few decades we have become increasingly aware of the need for any intervention to be acceptable to the public, as well as it being effective and efficient. This first came to prominence with the realization that many effective drugs prescribed by doctors are not taken by the patients – opening up research on what is now called adherence. This realization has turned into a modern movement in health care with increasing emphasis given to patient choice, patient-centred care and the empowerment of the public and patients to take control of their health and health care. The lesson for HSR is that it needs to make sure that any recommended new approach to health care is acceptable: qualitative research methods are particularly valuable in establishing this.

Implementation

Once we have an intervention, strategy or policy that is clearly effective, efficient and acceptable, our problems are still not over. We then have to implement it. In other words, we have to find ways of ensuring that the health care professionals, managers or policy-makers take up the options that research findings find most appropriate. A lot of work has been undertaken on the production of evidence-based guidelines and protocols, in the naïve belief that the production of a guideline would ensure good practice. HSR has shown that this is not the case – doctors, in particular, do not necessarily follow the guidelines of best practice. There are many good reasons for this. For example, guidelines are based on evidence from the mean of groups of people with well-defined problems, and may not be appropriate for an individual with a multiplicity of problems. An emerging challenge for HSR is to find ways of helping to individualize the care of people with chronic disease.

Another way of defining HSR is to say that it is about *appropriateness and quality* – the delivery of the most appropriate and highest quality interventions and health care services for individuals and populations respectively. Appropriateness means doing the things that are most likely to help and avoiding those that do not. Quality is more difficult to define – but has been said to encompass the domains of effectiveness, efficiency, equity and accessibility, plus acceptability as outlined above.

Doing research on these topics is difficult. That is what this book is about. An even greater challenge is to find ways of integrating the different aspects of HSR and achieving genuine interdisciplinarity. As shown in Figure 1.2, each of the key domains overlap. HSR is about trying to make sure that health care technology and services are effective, acceptable, efficient, equitable and that such services can be and are implemented – i.e. that interventions and services are appropriate and of

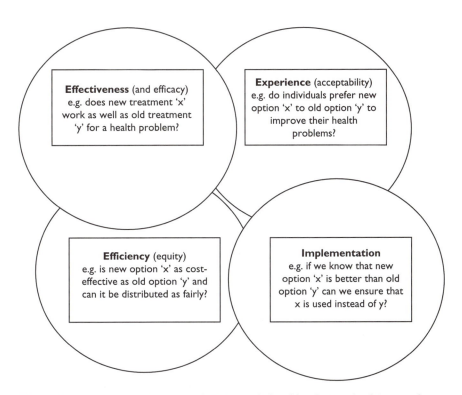

Figure 1.2   The main domains of HSR (as defined by the Medical Research Council and Health Services Research Collaboration)

high quality. These domains overlap and need integrating through multidisciplinary research.

HSR, clinical research, audit and quality assurance

HSR overlaps with clinical research, clinical audit and quality assurance, but there are distinctions between them.

Clinical research can be defined as any research that involves sick people. Such a definition would include things like clinical research, work on adherence and many other types of research also called HSR. But in addition, one of its most important functions is applied physiology: as we learn more about biology and disease processes from laboratory-based investigations, we have an increasing need to understand whether the mechanisms that have been uncovered are responsible for disease and illness in our patients, thus defining new targets for therapy. This involves careful observation of disease and the measurement of physiological and pathological variables in patients during the course of disease and before and after interventions – research activities not covered by the term HSR.

Audit is about maintaining high quality of care in health services. It involves the systematic analysis of procedures used and outcomes of all forms of health care delivered on a day-to-day basis by professionals and in medical institutions such as hospitals. It also has a major educational function, as it helps engender a critical and enquiring approach to health care delivery. The health care professionals generally carry it out.

Quality assurance can be defined as the definition of standards, the measurement of their achievement and the mechanisms employed to improve performance. It is more a managerial function than audit, and implies the presence of a planned service and agreed standards or targets.

Why do we need HSR?

During the nineteenth century and the first half of the twentieth, health research was dominated by the description of disease and clinical investigations. However, over the last 50 years there has been a huge shift to laboratory-based science. The vast majority of health research now involves genetic, molecular or cellular investigations in laboratories, predicated on the belief that a better understanding of the ways in which the body works in health and disease will lead to improved health. But the translation of knowledge gained in laboratories to the improved health of individuals and populations will not occur without HSR. HSR is a relatively new development within health research, and one of the main reasons for its recent and continuing growth is the huge expansion of the technological advances available to us. As more and more options become available it is increasingly important to assess them properly.

But there are many other reasons for expanding HSR, including:

- *The use of inappropriate care*: it is clear that interventions and systems of health care delivery that do not work, are inefficient or downright dangerous continue to be practised. We need to root out such practices and replace them with more appropriate ones.
- *Variations and inequities in health care*: although the UK National Health Service (NHS) and other health systems aspire to equitable care delivery this has not yet been achieved. Large variations in the delivery of health care occur, and the reasons for them need to be explored.
- *Limitation of resources*: the potential for health care to consume ever increasing

proportions of a country's gross national product became apparent in the USA towards the end of the last century, before the introduction of managed care and other mechanisms designed to reduce spending. No matter how much a community might wish to pay for good health care and health research for all its citizens, decisions have to be made, and HSR can inform these.

Multidisciplinarity and this book

This book is about the methods used in HSR and related applied health research. It focuses on the need for a multidisciplinary approach to the evaluation of health and health care. Research multidisciplinarity, or the involvement of people from more than one discipline or approach in a project, is an essential part of good HSR for the reasons outlined in the second section of this chapter. It has also been one of the principles behind the development of the Medical Research Council's (MRC) Health Services Research Collaboration (HSRC) (see www.hsrc.ac.uk), and the majority of the authors of the chapters that follow have been closely involved in the development of that organization. Most of the research that we currently undertake is led by one discipline, but involves others; in the future we need to do better than this and make sure that the design, management and execution of the research is interdisciplinary, i.e. that each discipline is of equal importance to the project.

Further reading

Bowling, A. (1997) *Research Methods in Health: Investigating Health and Health Services*. Buckingham: Open University Press.

Crombie, I.K. (1997) *Research in Health Care*. Chichester: Wiley.

Dieppe, P. (2000) To cure or not to cure, that is not the question, *Journal of the Royal Society of Medicine*, 93: 611–13.

Good, G.J. (1994) *Medicine, Rationality and Experience*. Cambridge: Cambridge University Press.

Medical Research Council (1998) *Health Services Research Collaboration*, www.hsrc.ac.uk.

Wade, D.T. and Halligan, P.W. (2004) Do biomedical models of illness make for good health-care systems?, *British Medical Journal*, 329: 1398–401.

References

Fabrega, H. (1997) *Evolution of Sickness and Healing*. Berkley, CA: University of California Press.

Kerlinger, F. (1986) *Foundations of Behavioural Research*. New York: Holt.

Skrabanek, P. and McCormick, J. (1998) *Follies and Fallacies in Medicine*, 3rd edn. Whitehorn: Tarragon Press.

WHO (World Health Organization) (1948) Preamble to the *Constitution of the World Health Organization* as adopted by The International Health Conference, New York 19–22 June 1946. Geneva: World Health Organization.

WHO (World Health Organization) (1999) International Classification of Impaired, Disability and Handicap. Geneva: World Health Organization.

2 Describing and evaluating health systems

Ellen Nolte, Martin McKee and Suzanne Wait

Introduction: what is a health system?

Before one can even begin to discuss evaluation of health systems, it is first necessary to decide what a health system is. There is, unfortunately, no simple answer. A pragmatic view interprets a health system as being 'made up of users, payers, providers and regulators [that] can be defined by the relations between them' (McPake *et al.* 2002), with 'relations' referring to four key functions of health systems: regulation, financing, resource allocation and provision of services (Mills and Ranson 2001). In practice, however, health care systems are often defined by national borders, exemplified by the remark made frequently by journalists since the publication of the *World Health Report* (WHO 2000) that 'the French health care system [is] judged by the World Health Organization . . . to be the best in the world' (British Broadcasting Corporation 2000). Yet within each country there is almost always a complex mixture of different systems, in which some people use different ways to pay for health care and in turn receive different benefits (McKee and Figueras 1997). For example, while many people would identify the British health system with its National Health Service (NHS), a system established in 1948 to provide universal coverage paid from general taxation, that interpretation would miss the growing differences in the way in which health care is organized in the four constituent parts of the UK, with Scotland, in particular, moving increasingly away from the model evolving in England. Similarly, it would miss the substantial volume of health care provided in the private health care sector, both to those that have private health insurance and, increasingly, for those who choose to pay directly. And the UK is, in comparison with some countries, remarkably homogeneous. What, for example, is meant by the term 'American health care system', with its myriad of payment plans for those in employment, superimposed upon Medicare, for the elderly, and Medicaid (with its many variations from state to state) for the poor, to say nothing of a range of other federally funded programmes such as those for the armed forces, for veterans and for native Americans? Even the Soviet health care system, which might be thought to have been more homogenous than most, contained a large number of parallel systems for those employed in the armed forces, the railways, Aeroflot (the Soviet airline), as well as the *nomenklatura* (the Communist Party elite).

Then there is the problem of defining the boundaries of a health system. There are many activities that contribute, directly or indirectly, to the provision of health care that, in different countries, may or may not be within what is considered to be the health system. The most obvious example is social care, especially for elderly people where it may be difficult, and indeed often inappropriate, to disentangle the provision of active health care (such as the investigation and treatment of chronic disorders) from more basic nursing care, to provision of appropriate living conditions. However, as health systems become increasingly complex, they depend ever more on a wide range of activities to generate and disseminate the knowledge required for effective health care, including basic and applied researchers and a growing body of 'knowledge brokers'. All contribute to the delivery of health care, yet they may be located in universities, industry, other branches of government, or one of the many charitable foundations working in the field of health. Similarly, does one include those involved in training health professionals? This role has often been linked closely with the provision of health care but, while remaining so, the nature of the association is changing. For example, in the UK, nurse training was until recently carried out by major hospitals but is now based in universities. The Soviet Union removed medical training from the universities in the countries of central and eastern Europe, placing them in institutions under the control of ministries of health, a policy that was reversed in many countries during the 1990s. Then there is the production, regulation and distribution of pharmaceuticals and medical technology, which like the training of professionals has, in some countries, moved across the interface that is commonly seen as the boundary of the health system, in particular in relation to products such as vaccines.

Yet it is not only diversity within the nation state that must be accommodated. Some countries operate health systems beyond their borders, most obviously in respect of troops deployed abroad but also, in a globalizing world, by corporations based in industrialized countries providing for their employees in other parts of the world. These may, *de facto*, owe more to the norms of the country from which they originate rather than the one in which they are located. Yet this is only one small effect of the process of globalization that – facilitated by agreements such as the General Agreement on Trade in Services that enable international corporations to move into the mainstream of health care delivery (Pollock and Price 2003) – means that the link between the nation state and the services it provides for its citizens becomes ever more tenuous.

Given this complexity, it is difficult to argue with Field's contention that the 'question of the drawing of the precise boundaries of [the health] system is an empirical and definitional one, and must, to some degree, remain arbitrary' (Field 1973). This, inevitably, leads to a situation in which different analysts choose different definitions. Thus, Anderson takes a narrow perspective, placing a health care system within the 'boundaries of a relatively easily defined system with entry and exit points, hierarchies of personnel, types of patients' (Anderson 1972). This health care system is 'the officially and professionally recognised "helping" services regarding disease, disability, and death'. More expansively, Field defines the health system as 'the aggregate of commitments and resources (human, cultural, political, and material) any society devotes to, or sets aside to, or invests into the "health" concern as distinguished from other concerns such as general education, defence, industrial production, communications, capital construction, and so on' (Field 1973). Yet he faces the problem of operationalizing this concept and, when developing it further using a structural-functional perspective, he proposes a more specific definition as 'that societal mechanism which transforms generalised resources or inputs (mandate, knowledge, personnel and resources) into specialised outputs in the form of health services aimed at the health problems of the society', with the 'health problems' being referred to as the five Ds: death, disease, disability, discomfort and dissatisfaction. A similar line of reasoning is followed by Roemer, who has arguably written more on health systems than any other individual, and who defines the health system as 'the combination of resources, organization, financing, and management that culminate in the delivery of health services to the population' (Roemer 1991). Yet both these authors define the health system in terms of the structures used to deliver health care. In contrast, Weinerman, drawing on the World Health Organization (WHO) definition of health as the 'state of complete physical, mental and social well-being and not merely the absence of disease or infirmity' (WHO 1948), defined the health system as 'any set of arrangements in a society . . . which assigns social roles and resources to achieve the goals of protecting or restoring health to the eligible population' (Weinerman 1971). Although his analysis, in practice, focuses mainly on personal health services, this definition embraces 'all of the activities of a society which are designed to protect or restore health, whether directed to the individual, the community, or the environment'. In a similar vein, Long argues that, if health is to be interpreted in accordance with the WHO definition, then 'any service designed to improve the physical, mental, or social well-being of one individual or groups of individuals must be considered a health service' (Long 1994). Consequently, health care also includes education, housing, nutrition, environmental monitoring and others. However, Long also takes issue with the common practice of using the term *health care* interchangeably with *medical care*; instead he defines medical care as being only one of several types of services identified as health care services. Hence, the medical care system – as opposed to the health care system – refers to the organization, financing and delivery of medical care services that comprise three major generic components: preventive care, acute care and long-term care (Long 1994). In this respect, Long's definition is actually rather narrow, focusing on the 'health care system' solely as a provider of health services.

In 1998, WHO began to develop its Health System Performance Assessment Framework (HSPAF). This led to the publication of the *World Health Report 2000*, which was the first attempt to provide a comprehensive assessment of the performance of health systems in the then 191 member states of WHO (Murray and Frenk 2000; WHO 2000). This approach adopted a very broad definition of what constitutes a health system. It considered that the crucial determinant of whether something is within or outside a health system is the intent to improve health. It includes 'all actors, institutions and resources that undertake health actions – where the primary intent of a health action is to improve health . . . It incorporates selected intersectoral actions in which the stewards of the health system take responsibility to advocate for improvements in areas outside their direct control, such as legislation to reduce fatalities from traffic accidents' (Murray and Evans, 2003). With this, WHO has arrived at one of the major challenges facing those seeking to evaluate health systems: even if one can reach a satisfactory definition of what a health system actually is, how does one disentangle its effects from the many other things that are taking place within the society in which it is embedded?

Yet there is another problem to be addressed. A frequent reason for assessing the performance of a health system or sub-system is to draw lessons from that assessment. Yet health systems exhibit strong path dependency. Many of the national specificities of each health system are determined by particular historical circumstances, such as the emergence of western European social insurance systems from strong sets of relationships between employers and employee associations in Germany and France following the industrial revolution, the rejection of centralized state control in the countries of central and eastern Europe that emerged from communist rule in the 1990s, the shared wartime experience that led to the creation of the British NHS, or the rugged individualism and non-conformism that characterizes much of American life, and by extension the delivery of health care. As a consequence, most analysts recognize that health systems cannot simply be relocated from one country to another (although unfortunately this understanding does not always extend to politicians and their advisers).

In summary, different authors have, at different times, employed quite different definitions of what a health system is. The lesson that can be drawn is that, whatever definition is being used, it is essential that it be defined explicitly and the means of evaluating this system are congruent with the definition. Yet beyond the question of which national system is best, there is the question of whether one type of system, such as one funded from taxation (often characterized as a 'Beveridge', system after the British architect of that country's NHS) or one funded by social insurance (often characterized as 'Bismarckian', after the German chancellor who introduced it in the latter part of the eighteenth century) is superior. To address this question it is first necessary to understand the various ways that have been used to classify health systems.

How does one classify health care systems?

For years, health policy researchers have asked 'Can one develop a classification of health care systems?' The way in which this quest has been pursued provides valuable insights into the difficulties involved and, in particular, the dangers of simplification.

Many of the most simple classifications, such as that containing the Bismarck and Beveridge models mentioned above, are derived from the concept used by Max Weber of 'ideal types' (Weber 1950). An ideal type refers to *an abstract model of a complex real phenomenon, which highlights its most significant features*. In this context, 'ideal' is not meant in the sense of desirable but in the sense of a pure, abstract construct, going back to the Platonic view that what one sees on earth is an imperfect representation of something that exists in some ideal world. This approach offers a series of hypothetical models that emphasize certain features that may have some explanatory power. Such models often reflect some underlying view about the way in which society is organized. It should also be noted that much of the literature that has adopted this perspective is concerned, at least implicitly, with one question, which has thus shaped its application; why, among industrialized countries, is the USA unique in not having developed a system of universal health care coverage?

One example is that developed by Field, who identified five ideal-type health systems that reflect the diversity of different patterns of health care organization (see Table 2.1) (Field 1978). In this typology, the key dimensions that define a health care system include the role of the state versus that of the market, as well as the position of the physician, the role of professional associations and the ownership of facilities.

An analogous approach is that developed by Roemer, who proposed a typology of health systems on two dimensions: the level of economic development, classified according to the gross national product (GNP), and political characteristics, namely the level of market intervention in health policy (see Table 2.2) (Roemer 1977, 1991). In this two-dimensional matrix, each dimension consists of four (originally three – Roemer 1977) levels, with the economic dimension distinguishing between 'affluent and industrialized', 'developing and transitional', 'very poor' and 'resource-rich'. The political categories include 'entrepreneurial and permissive', 'welfare-oriented', 'universal and comprehensive' and 'socialist and centrally planned'. Illustrative examples include an entrepreneurial system in an industrialized country,

Table 2.1 Types of national health systems, as classified by Field

	General definition	Position of physician	Role of professional associations	Ownership of facilities	Economic transfers	Prototypes
Type 1 Private	Health care as item of personal consumption	Solo entrepreneur	Powerful	Private	Direct	USA, Western Europe
Type 2 Pluralistic	Health care as consumer good or service	and member of variety of groups/organizations	Very strong	Private and public	Direct and indirect	USA in twentieth century
Type 3 National health insurance	Health care as an insured/guaranteed consumer good or service	and member of medical organizations	Strong	Private and public	Mostly indirect	Sweden, France, Canada
Type 4 National health service	Health care as a state-supported consumer good or service	and member of medical organizations	Fairly strong	Mostly public	Indirect	Great Britain
Type 5 Socialized health service	Health care as a state-provided public service	State employee and member of medical organizations	Weak or non-existent	Entirely public	Entirely indirect	Soviet Union

Source: adapted from Rodwin (1984)

Table 2.2 Types of national health systems, as classified by Roemer

		Health system policies (market intervention)			
		Entrepreneurial & permissive	Welfare-oriented	Universal & comprehensive	Socialist & centrally planned
Economic level (GNP/capita)	Affluent & industrialized	USA	West Germany Canada Japan	Great Britain New Zealand Norway	Soviet Union Czechoslovakia
	Developing & transitional	Thailand Philippines South Africa	Brazil Egypt Malaysia	Israel Nicaragua	Cuba North Korea
	Very poor	Ghana Bangladesh Nepal	India Burma	Sri Lanka Tanzania	China Vietnam
	Resource-rich		Libya Gabon	Kuwait Saudi Arabia	

such as the USA, a welfare-oriented system in a transitional country such as Brazil, and a socialist system in a poor country, as exemplified by Vietnam.

Arguing from a political-economic perspective and drawing on a Marxist interpretation, Elling (1994) proposed classifying countries' health systems in order of increasing strength of their labour movements. This yields five types of countries, and thus health systems:

1 core capitalist;
2 core capitalist, social welfare;
3 industrialized socialist-oriented;
4 capitalist dependencies;
5 socialist-oriented, quasi-independent.

Thus, *core capitalist* countries are characterized by low strength of workers' movements, a decentralized, fractionated authority structure, a market-oriented health system that may include elements of a national insurance system, and gross disparities in distribution of wealth, access to health services and levels of health in terms of class, ethnicity or gender. Examples include the USA, Switzerland and Germany. The second type, *core capitalist – social welfare*, includes countries with stronger workers' movements and a better developed welfare system, with either a regional or national health (insurance) system. Examples include Canada, the UK and the Scandinavian countries. The third type, *industrialized socialist-oriented*, has largely disappeared with the break up of the Soviet Union, with the most prominent features being that the workers' movements were subsumed within the Communist Party, there were fewer social and economic disparities than in types (1) and (4) and there were partially (administratively) regionalized national health services. *Capitalist dependencies* are characterized by the workers' movements being suppressed, with little or no collective provision of health and welfare services and 'obscene social and economic as well as healthy disparities' (Elling 1994) as in Brazil, India and the Philippines. Finally, the main features of the *socialist-oriented – quasi-independent* type include strong workers' and peasants' movements, regionalized health services and greater equity in the distribution and control of resources including health services (e.g. China, Cuba, Tanzania).

These approaches are purely illustrative as other writers have developed their own typologies, although most are variations on the same themes (e.g. Maxwell 1974; Terris 1978; Raffel 1984). From a contemporary perspective, as Sheaff notes, they largely reflect 'certain political preoccupations of [the cold war] time. Then, a touchstone of political and social analysis was where a society or an economic sector fell in terms of the global political division between fundamentally market-based and fundamentally state-managed social systems' (Sheaff 1998).

While political scientists continue to debate whether the world is unipolar (i.e. dominated by the USA) or multipolar, what is incontrovertible is that the world is no longer divided into two competing camps, capitalism and communism. As a consequence, 'taxonomies reflecting Cold War alignments have become unrealistically narrow' (Sheaff 1998) and ignore the multi-dimensionality that characterizes the provision of health care, a point developed by more recent commentators.

An example is the model developed by Frenk and Donabedian (1987). Rather than providing a typology of health systems, they developed a typology based on certain configurations of state intervention in health care in relation to specific principles for the population's eligibility to receive care. The original model focused on the supply side of services, which was categorized according to, first, the degree of ownership – whether the state limits its role to the financing of care or also assumes the role of a health care provider – and, second, the administrative structures, reflecting the concentration of control – i.e., is control concentrated in a

Table 2.3   Typology of health care modalities

		Basis for population eligibility			
		Purchasing power	*Poverty*	*Socially perceived priority*	*Citizenship*
Mechanism for state intervention (degree of control)	*Regulation*	Private enterprise	Private charity	Company-based services	Social insurance (German model)
	Financing	–	Medicaid (USA)	Incipient health insurance	National health insurance
	Delivery	–	Public assistance	Social security (Latin American model)	Socialized (national health service)

Reprinted from Health Policy, v.27:19–34, Frenk: Dimensions of health system reform, c 1994, with permission from Elsevier.

single agency or programme or is it dispersed among several agencies. This model was subsequently expanded to also include aspects of financing and regulation (see Table 2.3) (Frenk 1994).

For example, a characteristic feature of the German model is that financing is operated by private, non-profit funds that contract private providers. The role of the state is largely restricted to regulating these groups and to establishing a regulatory framework that guarantees minimum levels of benefits to which all citizens are entitled. In contrast, in countries such as the UK and Sweden, the state has been responsible for the delivery of most services.

This approach also makes it possible to disaggregate the various modalities of state intervention that may coexist in any given country, such as the multiple elements of the American system. Thus, company-based services, under which private employers organize the financing and delivery of services for their workers, exist alongside state financing of health services for the poor (Medicaid) alongside state provision of services to particular sub-groups of the population (e.g. veterans).

Another approach is to step down a level further to classify countries on the basis of more specific aspects of their health system. Thus, in 1992, the Organization for Economic Cooperation and Development (OECD) undertook a systematic analysis of health care systems that sought to identify the dominant mechanisms for funding, payment and regulation in seven OECD countries in western Europe (OECD 1992). It drew on earlier work by Evans (1981) who proposed distinct models that summarized interactions between five principal sets of actors in health care systems: (a) consumer/patient, (b) first-level providers (e.g. general practitioners, pharmacists supplying over-the-counter medicines), (c) second-level providers (e.g. hospital services, pharmacists supplying prescribed drugs), (d) insurers (or third-party payers) and (e) government in its capacity as regulator of the system. The main interactions include provision of services, referrals from first- to second-level providers, payment for services, payment for insurance, payment of insurance claims and various forms of regulation by government. Using this model, the authors then identified seven models to describe the sub-systems of finance and methods of paying providers (see Table 2.4). These models are further illustrated with diagrams depicting financial and patient flows and the relationships between patients, providers and third parties, in each case following a standardized, highly structured format.

In this, and in its other work, in particular in developing national health accounts,

Table 2.4 Sub-systems of finance and provider payments

Model	Example
Voluntary, out-of-pocket payment	Supporting role only, e.g. purchase of over-the-counter medicines, cost-sharing for prescribed medicines
Voluntary (insurance with) reimbursement of patients	Private sector in UK and Netherlands
Public (compulsory insurance with) reimbursement of patients	Elements retained in the social health insurance systems in France and Belgium
Voluntary (insurer/provider) contract	Individual Practice Association and prepaid group practices in Spain (private sector)
Public (insurer/provider) contract	Primary care in Germany, Netherlands, Ireland, UK; hospitals in Belgium, Germany, Netherlands, UK
Voluntary insurance with integration between insurers and providers	USA: Health Maintenance Organizations
Compulsory insurance with integration between insurance and providers	Spain; public hospitals in France and Ireland (previously public hospitals in UK)

Source: OECD (1992)

the OECD has made important contributions to the comparison of health systems, not least in highlighting the need for a systematic approach and, in particular, the use of agreed definitions. However it also illustrates the complexity involved, as this classification based on systems of financing deals solely with revenue, while a classification based on capital financing (e.g. funding and ownership of hospitals and other health care facilities) would look quite different (Thompson and McKee 2004).

A completely different approach has emerged from work on complex adaptive human systems, based on soft systems theory (Checkland 1981). This approach implicitly rejects the concept of ideal types and sees the health system, like any other system, as somewhat more complicated. The health system is a complex 'whole' that is made up of a hierarchy of levels of organization, or sub-systems, with higher levels becoming progressively more complex. According to Checkland (1981), the leading exponent of soft systems theory, a system has certain features:

- it has a purpose or mission and its performance can be measured;
- it contains decision-making processes that are themselves systems and these interact so that their effects can be transmitted throughout the system;
- it exists in wider systems and/or environments with which it interacts but from which it is separated;
- it has resources that can be used by the decision-making process;
- it has some degree of continuity.

Furthermore, unlike the implication of some other approaches that also break health systems into their constituent parts, this approach rejects the idea that the characteristics of a system, analysed on a given level, can be predicted from knowledge of the sub-systems that contribute to it, as each level displays emergent properties that do not exist at lower levels. An analogy is that of a living organism, such as a human in which, as identical twins demonstrate, even a complete knowledge of the constituent genes does not allow the investigator to predict with certainty all the characteristics of the individual twin.

For the analyst, the key issue is that the appropriate level at which evaluation should take place is determined by the question being asked. Each level of complexity is characterized by specific features that require specific approaches and techniques for analysis. Wilson and Holt (2001) illustrated this, although not explicitly referring to soft systems theory, in relation to human beings who, they argue, can be considered as composed of and operating within multiple interacting and self-adjusting systems. Looking at human health and illness, they identify several levels of 'systems', each requiring specific approaches of analysis. The human body, for example, is composed of multiple interacting and self-regulating physiological systems whose interactions and functioning can be investigated by using a variety of biochemical and physiological techniques. The next level is the behaviour of the individual that is determined by a complex set of rules based on past experience and responses to environmental stimuli whose complexity may be understood more closely by applying techniques derived from psychology and related disciplines. The set of rules and experiences determining individual behaviour itself is largely influenced by relationships the individual is embedded in and which impact their beliefs and expectations. Appropriate methods to understand these interdependencies would be derived primarily from the social sciences, such as social psychology. However, individuals and their immediate social relationships are further embedded within wider social, political and cultural systems that 'can influence outcomes in entirely novel and unpredictable ways' (Wilson and Holt 2001). Potential approaches to interpreting this level of complexity would involve a variety of disciplines including anthropology, social sciences, political sciences and economics.

It should, however, be recognized that, rather like complexity theory, which has been shown to explain such diverse phenomena as the pattern of migrating birds, the population of wild animals and the behaviour of stock markets (Lewin 1992), soft systems analysis suffers from a major limitation, and one that diminishes it in the view of many politicians: it cannot *predict* what will happen. A health system, like a living organism, contains processes of communication and control that enable it to adapt in response to environmental pressures. In other words, it cannot be assumed that an intervention that was successful in one setting will necessarily work in another. Whether such outcomes are actually predictable is, of course, another matter (McKee 1995).

As both the OECD model and the applications of soft systems theory show, there has been a move away from the evaluation of the system as a whole (with the notable exception of the 2000 *World Health Report*) to assessments of different ways of achieving some of the many functions that contribute to the overall health system or, put another way, to the evaluation of sub-systems.

Getting inside the system: a framework for assessment

The levels within a health care system are potentially almost infinite, reflecting the very many questions that it is possible to ask about a system and its components, and taking account of the many problems in defining the boundaries of the system discussed earlier. One simplified approach is to look at the different levels of decision-making within a health care system: the *primary process of patient care* (micro level); the *organizational context* (meso level); and the *financing and policy context* (macro level) (Plochg and Klazinga 2002). Each level is characterized by distinct rationales, addressing different dynamics in the health care system; for each level it is thus possible to identify specific issues that ultimately shape the health care system, for example:

- *Micro level* – what is the nature of the interaction between health service users and professionals?
- *Meso level* – what is the most effective balance between inpatient and ambulatory (outpatient) care?
- *Macro level* – how are health services financed?

The model underpinning the HSPAF, as set out in the *World Health Report 2000*, is more complex (WHO 2000). As already noted, the framework identifies three major social goals to which health systems contribute, namely health attainment, responsiveness to the expectations of the population and fairness of financial contribution. However, in order to achieve these goals or objectives the health system has to fulfil certain key functions; these are identified as *financing*, *provision* of personal and non-personal health services, *resource generation* and *stewardship*, or the oversight function of the health system (see Figure 2.1).

Each function can be further divided into distinct sub-functions that can be analysed separately. Thus, financing involves the components revenue collection, fund pooling and purchasing (see Box 2.1). In brief, revenue collection refers to the process of mobilizing resources (i.e. money), usually from households or corporate entities but also from governments and external donors. Fund pooling refers to the spreading of financial risk across the population through the accumulation of pre-paid health care revenues, while purchasing is the process through which revenues that have been collected are allocated to providers who must deliver a package of services.

Similarly, the function 'provision' can be subdivided into personal health services, i.e. services that are consumed directly by an individual, and non-personal health services, i.e. actions that are applied either to collectives (e.g mass health education) or to the non-human components of the environment, such as basic sanitation. Box 2.1 illustrates the wider implications of the health system functions as outlined by the *World Health Report 2000*. Thus, it is important to stress that resource generation is much more than collecting money. It also involves forward planning to ensure there is something to buy with the money and which not only relates to human and physical resources but also to intellectual and social resources.

This approach offers a basis for categorizing the various elements within a health system. A next step is to describe how they operate. Here it is possible to derive

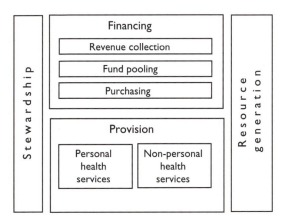

Figure 2.1   Functions of health systems

Source: Murray and Frenk (2000). Reproduced with kind permission of the publisher.

Box 2.1   Functions and sub-functions of health systems

Financing

Revenue collection: establishing prepayment systems and protecting the poor from catastrophic illness
Fund pooling: maintaining equity between generations, social groups etc.
Purchasing: making sure the money is used appropriately

Provision

Provision of care for the right people, in the right place, in the right way
Balancing strategic purchasing with provider autonomy
Linking quality with control over resources

Resource generation

Physical capital: investment in high-quality, appropriate facilities
Human capital: investment in trained, motivated people with the appropriate mix of skills
Intellectual capital: investment in research and development
Social capital: investment in networks and relationships

Stewardship

Health policy formulation: defining the vision and direction for the health system
Regulation: setting fair rules of the game with a level playing field
Intelligence: assessing performance and sharing information

Source: adapted from Murray and Frenk (2000), World Health Organization (2000)

---

some insights from soft systems theory (Checkland 1981). This is based on an acronym – CATWOE – which describes any form of human activity and the circumstances that surround it (see Box 2.2). A certain *transformation* (process) is performed for clients (those who more or less directly benefit – *customers* – or suffer) by *actors*. The activity is ultimately 'controlled' or paid for by *owners*, and its implementation is influenced by the *environment* within which it is located. This all takes place against a background of various beliefs or values, in this case termed *Weltanschauung*, or world view.

For example, one might describe the British NHS as 'a system for meeting the health needs of the entire population (*transformation, customers*) through the activities of those working in the NHS (*actors*, implied *ownership* by government), within limited resources (*environmental constraints*) and in the belief that health care free at the point of delivery is a good thing and most health professionals are essentially altruistic (*Weltanschauung*)'. Going down a level, its system of financing could be described as 'a system for distributing money collected for health care to hospitals and health care workers (*transformation, customers*), in a way determined by government, advised by review bodies (*ownership, actors*), in the light of competing claims on government expenditure (*environmental constraints*), in the belief that rewards to

---

Box 2.2 CATWOE model

Customers	beneficiaries of the system
Actors	who carry out, or cause to be carried out, the transformation
Transformation process	the means by which defined inputs are transformed into defined outputs
Weltanschauung	vision of the world assumed for the system to function
Ownership of the system	someone with prime concern for it and the power to cause it to cease to exist
Environmental constraints	in the environment (geography, national wealth) or related systems (educational, legal, governmental, financial)

Source: Checkland (1981)

---

staff in the health care sector should be commensurate with those in other sectors (*Weltanschauung*)'.

While this provides a structured, systematic approach to describing health systems and the various elements that make them up, it does not say anything about how they are performing. At all levels of a health system, this can be assessed in terms of what is actually achieved, how it is achieved, and whether there are the prerequisites available for the system to achieve. Put another way, and adopting the approach first developed by Avedis Donabedian in his work on quality of care (Donabedian 1966, 1980), a system can be evaluated according to *structure, process* and *outcome*. Donabedian argued that 'good structure increases the likelihood of good process, and good process increases the likelihood of good outcome' (1988). The approach has subsequently been adopted widely within health services research and, in the specific context of evaluation of health systems, to include *outputs,* referring to the throughput or productivity of the health care system, i.e. the immediate result of professional or institutional health care activities, usually expressed as units of service (see Box 2.3) (Last 2001).

In summary, although it is common for media commentators (and some politicians) to speak of the British or the American or French health system, a rather more sophisticated approach is required. Several steps are needed. The first is to decide the precise nature of the question being asked. Is the subject of interest the overall health system, and if so, how are the boundaries of the system defined? If it is one element within the system, what is its purpose and what elements does it comprise? The framework set out in the *World Health Report 2000*, while not exhaustive, provides a useful starting point to think about the various elements that make up a health system. A second step is to describe the systems, or sub-systems being considered. The soft systems approach, using the CATWOE framework, may be of help here, not least because, in the area of comparative research, it will often highlight how like is not being compared with like. For example, during the 1990s, there was considerable enthusiasm from some politicians in the UK for the system of social insurance funding that exists in, for example, Germany. However, a simple application of this framework would have highlighted the very important role in Germany of employers' associations and trade unions, working through

---

Box 2.3   Dimensions of health services and health systems

- **Structure (input)**   *Attributes of the settings in which care occurs: resources needed for health care*

  Material resources (facilities, capital, equipment, drugs etc.)

  Intellectual resources (medical knowledge, information systems)

  Human resources (health care professionals)

- **Process**   *Use of resources: what is done in giving and receiving care*

  Patient-Related (intervention rates, referral rates etc.)

  Organizational (supply with drugs, management of waiting lists, payment of health care staff, collection of funds etc.)

- **Output**   *Productivity or throughput*

  Length of stay in hospital, waiting times, discharge rates, access, effectiveness, equity of care

- **Outcome**   *Effects of health care on the health status of patients and populations*

  Definite: mortality, morbidity, disability, quality of life

  Intermediate: blood pressure, body weight, personal well-being, functional ability, coping ability, improved knowledge etc.

---

well-established systems of industrial governance, a model that simply does not exist in the UK (Green *et al.* 2002).

Having defined the system of interest, the final step is to decide how to evaluate it. The model developed by Donabedian provides a basis for consideration, separating structures, processes and outcomes. The experiences of those undertaking evaluations of the performance of health systems will be examined later but, for now, it may be helpful to step sideways to review the history of international comparisons of health systems.

International comparisons of health systems

Learning about other countries is rather like breathing: only the brain dead are likely to avoid the experience.

(Klein 1997)

On any matter not self-evident, there are ninety-nine persons totally incapable of judging of it, for one who is capable.

(John Stuart Mill, *On Liberty*)

Interest in cross-national comparisons of health care systems can be traced back to the 1930s, with roots in an interest in the historical evolution of health care systems, as exemplified by the work of Sigerist (1943), much of which had the goal of informing developments in national health policy (Goldman 1946; Mountin and Perrott 1947). Cross-national comparisons received increasing attention from the 1960s onwards, the most influential examples being works by Abel-Smith (1963,

1967), Roemer (1960, 1969), Anderson (1963) and Mechanic (1975) to name but a few. Comprehensive overviews of work undertaken up to the 1960s and 1970s have been assembled by Weinerman (1971) and Elling (1980).

A key message of this chapter is that the approach taken in describing and analysing health systems depends critically on the question being asked. In judging what has been done previously, therefore, it is necessary to examine the background against which it took place. Much, though not all, of this research has its origins in the USA. This was a time when the economy was booming, and with it the health care system, in what Relman described as the 'era of expansion' (1988). Techno-logical developments seemed to offer boundless possibilities, echoed in another area by the successful quest to place a man on the moon. However, successive extension of coverage of population groups in insurance-based systems or, as in the USA, the introduction of Medicare and Medicaid in the mid-1960s, giving more citizens access to care, also led to an increase in demand and consequently rapid growth in health expenditure in many industrialized countries, by then entering a period characterized by Relman as the 'era of cost containment': 'Increasingly, health administrators have been called upon to explain their demands for more and more national resources' (Abel-Smith 1967).

In part reflecting the availability of data but also the political concern about health care spending, much work that has been undertaken subsequently was mainly from a health economics perspective, looking mostly at health care expend-iture and its determinants (Kanavos and Mossialos 1990). The most prominent examples include the work by the OECD since the 1980s in an effort to provide an empirical basis for a comparative understanding of the differences and similarities between OECD countries' health systems (OECD 1985; Schieber 1987). This emphasis on inputs into health care has changed only recently in the light of increasing pressures for reform of health care delivery, with many countries facing similar problems of rising costs, demographic changes, technological advances and increasing consumer expectations. There has been increasing interest in the possibil-ity of learning from the many experiences of others, drawing lessons on how to finance, manage and organize health care so as to improve the overall performance of health systems. This last point has gained particular momentum on national and international agendas with the publication of *The World Health Report 2000* and its ranking of the world's health systems (WHO 2000), stimulating a wide-ranging debate about approaches to assessing health system performance both nationally and internationally (OECD 2002), which will be examined in more detail in the final section of this chapter.

Approaches to health system comparisons fall broadly into one of three main groups: descriptive studies, quantitative approaches and focused analytical studies.

Descriptive studies

Descriptive studies are systematic, structured descriptions of health systems or their sub-systems that can provide a basis for subsequent analysis. The use of a clear structure identifies areas that are unclear or poorly thought out. Examples include the work by the OECD described above (OECD 1992). The OECD reports pro-vided a systematic assessment of the sub-systems of finance and methods of paying providers through the application of a standard and highly structured format.

This approach has been adopted by the European Observatory on Health Systems and Policies in its Health Care Systems in Transition (HiTs) documents (European Observatory on Health Systems and Policies, 2004), which provides a highly structured description of health care systems in Europe and other industrialized countries. Beginning with contextual information about the country, HiTs describe the entities involved in financing, paying for and delivering care, drawing out their often complex interrelationships. HiTs then conclude with an examination of trends in health system reform. Prepared by a team that includes authors from the country in question as well as the Observatory, HiTs go beyond the formal structures to reflect the often messy reality of relationships. HiTs are now available for over 40 European countries, as well as some exemplar countries in other parts of the world, such as Australia and New Zealand. While not intended as a means of comparing systems, HiTs do contain a number of comparative tables, looking at each country's position in terms of, for example, resources used and outputs achieved (while noting the limitations of the data).

Another example is the International Network for Health Policy and Reform, which draws on information gathered from currently 16 industrialized countries, building on the presence of a partner institution in each country, and using a biannual survey of health reforms and health policy developments. The survey follows a highly structured format with standardized definitions and the information is drawn together in the form of regular published and online reports (International Network for Health Policy and Reform 2004).

Other approaches make use of the wealth of quantitative data collected in a fairly standardized format by international organizations such as the OECD (2003) and the WHO Regional Office for Europe (WHO Regional Office for Europe 2004). One example is the Commonwealth Fund programme on multinational comparisons of health systems data, which compares the US health care system with those in 28 industrialized countries in terms of, variously, financing, expenditures, availability and use of services, responsiveness to patients, and health outcomes. These are published on an annual basis (Reinhardt et al. 2002). Although relatively easy to do, such comparisons face the obvious problem of comparability. Some of the difficulties will be discussed in detail later, but, fundamentally, these approaches suffer from the problem that what can be counted is not necessarily what is important.

Quantitative approaches

Quantitative approaches have most often evolved from the health economics perspective to assess the performance of health systems in international comparison. There is a large literature on international comparisons of health expenditure, exploring the relationship between national wealth (such as gross domestic product, GDP) and health expenditure (Parkin et al. 1987; Kanavos and Mossialos 1990; Milne and Molana 1991). These studies do, however, yield conflicting results and it has been argued that, because of the considerable challenges involved in measuring health expenditure and national wealth, the observed positive relationship between health spending and GDP is unhelpful and likely to be misleading for health policy development (see Box 2.4).

Other studies have employed a production function approach that describes 'the production of health in terms of a function of possible explanatory variables' (Buck et al. 1999), usually examining factors indicative of health care ('health care input') and other explanatory variables for their impact on some health measure ('health care output') through regression analysis. Examples include a series of studies by the OECD that examined the associations of a number of input and process indicators such as health care expenditure, number of physicians, type of provider payment or access to services with health outcomes such as premature mortality and infant mortality (Or 2000, 2001). Other studies examined the association between specific aspects of health care systems and selected health outcomes – for example, the strength of the primary care system in different countries as a predictor for health outcomes (see Box 2.5) (Macinko et al. 2003).

Box 2.4   International comparisons of health expenditure: how valid are they?

Cross-country comparisons of health expenditure require adjusting expenditure according to the relative cost of what is being purchased. This is done by means of purchasing power parity (PPP) adjustment, in which the price of a basket of goods in each country is compared. First, it is important to specify whether general or health-specific PPPs are being used, as changes in the two are only imperfectly correlated. Furthermore, there are different PPPs to chose from, calculated by different organizations, such as the OECD and EUROSTAT, the statistical office of the European Union, each covering their own member states. Second, even when using health PPPs, it is important to recognize their limitations as they are only recalculated every five years and they focus largely on internationally traded goods, and in particular on pharmaceuticals, largely ignoring the major cost of staff in most health care systems.

Box 2.5   The contribution of primary care systems to health outcomes

Starfield and colleagues undertook a series of studies assessing the contribution of primary care systems to health outcomes in various settings. Defining primary care as 'that level of a health service system that provides entry into the system . . . provides person-focused care over time, provides care for all but very uncommon or unusual conditions, and coordinates or integrates care provided elsewhere or by others', one study looked specifically at the relationship between primary care and health outcomes in 18 OECD countries for the period 1970–98 (Macinko *et al.* 2003). The strength of primary care (PC) was measured using a ten-component scale reflecting structural characteristics, for example financing, resource allocation and accessibility, and specific practice features of PC, such as gatekeeper function, comprehensiveness and coordination. These components were then scored according to predefined criteria and combined to form a summary score, ranging from 0 (no component defined as characteristic for PC present) to 20 (all components present). In applying this model to 1995 data, France was shown to score lowest (2) and the UK highest (19). The relationship between PC strength and mortality as health outcome was then assessed using a regression model.

This showed the strength of a country's primary care system to be significant and negatively associated with all-cause (premature) mortality and premature mortality from selected conditions including asthma and bronchitis, emphysema and pneumonia and cardiovascular disease even after adjustment for a number of health determinants such as national wealth (GDP) or alcohol and tobacco consumption. Keeping some limitations of the analysis in mind, such as its ecological design and the limitations inherent in the underlying data, the overall findings suggest that the financing, organization and delivery of primary care seem to have an important impact on population health.

In addition to the limitations of the data, some of these studies are problematic because the theoretical basis of the relationships is not set out clearly, often giving the impression that the model was driven by data availability rather than plausible mechanisms and, especially when studies use a measure of adult mortality (such as life expectancy) as a dependent variable, they fail to take account of the well-known lag effects between exposures and outcomes that affect many disease processes.

The work on the performance of health systems by WHO, set out in the *World Health Report in 2000*, offers a somewhat different approach. Drawing on the goals of the health system as set out in its performance assessment framework, WHO used three main indicators to measure performance: population health, responsiveness and fair financing. Overall health system performance was then assessed as a composite of these indicators, which was in turn compared with what might be expected given the country's level of economic and educational development. The 191 WHO member states were then ranked according to these performance measures, producing a highly controversial league table of the world's health systems. The report played an important role in stimulating a wide-ranging debate on health system performance, and the various criticisms that it engendered helped bring to light the methodological challenges inherent in conducting and interpreting international comparisons, which are discussed below.

Yet another approach has evolved from epidemiology, involving analysis of data on mortality at a population level that are routinely available in many countries. It is based on the concept that certain deaths should not occur in the presence of timely and effective medical care (Nolte and McKee 2004). This concept of 'avoidable mortality' was introduced in the 1970s as a means to assess the quality of health care (Rutstein *et al.* 1976) and was subsequently adopted by a wide range of researchers especially in Europe (Charlton *et al.* 1983), producing for example the *European Community Atlas of 'Avoidable Death'* (Holland 1988). Much of this work dates back to the 1980s and early 1990s; only recently has this concept been revitalized as a potential useful tool to assess the quality and performance of health systems (see Box 2.6) (Nolte and McKee 2003, 2004).

Box 2.6   Avoidable mortality

Nolte and McKee (2004) have undertaken a systematic review of empirical and methodological studies of the concept of 'avoidable' mortality and of studies of the attribution of outcomes to health care. Their study demonstrated that 'avoidable' mortality proved a valuable instrument for the detection of potential weaknesses in health care that could then be investigated in more depth, and that it continues to do so.

Building on this work, the authors used a modified version of the concept of avoidable mortality by updating the list of conditions considered amenable to health care in the light of advances in medical knowledge and technology and looking at deaths under 75 years of age. The concept was then applied to routinely available data from selected countries in the European Union to investigate the potential impact of health care on changing life expectancy and mortality in the 1980s and 1990s. This showed that, since 1980, all European countries experienced increases in life expectancy between birth and age 75, although the pace of change differed over time and between countries. Reductions in amenable mortality made substantial positive contributions in the 1980s in all countries. The largest contribution was from falling infant mortality but there were also improvements among the middle-aged, for example in Denmark, The Netherlands, the UK, France and Sweden. In many countries the pace of improvement slowed in the 1990s although not in the Mediterranean countries, a finding that would imply a continued catching up in the southern European countries. As a result, in the 1990s, differences in amenable mortality in the European Union had narrowed, although standardized death rates from amenable causes among Portuguese men remained three times higher than those among Swedish men (see Figure 2.2).

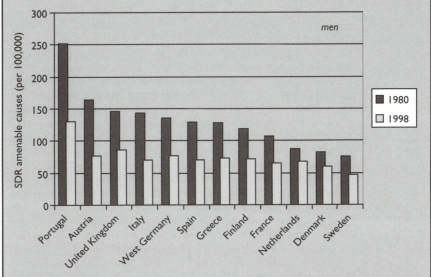

Figure 2.2　Age-standardized death rates (0–74) from causes amenable to health care in selected European Union countries, 1980 and 1998

Differences among women are less pronounced; but again, in 1998, amenable mortality was highest in Portugal (96.9/100,000) and lowest in Sweden (51.9/100,000) (not shown).

The findings support the notion that improvements in access to effective health care had a measurable impact in many countries during the 1980s and 1990s. However, the scope for improvement in amenable deaths was greatest in those countries where initial rates were highest. As a consequence, the extent of variation between countries will inevitably decrease as rates fall to low levels in all countries. It therefore seems that, in the twenty-first century, the ability to compare health system performance in industrialized countries using mortality data at the aggregate level may be limited.

Focused analytical studies

A third approach is the focused analytic study that takes a single issue and asks questions such as what are the strengths and weaknesses of different ways of funding health care systems? What are the lessons from experience of hospital reform? What are the challenges in regulating the medical profession?

There are many examples of this approach, such as the studies undertaken by the European Observatory on Health Systems and Policies on topics such as funding health care (Mossialos *et al.* 2002), the role of hospitals (McKee and Healy 2002), and regulating entrepreneurial behaviour in health systems (Saltman *et al.* 2002). This approach is based on the belief that benefits can be obtained by learning from best practice within health systems, in particular by looking at examples from other countries, while recognizing the importance of national specificities and path dependency noted earlier. It builds on a rich literature on lesson drawing, in particular the pioneering work by Rose (1993). This involves a series of questions. First, what policies, that are *already in operation* would work in the exporting setting, drawing on existing evaluative research? Note the emphasis on 'already in operation'. Too frequently, lessons are drawn from concepts that have yet to be put into practice, on the basis of beliefs about what they *might* achieve if ever implemented. This was a feature of much of the debate on quasi-markets in health care in the 1990s (Le Grand and Bartlett 1993). Second, what are the contextual factors that are necessary for it to work in that setting? Third, do those factors exist, to an extent sufficient for policy transfer to take place, in the setting into which the policy is being imported, and in what ways does the policy need to be modified? Fourth, once imported, does the policy work as intended, again introducing the need for evaluative research and thus closing the circle.

Lesson drawing can take a variety of forms, from direct copying, through adaptation, creation of hybrids and acting as a source of inspiration. However, it is also common for policies developed elsewhere not to be transferred but instead used as *post hoc* validation for decisions already taken (Bennett 1991). Clearly lesson drawing depends on both a detailed understanding of the policies being compared and a detailed understanding of the contextual factors that determine whether a policy works in different circumstances. A soft systems approach may be helpful in making explicit both of these elements. Leichter has proposed a framework for contextual analysis, incorporating situational (transient, impermanent, or idiosyncratic conditions or events that impact on policy-making), structural (relatively unchanging elements of the society and polity), cultural (the value system within society) and external (events, structures, and values that exist outside the boundaries of a political system, but that influence decisions in the system) factors (Leichter 1979). However, this remains a relatively under-researched area of comparative health systems research, not least because of its complexity and the need to draw on many areas of knowledge including comparative government, comparative law, anthropology and economics.

Assessing the performance of health services and health systems

The concern with measuring the performance of health services and health systems is not new. As long ago as the 1860s, Florence Nightingale was pioneering the systematic collection and reporting of hospital performance data. In the 1910s, Ernest Codman promoted the need for collection and public release of surgical outcome data. He recorded diagnostic and treatment errors and linked these to outcomes to improve services (Neuhauser 2002). However, it is only recently that

---

Box 2.7 Why study health system performance?

- *Accelerating advances in medical technology*
Potential for new interventions and methods for delivering and organizing health care, with consequences for health care expenditures, resulting in the need to ensure that innovations – of whatever sort – promote system objectives and avoid adverse side effects (Smith 2002a).

- *Evidence on variation in the use of services often with little variation in health outcomes*
Evidence of overuse, underuse and misuse of services; increase in available technologies and patient expectations (overuse); limited access, trust, fragmentation of services (underuse); and system failures (misuse) (Becher and Chassin 2001).

- *Growing uncertainty about the actual quality and outcomes of health services*
UK: Bristol Inquiry into the deaths of children undergoing heart surgery at the Bristol Royal Infirmary has highlighted the failings of existing internal quality assurance and professional regulation systems (Smith 1998).
USA: According to estimates by the Institute of Medicine at least 44,000 avoidable deaths are caused by medical errors in hospitals (2 per cent of all deaths), which is more than the number of lives lost by motor vehicle accidents per year (Kohn *et al.* 1999).

- *Rising public expectations*
Demand for 'value for money' as taxpayers or insured; increasing access to information, facilitated by the new electronic media such as the internet; increasing awareness of medical errors, and preparedness to challenge professional authority, to litigate and advocate.

- *New public management culture in publicly-funded health care systems*
Demand for public accountability of public services including financial transparency; creation of market and quasi-market mechanisms such as the introduction of competition between providers or, as in the UK in the early 1990s, the introduction of the internal market.

---

performance assessment has been put more firmly on the national and international agenda (see Box 2.7).

This section examines some of the main conceptual and methodological issues that underlie our understanding of performance initiatives in the field of health (Wait and Nolte in press). Most often these involve the use of performance indicators or, more broadly, measures that capture a variety of health and health-system related trends and factors. The terminology can, however, sometimes be confusing; Box 2.8 gives an overview of the most common definitions used in this field.

This terminology is common to assessments of individual clinical or organizational interventions and to health systems and their major sub-systems. Depending on the scope of the assessment, it may focus on the measurement of inputs (structure), process or outcomes, or combinations thereof, often subsumed under the heading 'performance indicator' (Wait and Nolte in press). However, when system-wide assessments are undertaken, they are often based on somewhat crude measures, for example health care expenditure, health care resources such as the number of

> **Box 2.8   Some definitions used is assessing health care performance**
>
> - **Indicator**
>   'Measurement tool used to monitor and evaluate the quality of important government, management, clinical, and support functions' (Joint Commission on Accreditation of Healthcare Organizations 1990).
>
> - **Performance indicator**
>   A 'quantitative measure of quality' (Ibrahim 2001).
>
> - **Quality**
>   '[T]he degree to which health services for individuals and populations increase the likelihood of desired health outcomes and are consistent with current professional knowledge' (Hurtado *et al.* 2001).
>
> - **Performance**
>   Multidimensional concept that 'along with efficiency [incorporates] dimensions of quality (in the sense of safety, effectiveness of care, quality of services rendered and quality as perceived by patients and the people around them) and equity' (Girard and Minvielle 2002).

physicians, nurses, facilities, etc. or summary measures of population health such as mortality or life expectancy (Hurst and Jee-Hughes 2000). Among the more advanced examples are, at the national level, the National Performance Assessment Framework (PAF) in the UK (Smee 2002; Smith 2002b) and, at the international level, the previously mentioned HSPAF developed by WHO (2000).

Given the broad definition of performance, the scope of performance indicators can potentially be enormous, ranging from assessing national health systems down to patient experience with an individual provider (Wait and Nolte in press). Assessments may thus involve indicators at the *micro level* describing the primary process of patient care, such as assessing or comparing the performance of individual surgeons. For example, the New York State Department of Health has operated a programme since 1989 that collects and makes public data on risk-adjusted mortality following coronary artery bypass surgery by hospital and by surgeon (see Box 2.9). In England, following the Bristol Inquiry in 2001, there have also been plans to publish performance data by individual surgeons and several specialist associations undertake analysis of especially collected data sets as a method of comparative audit. Also in the UK, an independent company, Dr Foster, published data on the mortality experience of hospitals, in collaboration with *The Times* newspaper, as well as a guide to individual specialists (Dr Foster 2004), although in this case looking only at measures of process such as waiting times.

The next level of assessment involves looking at the *meso, or organisational level*, for example, assessing the performance of a primary care team or a hospital. Examples include the public reporting systems in New York and several other American states (Hannan *et al.* 1997). Within the UK PAF, performance indicators of individual hospitals have been published since 2000. In 2001, this was complemented by a performance rating system in which the progress of NHS Hospital Trusts (health care delivery organizations) in England were assessed against nine key targets, 28 performance indicators and judgements of the Commission for Health Improvement (a health service inspectorate) and, based on this assessment, were awarded

> **Box 2.9   Measuring the performance of health care providers**
>
> Some areas in the USA have been publishing data comparing mortality rates accord-
> ing to individual surgeons over the last ten years. One example is New York State
> where the State Department of Health (DoH) has been collecting data to assess the
> quality of care provided to patients undergoing coronary artery bypass grafting
> (CABG) since 1989, using a registry (Hannan *et al.* 1997). Each hospital collects
> relevant data and forwards them to the DoH on a quarterly basis.
>
> The data are then processed to produce mortality rates for each hospital and
> surgeon that take into account the severity of each patient's presenting illness
> and coexisting conditions. In 1990, the DoH published data on crude, expected and
> risk-adjusted mortality rates and volume of CABG procedures performed at each
> hospital in New York State. Thus, while surgeon-specific death rates were also
> calculated, these were not published, the argument being that low volume of
> operations would lead to substantial variation in mortality rates and therefore be
> susceptible to misinterpretation. However, upon release of the hospital-specific
> death rates a newspaper, the *Newsday*, issued a lawsuit against the DoH under the
> Freedom of Information Law to also gain access to surgeon-specific data. The DoH
> lost the case and had to publish the data in 1991. Surgeon-specific death rates have
> now been published on an annual basis since 1992. A similar system is in place in
> Pennsylvania.

stars, with three stars relating to highest levels of performance down to zero stars,
indicating the poorest levels of performance (Department of Health 2002). Efforts
to evaluate performance in the ambulatory sector have been hindered mostly by
limited availability of appropriate information; however, in the UK performance
ratings have now been extended to include Primary Care Trusts, the organizations
that purchase health care (Commission for Health Improvement 2004).

Assessments at the *macro level* (regional, national) or the financing and policy
context of health care include the UK PAF as mentioned above and other national
initiatives seeking to provide a framework to assess the performance of the health
care system. A comprehensive evaluation of these national frameworks was recently
provided by Arah and colleagues (Arah *et al.* 2003).

Finally, it is important to define the actual objective of (public) reporting of
performance indicators. Objectives may include (i) accountability to funders and
other stakeholders; (ii) identification of areas of poor performance and centres of
excellence; (iii) facilitation of selection and choice of providers by consumer/
patients and purchasers of health care; (iv) provider behaviour change; and (v)
providing epidemiological and other public health data (Nutley and Smith 1998).
Depending on the objective(s) the target audience thus includes the general public,
health care providers, purchasers and policy-makers.

Conceptual problems

There are a number of challenges relating to the development, application and
reporting of performance indicators; the following section will reflect briefly on
some of the major issues including definitions, underlying data and selection of
indicators, methodological issues, interpretation of data and unintended
consequences.

Definitions

Some of the more fundamental challenges relate to the definitions underlying the process of performance assessment. Thus, in assessing the performance of health systems, be it at the national or international level, one important question is how one defines the health system, as this will define the performance measures being used. For example, as noted earlier, the *World Health Report 2000* used a rather broad definition of a health system that incorporated the importance of intersectoral action to promote health (WHO 2000). However, perhaps inevitably, as a report from an international organization whose constituents are individual countries, it adopted as its basis for comparison the health systems of those countries. This immediately created a problem. In some countries, as already noted, the financing and delivery of health care is the responsibility of a diverse array of organizations that can only loosely be considered to comprise a system. In other countries, such as Afghanistan, Sierra Leone or the Democratic Republic of the Congo, to take only three of the most obvious examples, it was difficult at that time to argue that there was anything in place that resembled a system of government, or at least one whose writ applied beyond the outskirts of the capital city.

Another important challenge relates to the ideological values underpinning any approach to assessing performance. For example, in their assessment of the world's health systems WHO weighted different indicators to reflect their perceived importance in the overall index of performance (WHO 2000). This raises the fundamental question about whose values count. The assessments published in the *World Health Report 2000* used key informants from around the world, but the case has been be made that other people, such as those who use the services, should decide which aspects of the health system matter most (Mulligan *et al.* 2000). Some of these issues have now been addressed in subsequent work by WHO, by undertaking large-scale (household) surveys to assess preferences for health system outcomes from the users' point of view (Murray and Evans 2003).

An equally great problem relates to the question of whether and how the measures adopted for assessing performance conform to the underlying definition of the health system. Again the *World Health Report 2000* provides an illustrative example of inconsistencies in this respect (see Box 2.10).

Other examples include the Commonwealth Fund International Working Group on Quality Indicators initiative (CMF QI) and the related OECD Health Care Quality Indicator Project (HCQI) (Nolte *et al.* 2003; Hussey *et al.* 2004). These initiatives aim at the development of a common set of quality indicators for use in cross-national comparisons of health systems. In its first stage the CMF QI initiative adopted a relatively narrow definition of a health system, focusing on the technical quality of health care, or, more specifically, the appropriateness and effectiveness of care (Hussey *et al.* 2004). Yet, the 21 indicators selected to reflect medical care in five countries also included smoking rates. The authors acknowledged that '[t]he health care system does not have perfect control over people's decision to smoke', but, they argued, 'advice and treatment provided by physicians' had been shown to have an impact on smoking cessation (Hussey *et al.* 2004). This line of reasoning seems, however, slightly at odds with the rather narrow objective of evaluating the technical quality of health care.

Selection of indicators and availability of data

Limited data availability and lack of uniformity of data across different settings pose substantial challenges to most initiatives seeking to assess health system performance. In many parts of the world even basic vital statistics are simply not available,

> **Box 2.10 The attribution of outcomes to activities in the health system**
>
> On the basis that a health system should improve health, should respond to the legitimate demands of those it serves, and should prevent families who suffer from illness becoming impoverished as a result, WHO (2000) defined three measures on which to assess health systems: *health attainment, responsiveness,* and *fairness of financing.* For the first two, both absolute levels and distribution, as a measure of equity, were assessed, with health attainment assessed as disability adjusted life expectancy (DALE). The overall performance of each health care system was then determined by combining the weighted scores on each measure.
>
> Yet immediately a paradox emerges. It is apparent that many of the determinants of aggregate health lie outside the health care sector. Thus, the measure of health attainment reflects not only those policies and resulting inputs whose primary intent is to improve health but also policies in a wide range of other sectors, such as education, housing and employment, where the production of health is a secondary goal. Yet the other parameters, responsiveness and fairness of financing, relate solely to the delivery of health care services.
>
> Nolte and McKee (2003) have thus examined how health systems perform when attainment can be more directly attributed to health care. Using the concept of 'avoidable mortality' (see Box 2.6), they have calculated standardized death rates from conditions considered amenable to health care for 19 OECD countries (1998) and generated rankings based on the level of amenable mortality. These rankings were then compared with the rankings produced by WHO based on DALE. This exercise showed that rankings changed for most countries that were included in the study, illustrating that the findings of any performance assessment very much depend on the concepts that underlie them.

because of fragmentary population registration systems and even in some industrialized countries significant gaps exist in coverage of some groups, for example native Americans or Australian Aborigines. Where data exist their usefulness may be restricted due to lack of comparability, which poses particular challenges to international comparisons. Thus, in parallel with its reports describing elements of health systems, the OECD (2003) has undertaken pioneering work in assembling an international database of inputs, processes and outcomes of health systems. In doing so, it has identified many weaknesses in the existing data. For example, figures for numbers of health professionals in some countries are based on head counts, taken from professional registers, while in others they are limited to numbers (or in some cases, whole-time equivalents) in employment (and in some cases, only those working in the state sector). Even the question of how much each country spends on health care is often difficult to answer. Most obviously, there is the problem of defining the boundaries of the system. However, even accurate figures for overall expenditure are themselves of limited use and they are frequently expressed in terms of measures of national wealth, such as GNP per capita. Knowledge of this figure is not always easy, especially in less developed countries where the size of the population may be uncertain.

This problem is further highlighted by the *World Health Report 2000* (WHO 2000). Assessing the performance of the health systems of 191 countries required many heroic assumptions, not least in relation to the virtual absence of data from a majority of the countries involved. In a recent critique, Musgrove showed that only 39 per cent of the indicator values included in the *World Health Report* were based on existing data, the remainder being estimates using regression analyses and other means (Musgrove 2003). Using complex models to generate estimates fails, however, to tackle the underlying problem.

Accurate collection of indicator data relies on the existence of reliable and well-established health information systems. However, most existing systems were originally devised for internal mechanisms of financial control, and their adaptation for purposes of performance assessment may not be straightforward. Problems with minimum data sets, inaccuracies in interpretation of aggregated data, failure to integrate population- and patient-level data and lack of linkage between diagnostic data and outcomes of care are some of the main drawbacks reported in existing health information systems (Shaw and Kalo 2002). With these caveats in mind, the value of performance initiatives can be greatly enhanced if target indicators are selected for their relevance and usefulness as evaluation tools rather than merely on data availability. Indeed, indicators often seem to be selected on the basis of what is available and practical rather than what is meaningful, such as areas that need improvement and require prioritization or health system goals and values (Walshe 2003).

Several groups have presented lists of desirable attributes for performance indicators. According to Pringle and colleagues these should be valid, communicable, effective, reliable, objective, available, contextual, attributable, interpretable, comparable, remediable and repeatable (Pringle *et al.* 2002). The CMF QI selected performance indicators based on (i) feasibility: indicators are already being collected by one or more countries; (ii) scientific soundness: indicators have to be reliable and valid; (iii) interpretability: indicators have to allow a clear conclusion for policymakers; (iv) actionability: measures can be directly affected by the health care system, and (v) importance: indicator reflects important health conditions in terms of burden of disease, cost of care or priorities of policy-makers (Hussey *et al.* 2004).

Methodological challenges

The methodological challenges to performance assessment or, more generally, evaluation of health systems are manifold and are related to the underlying data, variation in information needs of different users, questions about the actual link between specific inputs and processes of health care and health outcomes, possible time lags between interventions and outcome and the timing of measurements, etc. Also, not all outcomes that are valued by society are measurable – for example, how does one assess reassurance?

One example is emergency readmission to hospital, which is often used as proxy measure of avoidable adverse outcomes after initial admission to hospital, for example in the English NHS performance ratings mentioned above. The use of this indicator is usually justified because a high proportion of emergency readmissions should be preventable if the preceding care is adequate (Leng *et al.* 1999). The appropriateness of this measure, or of readmission to hospital more generally, as a quality or performance indicator has been questioned as other factors unrelated to the quality of hospital care can affect the likelihood of readmission, including patient factors such as severity and chronicity of the underlying condition or levels of co-morbidity, or hospital factors such as validity of administrative data. In addition, variation of (emergency) readmission rates between hospitals may be due to factors such as variation in population structure (ageing population, elderly living alone), falling length of hospital stay, variation among hospitals in case mix and severity, and issues such as random variation due to small numbers and problems in defining the denominator – again factors not related to the actual quality of care. This is further illustrated by a case study undertaken in Scotland that analysed emergency readmission rates in some detail (Leng *et al.* 1999). It showed that about 17 per cent of the emergency readmissions recorded were unrelated to the initial admission and therefore did not reflect the previous quality of care. The challenge is thus to establish a *causal relationship* between patient outcome and the actual process of care, or, as discussed in Box 2.10, between health outcome at the population level and elements of the health system.

Another issue relates to the use of composite measures. One example is the *World Health Report 2000*, which assessed overall health system performance as a weighted composite measure of health attainment, responsiveness and fair financing in relation to what might be expected given the country's level of economic and educational development (WHO 2000), another is the NHS star rating system described earlier (Department of Health 2002). The use of such measures has been challenged on conceptual and methodological grounds. Thus, referring to the methods employed by WHO, Naylor and colleagues argued that composite indices of health system performance are, at best, of 'dubious precision' for they 'combine uncertain weighing systems, imprecision arising from the potential non-comparability of component measures, and misleading reliability in the form of whole-population averages that mask distributional issues' (Naylor *et al.* 2002). Moreover, presentation of even disaggregated data as means and medians may be misleading since this is likely to conceal fluctuations at various levels within the health system. Naylor *et al.* thus concluded that '[H]ealth systems are extraordinarily complex. In consequence, one must beware of the seductive reductionism of devising a single measure to capture all dimensions of health status, let alone health system performance. A balanced approach with an array of indicators is desirable, as each set of stakeholders will need a different type of information to make better decisions' (2002).

Interpretation and unintended consequences

We have known incurable cases discharged from one hospital, to which the deaths ought to have been accounted and received into another hospital, to die there in a day or two after admission, thereby lowering the mortality rate of the first at the expense of the second.

(Florence Nightingale 1863)

A final question needing to be asked is whether national performance initiatives can contribute to improving the performance of the health care systems they are assessing (see also Box 2.11). Several scholars have expressed concern that the use of indicators has become an end in itself and have urged the evaluation of existing performance indicator systems (Goddard *et al.* 2000; Walshe 2003). Such evaluations are needed to assess the impact and validity of the indicator systems used, their contribution to increasing accountability through the performance management process and their ability to truly reflect the goals and objectives set out by the health care system.

The reporting of performance indicators can have different objectives, such as increasing consumer choice and facilitating change in provider behaviour and, ultimately, improving the performance of the health care system. There are, however, relatively few data to assess whether and how well performance indicator systems achieve any of these objectives. Evidence from the USA suggests that consumers as well as purchasers or payers rarely search out publicly available information and, if they do, do not understand or trust it (Marshall *et al.* 2000). Also,

---

Box 2.11   Advantages and disadvantages of league tables

League tables are increasingly being used to rank performance in many different sectors including health care and education (Nutley and Smith 1998; Adab *et al.* 2002). League tables are intuitively appealing, especially to politicians who are anxious to know how public funds are being spent. It is seen as a means to reduce a mass of complex information into a format that almost anyone can understand.

Advantages of performance league tables include that they may stimulate competition between providers and may consequently lead to service improvement as providers will adopt best practices. The New York experience has been listed as one example although the findings have been challenged (Chassin 2002). It was also argued that league tables may improve patient or consumer choice, which has been interpreted as a necessity for an efficient market economy. In addition, league tables have the potential to facilitate regulators to monitor and ensure accountability of providers. Regulators can use league table rankings to identify clinicians or hospitals with a high frequency of selected adverse outcomes as a starting point for further enquiry.

On the downside, however, the apparent simplicity of league tables can be quite misleading, and many commentators have drawn attention to the numerous technical problems as discussed in the main text. Also, the aspect of increased consumer choice will only be relevant in health systems where there is indeed a choice of provider and thus largely excludes countries like the UK where patients have relatively little choice when using an individual practitioner or hospital. Finally, while league tables may have the potential to improve quality of services by encouraging providers to put more emphasis on quality of care, they may also have unintended consequences such as distorting priorities by encouraging providers to focus on performance measures *per se* rather than quality improvement ('gaming'). A related problem is that with ranking performance there is an implicit assumption that providers located at the bottom of the table provide a poorer service. This gives way to the development of a culture of naming and shaming in which the blame is often apportioned to individuals.

---

physicians appear to be rather sceptical about the data and only a small proportion apparently uses them. The US experience thus seems to suggest that 'public disclosure of information about the quality of health care is a weak strategy for ensuring quality' (Schneider and Lieberman 2001). However, there is also evidence suggesting that managers and some providers do use comparative information, with data from the USA showing that hospitals appear to have been most responsive to publicized data with some evidence pointing towards improvements in care where public reporting occurred (Marshall *et al.* 2000; Chassin 2002). Based on this and experience elsewhere, Leatherman (2002: 329) thus concluded that '[t]he state of the art of performance measurement and reporting has made dramatic advances in the past decade but it is still deficient to support widespread diffusion, predictable systematic application, and routinely fair and accurate assessments'.

Conclusions

The quest for a means of evaluating an entire health system is far from simple. Health systems are intrinsically complex entities, with flexible boundaries, the definitions of which depend on the question being asked. While the main goals of a health system can easily be defined, it is more difficult to identify a way of assessing whether these goals are being achieved and the extent to which apparent progress can be attributed to the health system or to other factors. It is important not to overlook the many intermediate or subsidiary goals of a health system, as policies designed to achieve one goal may impact adversely on progress towards another. Health systems, like all human systems, are adaptable, so that the impact of an intervention designed to bring about change can be difficult to predict. They are also contextually bounded, so that something that works in one country may not work in the same way in another.

If there are key messages that can be taken from this chapter they are, first, that in evaluating some aspect of a health care system one must begin by defining the question being asked as precisely as possible and, second, that the evaluation must be informed by the context within which each system exists.

There is an inevitable tension between the simple answers often sought by politicians, such as whether the health system in country A is better than that in country B, and the messy complexity that gives rise to the analysts answer that 'it depends on what you mean'. Instead, by cataloguing the many challenges that exist, this chapter may act as a stimulus for both groups to come together in a constructive dialogue that will enable the former to define their questions more precisely and the latter to develop ways in which these improved questions can be answered.

Key points

- There are different definitions of what a health system is.
- The approach taken to describing and analysing health systems depends critically on the question being asked.
- In evaluating health systems, the question being asked must be defined as precisely as possible.
- Thus any definition used must be explicit and the means of evaluating the system must be congruent with the definition.
- The evaluation must be informed by the context within which each system exists.
- There has been a move away from the evaluation of the system as a whole towards the evaluation of sub-systems.
- Approaches to health system comparison fall broadly into one of three main groups: descriptive studies, quantitative approaches and focused analytical studies.
- Challenges to the development, application and reporting of performance indicators include: the definitions underlying the process of performance assessment; the ideological values underpinning any approach to this; limited data availability and lack of uniformity of data across different settings; and methodological issues, including the validity of proxy composite measures.

Acknowledgement

The work of Ellen Nolte and Suzanne Wait on international benchmarking in health is supported by fellowships from the Nuffield Trust.

References

Abel-Smith, B. (1963) Paying for health services: a study of the costs and sources of finance in six countries, *Public Health Papers*, 17: 1–86.

Abel-Smith, B. (1967) An international study of health expenditure and its relevance for health planning, *Public Health Papers*, 32: 1–127.

Adab, P., Rouse, A.M., Mohammed, M.A. and Marshall, T. (2002) Performance league tables: the NHS deserves better, *British Medical Journal*, 324: 95–8.

Anderson, O.W. (1963) Medical care: its social and organizational aspects. Health-services systems in the United States and other countries – critical comparisons, *New England Journal of Medicine*, 269: 839–43.

Anderson, O.W. (1972) *Health Care: Can there be Equity? The United States, Sweden and England*. New York: Wiley.

Arah, O.A., Klazinga, N.S., Delnoij, D.M.J., Ten Asbroek, A.H.A. and Custers, T. (2003) Conceptual framework for health systems performance: a quest for effectiveness, quality and improvement, *International Journal of Quality in Health Care*, 15: 377–98.

Becher, E.C. and Chassin, M.R. (2001) Improving the quality of health care: who will lead? *Health Affairs*, 20: 164–79.

Bennett, C.J. (1991) How states use foreign evidence, *Journal of Public Policy*, 11: 31–54.

British Broadcasting Corporation (2000) French health care 'best in world', http://news.bbc.co.uk/1/hi/health/799444.stm (accessed 8 May 2004).

Buck, D., Eastwood, A. and Smith, P.C. (1999) Can we measure the social importance of health care? *International Journal of Technology Assessment in Health Care*, 15: 89–107.

Charlton, J.R.H., Hartley, R.M., Silver, R. and Holland, W.W. (1983) Geographical variation in mortality from conditions amenable to medical intervention in England and Wales, *Lancet*, i: 691–6.

Chassin, M.R. (2002) Achieving and sustaining improved quality: lessons from New York State and cardiac surgery, *Health Affairs*, 21: 40–51.

Checkland, P. (1981) *Systems Thinking, Systems Practice*. Chichester: Wiley.

Commission for Health Improvement (2004) http://www.chi.nhs.uk/ratings/ (accessed 2 May 2004).

Department of Health (2002) *NHS Performance Ratings*. London: Department of Health.

Donabedian, A. (1966) Evaluating the quality of medical care, *Milbank Quarterly*, 44: 166–203.

Donabedian, A. (1980) *The Definition of Quality and Approaches to its Management*. Ann Arbor, MI: Health Administration Press.

Donabedian, A. (1988) The quality of care: how can it be assessed? *JAMA*, 260: 1743–8.

Dr Foster (2004) http://www.drfoster.co.uk/home.asp (accessed 2 May 2004).

Elling, R.H. (1980) *Cross-national Study of Health Systems: Concepts, Methods and Data Sources. Health Affairs Information Guide Series 2*. Detroit, MI: Gale Research Company.

Elling, R.H. (1994) Theory and method for the cross-national study of health systems, *International Journal of Health Services*, 24: 285–309.

European Observatory on Health Systems and Policies (2004) http://www.who.dk/observatory (accessed 30 April 2004).

Evans, R.G. (1981) Incomplete vertical integration: the distinctive structure of the health-care industry, in J. Van Der Gaag and M. Perlman (eds) *Health, Economics and Health Economics*. Amsterdam: North Holland.

Field, M.G. (1973) The concept of the 'health system' at the macrosociological level, *Social Science & Medicine*, 7: 763–85.

Field, M.G. (1978) *Comparative Health Systems: Differentiation and Convergence*. Washington: National Center for Health Services Research.

Frenk, J. (1994) Dimensions of health system reform, *Health Policy*, 27: 19–34.

Frenk, J. and Donabedian, A. (1987) State intervention in medical care: types, trends and variables, *Health Policy and Planning*, 2: 17–31.

Girard, J.-F. and Minvielle, E. (2002) Measuring up: lessons and potential, in *Measuring Up: Improving Health System Performance in OECD Countries*. Paris: OECD.

Goddard, M., Mannion, R. and Smith, P. (2000) Enhancing performance in heath care: a theoretical perspective on agency and the role of information, *Health Economics*, 9: 95–107.

Goldman, F. (1946) Foreign programs of medical care and their lessons, *New England Journal of Medicine*, 234: 156.

Green, D.G., Irvine, I., Mckee, M., Dixon, A. and Mossialos, E. (2002) For and against: social insurance – the right way forward for health care in the United Kingdom? *British Medical Journal*, 325: 488–90.

Hannan, E.L., Stone, C.C., Biddle, T.L. and Debuono, B.A. (1997) Public release of cardiac surgery outcomes data in New York: what do New York state cardiologists think of it? *American Heart Journal*, 134: 1120–8.

Holland, W.W. (1988) *European Community Atlas of 'Avoidable Death'*. Oxford: Oxford University Press.

Hurst, J. and Jee-Hughes, M. (2000) *Performance Measurements and Performance Management in OECD Health Systems*. Paris: OECD.

Hurtado, M.P., Swift, E.K. and Corrigan, J.M. (2001) *Envisioning the National Health Care Quality Report*. Washington: National Academy Press.

Hussey, P.S., Anderson, G.F., Osborn, R., Feek, C., Mclaughlin, V., Millar, J. and Epstein, A. (2004) How does the quality of care compare in five countries? *Health Affairs*, 23: 89–99.

Ibrahim, J.E. (2001) Performance indicators from all perspectives, *International Journal of Quality in Health Care*, 13: 431–2.

International Network for Health Policy and Reform (2004) http://www.health-policy-monitor.org/index.jsp (accessed 30 April 2004).

Joint Commission on Accreditation of Healthcare Organizations (1990) *Primer on Indicators Development and Application*. Oakbrook Terrace, IL: Joint Commission on Accreditation of Healthcare Organizations.

Kanavos, P. and Mossialos, E. (1990) International comparisons of expenditures: what we know and what we do not know, *Journal of Health Services Research and Policy*, 4: 122–6.

Klein, R. (1997) Learning from others: shall the last be first? *Journal of Health Politics, Policy and Law*, 22: 1267–78.

Kohn, L.T., Corrigan, J.M. and Donaldson, M.S. (1999) *To Err is Human: Building a Safer Health System*. Washington, DC: National Academic Press.

Last, J.M. (2001) *A Dictionary of Epidemiology*. Oxford: Oxford University Press.

Le Grand, J. and Bartlett, W. (1993) *Quasi-Markets and Social Policy*. London: Palgrave Macmillan.

Leatherman, S. (2002) Applying performance indicators to health system improvement, in *Measuring Up: Improving Health System Performance in OECD Countries*. Paris: OECD.

Leichter, H.M. (1979) *A Comparative Approach to Policy Analysis: Health Care Policy in Four Nations*. Cambridge: Cambridge University Press.

Leng, G.C., Walsh, D., Fowkes, F.G.R. and Swainson, C.P. (1999) Is the emergency readmission rates a valid outcome indicator? *Quality in Health Care*, 8: 234–8.

Lewin, R. (1992) *Complexity: Life at the Edge of Chaos*. Chicago: University of Chicago Press.

Long, M.J. (1994) *The Medical Care System: A Conceptual Model*. Ann Arbor, MI: AUPHA Press.

Macinko, J., Starfield, B. and Shi, L. (2003) The contribution of primary care systems to health outcomes within Organization for Economic Cooperation and Development (OECD) countries, 1970–1998, *Health Services Research*, 38: 831–65.

Marshall, M.N., Shekelle, P.G., Leatherman, S. and Brook, R.H. (2000) The public release of performance data: what do we expect to gain? A review of the evidence, *JAMA*, 283: 1866–74.

Maxwell, R. (1974) *Health Care, the Growing Dilemma: Needs Versus Resources in Western Europe, the US and the USSR*. New York: McKinsey & Co.

McKee, M. (1995) 2020 vision, *Journal of Public Health Medicine*, 17: 127–31.

McKee, M. and Figueras, J. (1997) Comparing health care systems: how do we know if we can learn from others? *Journal of Health Services Research and Policy*, 2: 122–5.

McKee, M. and Healy, J. (2002) *Hospitals in a Changing Europe.* Buckingham: Open University Press.

McPake, B., Kumaranyake, L. and Normand, C. (2002) *Health Economics: An International Perspective.* London: Routledge.

Mechanic, D. (1975) Ideology, medical technology, and health care organization in modern nations, *American Journal of Public Health*, 65: 241–7.

Mills, A. and Ranson, M. (2001) The design of health systems, in M. Merson, R. Black and A. Mills (eds) *International Public Health, Diseases, Programs, Systems, and Policies.* Gaithersburg, MD: Aspen Publications.

Milne, R. and Molana, H. (1991) On the effect of income and relative price on demand for health care: EC evidence, *Applied Economics*, 23: 1221–6.

Mossialos, E., Dixon, A., Figueras, J. and Kutzin, J. (2002) *Funding Health Care: Options for Europe.* Buckingham: Open University Press.

Mountin, J.W. and Perrott, G.S. (1947) Health insurance programs and plans of western Europe: summary of observations, *Public Health Reports*, 62: 369–99.

Mulligan, J., Appleby, J. and Harrison, A. (2000) Measuring the performance of health systems, *British Medical Journal*, 321: 191–2.

Murray, C.J.L. and Evans, D.B. (2003) *Health Systems Performance Assessment: Debates, Methods and Empiricism.* Geneva: WHO.

Murray, C.J.L. and Frenk, J. (2000) A framework for assessing the performance of health systems, *Bulletin of the World Health Organization*, 78: 717–31.

Musgrove, P. (2003) Judging health systems: reflections on WHO's methods, *Lancet*, 361: 1817–20.

Naylor, C.D., Iron, K. and Handa, K. (2002) Measuring health system performance: problems and opportunities in the era of assessment and accountability, in *Measuring Up: Improving Health System Performance in OECD Countries.* Paris: OECD.

Neuhauser, D. (2002) Ernest Amory Codman MD, *Quality and Safety in Health Care*, 11: 104–5.

Nolte, E. and McKee, M. (2003) Measuring the health of the nations: how much is attributable to health care? An analysis of mortality amenable to medical care, *British Medical Journal*, 327: 1129–32.

Nolte, E. and McKee, M. (2004) *Does Healthcare Save Lives? Avoidable Mortality Revisited.* London: The Nuffield Trust.

Nolte, E., Wait, S., Bain, C. and McKee, M. (2003) What can be measured or what is important? A critical analysis of international comparisons of health system performance. Poster presented at 5th International Conference on the Scientific Basis of Health Services, Washington, 20–3 September.

Nutley, S. and Smith, P.C. (1998) League tables for performance improvement in health care, *Journal of Health Services Research and Policy*, 3: 50–7.

OECD (1985) *Measuring Health Care: 1960–1983 Expenditure, Costs and Performance.* Paris: OECD.

OECD (1992) *The Reform of Health Care Systems: A Comparative Analysis of Seven OECD Countries.* Paris: OECD.

OECD (2002) *Measuring Up: Improving Health System Performance in OECD Countries.* Paris: OECD.

OECD (2003) *OECD Health Data 2003: A Comparative Analysis of 30 OECD Countries.* Paris: OECD.

Or, Z. (2000) Determinants of health outcomes in industrialised countries: a pooled, cross-country, time-series analysis, *OECD Economic Studies*, 30: 53–77.

Or, Z. (2001) *Exploring the Effects of Health Care on Mortality Across OECD Countries.* Paris: OECD.

Parkin, D., Mcguire, A. and Yule, B. (1987) Aggregate health care expenditures and national income: is health Care a luxury good? *Journal of Health Economics*, 6: 109–27.

Plochg, T. and Klazinga, N.S. (2002) Community-based integrated care: myth or must? *International Journal for Quality in Health Care*, 14: 91–101.

Pollock, A.M. and Price, D. (2003) The public health implications of world trade negotiations on the general agreement on trade in services and public services, *Lancet*, 362: 1072–5.

Pringle, M., Wilson, T. and Grol, R. (2002) Measuring 'goodness' in individuals and health-care systems, *British Medical Journal*, 325: 704–7.

Raffel, M.W. (1984) *Comparative Health Systems – Descriptive Analyses of Fourteen National Health Systems*. University Park, PA: Pennsylvania State University Press.

Reinhardt, U.E., Hussey, P.S. and Anderson, G.F. (2002) Cross-national comparisons of health systems using OECD data, 1999, *Health Affairs*, 21: 169–81.

Relman, A.S. (1988) Assessment and accountability: the third revolution in medical care, *New England Journal of Medicine*, 319: 1220–2.

Rodwin, V.G. (1984) *The Health Planning Predicament: France, Quebec, England, and the United States*. Berkeley, CA: University of California Press.

Roemer, M.I. (1960) Health departments and medical care – a world scanning, *American Journal of Public Health*, 50: 154.

Roemer, M.I. (1969) *The Organization of Medical Care Under Social Security*. Geneva: International Labour Office.

Roemer, M.I. (1977) *Comparative National Policies on Health Care*. New York: Marcel Dekker.

Roemer, M.I. (1991) *National Health Systems of the World*. New York: Oxford University Press.

Rose, R. (1993) *Lesson Drawing in Public Policy*. Chatham, NJ: Chatham House.

Rutstein, D.D., Berenberg, W., Chalmers, T.C., Child, C.G., Fishman, A.P. and Perrin, E.B. (1976) Measuring the quality of medical care, *New England Journal of Medicine*, 294: 582–8.

Saltman, R.B., Busse, R. and Mossialos, E. (2002) *Regulating Entrepreneurial Behaviour in European Health Care Systems*. Buckingham: Open University Press.

Schieber, G.J. (1987) *Financing and Delivering Health Care: A Comparative Analysis of OECD Countries*. Paris: OECD.

Schneider, E.C. and Lieberman, T. (2001) Publicly disclosed information about the quality of health care: response of the US public, *Quality in Health Care*, 10: 96–103.

Shaw, C. and Kalo, I. (2002) *A Background for National Quality Policies in Health Systems*. Copenhagen: WHO Regional Office for Europe.

Sheaff, R. (1998) Towards a global theory of health systems: Milton Roemer's *National Health Systems of the World*, *Health Care Analysis*, 6: 150–70.

Sigerist, H.E. (1943) From Bismarck to Beveridge: developments and trends in social security legislation, *Bulletin of the History of Medicine*, 8: 365–88.

Smee, C.H. (2002) Improving value for money in the United Kingdom National Health Service: performance measurement and improvement in a centralised system, in *Measuring Up: Improving Health System Performance in OECD Countries*. Paris: OECD.

Smith, P. (2002a) Editor's preface, in *Measuring Up: Improving Health System Performance in OECD Countries*. Paris: OECD.

Smith, P. (2002b) Performance management in British health care: will it deliver? *Health Affairs*, 21: 103–32.

Smith, R. (1998) Regulation of doctors and the Bristol Inquiry, *British Medical Journal*, 317: 1539–40.

Terris, M. (1978) The three world systems of medical care: trends and prospects, *American Journal of Public Health*, 65: 1125–31.

Thompson, C.R. and McKee, M. (2004) Financing and planning of public hospitals in the European Union, *Health Policy*, 67: 281–91.

Wait, S. and Nolte, E. (in press) Benchmarking health systems: trends, conceptual issues and future perspectives, *Benchmarking: An International Journal*.

Walshe, K. (2003) International comparisons of the quality of health care; what do they tell us? *Quality and Safety in Health Care*, 12: 4–5.

Weber, M. (1950) *On Methodology of Social Sciences*. New York: Macmillan.

Weinerman, E.R. (1971) Research on comparative health service systems, *Medical Care*, 9: 272–90.

WHO (World Health Organization) (1948) Preamble to the *Constitution of the World Health Organization* as adopted by The International Health Conference, New York 19–22 June 1946. Geneva: World Health Organization.

WHO (World Health Organization) (2000) *The World Health Report 2000: Health Systems, Improving Performance*. Geneva: World Health Organization.

WHO (World Health Organization) Regional Office For Europe (2004) *Health for All Database*. Copenhagen: WHO Regional Office for Europe.

Wilson, T. and Holt, T. (2001) Complexity and clinical care, *British Medical Journal*, 323: 685–88.

Part 2
Multidisciplinary methods of investigation

3 Evidence-based health care: systematic reviews

Paul Cullinan

Introduction

The term 'systematic review' means a succinct description of the methodical and deliberate survey and assessment of a body of evidence relating to a particular health issue. Health care professionals have always appreciated summaries of knowledge; traditionally these have been prepared by experts relying on their personal knowledge of, and expressing their opinions on, the evidence available to them. Such reviews remain the mainstay of most medical textbooks or 'review articles' and in many cases they provide a powerful – if polemic – resource.

However, narrative reviews like these face the risk of subjectivity in both the choice of reviewed material and in its interpretation. The danger was first recognized in the psychosocial literature but Archie Cochrane, in his call for the collection of *all* randomized trials relevant to the therapeutics of a particular specialty, was among the first to extend its recognition to medical issues (Cochrane 1979). Eight years later, Cynthia Mulrow described the many potential and actual pitfalls in traditional medical review articles (Mulrow 1987). Shortly afterwards, a much-quoted study highlighted the tardiness of expert opinion in comparison to systematic examination of the published evidence for thrombolytic therapy in acute myocardial infarction (Antman *et al.* 1992) – see Figure 3.1.

Systematic reviews of evidence were designed to overcome the deficiencies of subjectivity, selectivity and timeliness. Further justifications included the increasing demand and need for accurate, transparent but digestible summaries of an ever-burgeoning literature. Not only clinicians but also policy-makers increasingly use systematic reviews to inform their practice. For many interventions the evidence base is relatively weak, perhaps comprising a few small, randomized trials. When none is sufficiently powerful alone to provide a convincing estimate of effectiveness or harm, their systematic meta-analysis may provide a useful summary estimate. The combination of results from different centres may also improve the generalizability of their findings. Finally, systematic literature reviews often inform research priorities, usually by highlighting the lack of available evidence in a particular area.

A very large number of high-quality systematic reviews are undertaken every year. Many are published in abbreviated form in standard journals. A comprehensive list of those undertaken through the worldwide Cochrane Collaboration is freely available on the web (www.cochrane.co.uk).

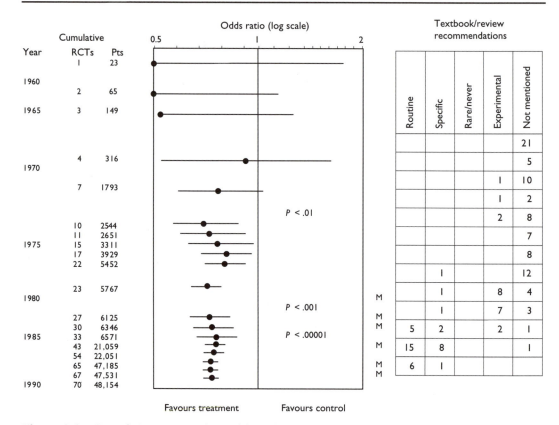

Figure 3.1   Cumulative meta-analysis of thrombolytic treatment for acute myocardial infarction

Source: adapted from Antman *et al.* Figure 2, *Journal of the American Medical Association,* 1992; 268(2): 240–8. Copyrighted © (1992), American Medical Association. All rights reserved. M = at least one meta-analysis was published that year.

Methodology: an overview

Conceptually, and for the most part, the methodology of systematic reviews is not difficult. For most types of review the necessary steps are explicit, widely agreed and are summarized in Box 3.1. While they appear mechanistic – and indeed they are intended to be so – a degree of judgement at each step is required. This is perhaps most important in the formulation of appropriate questions and in the interpretation of the findings. A systematic review should not be undertaken lightly; dependent on the size of the research base a properly conducted review will take up to two years and will very rarely be possible in under six months.

   Most systematic reviews are concerned with the effectiveness of medical interventions. Most of those for example prepared under the aegis of the Cochrane Collaboration are, in keeping with the interest of its namesake, explicitly so. There is increasing interest in, but far less experience of, reviews in other areas of health care such as disease aetiology, prognosis or the usefulness of diagnostic tests. Nonetheless the same principles apply. More recently there has been interest in the incorporation of qualitative data into systematic reviews of trials (Dixon-Woods and Fitzpatrick 2001).

Box 3.1   Steps in systematic reviewing

1   specification of question(s) to be answered
2   literature search (data collection)
3   selection of studies for review
4   data extraction
5   meta-analysis
6   sensitivity analysis
7   qualitative interpretation and summary of findings
8   summary and recommendations

Defining the question(s)

The best systematic reviews address problems that are both focused and relevant and ones that are amenable to change. Clearly focused questions are helpful for those who read the review and for those who wish to apply its findings, but they are also an essential guide to those undertaking the review. Only in this way can clear decisions later be made about which evidence to include in the review and about the most appropriate ways of summarizing it. 'Relevance' refers to issues that 'matter'. Systematic reviews that address issues that are not meaningful or practical or that concern outdated treatments or trivial outcomes are wasteful. Expensive interventions, those that are widely used and are therefore capable of causing widespread benefit or harm, and those that could be widely used because they are simple, are all examples of issues appropriate for systematic review (Counsell 1997).

Even so, some practices are so deeply embedded in medical practice that they are very difficult to influence even if they are demonstrably useless or even harmful. Some argue that in these cases the production of a systematic review indicating that it is useless is unlikely to alter the practice. This, however, has not stopped others: for example in recent years systematic reviews of such medical shibboleths as fluids for febrile children (Guppy *et al.* 2004), counselling for victims of trauma (Rose *et al.* 2003) and albumen infusion in critical care (Wilkes and Navickis 2001) have all appeared amidst some controversy.

There are several guides to the setting of appropriate questions (Cooper 1984; Counsell 1997). Questions that concern therapies are usually considered in three components and will include reference to each of them: the population, the intervention and the outcome. Thus the patient group will be described by age, sex, diagnosis and setting; and perhaps by other factors such as race or co-morbidity or socioeconomic status. The intervention under consideration will be clearly defined: 'angioplasty' rather than 'interventional cardiology' for example. Often most difficult at the start of the review process will be determining the focus of outcome(s). Published studies tend to employ and present a wide variety of related outcomes which themselves may be composites of separate outcomes and impossible to disentangle without reference to the original data. A narrow focus on a particular measure of outcome at the start of a systematic review may dramatically limit the subsequent selection of evidence. On the other hand, there are inherent difficulties in combining or comparing disparate outcome measures. Sadly there is only limited evidence relating to several important outcomes such as quality of life or employment and work performance.

Collecting the evidence

The arrival of electronic literature searching has been an undoubted benefit. The days of leafing through unwieldy, small print reference books are largely gone and, if done with care, a long list of appropriate, published references can be obtained at a desktop computer in a matter of days.

However, this convenience is deceptive and amassing the full available evidence remains the most laborious and time-consuming part of preparing a systematic review. It is also the part where many difficulties are likely to arise and where much controversy may be generated. Many more studies are conducted than will ever appear in print. The central issue is whether published studies are an unbiased sample of all studies conducted in a particular area. If they are not then their systematic review will produce a biased and possibly misleading picture. Unfortunately, it is probable that in many areas there is considerable bias arising in one or more of the following ways.

Publication bias

'Publication bias' refers to the tendency for authors to submit, and for journal editors to publish, studies whose findings are either positive or favourable or, more occasionally, controversial. 'Positive' in this sense generally equates with statistical significance. Where such bias exists, negative or, more generally, mundane findings are less likely to be published. Evidence for publication bias was first produced in 1959 when Theodore Sterling reported that studies of pschycological treatments were more likely to be published if their null hypothesis had been rejected (Sterling 1959). Subsequent studies have affirmed that:

- those with statistically significant findings are between two and three times more likely to be published than studies where the results are deemed not 'significant' (Dickersin 1997);
- authors are about ten times more likely to submit the findings of studies whose results are significant (Greenwald 1975);
- studies that 'merely confirm' earlier findings are less likely to be published (Zelen 1983).

Investigators as authors seek fame, and editors strive to enhance the impact of their journal. While such foibles are only human, the result is a published literature that is likely to favour the positive and the contentious above the negative and the prosaic. This is a particular problem with the therapeutic literature where such bias will overestimate the efficacy of a treatment.

Commercial interests

A high proportion of drug trials are sponsored by pharmaceutical companies with a vested interest in their findings. A particular example of publication bias may arise from their relative reluctance to encourage the publication of unfavourable findings (Lauritsen et al. 1987; Melander et al. 2003). This may lead to serious distortions in the available evidence base relating to a treatment, thus undermining any systematic review, a situation described by the editors of the *Lancet* as a 'disaster'. There are clear examples where this process has led to misleading conclusions (Jureidini et al. 2004; Whittington et al. 2004). Safeguards to ensure the independent rights of academic researchers to publish were introduced recently but cannot be assumed to have been in place previously.

Language

Most health-related research articles are published in English but it is important to remember that not all are. In some areas – for example, in complementary therapies – large proportions of studies are published in other languages. Nor can it be assumed that those studies reported in English-language journals are representative of the entire literature. Studies with positive findings are more likely to be published in English (Egger *et al.* 1997b). Inclusion of studies otherwise excluded on the basis of the language in which they were published may have important effects on the conclusions of a systematic review (Gregoire *et al.* 1995).

Multiple publication

Repeated publication of results from the same study may involve publication in more than one language but is not uncommon in a single language. Such 'salami science' (Huth 1986) may be difficult to detect (Huston and Moher 1996). Usually such publications present slightly different versions of a single study's findings or findings from a single centre within a multi-centre study. For the reviewer the difficulty is in establishing whether these represent genuinely separate studies.

In an attempt to compensate for some of these potential biases, attention has turned to studies that have not been formally published. These include doctoral theses, abstracts, conference proceedings and other types of 'grey literature'; and studies that have been completed but never submitted for publication at all. There is some concern that the information contained in sources such as these may be of lower quality than that published in peer-reviewed journals (Cook *et al.* 1993). Moreover, being poorly indexed or not indexed at all, the grey and otherwise unpublished literature is far harder to search in a systematic manner (McManus *et al.* 1998). Unpublished material that can be located may not be representative of all unpublished literature.

Several methods have been devised for assessing the existence and extent of any publication bias. The most commonly used is the 'funnel plot', a simple and rapid graphical technique (Light and Pillemer 1984). Because small studies are more subject to random error, their results (positive or negative) will be less precise and should be more widely distributed than those arising from large studies. A plot of 'effect estimate' against 'precision' (e.g. sample size or standard error) of all the published studies should, in the absence of bias, produce a scatter diagram that resembles a symmetric funnel whose wider end represents the scatter of results from smaller studies (see Figure 3.2). Funnel plots of a systematically biased evidence base will be skewed and appear to have a missing piece.

Funnel plots are useful only where there is a sufficient distribution of studies of different sample sizes. Their asymmetry may also arise from other causes than a biased publication base. Thus therapeutic studies may differ in the risk profile of their participants or the intensity with which an intervention has been applied. Nonetheless, funnel symmetry seems a good guide to the presence of bias in a systematic review – at least where this is expressed as agreement between a review and large randomized trials (Egger *et al.* 1997a). More complex methods of detecting 'missing' studies and of measuring their likely effects exist but have not been fully evaluated (Dear and Begg 1992; Givens *et al.* 1997).

Systematic literature searching is best left to an expert; or at least done in close collaboration with one. University librarians are often a helpful resource. Electronic searches should be sensitive and cover all relevant databases since there is variable and incomplete overlap between them. The more exhaustive a search the less likely

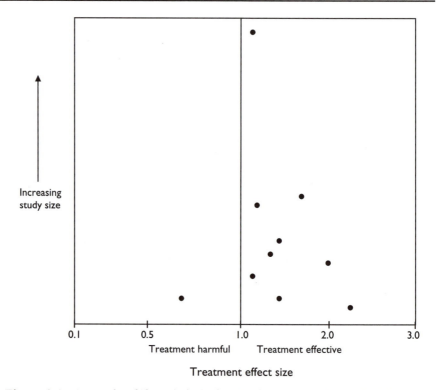

Figure 3.2   Example of 'funnel plot' of results from ten randomized trials suggesting important publication bias

it is that important data will be missed and the less likely that the review will be affected by any reviewer biases. Restriction to single (generally English) language publications is hard to justify except by a plea of expediency. Problems of locating all relevant studies may arise when the topic of interest is addressed not as a primary hypothesis but in a secondary analysis. Electronic searching should be augmented by a careful scan of the reference sections of located articles and may be supplemented by searches of the contents pages of suitable journals and by access to grey literature or by direct contact with leading researchers in the field. Although most reviewers will make these efforts, relatively few will subsequently include material found in this way (Cook *et al.* 1993).

Selecting studies for inclusion

A full literature search will uncover far more material than can or should be included in a review. The next step – that of selecting studies for inclusion – is again fraught with the potential for bias. In deciding which studies ought to be included, two criteria (at least) need to be considered.

The first is that studies to be included in a review should contain primary data that are pertinent to the subject and results that address one or more of the review questions. This is less obvious than it sounds, particularly with the issue of appropriate outcome measures. Just as there are many ways to 'skin a cat' there are dozens of ways of measuring, for example, the effects of a treatment or the prognosis of a disease. It may be necessary to select and then categorize studies by the measures included therein. This can be difficult or even impossible when composite measures alone are reported; in such cases an appeal to the authors for unpublished, disaggregated outcome measures may be fruitful.

Second, the methodological quality of the study should be noted. This is more straightforward for randomized and controlled therapeutic studies where there are several widely agreed quality standards. Appraisal of quality in this way allows several options in the eventual selection:

- Studies of low quality may be omitted altogether. At least one author has claimed that the 'inclusion of bad studies may completely subvert the true outcome of a[n] ... analysis' (Eysenck 1995). The selection of high-quality studies is, Eysenck argues, part of an expert reviewer's task. If this route is to be taken then it seems wise to establish a prior set of quality criteria – and to apply them without knowledge of a study's findings. More than one assessor for each study may be valuable at this stage.
- Others would argue that wholesale inclusion is the *raison d'être* of a systematic review and selection on the basis of quality, inevitably a qualitative process itself, may be a source of important bias.
- A third way, and one most widely advocated, is to use a quality assessment as part of a review's 'sensitivity analysis'. In this way the findings of a review may be compared when all studies are included, or when the 'good' and 'less good' are analysed separately (Blanc and Toren 1999).

Concerns are often expressed about the selection of studies for inclusion in a review, especially when they are few or when the review's conclusions are controversial. It is improbable, however, that high-quality reviews will omit important studies.

Extracting data

Once selected, studies need to be dissected and their data extracted onto what social scientists call a 'coding sheet' and others a 'data extraction form'. This will permit the synthesis of the studies' findings; or at worst establish that no synthesis is possible. Where there is a very large number of studies it may be helpful to devise an extraction form beforehand, after careful consideration of what information is going to be useful. Where there are few studies it may be simpler to read them repeatedly and decide then what information is available for coding.

Coding forms should include at least the following information:

- study reference including year of publication;
- study design;
- study population and setting;
- numbers of participants;
- details of intervention (if appropriate);
- statistical outcomes.

Anybody who has ever undertaken data extraction in this way will know the frustrations of what on paper appears to be a straightforward process. Difficulties arise when, as is all too frequent, published details are vague, missing or contradictory. Again, too, the problems with variable outcome measures become apparent. In some cases it may be necessary to abandon the ideal of a common measurement and rely instead on a synthesis of standardized measurements although this may be difficult to interpret clinically. The use of a field for 'miscellaneous notes' where the coder can note peculiarities of individual studies is generally helpful. Nonetheless, data extraction forms almost always include blank spaces beside coded studies: 'perfection is never achieved' (Cooper 1988).

Data are frequently missing from otherwise useful publications; or are presented in a form that makes it impossible to include them in a combined analysis. In these cases an appeal to the authors for the necessary figures is often made, albeit with mixed success.

Analysis

Meta-analysis is the systematic process whereby a single quantitative measure of effect is derived from the combination of effects from a number of separate studies. The term was first used in the psychological literature of 1976 (Glass 1978) and, helpfully, it is now a medical subject heading term within Medline. The statistical methods for meta-analysis range from the straightforward to the very complex; an increasing variety of software, much of it free, is now available.

'Vote counting' is the process whereby studies are categorized as 'positive' or 'negative', generally on the basis of their statistical significance. The numbers in each category are tallied and compared. Although very simple, this method gives equal weight to studies of (very) different sizes. Moreover, as with any technique reliant solely on 'p values' it fails to account for the range of outcomes that a summary measure encompasses.

Many outcome measures used in therapeutic or other research are of a 'binary' nature. Binary outcomes may take one of two values such as dead/alive, hospitalized/not hospitalized or cancer/no cancer. Other measures may be continuous; examples include absolute blood pressure or one of the many measurements of lung function. Ordinal outcomes include several 'ordered' categories, the intervals between each not necessarily being equal. Tumour stages or systems for the classification of chest X-rays in pneumoconiosis are examples of ordinal measures. For the purposes of meta-analysis, the method of expressing a single study's effects – therapeutic, preventive or aetiological – will depend on the type of outcome measure it has used. Meta-analysis can only be performed when there is a common outcome type.

- For studies with binary outcomes, effects are generally expressed as 'odds ratios' or 'risk ratios', the former especially in therapeutic studies. When such effects from several trials are to be combined then a normally-distributed variable can usually be obtained by using ln-transformed values. Other methods of expressing treatment effects include the 'numbers needed to treat' (NNT – the reciprocal of the risk difference) and the relative risk reduction. These are especially useful for clinical applications of research but are more difficult to combine in meta-analysis.
- Effects expressed through continuous outcome measures are generally summarized by mean differences between the study groups. In order to allow for the greater precision afforded by larger studies and to account for variation in absolute effects between studies of different groups, these differences are often 'standardized' by being expressed, for example, in units of standard deviation.
- Ordinal effect differences are more difficult to synthesize, especially where different scales are used in different studies (Whitehead and Whitehead 1991).

Statistical techniques for the meta-analysis of binary or continuous outcomes use either a 'fixed' or a 'random' effects approach.

- Fixed effects models assume that all the studies under analysis are estimates of a single population effect; or, in other words, if they each were sufficiently (infinitely) large then their results would be identical. The most simple fixed effects method (the 'inverse variance' method) estimates a mean effect size from the results of each component study after these have been weighted by their inverse variances. Alternative methods use a Mantel-Haenzal approach, with a continuity correction if necessary, or a modification described first by Peto *et al.* (1977). Further, more complex methods use maximum likelihood or exact estimations (Emerson 1994). The choice of method may not matter since in most cases they will produce very similar results. Meta-analysis of small numbers of studies with large sample sizes is best done using an inverse-variance method while Mantel-Haenzal techniques are to be preferred for combining the results of a large number of small studies (Sutton *et al.* 2001).
- Random effects models make no assumptions about the homogeneity of the effect estimates of the component studies and thus incorporate within them an additional source of variation expressing between-study differences. This variation is assumed to be random – an assumption that has been questioned. Using this method the weighting applied to larger studies is smaller – and that for smaller studies larger – than that with a fixed effect model.

If there is little heterogeneity between studies then meta-analysis using fixed- or random-effects methods will produce very similar results although the latter with somewhat lower precision. Nonetheless there has been a long-running debate over which is preferable (Thompson 1993). Frequently both methods are used and presented alongside each other. Some argue that differences found between the two methods should be viewed as an opportunity to explore the causes of any underlying heterogeneity.

The results are usually plotted on a 'forest plot' displaying the effect sizes for each study and separately the combined effect measure(s) estimated by meta-analysis. A (fictional) example is shown in Figure 3.3.

Other statistical approaches

Bayesian statistical methods work by making prior assumptions about the distribution of data; these are subsequently updated (to 'posterior' distributions) after analysis. In Bayesian meta-analysis a prior estimate of the mean effect size is specified, often empirically, along with estimates of the within-study and between-study variations depending on whether a fixed-effect or random-effect method is used (Eddy *et al.* 1998). The confidence intervals of a combined effect measure derived through Bayesian techniques are usually wider than those from more standard methods.

Heterogeneity

Studies under meta-analysis are said to be heterogeneous if their results differ strongly. Some would argue that the findings of such studies ought not to be included in any combined analysis; others that this is a *raison d'être* of meta-analysis and an opportunity to discover why different studies produce different results. An estimate of whether there is statistically significant heterogeneity can be made using a test first described by Cochran 50 years ago (Cochran 1954). If tests indicate no significant heterogeneity then the component studies may be assumed to refer to a

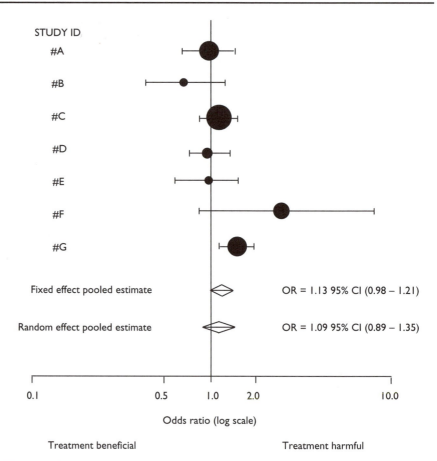

Figure 3.3 Example of 'forest plot' summarizing the meta-analysis of a systematic review of treatment. The horizontal bars depict confidence intervals; the circle diameters are proportional to study size.

single population, in which case a fixed-effects method of meta-analysis is appropriate.

Where there is heterogeneity, most experts would consider this an important finding that requires further examination in itself. Variation in study results often derives from differences in baseline risk between studies. Other common sources are in the intensity of application of the treatment, or other exposure, under study; in the setting in which they were applied or experienced; or in the control of various confounding exposures. Useful elaborations to basic meta-analyses may be made by separate ('sub-group') analysis of studies stratified by, for example, baseline risk (Smith *et al.* 1993) or study setting. 'Cumulative' meta-analyses are repeated analyses of accumulated data as they are published. They may point to important time shifts in treatment methods or highlight, albeit retrospectively, the time point at which an effect became 'significant' (Lau *et al.* 1992).

There are several methods for the statistical exploration of heterogeneity, especially when the number of component studies is high. These regression methods, which rely heavily on adequate information on relevant co-variables being available in each of the studies, include extensions of both the basic fixed-effects (meta-regression) and random-effects (mixed model regression) approaches.

Sensitivity analyses

The robustness of a systematic review is assessed through a 'sensitivity analysis' whereby its findings are repeatedly re-examined after changes in any underlying assumptions are made. Most often this involves including or excluding component studies on the basis of their quality or their publication status. Reviews whose conclusions are unstable in this manner should be interpreted with caution (Linde and Willich 2003).

Interpreting systematic reviews

Where one or more meta-analyses has been undertaken, the interpretation of a systematic review is straightforward – even if the findings may be unwelcome. Thus reviews of single treatments – usually pharmacological – derived from a reasonable number of well-conducted, randomized trials are relatively easy to interpret. Less easy is the interpretation of systematic reviews of small bodies of relatively poor studies; or of complex interventions or health-related and social policies. There the evidence base tends to be less firm, there tends to be considerable variation in outcome measures, making meta-analysis difficult or impossible, and a 'narrative' approach to interpretation is the only available option. Frequently, such reviews conclude that there is insufficient evidence to answer the original question(s). Indeed some have argued that such indecisiveness is inevitable (Petticrew 2003) and that this is likely to remain so until better methods of reviewing observational (non-trial) data are developed.

In the field of medicine, systematic reviews have been successful in at least two areas. The first, largely for the reasons given above, is in influencing drug prescribing for common diseases, and in particular cardiac diseases (Collins *et al.* 1997). Through the systematic review of small and medium-sized trials it has been possible to measure and implement simple treatments such as aspirin which produce moderate risk reductions that have important health benefits when applied to large populations. Even here, however, there are potential – and actual – pitfalls. Meta-analysis appears to be an imperfect predictor of the results of subsequent, large-scale (n > 1000) randomized trials, at least where these are categorized as 'positive' or 'negative' (Villar *et al.* 1995; LeLorier *et al.* 1997). Although clinically significant differences appear to be rare (Cappelleri *et al.* 1996) when this occurs it leads to considerable confusion and doubt about the value of meta-analysis. A notable example concerns the use of intravenous magnesium in the management of acute myocardial infarction where a positive meta-analysis was followed by a very large and essentially negative randomized trial (ISIS-4 (Fourth International Study of Infarct Survival) Collaborative Group 1995). A subsequent meta-analysis that incorporated the results of the new trial confirmed the ineffectiveness of the treatment. Such discrepancies are manna to those who are suspicious of systematic reviews (Eysenck 1995; Feinstein 1995). Further difficulties arise when separate systematic reviews of essentially the same evidence base reach opposite conclusions (Burge and Lewis 2003); fortunately this appears to be rare and usually arises from inadequate sensitivity analysis.

In contrast, the second area in which systematic reviews have proved valuable is where the evidence base is genuinely incomplete. Reviews here serve to establish the lack of any certainty – the 'research gap' – thus highlighting the need and direction of future primary research. The essentially negative conclusions of a systematic review of non-invasive ventilation in the treatment of sleep apnoea (Wright *et al.* 1997) was greeted with fury by specialist clinicians; but arguably provided the impetus for a subsequent, carefully designed randomised trial with positive findings (Jenkinson *et al.* 1999).

Conclusions

Dozens of high quality systematic reviews are carried out and published each year. Their approach offers considerable advantages – notably completeness, standardization and transparency – over the traditional, more subjective narrative review and is threatened only by an incomplete or distorted evidence base. As with all evidence derived from group data, their findings will continue to frustrate clinicians who seek answers at an individual level; and many important questions cannot be answered because there are not the data with which to do so. In these cases it is always worth recalling the adage that 'absence of evidence is not evidence of absence' (Hartung *et al.* 1983).

Key points

- Systematic reviews are a succinct description of the methodical and deliberate survey and assessment of a body of evidence on a topic.

- Non-systematic, narrative reviews risk subjectivity in the choice of reviewed material and in its interpretation.

- Amassing the full available evidence to review is laborious and time-consuming.

- A central issue is whether published studies are an unbiased sample of all studies on a topic. Potential biases include publication bias and exclusion of non-English papers.

- Electronic literature searches should be sensitive and cover all relevant databases, including other languages; the reference sections of included material should be scanned; the grey literature and the contents pages of relevant journals should be searched; contacts should be made with leading researchers in the field.

- The included studies should contain pertinent primary data and meet predefined standards of methodological quality.

- The data from included studies should be transferred to a 'data extraction sheet' to permit synthesis of their findings, or establish that no synthesis is possible.

- Where there is a sufficient distribution of studies with different sample sizes, the existence and extent of any publication bias can be assessed by constructing 'funnel plots', although their asymmetry may have other causes.

- Meta-analysis is the systematic process whereby a single quantitative measure of effect is derived from the combination of effects from a number of separate studies.

- The advantages of high-quality systematic reviews over more subjective narrative reviews are their completeness, standardization and transparency.

Further reading

Guides to systematic reviewing

Cooper, H. (1998) *Synthesizing Research: A Guide for Literature Reviewers.* London: Sage. Helpful guide intended for social, behavioural and medical researchers.

Deeks, J., Glanville, J. and Sheldon, T. (1996) *Undertaking Systematic Reviews of Research on Effectiveness: CRD Guidelines for those Carrying out or Commissioning Reviews.* York: CRD.

Khan, K.S., Kunz, R., Kleijnen, J. and Antes, G. (2003) *Systematic Reviews to Support Evidence-based Medicine: How to Review and Apply Findings of Healthcare Research.* London: Royal Society of Medicine.

The Cochrane Reviewers' Handbook (www.cochrane.co.uk). Very comprehensive.

Meta-analysis

Lipsey, M.W. and Wilson, D.B. (2001) *Practical Meta-analysis.* London: Sage.

Sutton, A.J., Lambert P.C., Hellmich M. *et al.* (2000) Meta-analysis in practice: a critical review of available software, in D.A. Berry and D.K. Stragl (eds) *Meta-analysis in Medicine and Health Policy.* New York: Marcel Dekker.

Resources

- Review Manager (RevMan) Version 4.2 for Windows. Cochrane Collaboration (www.cochrane.co.uk).
- WinPEPI programs such as Calculate2 are available through www.healthcarefreeware.com.

References

Antman, E.M., Lau, J., Kupelnick, B. *et al.* (1992) A comparison of results of meta-analyses of randomized control trials and recommendations of clinical experts. Treatments for myocardial infarction, *Journal of the American Medical Association,* 268: 240–8.

Blanc, P.D. and Toren, K. (1999) How much adult asthma can be attributed to occupational factors? *American Journal of Medicine,* 107: 580–7.

Burge, P.S. and Lewis, S.A. (2003) So inhaled steroids slow the rate of decline of FEV1 in patients with COPD after all? *Thorax,* 58: 911–13.

Cappelleri, J.C., Ioannidis, J.P., Schmid, C.H. *et al.* (1996) Large trials vs meta-analysis of smaller trials: how do their results compare? *Journal of the American Medical Association,* 276: 1332–8.

Cochran, W.G. (1954) The combination of estimates from different experiments, *Biometrics,* 10: 101–29.

Cochrane, A.L. (1979) 1931–1971: a critical review, with particular reference to the medical profession, in *Medicines for the Year 2000,* pp. 1–11. London: Office of Health Economics.

Collins, R., Peto, R., Gray, R. and Parish, S. (1997) Large-scale randomised evidence: trials and overviews, in A. Maynard and I. Chalmers (eds) *Non-random Reflections on Health Services Research.* London: BMJ Publishing.

Cook, D.J., Guyatt, G.H., Ryan, G. *et al.* (1993) Should unpublished data be included in meta-analyses? Current convictions and controversies, *Journal of the American Medical Association,* 269: 2749–53.

Cooper, H. (1988) *Synthesising Research: A Guide for Literature Reviewers,* 3rd edn. London: Sage.

Cooper, H.M. (1984) The problem formulating stage, in H.M. Cooper (ed.) *Integrating Research: A Guide for Literature Reviews*, pp. 19–37. Newbury Park, CA: Sage.

Counsell, C. (1997) Formulating questions and locating primary studies for inclusion in systematic reviews, *Annals of Internal Medicine*, 127: 380–7.

Davey Smith, G., Song, F. and Sheldon, T.A. (1993) Cholesterol lowering and mortality: the importance of considering initial level of risk, *British Medical Journal*, 306: 1367–73.

Dear, K.G.B. and Begg, C.B. (1992) An approach for assessing publication bias prior to performing a meta-analysis, *Statistical Science*, 7: 237–45.

Dickersin, K. (1997) How important is publication bias? A synthesis of available data, *AIDS: Education and Prevention*, 9: 15–21.

Dixon-Woods, M. and Fitzpatrick, R. (2001) Qualitative research in systematic reviews has established a place for itself, *British Medical Journal*, 323: 765–6.

Eddy, D.M., Hasselblad, V. and Schachter, R. (1992) *Meta-analysis by the Confidence Profile Method: The Statistical Synthesis of Evidence*. Boston, MA: Academic Press.

Egger, M., Davey Smith, G., Schneider, M. and Minder, C. (1997a) Bias in meta-analysis detected by a simple, graphical test, *British Medical Journal*, 315: 629–34.

Egger, M., Zellweger-Zahner, T., Schneider, M. *et al.* (1997b) Language bias in randomised controlled trials published in English and German, *Lancet*, 350: 326–9.

Emerson, J.D. (1994) Combining estimates of the odds ratio: the state of the art, *Statistical Methods in Medical Research*, 3: 157–78.

Everitt, B. and Dunn, G. (1998) *Statistical Analysis of Medical Data: New Developments*. London: Arnold.

Eysenck, H.J. (1995) Problems with meta-analysis, in I. Chalmers and D.G. Altman (eds) *Systematic Reviews*. London: BMJ Publishing.

Feinstein, A.R. (1995) Meta-analysis: statistical alchemy for the 21st century, *Journal of Clinical Epidemiology*, 48: 71–9.

Givens, G.H., Smith, D.D. and Tweedie, R.L. (1997) Publication bias in meta-analysis: a Bayesian data-augmentation approach to account for issues exemplified in the passive smoking debate, *Statistical Science*, 12: 221–50.

Glass, G.V. (1978) Primary, secondary and meta-analysis of research, *Educational Researcher*, 5: 3–8.

Greenwald, A.G. (1975) Consequences of prejudice against the null hypothesis, *Psychological Bulletin*, 82: 1–20.

Gregoire, G., Derderian, F. and Le Lorier, J. (1995) Selecting the language of the publications included in a meta-analysis: is there a Tower of Babel bias? *Journal of Clinical Epidemiology*, 48: 159–63.

Guppy, M.P., Mickan, S.M. and Del Mar, C.B. (2004) Drink plenty of fluids: a systematic review of evidence for this recommendation in acute respiratory infections, *British Medical Journal*, 328: 499–500.

Hartung, J., Cottrell, J.E. and Giffin, J.P. (1983) Absence of evidence is not evidence of absence, *Anesthesiology*, 58(3): 298–300.

Huston, P. and Moher, D. (1996) Redundancy, disaggregation, and the integrity of medical research, *Lancet*, 347: 1024–6.

Huth, E.J. (1986) Irresponsible authorship and wasteful publication, *Annals of Internal Medicine*, 104: 257–9.

ISIS-4 (Fourth International Study of Infarct Survival) Collaborative Group (1995) ISIS-4: a randomised factorial trial assessing early oral captopril, oral mononitrate, and intravenous magnesium sulphate in 58,050 patients with suspected acute myocardial infarction, *Lancet*, 345: 669–85.

Jenkinson, C., Davies, R.J., Mullins, R. and Stradling, J.R. (1999) Comparison of therapeutic and subtherapeutic nasal continuous positive airway pressure for obstructive sleep apnoea: a randomised prospective parallel trial, *Lancet*, 353: 2100–5.

Jureidini, J.N., Doecke, C.J., Mansfield, P.R. *et al.* (2004) Efficacy and safety of antidepressants for children and adolescents, *British Medical Journal*, 328: 879–83.

Lau, J., Antman, E.M., Jimenez-Silva, J. *et al.* (1992) Cumulative meta-analysis of therapeutic trials for myocardial infarction, *New England Journal of Medicine*, 327: 248–54.

Lauritsen, K., Havelund, T., Laursen, L.S. and Rask-Madsen, J. (1987) Withholding unfavourable results in drug company sponsored clinical trials, *Lancet*, 1 (8541): 1091.

LeLorier, J., Gregoire, G., Benhaddad, A. *et al.* (1997) Discrepancies between meta-analyses and subsequent large randomized, controlled trials, *New England Journal of Medicine*, 337: 536–42.

Light, R.J. and Pillemer, D.B. (1984) *Summing Up: The Science of Reviewing Research.* Cambridge, MA: Harvard University Press.

Linde, K. and Willich, S.N. (2003) How objective are systematic reviews? Differences between reviews on complementary medicine, *Journal of the Royal Society of Medicine*, 96: 17–22.

McManus, R.J., Wilson, S., Delaney, B.C. *et al.* (1998) Review of the usefulness of contacting other experts when conducting a literature search for systematic reviews, *British Medical Journal*, 317: 1562–3.

Melander, H., Ahlqvist-Rastad, J., Meijer, G. and Beermann, B. (2003) Evidence b(i)ased medicine – selective reporting from studies sponsored by pharmaceutical industry: review of studies in new drug applications, *British Medical Journal*, 326: 1171–3.

Mulrow, C.D. (1987) The medical review article: state of the science, *Annals of Internal Medicine*, 106: 485–8.

Peto, R., Pike, M.C., Armitage, P., Breslow, N.E., Cox, D.R., Howard, S.V., Mantel, N., McPherson, K., Peto, J. and Smith, P.G. (1977) Design and analysis of randomised clinical trials requiring prolonged observation of each patient II: analysis and examples, *British Journal of Cancer*, 35–39.

Petticrew, M. (2003) Why certain systematic reviews reach uncertain conclusions, *British Medical Journal*, 326: 756–8.

Rose, S., Bisson, J. and Wessely, S. (2003) A systematic review of single-session psychological interventions ('debriefing') following trauma, *Psychotherapy and Psychosomatics*, 72: 176–84.

Sterling, T.D. (1959) Publication decisions and their possible effects on inferences drawn from tests of significance – or vice versa, *Journal of the American Statistical Association*, 54: 30–4.

Sutton, A.J., Jones, D.R., Abrams, K.R. *et al.* (2001) Meta-analysis in health technology assessment, in A. Stevens *et al.* (eds) *Advanced Handbook of Methods in Evidence Based Health-care*, pp. 391–408. London: Sage.

Thompson, S.G. (1993) Controversies in meta-analysis: the case of the trials of serum cholesterol reduction, *Statistical Methods in Medical Research*, 2: 173–92.

Villar, J., Carroli, G. and Belizan, J.M. (1995) Predictive ability of meta-analyses of randomised controlled trials, *Lancet*, 345: 772–6.

Whitehead, A. and Whitehead, J. (1991) A general parametric approach to the meta-analysis of randomized clinical trials, *Statistical Methods*, 10: 1665–77.

Whittington, C.J., Kendall, T., Fonagy, P. *et al.* (2004) Selective serotonin reuptake inhibitors in childhood depression: systematic review of published versus unpublished data, *Lancet*, 363: 1341–5.

Wilkes, M.M. and Navickis, R.J. (2001) Patient survival after human albumin administration: a meta-analysis of randomized, controlled trials, *Annals of Internal Medicine*, 135: 149–64.

Wright, J., Johns, R., Watt, I., Melville, A. and Sheldon, T. (1997) Health effects of obstructive sleep apnoea and the effectiveness of continuous positive airways pressure: a systematic review of the research evidence, *British Medical Journal*, 314: 851–60.

Zelen, M. (1983) Guidelines for publishing papers on cancer clinical trials: responsibilities of editors and authors, *Journal of Clinical Oncology*, 1: 164–9.

4 | Critical appraisal

Alan O'Rourke

Introduction

What exactly is critical appraisal, and what is the difference between 'appraising' an article and simply reading it? If you have been conscientious enough to organize a literature search, go to the library and copy a promising article, why can't we leave you alone to read it? Why do we ask you to put it through some complex process called critical appraisal? Consider the situation outlined in Box 4.1.

Box 4.1   Dr Findlay's Monday morning surgery

Your first patient is a 47-year old woman, bearing a newspaper clipping given to her by a friend, reviewing a recent article from a national medical journal that warns against the use of hormonal replacement therapy because of links with breast cancer. You assess her risk of breast cancer as low, and she declines HRT. When you discuss with her the results of an article showing that postmenopausal use of oestrogen reduces the risk of coronary heart disease, she counters with another article from the same issue that concludes that cardiovascular mortality is increased in oestrogen users. As you review these studies, you fail to recognize that all have serious flaws. You feel confused about the overall benefit of HRT, and you make a mental note to read more about it.

Your next patient, a 28-year-old man with allergic rhinitis, hands you an internet download recommending the latest antihistamine as far superior to the commonly used varieties. As he asks you for this new prescription, you realize that this drug is not on your Primary Care Trust formulary list. You promise to review the article and call him later in the week, and discuss his treatment.

The mother of your next patient, a 12-year-old boy, requests a test that you have never heard of. She hands you yet another article, which suggests that physicians who do not offer this test are guilty of negligence. As you review this study, you wish that you remembered more about how to assess an article critically, and you hope that the rest of the day goes better!

Source: adapted from: Miser (1999)

Critical appraisal is a discipline for increasing the effectiveness of your reading, by providing a comprehensive checklist for examining the quality of a research report.

This includes screening questions to enable you to quickly exclude papers that are too poor in quality to inform practice, and then in-depth questions to systematically evaluate those that pass muster to extract their salient points. Critical appraisal specifically supports the processes of evidence-based medicine (EBM), evidence-based practice (EBP), evidence-based healthcare (EBHC) and clinical effectiveness, by encouraging systematic assessment of reports of research evidence, to see which ones can be used to answer clinical problems and inform 'best practice'.

With traditional paper based catalogues like *Index Medicus* it could take all day to find just a few articles. But, thanks to the development of modern electronic databases like Medline, CINAHL and PsychLIT, in a matter of minutes you can now have a printout of thousands . . . but will they be the right sort of articles? In fact, it is now easy to find too many references, and this produces its own specific problems:

- the sheer volume of material now being published ('information overload');
- that much of the literature is of limited use, or even misleading (the 80/20 rule: 80 per cent of what you want to know is contained in 20 per cent of the total literature: you'll never need the rest!);
- the retort that all studies have flaws, albeit often minor, or are too 'ivory tower' to make much difference to 'real life' ('nihilism').

Critical appraisal provides useful tools for:

- systematically evaluating scientific literature;
- sifting the 'wheat' from the 'chaff' when you have conflicting studies;
- filtering out original research or meta-analyses which are methodologically sound;
- deciding which papers are going to influence what you do in your daily work;
- breaking down barriers between research (pure science) and practice (applied science).

Unfortunately, it cannot overcome the problem of publication bias and the 'grey literature', and indeed the increasing importance of meta-analyses and systematic reviews may make these more significant problems in the future.

Although the finer points depend on what sort of article you are appraising, there are always three basic stages:

A. The message
What are the findings of this article? Is there a message, what are the conclusions, what questions has the study raised and answered?

B. The validity
Are the conclusions justified by the description of the methodology and the findings? Is the methodology sound, have the authors made reasonable assumptions, are there confounding factors they have failed to consider? If they are using a sample, have they justified its size and composition?

C. The generalizability (sometimes called applicability or utility)
Are the problems I deal with sufficiently like those in the study to extrapolate the findings? Can I generalize from this study to my workplace?

Generalizability is in some ways the hardest to be rigidly scientific about, and making decisions here may still be an art. For instance, even if a doctor locates a paper that is scientifically faultless, he may be left pondering questions like:

- If the selection criteria included 'age 70–80' can I use the conclusions for patients in the 65–70 age groups, and what about the relatively fit and 'biologically young' 81-year-olds?
- Can studies on urban Americans be extrapolated from say Birmingham, Alabama, to Birmingham, West Midlands, and are rural subjects in Norway different to those in Wales?

At the end of this chapter, you should, be able to critically appraise a research paper to decide if its contents could be used to improve your practice, to help you make informed decisions, or be incorporated into the write-up of your own literature review.

Problem formulation and identifying research studies

The first stage in using the literature to answer a specific question is to convert your practice problem or research question into a search strategy, which will allow you to effectively search databases. In the modern world, that will almost certainly mean running your search strategy on an electronic database like Medline. In many health-related problems, the question can be resolved to three (or sometimes) four key components:

- **The population of interest (P):** this should be defined as accurately as possible in terms of age, sex, ethnic and social group, condition and illness severity.
- **The intervention (I):** usually this is something whose impact on the population you wish to explore. So it could be a drug (for high blood pressure), a surgical procedure (for a deformed joint), an educational programme (to alter risk factors), or a diagnostic test (such as blood screening for prostate cancer). We usually think of such 'interventions' as intended to produce benefit, but for epidemiological work they can include exposure to risk factors, such as radiation or cigarette smoking.
- **The outcome (O):** this includes any end-points you may measure to see what effect your intervention has, such as reducing blood pressure, restoring mobility, confirming or excluding a provisional diagnosis or changing lifestyle. Although most researchers can define their population and intervention quite easily, it can be salutary to force them to think of outcomes.

Sometimes, if there is more than one option, there may be a fourth component:

- **The comparison (C):** this may simply be with a control group, who receive no intervention (or, increasingly for ethical reasons, the current standard or best intervention), or there may be several groups receiving quite different management (e.g. a comparison of drug therapy, angioplasty via a catheter or major surgery and coronary artery bypass for ischaemic heart disease).

This three- or four-part structuring of the problem or research question to make a search strategy is sometimes called the PIOC or PICO format. The next stage is to think of any acronyms, synonyms, abbreviations or alternative terminology used to describe the three or four concepts you have identified. This provides you with a full range of subject headings to use for your literature search. Exactly how you run this depends on which databases you are using, and the best way to learn is to do some searches, initially with guidance from an experienced member of the library staff. Further discussion of the techniques of literature searching is beyond the scope of this chapter.

Suppose your research question is 'Does early discharge of stroke patients into

Table 4.1 Translating a research question into a search strategy, showing the Boolean operators (in bold) which would be used to combine the search terms when running the search

Concept 1: population	Concept 2: intervention	Concept 3: outcome	Concept 4: comparison
Patients suffering strokes **or** cerebro-vascular accidents **or** cerebral haemorrhage **or** cerebral emboli **or** sub-arachnoid haemorrhage (SAH)	**and** Community health services **or** discharge **or** early discharge **or** length of stay **or** ambulatory care	**and** Mobility **or** survival **or** self-caring **or** independence **or** activities of daily living	**and** Hospitalization **or** stroke unit **or** rehabilitation **or** orthodox care

the community produce better results than standard hospital care?' Table 4.1 shows how you might structure the problem.

Assuming that you have run your search and retrieved some papers, we will now consider critical appraisal of some of the main types of research study.

Appraisal of original quantitative research

This model applies to primary studies and pieces of original research using quantitative methodologies. Start by skim reading to get the flavour, and then analyse more slowly, beginning with three screening questions to see if the research passes muster for closer scrutiny. Also, is it from a peer-reviewed journal? Look at the instructions to authors if in doubt: this should suggest quality, but it is no absolute guarantee of scientific rigour. Appropriate critical appraisal questions are shown in Figure 4.1.

Specifically, you need to address the following questions in appraising the article:

A. The message
What is the bottom line to extract to inform your practice? What, in one sentence, are the findings and conclusion of this study?

B. The validity

Screening questions:

1 Did the trial address a clearly focused issue/research question?
2 How was the sample selected? Is it big enough (look for a power calculation), and is it representative? Was the assignment of subjects to interventions randomized?
3 Were all the subjects who entered the study properly accounted for at its conclusion?

If you get a 'yes' to all these three, then continue to tease out the meaning of the article by looking for answers to the following questions:

Are there any differences between the two groups in terms of selection bias or confounding variables which could explain the differences between them (factors like age, sex, social class)?

4 Blinding: were the subjects, researcher and other study personnel 'blind' to the intervention? Beware of potential breaches of blinding (e.g. if an active drug with a bitter taste and an insipid placebo are used).
5 Were the groups similar at the start of the trial?
6 Excepting the experimental intervention, were the groups treated equally?

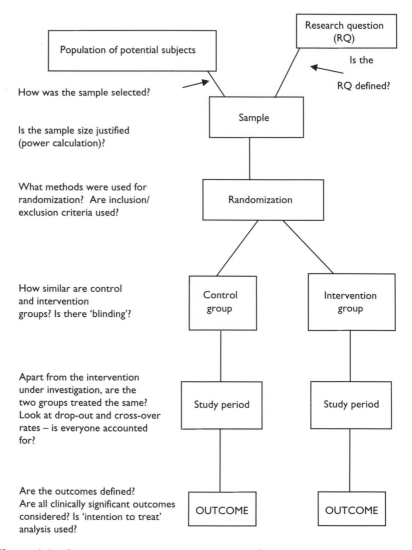

Figure 4.1   Stages in primary quantitative research, and appropriate critical appraisal questions

So, what are the results?

7 How large was the treatment effect? (Consider what outcomes were recorded, and how the differences between the groups were expressed.)
8 How precise was the estimate of the treatment effects? (Hint: look for confidence intervals – see below for an explanation of these.)

Other points worth considering include:

• declaration of outside interests or commercial sponsorship;
• ethics committee approval as indicated;
• if the authors have included a literature review to put the study in context, the review should be current, comprehensive and balanced.

C. The generalizability

9   Can the results be applied to the local population? (Or, how different are the subjects in the study population from the situations you deal with?)
10 Were all the important outcomes considered? (And if any were neglected, the effect that may have on the interpretation.)
11 Are the benefits worth the harms and costs? (This is a bit of an 'extra' and much research will not include cost-benefit analyses, but if looking at how to choose different management options, and stick within budgets, such costings may be useful.)

Appraisal of reviews

This format is suggested for secondary studies that synthesize or integrate information from multiple primary studies. These may be meta-analyses, systematic reviews, guidelines or economic analyses. A systematic review is an overview of primary research studies that reach specific standards in terms of methodology (see chapter 3). A meta-analysis is a mathematical re-analysis of the combined raw data from two or more primary studies that addressed the same research question, and used comparable methodologies. Unfortunately, these techniques cannot overcome the problem of publication bias. Papers with 'exciting' positive conclusions are more likely to be published than ones with 'boring' conclusions, that accept the null hypothesis, or reinforce current practice. However, when people produce a meta-analysis of all studies on a particular topic, because unpublished or un-indexed studies in the 'grey literature,' are harder to find, the meta-analysis may be over-optimistic about new therapies. Positive studies may also produce duplicate publications, with no clear acknowledgement that they are analysing the same group of patients several times (Tramèr *et al.* 1997). Again, a systematic approach to assessing these articles is recommended:

A. The message

1   Does the review set out to answer a precise question? (i.e. it is something more scientific than an attempt to gather everything written about fungal skin diseases).

B. The validity

2   Have the authors sought out studies thoroughly, including the following sources:

- relevant bibliographic database (e.g. Medline and Cochrane for medical topics);
- foreign language literature;
- 'grey literature' (unpublished or un-indexed reports: theses, conference proceedings, internal reports, non-indexed journals, pharmaceutical industry files);
- reference chaining from any articles found, and citation searches;
- personal approaches to experts in the field to find unpublished reports;
- hand searches of the relevant specialized journals (for meta-analysis, it may be important to track down the raw study data for re-analysis, rather than the final report alone).

3   Have the authors included explicit inclusion and exclusion criteria for studies, taking account of the subjects in the studies, the interventions used, the outcomes recorded and the methodology?

4 For a meta-analysis, how are the results presented? In practice the results are often displayed graphically as the 95 per cent confidence intervals of the effect of each trial (see below).

5 Have the authors considered the 'homogeneity' of the individual studies: the idea that the studies are sufficiently similar in their design, interventions and subjects to merit combination? (If you were looking at the effect of *fruit* consumption on cancer, you could combine studies about apple, pear, orange and grapefruit consumption, but if you were only interested in the effect of *citrus fruit*, you wouldn't want the apple or pear studies). In meta-analysis, this is done either by eyeballing graphs like the Forrest Plot of the confidence intervals, by applications of chi-square tests (Thompson 1995) or by plotting effect estimates against sample size and looking for a symmetrical 'funnel plot' – a shape like an inverted filter funnel (Egger *et al.* 1997).

C. The generalizability

6 In some ways this may be easier than for a piece of original research. The various studies may have used patients of different ages or social classes, but if the treatment effects are consistent across the studies, then generalization to other groups or populations is more justified.

Appraisal of qualitative studies

At first sight, appraisal of qualitative studies seems more intuitive and less deductive; less of a science and more of an art. There may be lots of quotes and summaries of interviews, rather than columns of numbers; the outcomes may be more subjective and multi-faceted than 'absent/present' dichotomies. The tools for data collection (interviews, focus groups and surveys) may sound more at risk of observer effect and bias than blood pressure cuffs and weighing scales. The emphasis may be less on rigid replicabilty with control of all but one variable, and more on the richness of one unique, but illuminating, situation. Generalizability may be at risk from complex factors like secular trends and individual motivation. There may be an uneasy suspicion that the authors, however subconsciously, have been 'selective' in their choice of quotes to support conclusions: the reader may even interpret the quotes differently. Students used to the impartial observer model of the researcher, however far from the truth that actually is, may be unsettled by the ethnographer expressing understanding, sympathy and even empathy for the predicaments of their 'participants'. In critical appraisal of such papers, however, essentially you must still pose and answer the same three questions: what is the message; can I believe it; can I generalize? For qualitative work to pass muster, the authors must still demonstrate:

- A clear aim for their project, not just an attempt to gather masses of data and then impose some 'order' on it.
- Choice of an *appropriate* methodology.
- Justification for who *was* and who *was not* included, and some discussion of the effect of drop-outs and non-responders. It may be more important to employ *purposive* sampling to gather the whole range of possible opinions and experiences, rather than random sampling to produce a representative study group.

There is also an extra appraisal question, specifically pertinent to qualitative work:

- What is the relationship between investigators and subjects and has this introduced any biases to the study?

Worked examples

Below are three specimen research papers, with reasonably in-depth critical appraisals of each. Although they cover different topics, between them they illustrate the principals of appraising original quantitative, original qualitative and review papers. Before reading this section, you may like to retrieve one or more of the papers from your local library (or the two from the *British Medical Journal* can be downloaded from its website: http://bmj.bmjjournals.com/), and sketch out your own appraisal.

Critical appraisal of a randomized controlled trial (primary quantitative work)

Rudd, A.G., Wolfe, C.D.A., Tilling, K. and Beech, R. (1997) Randomised control trial to evaluate early discharge scheme for patients with stroke, *British Medical Journal*, 315: 1039–44.

This study adheres to the CONSORT statement that lays down standards for the reporting of clinical trials, and so the illustration on page 1040 makes it easier to follow the pathway of patients through the trial. The study reports baseline data in Table 1 which makes it easier to make comparisons between the subjects at entry into each arm. Graphical and tabular presentation are useful means of navigating one's way around a study. However, the study covers a bewildering array of outcomes ('the kitchen sink' approach) and so interpretation is easier if one focuses on the primary outcome. Tables present data at two endpoints (discharge from hospital and one year after stroke), but for appraisal you may need to think about which of these represents the most appropriate time scale.

A. Are the results of the trial valid?

1 Did the trial address a clearly focused issue?

The structured abstract helps us to identify the *population* (setting/subjects): '331 medically stable patients who lived alone and were able to transfer independently or who lived with a resident carer and were able to transfer with help'. These are patients presenting to 'two teaching hospitals in inner London'. However, this means excluding a large number of patients who might benefit from stroke care interventions. It is also likely that incidence of cardiac or respiratory problems might be lower than in an area of heavy industry, and the pattern of social support may well be different for an inner city than for a more family-oriented community. These are however questions about generalizability, rather than clarity in the definition of the population, so they need not be answered fully at this stage.

The *intervention* is described as 'specialist community rehabilitation' as compared with 'conventional hospital and community care'. There are at least two problems with this definition. First, 'conventional care' may cover significant variation in the quality and extent of what is provided in different institutions and teams. A second problem relates to the fact that we are dealing here with 'packages of care' with a number of indistinguishable elements. Given this latter problem, one has to employ a pragmatic approach to this study in that, if one can establish that some undefined ingredient of this package is effective, further research can be employed to identify its exact nature and the mechanism of its benefit. The authors have to establish what the principal outcomes are and over what period of time they are to be measured; in this case, they use the 'Barthel score' at 12 months. The appraisers subsequently face two decisions:

- Is this particular outcome measure valid and meaningful?
- Is the period over which it has been measured valid in terms of the clinical context?

No doubt those who do not have a background in rehabilitation will find it difficult to comprehend the significance of the Barthel score. However, assistance is on hand in the article on page 1040, column 2, which indicates that the score is a measure of disability and that it is orientated such that low numbers are bad and high numbers are good (contrast the Glasgow Coma score). Also, for the purposes of this study, 0–14 equates to 'severe disability', 15–19 to 'moderate disability' and 20 (by implication) to normal function. Clinical knowledge is not required to judge whether outcome at time of discharge is more appropriate than outcome at one year. It is intuitive to think that, where the desired outcome is return to normal function (or as near as physical circumstances will allow), outcome one year after discharge would be more important clinically (hence the programme of community rehabilitation). In summary then, although large numbers of patients are being excluded from the study, the research question is well focused.

2 Was the assignment of patients to treatments randomized?

Details of randomization are contained in a separate paragraph in the left column of page 1040. We learn that 'randomisation was restricted in permuted blocks of ten with random number tables provided in blank sealed opaque envelopes'. High-quality randomization will be characterized by a method of allocation that is not open to manipulation or statistical artefact. Methods you should look out for are randomization using a computerized 'random number generator' or, as in this case, 'random number tables', both of which are regarded as high quality. 'Permuted blocks' are often used where a multi-centre trial is being conducted (e.g. numerous GP clinics), usually to ensure that there is not too great an imbalance between numbers in each arm and to allow independent allocation, usually for practical reasons. The reference to 'blank sealed opaque envelopes' is not a feature of the randomization itself but refers instead to the difficulty that participants would have in 'cracking the code' of allocation.

3 Were all of the patients who entered the trial properly accounted for at its conclusion?

Completion of follow up is always going to be problematic in a population with such disease severity, particularly with an average age of 71. Death at 12 months affected 16 and 21 per cent respectively of the patients in the two groups. Loss to follow up affects 3 and 2 per cent respectively with five patients in the community therapy group lost due to refusal to participate and emigration, and four from the conventional group. In making allowances for the severity of the condition one is not only looking at the absolute numbers lost to follow up but also whether there is any significant imbalance between the two groups. Although the numbers are high there is not a significant difference between losses to the two groups.

At this point we are introduced to the concept of the 'intention to treat' analysis: 'were patients analysed in the groups to which they were randomised?' This very often appears counterintuitive to those appraising an article – i.e. even were a participant to cross over to the alternate treatment group they would still be analysed according to their original group. However, this reflects the pragmatic nature of health service trials. In judging the overall effectiveness of an intervention one needs to be able to account for all those who could possibly benefit. This can be illustrated by the example of a drug that has a taste that is extremely unpleasant. The overall effectiveness of this drug would be measured by including those who stopped taking it because of its taste or those who switched to another drug and not only those who persist with it. The study does not specifically mention an 'intention to treat' analysis although one would assume that this type of analysis was used in this instance.

4 Were patients, health workers and study personnel 'blind' to treatment?
Patients were clearly aware of which group they were in: 'occasionally the patient did make clear which group they had been in' (p. 1040). In a health service context, as opposed to investigation of drugs, it can be extremely difficult to establish complete blinding to all parties. Health workers could not be blinded because of the locus of care and intensive nature of the intervention. Study personnel fall into two groups – those collecting the data and those analysing it. The research associate that conducted the assessment at 12 months, usually in the patient's home, was blind to treatment but occasionally might find out from the patient. Equally important, however, is whether those doing the analysis were aware of the identity of either group. Somewhat typically these details are not given.

5 Were the groups similar at the start of the trial?
Suppose that initially the imbalance between the two groups is contrary to the study hypothesis: the intervention group is worse for some important variable than the control, and is effectively 'handicapped'. If the outcomes or end points show that the intervention group fares at least as well as the control group in this situation, the magnitude of effect must be even greater for the experimental intervention. Such a situation modifies the interpretation but does not negate it. If, however, the direction of imbalance favours the experimental intervention, then it would confound the study, because then the intervention group is 'handicapped'. In fact, judging from the baseline data in Table 1 the groups were remarkably similar at initiation of the trial. But of concern is the wide range of length of stay before randomization in the community therapy group: the potential to benefit from conventional therapy prior to randomization may be considerable. There is a slightly higher proportion of dysphasic patients in the community therapy group, perhaps indicating that they might be more severely affected by their strokes. Both groups are matched quite well for the most relevant analyses, namely previous Barthel score and Barthel score at randomization.

6 Aside from the experimental intervention, were the groups treated equally?
This question addresses both whether the experimental conditions created for the investigation were preserved for the duration of the study and also whether any procedures carried out for the purposes of the study might have contributed to a differential effect. For example, if one group saw a researcher on a monthly basis but the other only saw them six-monthly then it is possible that the interaction with the researcher may have contributed to their rehabilitation, especially socially. In this case the study specifically states that 'All other services apart from therapy were as described for the conventional group' (p. 1040).

B. What are the results?

7 How large was the treatment effect?
The study was looking for a '3.5 difference in Barthel score' at one year based on 130 patients in each group. In fact there was no difference and the conventional group fell slightly short (126) of the required number. The treatments are therefore not significantly different from each other in terms of relative effectiveness. Taking

statistical significance at the level of p < 0.05 and looking at the other recorded outcomes we see that the community therapy group had a higher level of abnormal anxiety (p = 0.02) on the hospital anxiety and depression scale and had a higher level of satisfaction with their hospital care (p = 0.032) than the conventional group. No other measurements at one year reached statistical significance. Whether such differences went further to reach 'clinical significance' is debatable in both the above instances.

8 How precise was the estimate of the treatment effect?

Given the lack of statistical significance mentioned above this is something of an academic point. Nevertheless we see that the 95 per cent confidence interval for the Barthel score is 0 to 1 indicating no more than a one-point difference between the groups.

C. Will the results help locally?

9 Can the results be applied to the local population?

The study has the virtue of being conducted in a UK health care setting. However, the use of inner-city teaching hospitals is not typical of the wider National Health Service (NHS). One cannot be sure either that the contents of a rehabilitation package would be common to both the study population and your own population. Of course you must be reasonable in considering applicability, otherwise you end up with the *reductio ad absurdem* that only studies conducted in one's own organization can be applied to the local population. There is a virtue in an effect being proved regardless of setting (e.g. the rationale for systematic reviews), as this strengthens its universality. The burden of proof should therefore rest on those in a local setting to establish any factors that might make this study result less applicable. The main problem with this study as mentioned earlier is that a high proportion of stroke patients would be excluded by applying the study's strict inclusion criteria. However, a valid conclusion from critical appraisal might be that a certain subgroup might benefit from implementation of a policy or guideline based on this evidence if the whole potential population is unable to benefit.

10 Were all important outcomes considered?

It is helpful to think of three overlapping dimensions to outcomes:

* clinical effectiveness (clinician);
* cost effectiveness (manager);
* patient satisfaction/acceptability (patient).

Typically a study is unlikely to address all three dimensions to a satisfactory degree. This study has established that with regard to clinical effectiveness there is apparently little if anything to choose between the interventions. Evidence concerning the effect on patients is equivocal with apparent improved satisfaction with hospital care but higher anxiety in the community therapy group. In connection with cost, the study becomes particularly interesting. In Table 5 the authors have collected a number of resource elements, but apparently not in a systematic or comprehensive manner. It appears that they have tacked on a crude economic analysis to the study, although never identified as an original intention for the study: one must be extremely cautious if material that is extraneous to the original research question is introduced later in support of the authors' arguments.

11 Are the benefits worth the harms and costs?

The crude nature of the cost analysis makes such a bottom-line evaluation difficult.

At most one might conclude that in the absence of evidence to the contrary there may be reasons to investigate early discharge, particularly in those sub-groups of patients who are most likely to benefit. Clearly further research is required to conduct a full economic analysis alongside a randomized controlled trial with a determined effect to include all relevant cost factors. At a local level one would perhaps wish to obtain an accurate profile of the stroke population and attempt to model the possible effects of a change to policy on costs and inpatient/outpatient numbers. Other considerations might include transfer of costs between organizations (e.g. from acute trusts to community trusts) or between sectors (e.g. from health service to social services) which might make management of such change difficult to effect.

What can we therefore conclude?

Critical appraisal of an individual article is not always going to yield definitive answers to a problem or scenario. However, it will help to reduce uncertainty and to clarify and prioritize further questions for investigation. It also acts as a defence against using articles for purposes for which they are unsuitable or not originally intended. And it helps to identify where authors have gone beyond the limits of their own research study in drawing conclusions for clinical practice. Outstanding issues for consideration include:

- How can one further decrease uncertainty and extend applicability beyond the coverage of a single study?
- What does one do when two or more studies in the same area apparently reach different conclusions?

This takes us in turn to the need to identify and critically appraise systematic reviews of the literature.

Appraisal of a systematic review

Smeenk, F.W.J.M., van Haastregt, J.C.M., de Witte, L.P. and Crebolder, H.F.J.M. (1998) Effectiveness of home care programmes for patients with incurable cancer on their quality of life and time spent in hospital: a systematic review, *British Medical Journal*, 316: 1939–44.

A. Are the results of the review valid?

Screening questions

1 Did the review address a clearly focused issue?

Yes. This is clearly stated as: to examine if a comprehensive home-care programme (intervention) is more effective than standard hospital based care for patients with terminal cancer (population), in terms of maintaining quality of life and reducing time as an in-patient (outcomes). Although a 'comprehensive home care programme' is defined as something more than an intervention aimed at a single aspect of care at home, there still seems to be a degree of subjectivity about 'comprehensive' which the authors solved by establishing an internal consensus.

2 Did the authors look for the appropriate sort of papers?

Partly: see question 3 below. Is it worth continuing? There is a risk that the authors' literature search, although well constructed, may not be wide-ranging enough. However, unless you can find a study with a more extensive exploration of material outside the main databases, it seems worth persevering.

Detailed questions

3 Do you think the important, relevant studies were included?

Partly: there was an explicit search of databases, with defects addressed in the first paragraph 'Shortcomings' on p. 1942, but little evidence of grey literature search. The authors did not apply language restrictions (i.e. they did not attempt to discriminate against non-English papers in their trawl of the databases). However, these databases themselves may have a bias in favour of English language publications, necessitating a wider trawl. The search strategy seems to have been appropriate for retrieving pertinent papers but insufficiently thorough and wide-ranging.

4 Did the review's authors do enough to assess the quality of the included studies?

Yes: studies were scored by methodology, which was used to weight them later. Explicit inclusion/exclusion criteria cut out most identified studies (only 9 of 348 got through). Two investigators independently ranked studies for quality, and anonymized the articles by removing authors, titles and journal name. This would reduce bias towards certain well-respected authors or publications, and use of a third investigator to adjudicate over differences would deal with inter-observer differences. In such a small research group, some external advice on differences would be ideal. However, the resources and timescale of the study may have precluded this refinement. The criteria for inclusion of studies (study population and sampling, dropouts, description of intervention, outcome measures, and data handling and presentation) are comprehensive and relevant. The overall score for methodology is only 'moderate' for the papers used in the study.

5 If the results of the review have been combined, was it reasonable to do so?

There is no formal meta-analysis. Such is not practical, as the studies have different backgrounds (three hospital-based, two hospice-based, one in a rehabilitation centre). The studies also use different tools to measure outcomes. Four report improvements in all the scales they used; two deterioration in the scales used; one no significant change; and one shows improvements in two scales and deterioration in another. For some but not all studies more information is provided on two other outcomes: readmission rates and survival. Inclusion of this data is erratic, and the only significant differences are two studies which show reduced readmission rates in intervention group. The information on the interventions used by each study (Table 3) is also incomplete. There was variable use of interventions like home visiting, technical care and team meetings. It is not so much that some studies specifically did not employ these methods, but for many the tables show 'not stated' (i.e. not clear from the description of the methodology) or 'some' (i.e. not applied consistently to all subjects), and therefore introduce an extra variable into the study.

B. What are the results?

6 What is the overall result of the review?

No clear benefit is demonstrated for comprehensive home programmes over current 'standard provision'. Readmission rates were lower in the intervention groups, and significantly so for two studies, and five showed some evidence of physical improvement. However, these benefits are not consistent across the eight studies. Rather as a footnote, the authors seem to favour home visits and multidisciplinary team meetings as improving patient satisfaction. These interventions were used in some (but not *all* of the studies), and to back this up the authors cite three more studies, all of which describe themselves as randomized trials!

7 How precise are the results?
The results are summarized, rather than being presented mathematically.

C. Will the results help locally?

8 Can the results be applied to the local population?
The sort of home care programmes this study investigates may be seen as socially desirable and fitting in with the move from hospital to community care, or attractive to hard pressed hospital managers, wary of 'bed blocking cases' (two studies suggested significant reduction in readmission rates). But, moving such care into the community is not without resource implications, and this review does not come up with much rigorous evidence that such home care programmes deliver significant improvements. Generalizability seems weak: there were eight US studies and one UK study so one would have to consider the relative strengths of primary care in these countries: in the USA, primary care is not so comprehensive and well developed as in most of Europe.

9 Were all important outcomes considered?
One problem is the use of many evaluation scales, over 20 in various combinations across the eight studies. It is not clear which end points each scale measures: one suspects that there may be a degree of overlap in the end points measured by say P&S (Pain and Symptoms); MMPQ (McGill-Melzack Pain Questionnaire); MHI (Mental Health Index); and the PD (Psychological Distress) scales. In some ways, the studies have set themselves too many outcomes (physical and psychological well-being, ability to self-care, patient satisfaction; readmission rates; and survival). It would have been more useful to separate the softer issues (patient satisfaction) from the harder ones (readmission and survival).

10 Are the benefits worth the harms and costs?
There is no attempt to cost out care in hospital and care at home for cancer patients. The review is inconclusive as to whether care at home provides benefits. The authors do not seem to have gleaned financial information from the studies (it may not be there, or their criteria may not have included asking such questions). This would be problematic for the American studies, where free public access to health care is far from universal. One would need to have information on the patient mix, as to which were eligible for free care (under the Medicare and Medicaid schemes), and which were covered by private or occupational insurance, and how comprehensive the various schemes were for terminal care.

Appraisal of a qualitative study

Reed, J. and Morgan, D. (1999) Discharging older people from hospital to care homes, *Journal of Advanced Nursing*, 29: 819–25

Screening questions

1 Was there a clear statement of the aims of the research?

Yes. There is a clear aim identified: to explore the experiences of older people discharged from hospital into nursing and residential care, and identify possible forms of support.

2 Is a qualitative methodology appropriate?

Yes: a qualitative methodology is appropriate as the study considers the experiences of the subjects through their own eyes and those of staff.

Detailed questions

3 Sampling strategy

a. From where was the sample selected and why?

The sample were identified from hospital records for an acute Trust in the north-east of England, which was the study setting. The samples were discharged patients from hospital, nominated family members, and hospital and residential home nursing staff.

b. Who was selected and why?

They were selected to provide as wide a range of experiences as possible.

c. How were they selected and why?

A purposive sample of 20 older adults discharged from hospital. Of an original sample of 48, 19 were excluded because of frailty or cognitive impairment; others declined to take part, had left the area or died. The subjects nominated 17 family members. Twenty-four staff were interviewed, plus six written responses submitted, although the report states that this amounts to a total of 29 respondents.

d. Was the sample size justified?

No justification of sample size is offered, and there is no indication if there was data saturation.

e. Is it clear why some participants chose not to take part?

It is not clear why three patients did not participate. Staff responses were reported to be reduced as a consequence of work commitments, and the report indicates a range of efforts which were made to increase staff responses.

4 Was the sampling strategy appropriate to address the aims?

Overall, the sampling strategy was compromised by problems in sampling appropriate staff and a high attrition rate among eligible patients.

5 Data collection – is it clear:

a. Where the setting of the data collection was, and why that setting was chosen?

There is a clear description of the setting, but it is unclear why this setting was chosen.

b. How the data were collected and why?

Patients and family were interviewed individually, while staff were interviewed in focus groups, with one individual interview and six responses to a questionnaire. It is unclear why focus groups were the method of choice for staff, and other methods were used with this group on an *ad hoc* basis.

c. How the data were recorded and why?

Semi-structured interview schedules were used: no description of data-recording method.

d. If the methods were modified during the process and why?
The methods of collection of staff data were modified to increase the sample size.

e. If the data were collected in a way that addresses the research issue?
Overall, data collection methods addressed the research question.

6 Data analysis – is it clear:

a. How the analysis was done?
There is no discussion of how data analysis was undertaken.

b. If the data analysis was sufficiently rigorous?
It is not possible to tell if the analysis was sufficiently rigorous. There are questions about the validity and reliability of the analysis.

7 Research partnership relations – is it clear:

a. If the researchers critically examined their own role, potential bias and influence?
The study claimed to be an action research approach, working in collaboration with staff. However, this seems to be tokenistic, and there is no indication of how the research team worked with staff to address the findings. Patients and families appeared to be used as 'response fodder' with little or no feedback.

b. Where the data were collected and why that setting was chosen?
There is no discussion of why the particular research setting was chosen.

c. How the research was explained to the participants?
There is no description of how the research was explained, and it is unclear on what basis patients were given an opportunity to refuse to take part. There is no discussion of the ethics of interviewing older people about their experiences.

8 Has the relationship between researchers and participants been adequately considered?
Overall, there is inadequate discussion of the research relationships.

9 Findings
The findings are presented clearly, but the findings from the different groups of respondents address different themes, and there is little effort to bring these together.

10 Justification of data interpretation

a. Is there sufficient data presented to support the findings?
There is not sufficient data presented as direct quotations to justify the findings. This is particularly the case for the patient group, in which quotations are brief and infrequent.

b. Do the researchers explain how the data presented in the paper were selected from the original sample?
The researchers do not explain how the quotations presented were selected.

11 Transferability

The setting is described adequately to enable judgements of transferability; however this may be compromised because of threats to validity. In particular, the response rate was under 50 per cent and the study is limited to the cognitively intact – i.e. it excludes any with dementia or confusion.

12 What is the relevance and usefulness of the study:

a. In terms of addressing the research aim?

The study is relevant to the aim.

b. In terms of contributing to new understanding, insight or perspectives?

The study offers new insights.

c. In terms of suggesting further research?

The study offers potential for further research.

d. In terms of impacting on policy/practice?

There are policy and practice implications.

13. How relevant is the research? How important are these findings to practice?

Overall, and given the reservations about internal validity, the study is relevant and useful to people being discharged into care. It has important implications for practice. The study puts a neglected area (discharge to residential care) in context, especially as changing demographic factors (an ageing population, smaller families), social changes (greater mobility, more women in the workforce), and economic pressures (the rundown of NHS long-term beds) make for increasing use of this option to care for the frail elderly. There is evidence of wide reading, but not of a systematic literature review. A study like this seems to have ethical dimensions (on p. 822 the authors discuss the risk of 'exhausting the subjects'), but there is no evidence of ethics committee approval. There is no evidence of blinding: the observers are colleagues and staff. Is this what they mean by 'modified action research'? The main finding is that older people are passive in the process of selecting and moving to care homes and staff need to be more proactive in eliciting their views and preferences.

Appraisal of websites

Much research is now published on the internet. It is a valuable source or information, and it is academically respectable to cite web pages as well as journals and books as supporting evidence (make sure you include the full URL and the date you last visited the page in your citation). Evaluation or appraisal of websites is however still in its infancy: the basic rule is still '*caveat lector!*' – 'let the reader beware!' The very nature of the web, the ease of posting material and obtaining a site mean that there is little guarantee about the truth, validity or reliability of what you find. Among the questions you can use in evaluating a website are:

• Is it clear who maintains this website: government or university body, commercial company, religious group, a private individual? Is there evidence that the website depends on sponsorship, or generates financial gain?

- What is the purpose of this page: to inform me; to persuade me; to sell me something?
- What is the overall quality of the information?
- Do the references and hypertext links substantiate the claims and lead to relevant sites? Beware of impressive lists of references, all featuring the page owner as an author, and published in journals you have never heard off.
- Are there mechanisms for feedback and contacting the owners?
- Does the site breach ethical codes? Do you feel uneasy about its approach to confidentiality and privacy? (For further information on ethics and the internet see the *e-Health Code of Ethics*, www.ihealthcoalition.org/ethics/ethics.html from the *Journal of Medical Internet Research's* e-Health Ethics Initiative, www.jmir.org/2000/2/e9/.)
- Is the content kept up to date (look for 'last updated' entries at the bottom)?

Some high-level domain names may help identify the authority of the site: .com and .co addresses suggest commercial bodies; .org suggests non-profit making sites; .edu and .ac suggest academic institutions; gov., doh etc. suggest government departments; .nhs.uk suggests an NHS-sponsored page. The World Health Organization (WHO) wished to establish a top-level domain, .health, for sites it approved, but the American Internet Corporation for Assigned Names and Numbers (ICANN) rejected the proposal as being too prescriptive over 'content control'. The Americans seem unhappy about granting a single body such powers.

The following tools set out to evaluate websites:

- **The Distributed National Electronic Network:** a managed environment for accessing quality assured information resources on the internet which are available from many sources: journals, monographs, textbooks, abstracts, manuscripts, maps, music scores, and audio-visual – www.jnug.ac.uk/jisc/services.html.
- **DISCERN:** a checklist of 16 questions for users to evaluate websites, developed, standardized and validated by working with 13 national self-help groups. May be very time-consuming and subjective. Also, seems to assume that consumers accept that interventions should be based on objective studies and understand principles of 'evidence-based' practice – www.discern.org.uk/discern__about_this_site.htm.
- **Health On the Net (HON) Foundation:** an international, charitable body based in Geneva, it provides a database of evaluated health materials and also promotes the use of the HON code as a self-governance initiative to help unify the quality of medical and health information available, and the use of its logo as a kite-mark of adherence to these guidelines – http://www.hon.ch/.

For a personal view of quality evaluation of websites, in this case in the medical area, see Delamothe (2000).

Presentation of the results and some pitfalls

The impact of a piece of research can be highly dependent on how the results are presented. Bucher *et al.* (1994) showed that when two groups of doctors were presented with results of the same study of drugs to lower blood cholesterol, those shown the relative risk reduction were more likely to favour prescription than those shown absolute risk reductions. Especially for meta-analyses, results are now often shown as confidence intervals (CIs). Strictly: if the rate and the 95 per cent CIs were estimated from 100 different samples for the same population, then 95 per cent of the CIs would contain the true rate. A slightly less rigorous, but more useful 'lay' definition is: you can be 95 per cent sure that the true rate lies between the confidence intervals.

Consider a series of five independent studies exploring an intervention in several study populations. A team of reviewers then collate the data from all five studies for a meta-analysis. They can present results of the five primary studies and their meta-analysis as a forest plot diagram. The horizontal line represents the confidence intervals of each study, the 'blob' in the middle represents single best estimate of that study and the results of the meta-analysis are represented by a diamond (see Figure 4.2).

In interpreting numerical analyses, beware of very obscure statistical tests, or the use of parametric tests where the data does not justify them. Beware of 'statistically significant' results which are not 'clinically significant'. For instance, a new bronchodilator may show a 'very significant' improvement in asthmatics early-morning peak expiratory flow rates ($p < 0.001$), but that difference may be only 20 L/min, which is unlikely to make much difference to their quality of life! Also, more impressive p-values do *not* imply a bigger treatment effect: a p-value of < 0.001, compared to a < 0.05 does *not* mean a greater treatment effect: it means that it is *more likely* that there is a difference between the control and intervention groups. Hence, the move to confidence intervals (see above).

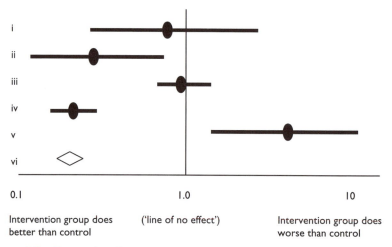

Figure 4.2   Forest plot diagram

i   Probably a small study, with a wide confidence interval, crossing unity (i.e. unable to say if the intervention is either beneficial or harmful).
ii   Probably another small study, with a wide confidence interval, but does not cross unity, so suggests that the intervention is beneficial, but only provides weak evidence.
iii   Larger study, so has a narrower confidence interval, but again crosses unity, so it is equivocal about the impact of the intervention.
iv   Again, probably a large study, entirely to the left of unity, so providing quite good evidence that the intervention is beneficial.
v   Probably another small study, with wide confidence interval, but entirely on the right of unity, suggesting, but not very conclusively, that the intervention may be harmful.
vi   Meta-analysis of the five smaller studies, providing more rigorous evidence of effectiveness.

The x-axis is usually on a logarithmic scale, and measures the odds ratio:

$$\frac{\text{odds of an event in the intervention group}}{\text{odds of an event in the control group}}$$

Table 4.2   Beta-blocker effect on mortality after myocardial infarction (MI)

	Study 1: beta-blockers after MI		*Study 1: beta-blockers after MI*	
	Control	*Intervention*	*Control*	*Intervention*
Intervention	No beta-blockers	Beta-blockers with ISA*	No beta-blockers	Beta-blockers without ISA*
Outcome	Mortality rate	Mortality rate		

*ISA = intrinsic sympathomimetic activity (when blocking the beta-receptors, the drug exerts a slight stimulation of the receptor, those without ISA block the receptors without any stimulation).

Also, be wary of conclusions derived from sub-group analysis, where the authors attempt to draw new conclusions by comparing the outcomes for patients in one study with the patients in another, rather than trying to draw together the patients in the control and intervention groups in each study. Such conclusions have often later been shown to be artefacts and not justified. For example, a meta-analysis of beta-blockers after myocardial infarction included the two studies in Table 4.2. The meta-analysis confirmed that beta-blockers improved survival after a myocardial infarction. A sub-group analysis of the intervention groups in the two studies concluded that beta-blockers without intrinsic sympathomimetic activity (ISA) were more effective than those with. In fact, a new randomized clinical trial would be needed to decide this issue conclusively, and the finding of this sub-group analysis was later disproved (Freemantle *et al.* 1999).

Also, be wary of 'data-dredging' exercises, testing multiple hypotheses against the data, especially if the hypotheses were constructed after the study had begun data collection.

Resources for critical appraisal

In some cases, you can save a lot of work by tapping into a collection of 'pre-appraised' articles, where experts in the field have already produced a formal critique of original research papers, often including a commentary on the application to daily practice:

- **The CAT Bank:** the Oxford Centre for Evidence-based Medicine's bank of Critically Appraised Topics (CATs), which also includes tables of numbers needed to treat (NNTs): www.cebm.net/cats.asp.
- **POEMS for primary care:** a POEM in this context is a piece of patient oriented evidence that matters. Each month this site draws on over 90 peer-reviewed journals to identify quality clinical information, which passes muster on criteria of both validity and relevance to primary care use. The material is presented as a 300 word synopsis: www.InfoPOEMS.com/.
- **Journal Club on the web:** provides access to a selection of critically appraised papers, with expert commentary on both the authors' methodology and the clinical applications, and a subject index of the archive. Some also include notes on interpreting the statistics used in the write-up: www.journalclub.org/.
- *American College of Physicians Journal Club: ACP Journal Club* is published bi-monthly by the American College of Physicians. It contains reviews of research papers where experts in that field discuss the validity and applicability of the

work. Essentially, it is the US version of *Evidence-Based Medicine*. The website includes the contents of the latest issue and one or two full text articles as tasters, but you will need to get hard copy for most of the content: www.acpjc.org/.

- *Evidence-Based Medicine:* sister publication to the *ACP Journal Club*, from the BMJ Publishing Group. More web content but still not quite everything which appears in the paper version: www.bmjpg.com/template.cfm?name=specjou_be.
- *Evidence-Based Mental Health:* a secondary publication journal aimed at keeping mental health professionals up to date with the latest high-quality research evidence: www.bmjpg.com/template.cfm?name=specjou_mh.
- *Evidence-Based Nursing* www.bmjpg.com/template.cfm?name=specjou_nu.
- **The PedsCCM Evidence-Based Journal Club:** includes an archive of structured critical appraisals. These also tend to be updated with further comments, to produce a discussion of the usefulness of the article to clinical practice in child health: http://PedsCCM.wustl.edu/EBJournal_Club.html.
- **ARIF:** Aggressive Research Intelligence Facility, from Birmingham University, largely concerned with critical appraisal of reviews to help purchasers make decisions, and including advice on finding and appraising review articles and summaries of commissioned work to date: www.bham.ac.uk/arif/.

Points to ponder

Critical appraisal is a mixture of the science of examining validity and the art of assessing utility. There are a number of unresolved questions you might like to think about:

- **Declaration of outside interests or commercial sponsorship:** how would you regard the report of a project funded by a pharmaceutical company who marketed some of the drugs involved?
- **Ethical reservations:** would you use the results of studies which were sound in methodology, but where you felt there were ethical problems, and no explicit evidence of ethics committee approval?
- **Using meta-analysis:** how 'applicable' are the results of studies like meta-analyses, which reduce subjects to 'average patients' in the care of often idiosyncratic individuals? How do you 'square the circle' when a meta-analysis and a randomized controlled trial in the same subject area produce conflicting results or, worse still, two meta-analyses disagree?

Conclusions

Critical appraisal is a systematic technique for filtering and analysing retrieved papers. All critical appraisal is based on three main steps: extracting the main message of the paper; establishing the rigour of the methodology used in the study; and assessing how generalizable the study findings are to wider populations.

For primary quantitative studies, key questions relate to the size and selection of the study population, randomization, potential biases and completeness of follow up, while for primary qualitative studies, key questions relate to the range of subjects used, appropriateness of the methodology and the relationship between the researchers and the subjects. For secondary studies (meta-analyses and systematic reviews), key questions relate to the rigour of the techniques used to locate primary studies, exclusion and inclusion criteria and the quality of the individual studies. As yet, rigorous criteria for the appraisal of websites are lacking, but some 'rules of thumb' are emerging for assessing the quality of internet-based information

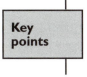

Key points

- Modern electronic databases mean that with a comprehensive search strategy, it is easy to retrieve many papers for a research or practice question.

- Critical appraisal is a systematic technique for filtering and analysing research papers.

- The three main steps of critical appraisal are: extracting the main message of the paper; establishing the rigour of the methodology used in the study; assessing how generalizable the study findings are to wider populations.

- For meta-analyses, forest plots and confidence intervals are good ways to summarize the findings of the individual and combined studies.

- Be wary of conclusions produced from data dredging, secondary analyses and obscure statistical tests.

- Some 'rules of thumb' are emerging for assessing the quality of internet-based information.

Acknowledgements

Some of the material and examples used in this chapter were originally jointly written with Dr Nick Fox, Andrew Booth, Deborah Hornby and Louise Falzon for a training programme in literature reviewing and critical appraisal for PhD students at Sheffield University, and that material is used here with the permission of my co-authors for that course.

Further reading

Avis, M. (1994) Reading research critically: an introduction to appraisal; designs and objectives, *Journal of Clinical Nursing*, Part 1: July, 3(4): 227–34; Part 2 Sept, 3(5): 271–7.

Eysenbach, G., Diepgen, T.L., Gray, J.A.M. *et al.* (1998) Towards quality management of medical information on the internet: evaluation, labelling and filtering of information, *British Medical Journal*, 317: 1496–1502.

Haynes, R.B., McKibbon, K.A., Fitzgerald, D. *et al.* (1986) How to store and retrieve articles worth keeping, *Annals of Internal Medicine*, 105: 978–84.

Jones, R. and Kinmouth, A.L. (1995) *Critical Reading for Primary Care*. Oxford: Oxford University Press.

Thomas, C. (1997) Critical appraisal, in Y. Carter and C. Thomas (eds) *Research Methods in Primary Care*. Oxford: Radcliffe Medical Press.

The *British Medical Journal* 'How to read a paper series', edited by Trisha Greenhalgh, and originally published in the *British Medical Journal* in 1997, volume 315, contains the following useful articles, with page numbers shown in brackets:

- Getting your bearings (deciding what the paper is about) (243–6)
- Assessing the methodological quality of published papers (305–8)
- Statistics for the non-statistician, I: statistical tests (364–6)

- Statistics for the non-statistician, II: 'significant' relations (422–5)
- Papers that report drug trials (480–3)
- Papers that report diagnostic or screening tests (540–3)
- Papers that tell you what things cost (economic analyses) (596–9)
- Papers that summarize other papers (systematic reviews/meta-analyses) (672–5)
- Papers that go beyond numbers (qualitative research) (740–3)

Collectively these are also available in book form in Greenhalgh, T. (2001) *How to Read a Paper : The Basics of Evidence Based Medicine*, 2nd edn. London: BMJ publishing Group.

Resources

- **Critical Appraisal of Bio-medical Literature:** online tutorial from the Wisdom Centre: www.wisdom.org.uk/ebpsem2.html.
- **The Critical Appraisal Skills Programme (CASP):** from the NHS Public Health Resources Unit: www.phru.nhs.uk/casp/casp.htm.
- *The Users' Guides to Evidence-based Practice:* a very good set of guides to using the literature were published in the *Journal of the American Medical Association* a few years ago, and these are now available on the web with clinical scenarios and worked examples of question answering at: www.cche.net/principles/content_all.asp.
- *The Evidence Based Medicine Tool Kit:* basically a simpler version of the users' guides: www.med.ualberta.ca/ebm/ebm.htm.

References

Bucher, H.C., Weinbacher, M. and Gyr, K. (1994) Influence of method of reporting study results on decision of physicians to prescribe drugs to lower cholesterol concentration, *British Medical Journal*, 309: 761–4.

Delamothe, T. (2000) Quality of websites: kitemarking the west wind, *British Medical Journal*, 321: 843–4.

Egger, M., Smith, G.D., Schneider, M. and Minder, C. (1997) Bias in meta-analysis detected by a simple, graphical test, *British Medical Journal*, 315: 629–34.

Freemantle, N., Cleland, J., Young, P., Mason, J. and Harrison, J. (1999) β-blockade after myocardial infarction: systematic review and meta regression analysis, *British Medical Journal*, 318: 1730–7.

Miser, W.F. (1999) Critical appraisal of the literature, *Journal of the American Board of Family Practice*, 12(4): 315–33.

Thompson, S.G. (1995) Why sources of heterogeneity in meta-analysis should be investigated, in I. Chalmers and D.G. Altman (eds) *Systematic Reviews*. London: BMJ Publishing Group.

Tramèr, M.R., Reynolds, D.J.M., Moore, R.A. and McQuay, H.J. (1997) Impact of covert duplicate publication on meta-analysis: a case study, *British Medical Journal*, 315: 635–40.

5 Features and designs of randomized controlled trials and non-randomized experimental designs

Kate Tilling, Jonathan Sterne, Sara Brookes and Tim Peters

Introduction

Randomized controlled trials are the gold standard study design for evaluation of health care interventions. However, the quality of many randomized controlled trials remains poor, and there is clear evidence that poor methodological quality is associated with biased estimates of the effect of interventions (Schulz *et al.* 1995; Moher *et al.* 1998). The purpose of this chapter is to present the basic principles of design and conduct of trials, including coverage of more complex designs. We will also discuss the role of non-randomized studies in evaluating the effect of health service interventions.

Types of randomized and non-randomized experimental design

A clinical trial (Meinert 1986) has been defined as 'a planned experiment designed to assess the efficacy of a treatment . . . by comparing the outcomes in a group of patients with the test treatment with those observed in a comparable group of patients receiving a control treatment'. The main types of experimental design are described in Table 5.1: the gold standard of evidence is the randomized controlled trial. Non-randomized experimental designs are available, although these have been shown to be prone to bias (Kunz and Oxman 1998). However, they may be useful in situations where clinicians refuse to participate in trials because of lack of individual uncertainty (see p. 91), or where there are practical obstacles or ethical objections to randomization (Black 1996). Practical obstacles include the large sample size required in a trial to detect long-term or rare events (where a case–control or cohort study may be more practicable, see Chapter 6). Ethical objections would be raised, for example, to randomized trials comparing intensive care with general ward care, leaving such interventions unevaluated unless non-randomized designs are used (Black 1996).

Table 5.1   Randomized and non-randomized experimental designs

Design	Key features	Advantages	Disadvantages
Randomized controlled trial	Participants randomly assigned to intervention or control arm	Groups balanced in everything except treatment received. If randomization concealed, can prevent selection bias	Time and effort required to design and carry out effectively
Cluster randomized controlled trial	Groups of participants (e.g. families, GP practices) randomized to intervention or control	May be logistically easier than individual randomization. More suitable for some interventions (e.g. community education programmes)	Need larger sample size than individually randomized trials. More complex analysis
Controlled trial	Participants non-randomly assigned to intervention or control arm (e.g. by day of week, even/odd birth date, etc.)	Easier to carry out than a randomized trial, as no need to prepare and conceal randomized allocation schedule	Allocation schedule can't be concealed, so selection bias may occur
Before/after comparison	Data collected before and after an intervention on a group of participants, and a paired comparison made	Reduces variability by using paired data	Changes other than the experimental intervention may occur over the time period
Randomized crossover trial	As above, but each participant receives control and intervention treatment in random order. Paired comparison made	Reduces variability by using paired data	Unsuitable for interventions with long-term effects, or conditions that change over time
Historical controlled study	Data collected after an intervention, and compared to data collected on some other group which did not experience the intervention. Unpaired comparison made	Requires minimal data collection	There may be differences between the intervention arm and the historical controls other than the experimental intervention

Any clinical trial requires choice of the intervention and control treatments (see below) and one or more outcome measures to be used in evaluating the effect of the intervention compared to the control (Meinert 1986).

Key features of randomized controlled trials

The randomized controlled trial is the key clinical trial design, because randomization ensures that the intervention and control groups do not differ systematically with respect to known or unknown prognostic factors. The quality of a randomized controlled trial has been defined as 'the likelihood of the trial design to generate unbiased results, that are sufficiently precise and allow application in clinical practice' (Verhagen *et al.* 2001). Many scales and checklists have been developed to assess the quality of randomized controlled trials (Moher *et al.* 1995), with two commonly used scales being the Jadad (Jadad *et al.* 1996) and the Delphi (Verhagen *et al.* 1998). However, it is now recommended that relevant methodological aspects should be assessed individually rather than by using an overall scale (Juni *et al.* 1999).

The CONSORT statement was developed to assess quality of reporting of randomized controlled trials, but inevitably also includes items thought to be important components of the quality of a trial, based on empirical evidence (Moher *et al.* 2001). Table 5.2 lists some of the key aspects of design of randomized controlled trials appearing in the Consolidated Standards of Reporting Trials (CONSORT) statement, or in quality scales or checklists.

Randomization

Most disease states have factors known to influence the outcome of treatment, called *prognostic factors*. The purpose of randomization is to ensure that the groups do not differ systematically with respect to known and unknown prognostic factors. As the total number of subjects in the trial increases, the balance of characteristics of subjects between the groups improves. Appreciable imbalances in prognostic factors may be particularly important in a multi-centre study where imbalances in assignment can occur within individual institutions. Balance of prognostic factors is also often an issue in cluster randomized trials, where the number of clusters may be low.

Table 5.2 Key aspects of design of randomized controlled trials

Feature	Reason	Practicalities
Randomization of participants to control or intervention	Ensure comparability of the two groups	Ranges from simple designs (see below) to more complex adaptive schemes (Meinert 1986)
Patient allocation – concealment of allocation schedule	Avoid selection bias	Centralized randomization (e.g. by telephone) should be used to ensure that patients and study personnel cannot know randomization allocation in advance
Blinding	Avoid respondent bias, where patients may report changes in self-assessed outcome because they know they are in the intervention arm. Also avoid interviewer/observed bias in those assessing outcome	Where possible, the trial should be double-blind (i.e. patient and study personnel responsible for outcome measurement are blind to the treatment allocation). Placebo controls (identical to the intervention treatment in all but active ingredients) are one method used to achieve this. Blind outcome assessment is often possible even when blinding of the participant is not (a single-blind trial), and is particularly important for subjective outcomes
Power calculation	Avoid either a trial that is too small to detect a clinically important effect, or too large (thus exposing too many patients to the non-effective treatment, when a smaller trial could have answered the clinical question)	Identify the sample size needed to detect a clinically important effect and/or to achieve an adequate level of precision. Inflate this to allow for eligibility criteria and patient dropout and, where appropriate, clustering effects. For example of power calculations see standard statistical texts (e.g. Kirkwood and Sterne 2003)
Intention to treat	Avoids bias due to dropout or non-adherence to protocol	Maximize follow-up rates, irrespective of arm of trial or adherence to treatment (see Chapter 21)

The randomization scheme prepared for the trial should be reproducible (Meinert 1986). Thus, schemes such as tossing a coin are unacceptable, as they cannot be reproduced. Computer-generated random numbers or tables of random numbers can be used. Four common methods of randomization are:

- *Simple randomization*: this can use computer-generated random numbers, either prepared specifically for the trial or using existing tables of random numbers where the digits of 0–9 appear with equal likelihood in each entry. Treatments are assigned to odd or even numbers (Altman and Bland 1999).
- *Block randomization*: this is one method used to prevent imbalances in subject numbers assigned to each group, particularly when the number of subjects in the trial is small. With block randomization, the total sample size is divided into blocks of a given size. Within each block, the group is assigned so that there are equal numbers allocated to each group. To prevent investigators from learning the block size and being able to guess order of assignment, the block size can be varied, usually at random from a small number of alternatives (Schulz and Grimes 2002). When used in conjunction with stratification (as described below), blocking prevents serious imbalances in characteristics across groups.
- *Stratified randomization*: stratified randomization ensures equal distribution of subjects with a particular characteristic in each group when, in addition, blocking is employed within strata (Kernan *et al.* 1999). Stratification is usually restricted to a small number of prognostic factors. Despite its complexity, stratified randomization is usually helpful in a multi-centre trial, so that both the numbers of subjects in each group and the important prognostic factors can be balanced within each site.
- *Minimization*: an alternative method to cater for more factors at once, where the characteristics of individuals already randomized alter in a systematic manner the chances of a given subject being allocated to the different trial groups, so as to maximize the resulting balance of these factors.

Statistical issues in design and analysis

Design of randomized controlled trials

Research must not only be planned early, but also planned often. All issues should be addressed at the start of the planning process, and many will need to be revisited at suitable times throughout the project. The protocol for a clinical trial will include some (and probably all) of the factors outlined in Table 5.3 (Meinert 1986). Many of these issues are statistical; indeed, the major statistical input to a study should be at the design stage, including planning the data analysis in advance. Leaving this until the end of a study will usually lead to difficulties that cannot be resolved, resulting in a study which is at best inefficient, and at worst inconclusive. The analysis plan should be laid out before the trial begins, and may include the following:

1 *Generalizability* – including total number of subjects approached, total number eligible, reasons for ineligibility, number consenting to randomization, reasons for refusal and other information reported in the CONSORT flow diagram (see Figure 5.1) (Moher *et al.* 2001). Data on those ineligible or refusing to take part in the trial should be collected and presented where possible.
2 *Baseline comparability of the two groups* – descriptive statistics only (p-values for these comparisons should not be presented).
3 *Process data* – including (where relevant) details of what constitutes 'usual care', and details of the intervention and care given to those in the intervention arm.

Table 5.3 Factors to be included in the protocol of a clinical trial

Factor	Statistician's role

Randomization plan – including generation of schedule and details of how schedule will be concealed from those involved in recruitment	Where applicable:
	    stratification
	    block randomization
	    more advanced randomization designs – e.g. minimization
	 Generation of random number schedule

Sample size calculation	Assist clinician(s) in:
	    developing precise research question
	    identifying and justifying clinically relevant effect size
	    estimating standard deviation
	 Carry out and explain sample size calculation

Inclusion/exclusion criteria and recruitment schedule	Adjust sample size for likely proportion of patients eligible and consenting to randomization Develop realistic recruitment plan Ensure information recorded to complete trial profile figure
Primary and secondary outcomes	Advise on validity, reliability and sensitivity of proposed outcomes

Patient follow-up plan	Advise on:
	    inter- and intra-observer measurement error, how to monitor and minimise it
	    minimizing missing data/dropout and its impact on analysis (e.g. ensuring interviewers ask for reasons when patients refuse further participation)
	    patient follow-up time(s)

Analysis plan	Develop analysis plan

4 *Primary analyses* – intention to treat (see Chapter 21) analyses of the primary outcome(s) (e.g. the primary outcome in a trial of care after stroke might be mortality at three months post-stroke). Should adjust for any stratification/minimization and for any baseline measurement of the outcome variable.

5 *Primary analyses of secondary outcomes* – intention to treat (see Chapter 21) analyses of secondary outcomes (e.g. a secondary outcome in a trial of care after stroke might be handicap at three months post-stroke). Should adjust for any stratification/minimization and for any baseline measurement of the outcome variable.

6 *Secondary analyses* – including some or all of the following:
   a) adjustment for baseline imbalance (see Chapter 21);
   b) explanatory analyses such as per protocol analyses or analyses including process measures (see Chapter 21);
   c) sub-group analyses (see Chapter 21).

Interim analyses

These are analyses carried out before the trial has finished, either as part of the protocol or at the request of the data monitoring committee (also commonly called the data and safety monitoring committee, or the data safety monitoring board) (Wilhelmsen 2002). In many trials, the study statistician performs the interim analyses and presents them to the data monitoring committee, which includes an independent statistician. In a variation on this model, the statistician performing

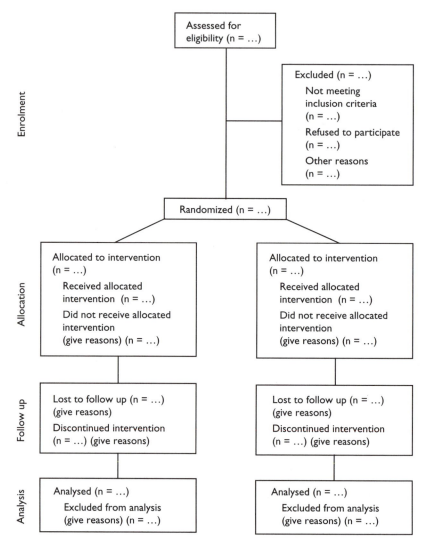

Figure 5.1   Revised template of the CONSORT diagram showing the flow of participants through each stage of a randomized trial (Moher *et al.* 2001)

these interim analyses is independent of the study statistician. The argument for this strategy is that the interim analyst must be unblinded to the treatment allocation code, and using an independent statistician preserves blinding of the study statistician in performing the final analyses (DeMets and Fleming 2004; Pocock 2004). It may be difficult to find an independent interim analyst in practice, partly because they would get little recognition for their work.

Interim analyses (where relevant) should be part of the pre-specified analysis plan, with statistical stopping rules built into the protocol (Meinert 1986). Issues may also arise during the course of the study that require *ad hoc* interim analyses, for example, concerns over safety, problems with recruitment and unexpected side-effect/ mortality rates for one or other of the arms (Collins 2003).

Final reports

Regarding presentation, the CONSORT statement provides guidelines for reporting the design, detailed methods and results of randomized controlled trials (Moher *et al.* 2001). Figure 5.1 is a CONSORT diagram showing the flow of participants through each stage of a randomized trial.

It has been argued that the statistician performing the final analyses and writing the report should (where possible) be blinded to the treatment allocation code until the final report has been prepared (Meinert 1986; Pocock 2004). This may help to prevent biases arising from additional (non-planned) analyses of secondary outcomes or time-points, or emphasis of 'statistically significant' results over 'non-significant' results. However, careful specification of the analysis plan before the study begins could have the same effect. In addition, the analyst may need to be unblinded for some secondary analyses (e.g. per protocol analyses). Issues concerning the analysis of randomized controlled trials are discussed in Chapter 21.

More detailed information on the design of clinical trials is available elsewhere (e.g. Meinert 1986; Pocock 1987; Kirkwood and Sterne 2003).

Choice of intervention and control

One of the key issues in the design of a clinical trial is choice of the intervention and control treatments (Meinert 1986). An ethical clinical trial requires there to be uncertainty before the trial starts as to which of the intervention and control treatments would be the 'best' treatment. There is debate over whether 'clinical equipoise' or 'uncertainty' is the best requirement for this pre-trial uncertainty (Weijer *et al.* 2000). Clinical equipoise occurs where there is uncertainty in the medical/scientific community about the best treatment to be given in a specific circumstance. Uncertainty occurs where each individual doctor recruiting to a trial is uncertain as to which is the best treatment to be given – he or she is then in a position ethically to randomize patients. The uncertainty principle has been advocated as a way to simplify entry criteria for randomized clinical trials (Peto and Baigent 1998).

A common choice for the control group of a clinical trial is a completely inactive placebo. However, it may not be ethical to use a placebo as the comparator, if an active treatment that is known to be effective exists. The *Declaration of Helsinki* (World Medical Association 2004), paragraph 29 states: 'The benefits, risks, burdens and effectiveness of a new method should be tested against those of the best current prophylactic, diagnostic, and therapeutic methods. This does not exclude the use of placebo, or no treatment, in studies where no proven prophylactic, diagnostic or therapeutic method exists'. A note of clarification on paragraph 29 continues:

> 'However, a placebo-controlled trial may be ethically acceptable, even if proven therapy is available, under the following circumstances:
>
> - Where for compelling and scientifically sound methodological reasons its use is necessary to determine the efficacy or safety of a prophylactic, diagnostic or therapeutic method; or
> - Where a prophylactic, diagnostic or therapeutic method is being investigated for a minor condition and the patients who receive placebo will not be subject to any additional risk of serious or irreversible harm.'

Alternatives to the placebo-controlled trial include:

- *Usual care*: this is commonly used in health services research. However, the components of usual care may be difficult to define for some research questions, and the estimated effect of the intervention may vary depending on the constituents of usual care.

- *Attention control*: this control group aims to balance the effects of contact/attention in the intervention group, by providing these to the control group whether in person or using written information.
- *Active control*: in an active controlled trial, the control group is given an intervention that has a therapeutic effect, such as an established drug or other treatment. Some 'usual care' and 'attention control' trials could be thought of as 'active control' trials. Trials with active controls tend to be larger than placebo-controlled trials, as the expected difference in effect of the active and intervention treatments is smaller than that between a placebo and an intervention (Emanuel and Miller 2001). Some studies of this type are 'non-inferiority' trials, where the null hypothesis (see Chapter 21) is that the intervention is not inferior to the active control (D'Agostino, Sr *et al.* 2003). 'Non-inferiority' or 'equivalence' trials tend to be larger than the more usual superiority trials because the aim is to have the entire confidence interval for the difference between the two arms of the trial within a range specified as part of the sample size calculation.

Types of randomized controlled trial

Parallel group trials

The most common type of randomised controlled trial is a *parallel group trial*, where two (or more) groups of patients are treated and followed up in parallel. The primary analysis is a comparison of the primary outcome(s) in the two different groups. The sample size for the trial depends on the size of the minimum clinically important difference and (for numerical outcomes) the standard deviation of the primary outcome in the study population (Kirkwood and Sterne 2003).

Crossover trials

In a *crossover trial*, every person experiences both interventions under comparison, with the two randomized groups receiving them in a different order, as shown in Figure 5.2. The primary analysis is a between-individual comparison of the difference between outcomes in the first and second half of the trial in the two arms of the trial (a comparison of $d_{12}-d_{11}$ with $d_{22}-d_{21}$, Figure 5.2). The sample size for the trial depends on the size of the minimum clinically important difference and the standard deviation of the *within-person differences* in the primary outcome in

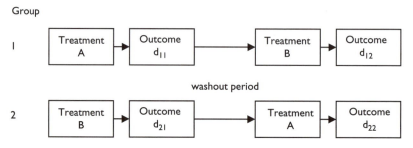

Figure 5.2   Schematic representation of a crossover trial

the study population. A crossover trial will usually be smaller than the equivalent parallel group trial, as it takes advantage of the fact that there is more variation in an outcome between people than within people. However, crossover trials are only suitable for cases where the treatment can be applied for a relatively short period of time, with a measurable outcome immediately afterwards. The effect also needs to be short-term, as the person then carries on to test the other treatment. For this reason there is often a break of a few days or weeks between treatments (the washout period, Figure 5.2) to allow the effects of the first treatment to wear off. Thus crossover trials are mostly used to study the short-term effects of treatments in chronic diseases (Sibbald and Roberts 1998).

Cluster randomized trials

In most randomized trials, the unit of randomization (and hence of analysis) is the individual – for example, individuals are randomized to receive care either in a stroke unit or a general medical ward. However, in some cases, randomization is applied to groups of people (clusters), rather than individuals (Ukoumunne et al. 1999; Donner and Klar 2000, 2004; Kirkwood and Sterne 2003). This might be because of the nature of the intervention: for example, to evaluate an intervention designed to improve GP management of patients after stroke, the unit of randomization is the GP, and thus the intervention would be applied to groups of patients. A cluster randomized trial might also be required for logistical reasons: for example, where it is thought that there might be contamination (members of the control group receive some or all of the intervention) between individuals within the same 'cluster' but different arms of an individually-randomized trial. Contamination might occur if a trial of an educational intervention randomized individuals rather than families, and members of the same family discussed the interventions they were receiving.

Cluster randomized trials require special methods of analysis, as detailed in Chapter 21. A cluster randomized trial also needs to include more individuals than the corresponding individually randomized trial. The inflation of the sample size over that required by a non-cluster randomized trial increases as the degree of similarity of people within a cluster increases and also as the cluster size increases (Hayes and Bennett 1999; Kirkwood and Sterne 2003; Donner and Klar 2004). Indeed, even if the degree of intra-cluster correlation is low, if the clusters are large then the inflation factor may still be appreciable. Other drawbacks of cluster randomized trials include: problems balancing baseline characteristics at both individual and cluster level (see 'Randomization', p. 87); increased difficulty with concealment (because individuals may be recruited after their cluster allocation is known); and problems with recruiting/retaining controls. Thus there should always be a clear and explicit rationale for opting for a cluster randomized trial, for reasons including efficiency and ethics.

N-of-one trials

In an n-of-1 or single patient trial the individual is recruited to their own individual trial, that is, to a trial containing a single person. This provides the unique opportunity to measure the effect of treatment on the symptoms that matter to that individual. In an n-of-1 trial the individual serves as his or her own control, receiving all treatments under investigation (Guyatt et al. 1988). Generally, comparisons will be made between a single new therapy and a current standard therapy or a placebo. However, as with traditional randomized controlled trials it is also possible to compare more than two treatment options.

The experimental unit, and therefore the unit of randomization, is the treatment period. Ideally such a trial is conducted as a double-blind (both the individual and outcome assessor blind to allocated treatment in any treatment period), multi-crossover trial with three or more periods for each treatment. The trial design will, however, be tailored to the clinical entity and therapies involved.

Sample size or power calculations used with classical randomized controlled trials can also be used to determine the appropriate number of treatment periods for an n-of-1 trial. While a large number of treatment periods would increase the statistical power, the natural course of the clinical entity, therapy characteristics and patient compliance will generally put an upper limit on this number, and thus statistical power will generally remain low unless treatment effects are large. The most commonly recommended design when comparing two treatments is random allocation within pairs of treatment periods (Johannessen and Fosstvedt 1991). For example, for the comparison of treatment A versus treatment B over eight treatment periods, the following randomization schedule might be generated: AB AB BA AB. This approach avoids the possibility of several consecutive treatment periods with the same treatment.

The duration of an n-of-1 trial will largely depend on the nature of the condition and the treatments under investigation, but is likely to be for several months. Hence, such trials are only effective for chronic and stable conditions where the natural history of the condition is unlikely to change dramatically over the course of the trial. To minimize potential carry-over effects between treatment periods the therapies under investigation should have a rapid onset and cessation of effect (Guyatt *et al.* 1988). In addition, a washout period between treatments can be incorporated into the trial or a run-in period, where the first few days on each treatment are not evaluated. Examples of clinical areas in which n-of-1 trials have been performed include osteoarthritis (March *et al.* 1994), gastroesophageal reflux disease (Wolfe *et al.* 2002), attention deficit hyperactivity disorder (Duggan *et al.* 2000) and chronic airflow limitation (Mahon *et al.* 1999).

The n-of-1 trial provides an alternative approach to clinical practice when the results of large-scale randomized trials are not available or may not be relevant to the individual. Within the context of the hierarchy of evidence-based study designs, it has recently been suggested that n-of-1 trials deliver the highest strength of evidence for making individual patient treatment decisions (Guyatt *et al.* 2000).

Patient preference trials

An extension to a randomized controlled trial is to allow patients who refuse randomization to choose which treatment they would like to receive (Torgerson and Sibbald 1998). This design combines the randomized controlled trial with a non-randomized experiment, and thus loses some of the advantage of randomization in protecting against confounding. A patient preference trial of intervention (I) against control (C) contains four arms: those randomized to I and C, and those allocating themselves to I and C. However, analysis of such trials is still under debate. A main comparison of the two randomized groups should certainly be made (Torgerson and Sibbald 1998). However, in using all four arms of the trial, there is likely to be confounding due to differences between patients with and without strong preferences for treatment.

Alternatives to the patient preference trial include: eliciting opinions from participants before randomization as to which would be their preferred options, but randomizing all consenting subjects; randomizing first and then only asking for consent from those randomized to the intervention arm (Zelen randomization);

and 'double randomisation' where the randomization is carried out first and then consent is asked from all participants (Lambert and Wood 2000).

The idea behind the patient preference trial is that an individual's treatment preference may alter their outcome, and so alter the results and conclusions of the trial, making generalizability questionable (Janevic *et al.* 2003). In many randomized trials, patient preferences, as with other confounders, will be balanced by randomization between the two arms of the trial. However, there may be cases where one treatment is preferred over another because of perceived side-effects or a perception that the new treatment 'must' be better than the control (Janevic *et al.* 2003). If strong preferences lead to patients not consenting to inclusion in randomized trials, this will lead to smaller (and less powerful) trials that also have questionable generalizability (Janevic *et al.* 2003).

Example – a patient preference trial in general practice

A randomized trial with patient preference arms was carried out to compare efficacy of antidepressant drugs and counselling for mild to moderate depression (Chilvers *et al.* 2001). Three hundred and twenty-three patients agreed to participate, with 103 (32 per cent) consenting to randomization. In the patient preference arm, 140 patients (64 per cent) chose the counselling intervention. Those choosing counselling were less severely depressed than those choosing antidepressant drugs, and than those consenting to randomization. There was some evidence that counselling showed a greater benefit in those who chose it than in those who were randomized to it, but the possibility of confounding (see Chapter 21) is hard to rule out here. The authors recommended that depressed patients should be allowed to choose between counselling and antidepressant drugs, but that those with no preference should be prescribed antidepressants.

Conclusions

The rationale for randomized controlled trials is to avoid the confounding inherent in observational research. However, simple randomized controlled trials are not common in health services research. Therefore, appropriate conduct of randomized controlled trials requires involvement of a multidisciplinary team including, for example, trialists, statisticians, clinicians and experts in outcome measurement.

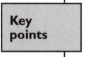

Key points

- Randomized controlled trials are the 'gold standard' for evaluating health service interventions.

- Careful study design is essential – most flaws in design cannot be corrected at the analysis stage.

- Randomization schemes should always be concealed from study personnel.

- Choice of control group will vary between studies, and components of care received should always be carefully described.

- Crossover trials may be useful in assessing the efficacy of short-term interventions in chronic disease.

- The decision to randomize clusters (rather than individuals) may be taken because of logistics, ethics or the nature of the intervention, and will affect both sample size calculations and analyses.

- The n-of-1 trial provides an alternative approach to clinical practice when the results of large-scale randomized trials are not available or are not relevant to the individual.

- Specifying the analysis plan carefully in advance will avoid bias at the analysis stage, and obviate the need to blind the statistician carrying out the final analyses.

References

Altman, D.G. and Bland, J.M. (1999) How to randomise, *British Medical Journal*, 319: 703–4.
Black, N. (1996) Why we need observational studies to evaluate the effectiveness of health care, *British Medical Journal*, 312: 1215–18.
Chilvers, C., Dewey, M., Fielding, K. *et al.* (2001) Antidepressant drugs and generic counselling for treatment of major depression in primary care: randomised trial with patient preference arms, *British Medical Journal*, 322: 772–5.
Collins, J.F. (2003) Data and safety monitoring board issues raised in the VA Status Epilepticus Study, *Controlled Clinical Trials*, 24: 71–7.
D'Agostino, R.B., Sr, Massaro, J.M. and Sullivan, L.M. (2003) Non-inferiority trials: design concepts and issues – the encounters of academic consultants in statistics, *Statistics in Medicine*, 22: 169–86.
DeMets, D.L. and Fleming, T.R. (2004) The independent statistician for data monitoring committees, *Statistics in Medicine*, 23: 1513–17.
Donner, A. and Klar, N. (2000) *Design and Analysis of Cluster Randomized Trials in Health Research*. London: Arnold.
Donner, A. and Klar, N. (2004) Pitfalls of and controversies in cluster randomization trials, *American Journal of Public Health*, 94: 416–22.
Duggan, C.M., Mitchell, G., Nikles, C.J. *et al.* (2000) Managing ADHD in general practice. N of 1 trials can help! *Australian Family Physician*, 29: 1205–9.
Emanuel, E.J. and Miller, F.G. (2001) The ethics of placebo-controlled trials – a middle ground, *New England Journal of Medicine*, 345: 915–19.
Guyatt, G., Sackett, D., Adachi, J. *et al.* (1988) A clinician's guide for conducting randomized trials in individual patients, *Canadian Medical Association Journal*, 139: 497–503.
Guyatt, G.H., Haynes, R.B., Jaeschke, R.Z. *et al.* (2000) Users' guides to the medical literature: XXV. Evidence-based medicine: principles for applying the users' guides to patient care. Evidence-Based Medicine Working Group, *Journal of the American Medical Association*, 284: 1290–6.
Hayes, R.J. and Bennett, S. (1999) Simple sample size calculation for cluster-randomized trials, *International Journal of Epidemiology*, 28: 319–26.
Jadad, A.R., Moore, R.A., Carroll, D. *et al.* (1996) Assessing the quality of reports of randomized clinical trials: is blinding necessary? *Controlled Clinical Trials*, 17: 1–12.
Janevic, M.R., Janz, N.K., Dodge, J.A. *et al.* (2003) The role of choice in health education intervention trials: a review and case study, *Social Science and Medicine*, 56: 1581–94.
Johannessen, T. and Fosstvedt, D. (1991) Statistical power in single subject trials, *Family Practice*, 8: 384–87.
Juni, P., Witschi, A., Bloch, R. and Egger, M. (1999) The hazards of scoring the quality of clinical trials for meta-analysis, *Journal of the American Medical Association*, 282: 1054–60.
Kernan, W.N., Viscoli, C.M., Makuch, R.W. *et al.* (1999) Stratified randomization for clinical trials, *Journal of Clinical Epidemiology*, 52: 19–26.
Kirkwood, B.R. and Sterne, J.A.C. (2003) *Essential Medical Statistics*, 2nd edn. Oxford: Blackwell Science.
Kunz, R. and Oxman, A.D. (1998) The unpredictability paradox: review of empirical comparisons of randomised and non-randomised clinical trials, *British Medical Journal*, 317: 1185–90.

Lambert, M.F. and Wood, J. (2000) Incorporating patient preferences into randomized trials, *Journal of Clinical Epidemiology*, 53: 163–66.

Mahon, J.L., Laupacis, A., Hodder, R.V. *et al.* (1999) Theophylline for irreversible chronic airflow limitation: a randomized study comparing n of 1 trials to standard practice, *Chest*, 115: 38–48.

March, L., Irwig, L., Schwarz, J. *et al.* (1994) N of 1 trials comparing a non-steroidal anti-inflammatory drug with paracetamol in osteoarthritis, *British Medical Journal*, 309: 1041–5.

Meinert, C.L. (1986) *Clinical Trials: Design, Conduct and Analysis.* New York: Oxford University Press.

Moher, D., Jadad, A.R., Nichol, G. *et al.* (1995) Assessing the quality of randomized controlled trials: an annotated bibliography of scales and checklists, *Controlled Clinical Trials*, 16: 62–73.

Moher, D., Pham, B., Jones, A. *et al.* (1998) Does quality of reports of randomised trials affect estimates of intervention efficacy reported in meta-analyses? *Lancet*, 352: 609–13.

Moher, D., Schulz, K.F. and Altman, D.G. (2001) The CONSORT statement: revised recommendations for improving the quality of reports of parallel-group randomised trials, *Lancet*, 357: 1191–4.

Peto, R. and Baigent, C. (1998) Trials: the next 50 years. Large scale randomised evidence of moderate benefits, *British Medical Journal*, 317: 1170–1.

Pocock, S.J. (1987) *Clinical Trials: A Practical Approach.* New York: Wiley.

Pocock, S.J. (2004) A major trial needs three statisticians: why, how and who?, *Statistics in Medicine*, 23: 1535–39.

Schulz, K.F., Chalmers, I., Hayes, R.J. and Altman, D.G. (1995) Empirical evidence of bias. Dimensions of methodological quality associated with estimates of treatment effects in controlled trials, *Journal of the American Medical Association*, 273: 408–12.

Schulz, K.F. and Grimes, D.A. (2002) Generation of allocation sequences in randomised trials: chance, not choice, *Lancet*, 359: 515–19.

Sibbald, B. and Roberts, C. (1998) Understanding controlled trials. Crossover trials, *British Medical Journal*, 316: 1719.

Torgerson, D.J. and Sibbald, B. (1998) Understanding controlled trials. What is a patient preference trial?, *British Medical Journal*, 316: 360.

Ukoumunne, O.C., Gulliford, M.C., Chinn, S. *et al.* (1999) Methods for evaluating area-wide and organisation-based interventions in health and health care: a systematic review, *Health Technology Assessment*, 3(5).

Verhagen, A.P., de Vet, H.C., de Bie, R.A., *et al.* (2001) The art of quality assessment of RCTs included in systematic reviews, *Journal of Clinical Epidemiology*, 54: 651–4.

Verhagen, A.P., de Vet, H.C., de Bie, R.A., Kessels *et al.* (1998) The Delphi list: a criteria list for quality assessment of randomized clinical trials for conducting systematic reviews developed by Delphi consensus, *Journal of Clinical Epidemiology*, 51: 1235–41.

Weijer, C., Shapiro, S.H. and Cranley, G.K. (2000) For and against: clinical equipoise and not the uncertainty principle is the moral underpinning of the randomised controlled trial, *British Medical Journal*, 321: 756–8.

Wilhelmsen, L. (2002) Role of the Data and Safety Monitoring Committee (DSMC), *Statistics in Medicine*, 21: 2823–9.

Wolfe, B., Del Rio, E., Weiss, S.L., *et al.* (2002) Validation of a single-patient drug trial methodology for personalized management of gastroesophageal reflux disease, *Journal of Managed Care Pharmacy*, 8: 459–68.

World Medical Association (2004) *Declaration of Helsinki* (as revised). http://www.wma.net/e/policy/b3.htm (accessed 1 June 2004).

6 Epidemiological study designs for health care research and evaluation

Richard M. Martin

Introduction

Epidemiology is the study of how often health-related events occur in different groups of people, why variations in the pattern of health and disease exist between populations, and the application of this study to the control of health problems. In the pioneering epidemiology texts of the early twentieth century, authors were largely concerned with infections and the aetiology of chronic disease. More recently, epidemiological study designs have been increasingly used in the evaluation of interventions and in assessing the provision and impact of health services (see Table 6.1). This evidence base can be obtained from routinely available statistics or by the use of specific epidemiological study designs.

In the hierarchy of research designs, the results of randomized controlled trials (RCTs) are considered to provide evidence of the highest grade. This is because if the investigator is successful in randomly assigning the intervention, the groups being compared should be similar with respect to all (known and unknown) factors related to the outcome, except for the intervention. Unpredictable random allocation, combined with blinding and intention to treat analysis, helps to ensure an unbiased estimate of the effect of an intervention (see Chapter 5). In contrast, the observational studies described in this chapter are often viewed as having less validity, since the potential biases known to afflict such studies could unquantifiably obscure, inflate or even reverse the real effects of treatment (MacMahon and Collins 2001). That is, the results may have arisen as a result of chance, bias, reverse causality or confounding (see Box 6.1 for definitions and later sections for elaboration).

RCTs, however, are often of poor quality, frequently provide conflicting evidence on the same question and are commonly based on highly selected populations (Concato *et al.* 2000). There are numerous situations in health services research when investigators will need to test hypotheses using observational studies where experimentation is unethical, difficult to implement, unnecessary, inappropriate or difficult to generalize, and researchers may undertake observational studies to generate hypotheses (Black 1996), identify rare but serious adverse effects (Jick *et al.* 1998), test the effects of interventions in a broad representation of the population at risk (Concato *et al.* 2000) and evaluate complex systems (Rychetnik *et al.* 2002) (see Box 6.2 for examples).

Table 6.1 Some uses of epidemiology in health services research

Issues investigated by epidemiological studies	Examples in the literature
Assessing population requirements for health care	Population requirement for primary hip replacement surgery: cross-sectional study (Frankel *et al.* 1999)
Evaluation of health care programmes	Effect of the transformation of the Veterans Affairs health care system on the quality of care: descriptive study (Jha *et al.* 2003)
Improving patient care	Optimum decision to delivery intervals for emergency caesarean section: cross-sectional study (Thomas *et al.* 2004)
To monitor implementation of guidance	Impact of NICE guidance on laparoscopic surgery for inguinal hernias: analysis of interrupted time series (Bloor *et al.* 2003)
Monitoring health care utilization	Equity in the use of coronary revascularisation by gender, age, deprivation and geography in the South West region, 1991–2000: database study (Ebrahim *et al.* 2002)
Investigating the impact of inequality in access to health care	Deprivation and late presentation of glaucoma: case-control study (Fraser *et al.* 2001)
Evaluating the organization of health care services	An inner city GP unit versus conventional care for elderly patients: cohort study (Boston *et al.* 2001)
Assessing the impact of overuse or underuse of health care interventions	Underuse of coronary revascularization procedures in patients considered appropriate candidates for revascularization: cohort study (Hemingway *et al.* 2001).
Surveillance and analysis for the detection of rare adverse effects of drugs (pharmaco-epidemiology)	Risk of non-fatal cardiac failure and ischaemic heart disease with long acting beta2 agonists: cohort study (Martin *et al.* 1998)
Investigating long-term outcomes, including those that are transgenerational	Parents' growth in childhood and the birth weight of their offspring: cohort study (Martin *et al.* 2004a)
Evaluating the health effects of social interventions	Evaluating a nurse-led attendance allowance screening service in general practice: uncontrolled cohort study (Thomson *et al.* 2004)
Understanding contextual effects (e.g. social participation) on individual health and health care utilization	Effect of neighborhood social participation on individual use of hormone replacement therapy and antihypertensive medication: cross-sectional study (Merlo *et al.* 2003)
Assessing the acceptability of health care interventions	Rates of continuation with newly prescribed antihypertensive drugs: cohort study using automated data (Jones *et al.* 1995)
Monitoring regional variations in provision of services	Regional variation in case fatality of myocardial infarction among young women (Dunn *et al.* 2000)
Evaluating quality of care	Quality assessment of 26304 herniorrhaphies in Denmark: database study (Bay-Nielsen *et al.* 2001)
Generating hypotheses	Cyclo-oxygenase 2 inhibition (a novel class of non-steroidal anti-inflammatory drug) and breast cancer prevention (Vainio and Morgan 1998)

The ubiquitous presence of a number of sources of bias in the conduct and interpretation of observational research (Davey Smith and Ebrahim 2002) requires that the design of such studies adheres to fundamental epidemiological principles to minimize the effects of bias. While epidemiologists seek to obtain valid (unbiased) evidence about the hypothesis under study, it is not always feasible (e.g. for logistical or ethical reasons) to conduct the ideal research study. When planning a new study

Box 6.1   Definitions of non-causal explanations of associations

- **Bias:** a departure from the *true* value when one observes an association between an exposure and an outcome.
- **Chance:** variation due to random fluctuations.
- **Confounding:** a situation in which a measure of the effect of an exposure is distorted because of the association of exposure with other factor(s) (*confounders*) that influence the outcome under study.
- **Reverse causality:** this term is applied to an exposure-outcome association which is thought to be due to the outcome actually causing the exposure rather than the other way round.

Source: Last (1995)

Box 6.2   Examples of reasons to conduct observational rather than experimental studies

- To study the effects of radioactivity it would be *unethical* to allocate individuals to be exposed or unexposed. Instead we have to observe subjects who have been exposed, either through some natural experiment (e.g. survivors of atomic bombs) or cancer patients treated with radiotherapy.
- Some interventions are theoretically possible but *difficult to implement*. For example, in order to study the long-term effects of exposure to having been breast-fed it is unlikely that many new mothers would accept random allocation to breast-feed or bottle-feed. Instead we have to observe subjects who were breast-fed as infants.
- If the effect of an intervention is dramatic and the likelihood of confounders small (e.g. penicillin for bacterial infections or insulin therapy for insulin dependent diabetes), experimentation may be *unnecessary*.
- Trials, even large ones, are often too small to detect rare events or outcomes that occur many years after the trial has ended – i.e. trials may be *inappropriate*. This is why all suspected adverse reactions to newly-marketed drugs have to be reported to national drug regulatory bodies.
- If trials recruit atypical subjects, their results may not be *generalizable* (Padkin, *et al.* 2001). It is known that subjects entering disease intervention trials are often different from all subjects with that disease (e.g. they may be more likely to adhere to therapy). The health care professionals or the trial setting may also be atypical or patients may receive better treatment or more rigorous monitoring and follow-up simply because they are in a trial. To investigate whether a treatment has a similar effect in routine clinical practice to that observed in a trial, one could examine a large observational dataset with data on a representative sample of patients.
- Observational studies may be used to *generate hypotheses* that are subsequently tested in randomized trials. For example, associations between diet and cancer seen in observational studies have subsequently been tested in randomized trials of food supplements.

or critically appraising the published literature, therefore, it is important to be aware of both the scope and limitations of each type of epidemiological study design. The main aims of this chapter are twofold: firstly, to provide a methodological overview of the major observational epidemiological study designs; and secondly, to describe the threats to the valid conduct and interpretation of observational studies and how these may be dealt with in the design and analysis of studies. The chapter addresses measures of occurrence of health-related events, epidemiological study designs, relative and absolute measures of exposure effect, interpretation of epidemiological studies and their conduct. RCTs are addressed in detail in Chapter 5 and are not considered any further in this chapter.

Overview of study designs

A broad distinction can be drawn between two types of study design: (a) *interventional* and (b) *observational* (see Figure 6.1). An interventional or experimental study is when the investigator tests whether modifying or changing something about the study participants alters the development or course of the outcome. For example, if a random half of smokers were given free nicotine patches and the other half were not, an investigator could determine whether free nicotine patches increased the proportion of participants who quit smoking over the subsequent year. The essence of an interventional study is that the investigator has the power to randomly assign exposures in a way that enhances the validity of a study.

Observational studies involve the investigator collecting data on factors (exposures) associated with the occurrence or progression of the outcome of interest, without attempting to alter the exposure status of participants. For example, a study could observe whether smokers are more likely to have a heart attack than non-smokers. The investigator does not intervene or manipulate the situation in any way, he or she simply *observes*. The essence of an observational epidemiological study is neatly captured in a quote by the baseball player, Yogi Berra: 'You can observe a lot just by watching.' However, since the investigator does not control the circumstances of the exposure, a simple comparison of exposed and unexposed will not accurately reflect the effect of the exposure if those who are exposed differ from those who are unexposed in other ways that are related to the outcome.

The principal observational epidemiological methods are *cohort studies*, in which participants are classified (and possibly selected) according to the presence or

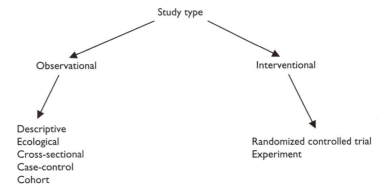

Figure 6.1 Overview of design strategies in epidemiology

absence of an exposure and followed up over time to ascertain the incidence of the outcome of interest; *case-control studies*, in which participants are selected according to the outcome of interest, and further classified according to their exposure status; *cross-sectional* (prevalence) *studies*, which describe the health of populations; and *ecological studies*, in which the units of observation are groups of people. *Case series* describe the characteristics of a number of patients with a given disease, but are usually based on a single clinician's experience and lack an appropriate comparison group. A search using the search engine of the BMJ publishing group website for the phrases 'case series', 'cohort study', 'case-control study' and 'cross-sectional study' in the title or abstract between January 2000 and May 2004 suggests that cohort studies (2970 hits) and case–control studies (2024 hits) are the most popular study designs, followed by cross-sectional studies (1217 hits) and case series (1009 hits). It is likely that case series are still overused and frequently overinterpreted in the medical research literature.

Some authors broadly classify observational studies as either *descriptive*, presenting the occurrence and distribution of an outcome, or *analytic*, which test hypotheses about disease causation (Hennekens and Buring 1987). Analytic studies usually demand the use of controls (exposed versus unexposed or case versus control), whereas descriptive studies do not (Grimes and Schulz 2002). The distinction is not always clear (Bhopal 2002), however, since descriptive data can be used to generate and explore hypotheses and analytic studies contain descriptive data. For example, a case–control study was established with the aim of investigating associations of different types of the oral contraceptive pill with the occurrence of heart attacks in young women (Dunn *et al.* 1999). Since the study identified all young women with a first heart attack presenting to National Health Service (NHS) hospitals in England and Scotland in a defined period of time, the investigators were also able to examine regional variations in the incidence and case fatality of heart attacks among young women (Dunn *et al.* 2000).

Measures of the occurrence of health-related events

A fundamental task in epidemiology is to quantify the occurrence of health-related events with reference to the size of the population (the population at risk) during specified points or periods of time. Outcomes of interest can include a wide range of events, such as disease, disability, death, recovery and use of health services. The importance of defining occurrence in relation to a population at risk is illustrated in the following example. If a GP had seen three male cases of Parkinson's disease over the last year and all had worked in the local pesticide factory, he may suspect a toxic aetiology. If 95 per cent of his male catchment population worked at the factory, this would be less suspicious. The two main measures of occurrence are *prevalence* and *incidence*. Prevalence quantifies existing cases while incidence quantifies the occurrence of new cases.

Prevalence

Prevalence is defined as the number of instances of a given disease or other condition in a given population at a designated time (Last 1995):

Number of existing cases in a defined population at a given point in time

Number of people in the defined population at the same point in time

For example, among 301 randomly selected Canadian Aboriginal people aged

35–75 living in Canada's Six Nation's Reserve between 1998–2000, 45 had coronary heart disease (Anand *et al.* 2001). The *prevalence* of coronary heart disease is $45/301 = 15$ per cent. Although prevalence has no time units, the point in time to which it refers must be specified.

The *point prevalence* is the prevalence based on a single examination at a fixed point in time. If repeated or continuous assessments of the same individuals are possible the *period prevalence* can be calculated, defined as the prevalence over a stated period of time (e.g. a week, a month or a longer time interval). Period prevalence represents the number of people who were counted as cases at any time during a specified period divided by the total number of people in that population during that time. For example, the proportion of people aged over 65 who have used painkillers at any time during a 12-month study is a period prevalence.

Incidence

Incidence is defined as the rate at which new events occur in a population during a specified period (Last 1995). Two distinct measures of incidence may be calculated: incidence risk and incidence rate. The *incidence risk* is:

$$\frac{\text{Number of new events in a defined population over a specified period}}{\text{Number of disease-free people in that population at the start of the time period}}$$

For example, a total of 5632 women aged 55–64 attended their local breast cancer screening service during 1990 and were found to be free of breast cancer. Over the next five years, 58 were diagnosed with breast cancer. The *incidence risk* of breast cancer over the five-year period was therefore $58/5632 = 0.0103$ (1.0 per cent).

Risk is a probability (so can never be more than 1 or 100 per cent) and is usually applied to non-recurrent disease or the first episode of an event. The denominator (number of persons at risk) has to be carefully defined. For example, for endometrial cancer (cancer of the lining of the womb) or cervical cancer the denominator is not all women but all women who have not had a hysterectomy. This is because a hysterectomy operation removes the womb and such women will no longer be at risk of endometrial or cervical cancer. Although risk has no time units, the time period to which it relates must be specified as its value increases with the duration of follow-up.

Incidence rate

Sometimes measurement of incidence is complicated by changes in the population at risk during the period when the cases are ascertained. This can occur because some participants enter the study some time after it begins (e.g. by birth, migration to the study area or recruitment into the study) or because some are lost during follow-up (e.g. through deaths, emigrations, refusals or other losses to follow-up). Events that 'compete' with the outcome of interest (deaths or other causes) to remove people from the population at risk are sometimes referred to as *competing risks*. To account for varying lengths of follow-up when calculating incidence rates, the number of new cases is related not to the number initially at risk but to each individual's time at risk (the *person-time at risk*), computed by adding together the lengths of time during which each individual member of the population is at risk during the measurement period. This is the *incidence rate*, defined as:

$$\frac{\text{Number of new events in a defined population over a specified time period}}{\text{Total person-time at risk during the specified time period}}$$

Rates are not probabilities and can be used to estimate the incidence of recurrent events. For example, general practice consultation rates in men aged 16–24 years were 2.21 per person per year, and were 2.52 per person per year in men aged 25–39 years (Martin *et al.* 2001). When presenting an incident rate, the time units must be specified (e.g. person–years at risk, person–days at risk etc.).

Person-time at risk is equivalent to the number at risk during the period of observation, multiplied by the mean period of observation. To illustrate how to calculate incidence rates, Table 6.2 shows data for five people who are part of a long-term follow-up study, the Boyd Orr cohort study (Gunnell *et al.* 1996). In this study 4999 children took part in a survey of diet and health between 1937–9. They were followed up until 28 February 2003 by linking of their survey records with information on their death certificates supplied by the NHS Central Registry in England and Scotland. There are three ways in which follow-up can end: (i) the person can be followed-up to the end of the follow-up period (28 February 2003); (ii) the person can be lost to follow-up; (iii) the person can experience the outcome of interest. Once a person is classified as a case, he or she is no longer at risk of becoming a new case, and therefore should not contribute further person-years at risk. Suppose we wish to calculate the incidence rate of coronary heart disease (CHD) during the long-term follow-up of these five people. From the table, the five exposed people have follow up times of 55.16, 54.03, 10.67, 29.03 and 54.92 years, which add up to 203.81 years. In these 203.81 years, there were two deaths from coronary heart disease, for an incidence rate of 0.0098 cases per year. This can be expressed as 9.8 cases per 1000 person-years.

In a published example, researchers investigated the risk of cardiovascular death and non-fatal venous thromboembolism (VTE, a blood clot in the venous circulation) in women using oral contraceptives with differing progestagen components (Jick *et al.* 1995). The study was conducted on a computerized general practice database, holding a longitudinal record for each patient of their medical and prescribing history. Women who had ever been prescribed one of the study oral contraceptive pills (OCPs) in the past were retrospectively identified, and entered the study on the date of their first prescription. The womens' records were retrospectively reviewed for the occurrence of VTE, while on the OCP between 1991–4. Women who discontinued the OCP, or were prescribed a different OCP, or who died or transferred out of the practice were considered no longer at risk of developing an event.

Since women were followed for variable lengths of time, it would not have been reasonable to calculate risks of VTE (as this would require a fixed length of follow-up for all women in the cohort). Instead the investigators measured the *incidence rate* of VTE among women with exposure to the study OCPs (either one of the newer third generation pills or one of the older second generation pills). To estimate person-time at risk for each study drug, the investigators accumulated the time from the date of the first study OCP until the first of the following occurred: the OCP

Table 6.2 Follow-up data for five participants in the Boyd Orr cohort study

ID	Date entered study	Date follow-up ended	Reason follow-up ended	Years of follow-up
1	13/10/1938	28/02/2003	End of study	55.16
2	03/11/1937	03/11/2002	Death other than CHD	54.03
3	14/10/1937	01/09/1958	Emigrated	10.67
4	04/12/1937	12/01/1997	Died of CHD	29.03
5	03/04/1937	03/12/2002	Died of CHD	54.92

was discontinued, a different OCP was prescribed, the woman died or transferred out of the practice or the study period ended. The 'number of women-years at risk' was thus the number of years each woman contributed to follow-up, summed for all the women in the study.

Rates of VTE were calculated by dividing the number of cases in each category of OCP (second or third generation pills) by the number of women-years at risk in each category of OCP. The data in Table 6.3 show that the women on third generation pills had nearly twice the incidence rate of VTE compared with women on a second generation pill.

Rates can be estimated from routinely collected data (e.g. vital statistics or cancer registration data) even though direct measures of person-time at risk are unavailable. An estimate of the person-time at risk during a specified time period is given by the size of the population at the mid-point of the calendar period of interest multiplied by the length of the time period.

Relationship between incidence and prevalence

Both incidence and duration of disease influence prevalence. Each incident case enters a prevalence pool and remains there until either recovery or death. If recovery and death rates are low (e.g. as in chronic diseases such as diabetes mellitus and multiple sclerosis), prevalence will be high even if incidence is low. Conversely, diseases with a short duration may have a low prevalence even if the incidence is high. The short duration may be either because the disease leads to rapid death (e.g. dissecting aortic aneurysm) or because recovery is prompt (e.g. appropriately treated appendicitis). The low prevalence implies that at any one moment a small proportion of people are suffering with, for example, dissecting aortic aneurysm. Prevalence may vary from one population to another because of variations in survival and recovery, as well as incidence. In general, prevalence is approximately equal to incidence multiplied by the mean duration of illness as long as the incidence and duration of disease are constant, and the prevalence low (less than 10 per cent).

Uses of incidence and prevalence

Incidence is most useful in studies of disease aetiology because prevalent cases are either a select group of survivors or chronic sufferers, and long-standing disease may modify people's behaviour and hence exposure to risk factors. Prevalence measures the burden of disease in a population and is a useful measure for public health professionals assessing a population's requirements for health care resources. For example, when need is greater than supply the prevalent number of people in the population with angina and who meet certain specific criteria predicts the need in that population for coronary revascularization (Martin *et al.* 2002). Prevalence is often used as an alternative to incidence in the study of the aetiology of rarer

Table 6.3   Results of cohort analysis on risk of venous thromboembolism

Type of OCP	No. with VTE	Women-years at risk	Incidence rate per 100,000
2nd generation	23	143,255	16.1
3rd generation	52	180,633	28.8

Source: Jick *et al.* (1998)

chronic diseases or events with an indefinite time of onset (such as occurs in mental illness), but differences in prevalence between populations may reflect differential survival rather than incidence. Mortality is the incidence of death from a disease. Mortality is only a satisfactory proxy for incidence, however, if survival is not related to the factors under investigation. For example, the decline in mortality from testicular cancer since 1970 is due to improved treatment efficacy, and does not reflect a fall in incidence (Brown *et al.* 1986).

Crude, specific and adjusted rates

A crude incidence or prevalence rate is one that relates to a whole population without any adjustment for the population age/sex structure. Crude rates may, therefore, mask differences in rates between various age and sex groups. For this reason it may be appropriate to present rates according to specific age and/or sex groups. When comparing rates in different populations, differences in the age/sex structure of the population may need to be taken into account by the calculation of *age-* and/or *sex-standardized rates.* Age and/or sex standardized rates are the number of events occurring in a defined population over a period of time, with adjustment for the age/sex structure of the population. Comparing rates that have been adjusted for age and sex ensures that differences in the age/sex structure of the population are not the explanation for observed differences in event rates between populations. Details of the methods used to calculate standardized rates are given by dos Santos Silva (1999: Chapter 4).

Routine sources of data

Routine sources of data serve a number of important roles in epidemiology. Firstly, they are a major source of data in descriptive studies which describe the distribution of a characteristic of interest in terms of time, place (e.g. between and within countries, urban versus rural) or person (e.g. age, sex, ethnicity, marital status, occupation). Secondly, they can be used to identify exposed and unexposed participants in cohort studies or cases and controls in case-control studies; thirdly, they can be linked to participants in cohort studies to provide outcome data (record-linkage studies).

Routine data are those that are routinely collected and are therefore often less time-consuming and less expensive to acquire. They typically cover large populations, sometimes millions of people, followed up for several years. There are, however, a number of disadvantages. Firstly, since they are usually not collected for specific epidemiological purposes, data are frequently of worse quality and accuracy than studies that are specifically established to test particular hypotheses. Secondly, information on confounding factors is generally not available. Thirdly, appropriate denominators to calculate measures of the occurrence of outcomes and the effect of exposures may be difficult to define. For example, in a routine database study of factors associated with prolonged waiting for elective surgery, the outcome was the rate of waiting, in which the numerator was the number of people waiting six months or more in a particular specialty and the denominator was the specialty-specific numbers of finished consultant episodes for each Trust, a proxy for the catchment population of each specialty in each Trust (population at risk) (Martin *et al.* 2003). If the denominator did not fully capture the size of the catchment population, comparisons of rates of prolonged waiting by factors related to the catchment population (such as numbers of consultants or hospital beds) may be biased (numerator/denominator bias). Finally, the number of variables available from routine data systems is generally limited. The variables that are available may therefore be used as proxy measures of more relevant exposures. In an example given in more detail below, differences in prostate cancer incidence were used as a proxy measure of the intensity of prostate specific antigen (PSA) screening (Coldman *et al.* 2003).

Several routine data sources, their uses and disadvantages are summarized in Table 6.4. There is increasing interest in the potential for a wide variety of routine databases, particularly those that are electronic, to provide evidence to plan and monitor health services, measure quality of care and undertake population-based research (Majeed 2004). However, it is important that the investigator is fully aware of the way the data were collected and processed so that all possible sources of data artefacts, bias and confounding are considered in the interpretation of the findings. The problems of analysing routine data have recently been highlighted by two studies from different investigators using the same dataset (General Practice Research Database) which reached opposite conclusions on the relation of third generation contraceptive pills and the risk of VTE (Skegg 2000). Several initiatives to improve the quality and completeness of electronic data recording in specific settings, such as in primary care (de Lusignan *et al.* 2004), are now being reported.

Descriptive studies

Descriptive studies are used by public health specialists, health protection agencies and health care providers for the surveillance of communicable and non-communicable diseases, to decide on the allocation of resources and to plan prevention or health promotion programmes (Grimes and Schulz 2002). Epidemiologists also undertake descriptive studies to identify clues as to possible determinants of diseases or disease risk factors, to identify potential modifiable environmental factors or to test particular hypotheses.

Analyses by time

The frequency of diseases, health events or risk factors may increase, decrease or stay constant over time. These trends can provide clues as to what might cause changes in health-related factors or events, or whether attempts at prevention have been successful. For example, declines in blood pressure levels among students entering university between 1948–68 suggested hypotheses about environmental contributions to elevated blood pressure (McCarron *et al.* 2001). In another study, researchers used data from prostate cancer cases and deaths reported to the British Columbia Cancer Registry during 1985–99 to test whether intensive prostate cancer screening using PSA is linked to reductions in prostate cancer mortality (Coldman *et al.* 2003). The hypothesis was tested by comparing changes in mortality between 1985–9 and 1990–4 in geographic areas defined as having low, medium or high levels of screening intensity (see Table 6.5). As the study was based on routine data, the level of PSA testing could not be directly determined. The authors reasoned, however, that differences in the incidence of prostate cancer between areas are likely to reflect differences in the detection of preclinical prostate cancer through PSA screening. Differences in prostate cancer incidence were therefore used as a proxy measure of the intensity of PSA screening. The table shows that mortality declines were greatest in those areas with low screening levels and vice versa, suggesting no association between intensity of PSA screening and prostate cancer mortality.

Table 6.4 Sources of routine statistics

Source	Description	Limitations
Census and population statistics	A population census is a periodic (often decennial) count of the number and characteristics (geographic, demographic, health-related, occupational, educational and economic) of people and households in a given area. Data provide denominators in routine health statistics and measures of population density and deprivation (e.g. Townsend Deprivation Score) at small area level.	The data are incomplete for some population sub-groups (very young children, young males, the homeless, armed forces). Statements (e.g. about age, marital status, occupation) may be inaccurate or vague. The data can become out of date rapidly. Population estimates are made between census points, using the last census as a baseline, but become less reliable over time.
Mortality statistics	Death certificates contain information on the immediate, underlying and contributory causes of death. National statistics bodies code the underlying cause of death according to the International Classification of Diseases, currently in the tenth revision. Other information includes place and date of birth, age at death, address, occupation. Such data allow record linkage (see below) and analyses of occupational mortality (e.g. Aylin et al. 1999).	Statements of cause of death may reflect fashions in diagnosis or differences in coding, distorting secular and geographical trends. At any time point, mortality data are subject to errors in diagnosis of cause of death or omissions in completing death certificates, which may vary by social class, age or sex. Classification and coding rules change over time, also distorting secular trends. There may be errors in selecting an underlying cause of death when several pathological conditions exist.
Cancer registers	Population-based cancer registries have been established in a number of countries. They record details of all people diagnosed with cancer to provide information on cancer frequency by time, geography and within population sub-groups. They allow comparison of survival rates by cancer stage or cancer type over time (e.g. disease-specific mortality rates for conservatively treated localized prostate cancer, stratified by histology, were estimated in the Connecticut Tumour Registry) (Albertsen et al. 1998).	Rely on voluntary notification and considerable under-registration has been found. The delay between the diagnosis of incident cancer and entry onto the register may be considerable, reducing the usefulness of such registers to identify incident cases (e.g. for case-control studies). Other problems are incomplete, inaccurate or missing records, duplicate entries, incomparability of diagnosis and coding over time and geographically, and inaccurate enumeration of the population. Disease patterns may reflect differences in health service access (including screening).
Other registers	Population-based registers have been established for other conditions (such as myocardial infarction, asthma, diabetes, new variant CJD, renal transplant, coronary artery bypass surgery, caesarean section, blindness, disability and congenital malformations) and are widely used for health services research.[1]	The limitations given above for cancer registers also apply to other registers. Registers based on highly select groups, such as people with asthma attending a particular hospital, are of limited usefulness in population-based research.
Hospital-based data	Computerized hospital discharge registers are available in some countries (e.g. in England, the Hospital Episodes Statistics (HES) database captures all episodes of inpatient care in the NHS, and records administrative, admission and clinical details). An example of the use of such data in assessing gender inequalities in coronary revascularization is given in Ebrahim et al. (2002). Similar systems exist in Scotland, where hospital-based data have been linked to other routine sources of data, such as community-based prescribing records (MEMO database).[2]	Variations in routine hospital data could reflect differences in recording practices and referral/admission/surgical policies rather than true variations in disease incidence. The data can rarely be linked to other records (MEMO is an exception).[3] Largely limited to descriptive and ecological analyses. Limitations in completeness and accuracy of the data, although data quality may improve with more use. Multiple occurrences of one individual can occur when they are referred from specialist to specialist. Defining the catchment populations of hospitals is problematic, making it difficult to provide a denominator for these data.

Morbidity statistics in general practice	Much information on morbidity, treatment, outcomes and health care utilization is routinely recorded by GPs and is often computerized. Data are population-based. In the UK, where GPs are responsible for a defined list of people, data on numbers of consultations for different disorders are readily converted to morbidity rates[4] and general practice data has been extensively used for health services research and pharmaco-epidemiology.[5]	GP records are often incomplete and inaccurate. Information on ethnic group and socioeconomic status is generally absent. The commonly used datasets (such as the General Practice Research Database, the National Survey of Morbidity in General Practice and the communicable diseases returns service) are based on volunteer practices which may systematically differ from practices that do not volunteer to provide data.
Infectious disease notifications	In many countries certain communicable diseases must be notified. Changes in notifications can lead to immediate action to control outbreaks. The data can be used to evaluate public health interventions (e.g. following the introduction of specific meningitis vaccines there were sharp declines in the numbers of children with *Haemophilus influenzae* b meningitis and meningitis C).	The completeness of notification varies (rarer diseases are more likely to be notified than common diseases) so the data are limited for calculating absolute disease frequency. The data can be supplemented from other sources, such as specific reporting systems for HIV, AIDS and sexually transmitted diseases, and returns on selected communicable diseases from volunteer general practices.
Other sources of morbidity data	Data may be available from health authorities, and local and national government departments. Specifically, health visitor and school health service records are local sources of data on routine examinations of schoolchildren; medical sickness certifications provide data on sickness absence from work; the Health and Safety Executive have information on industrial diseases; drug regulatory agencies and pharmaceutical companies hold records of suspected adverse drug reactions reported by health professionals (e.g. the Yellow Card scheme in the UK).	Concerns include the completeness and accuracy of data, and lack of standardization of clinical examinations and diagnoses leading to misclassification of data. There may be problems identifying the population-based denominator (e.g. there are difficulties comparing reports of drug reactions between different drugs because the total number of people taking each drug is not directly known).
Health service capacity	Many countries record hospital and community health service capacity such as numbers of people waiting for elective surgery, numbers of specialists and GPs, numbers of operating and dedicated day-case theatres, bed occupancy rate, activity associated with paramedical services, health visiting and community nursing, and numbers of independent sector hospitals and clinics.	Use of these data is limited to descriptive and ecological analyses as they cannot be linked to individuals. There are problems defining a population denominator for these data (e.g. see paper by Martin *et al.* (2003)).
Special health and lifestyle surveys	Countries often undertake regular routine surveys to describe lifestyle and other factors which influence a population's health (e.g. the National Health and Nutrition Examination Survey (NHANES) in the USA and the Health Survey in England). Data are collected by means of questionnaires, physical examination and blood tests. Datasets can be downloaded for analysis (e.g. www.data-archive.ac.uk/; www.cdc.gov/nchs/nhanes.htm).	Data collection is based on rigorous epidemiological survey methods so suffer from fewer problems than other routinely available data. Investigators planning to analyse these data need to be aware of the sampling methods used and how to take account of sampling strategies in the analyses.

[1] For example, the MONICA project on trends and determinants in cardiovascular disease (Tunstall-Pedoe et al. 1999); a study using an obstetric register to examine decision to delivery interval in emergency caesarean section (Thomas et al. 2004).[2,3] For further information, see www.dundee.ac.uk/memo/.[4] For example, national morbidity surveys (Office of Population Censuses and Surveys, Department of Health, and Royal College of General Practitioners 1995).[5] For a comprehensive review of sources, strengths and limitations of primary care data in England, see Majeed (2004).

Table 6.5   Mortality of prostate cancer among men aged 50–70 years by intensity of PSA screening

Screening intensity	% increase in prostate cancer incidence 1985–9 to 1990–4	% decrease in prostate cancer mortality 1985–9 to 1990–4
Low	5.4	28.9
Medium	53.6	18.0
High	70.5	13.5
Total	53.2	17.6

Source: Coldman *et al.* (2003)

One limitation of this study is the phenomenon of the 'sticking diagnosis' leading to attribution bias. Men with a screen-detected prostate cancer are more likely to have prostate cancer recorded on the death certificate and to have this coded as a cause of death or contributing factor, even if it was an indolent cancer which would not have been detected in areas with low screening rates. This bias would lead to an apparent increase in prostate cancer deaths in areas with intensive screening. Other explanations that need to be considered to explain temporal trends are listed in Box 6.3.

Box 6.3   Explanations for temporal trends

- **Chance:** variations may be due to *random* fluctuations.
- **Case ascertainment:** change in *diagnostic* techniques so that disease is more likely to be diagnosed (e.g. increase in diagnosis of brain tumours with introduction of CT brain scanning) or changes in *diagnostic fashion*.
- **Demography:** change in *age distribution* of population. An ageing population will result in an apparent increase in crude disease rates but will not alter *age-specific rates*.
- **Coding:** changes in the rules by which mortality is coded (International Classification of Diseases, ICD) can produce spurious effects. This can be demonstrated by use of bridge coding (i.e. compare new rates using the old coding rules).
- **Treatment effects:** new medical therapies may have a beneficial effect on disease frequency (e.g. changes in coronary care and secondary prevention were linked with temporal declines in coronary events (Tunstall-Pedoe *et al.* 2000)) or rarely actually result in an increase in mortality due to iatrogenic causes (e.g. isoprenaline inhalers were associated with increased asthma mortality in New Zealand and other countries in the 1960s and 1970s – Beasley *et al.* 1990).
- **True changes in incidence:** changes in risk factors may have resulted in a true increase or decrease in the *incidence* of the disease. This suggests the potential role of prevention by altering these risk factors.

Patterns of disease mortality or incidence over time change (normally increasing) with age (*age effects*), vary by when a person was born (*cohort effects*; e.g. due to early nutritional and lifestyle exposures) and are related to the time a person was diagnosed (*period effects*; e.g. because the effectiveness of treatments changes over time).

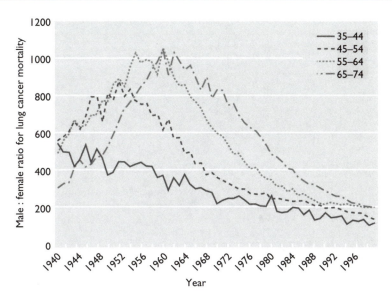

Figure 6.2 Secular trends in male : female ratio (expressed as a percentage) for lung cancer mortality for different generations in ten-year age bands, 1940–98, England and Wales

Source: Lawlor *et al.* BMJ 2001, 323: 541-5. Reproduced with permission from the BMJ Publishing Group.

Analyses should aim to separate out these three factors. For example, Lawlor *et al.* (2001) examined temporal trends in lung cancer among men and women using year of birth specific rates (see Figure 6.2). The male:female ratio for lung cancer mortality showed a clear cohort effect, with the peak occurring in later years for each successively older cohort. The cohort effect suggests an environmental exposure influencing successive generations – secular changes in sex differences in smoking behaviour is the likely exposure.

Analyses by place

Geographical studies compare health-related events in defined populations either between countries (international studies) or within countries, such as between regions or districts. The unit of observation is a population – for example, all people living in a country or town. Other populations can be analysed, such as a population of people within a hospital catchment area. Martin *et al.* (2003) plotted the geographic distribution of NHS Hospital Trusts with the most (top 25 per cent of the distribution) numbers of people waiting a prolonged length of time (at least six months) for elective surgery in 1999. Those Trusts with the highest number of prolonged waiters were generally clustered along the south coast, London, and in the North West of England (see Figure 6.3).

Analyses by person

Analyses can be undertaken according to personal characteristics such as gender, age, ethnicity or deprivation. For example, Ebrahim *et al.* (2002) investigated gender inequalities in the provision of coronary revascularization procedures. In

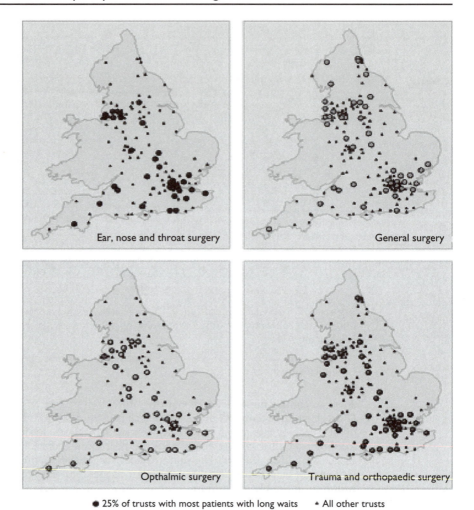

● 25% of trusts with most patients with long waits   ▲ All other trusts

Figure 6.3   Geographical distribution of Trusts with the most (top 25 per cent of the distribution) patients with prolonged waits in relation to all other Trusts: England, 1999 – inpatient elective surgery

Source: Martin *et al.* BMJ 2003, 326: 188-192. Reproduced with permission from the BMJ Publishing Group.

age-adjusted analyses, they found that men were twice as likely to be admitted to hospital with a diagnosis of acute myocardial infarction or unstable angina, but they were between three and five times more likely than women to have a coronary revascularization operation. Assuming admission due to acute myocardial infarction or unstable angina is a reasonable proxy for need for revascularization, and that women are as likely as men to benefit from the operation, a three- to fivefold difference is likely to reflect gender inequality in access to coronary revascularization.

Clinical case series

Clinicians may collect a series of cases that they have seen in the course of their clinics or ward work (clinical case series). Such case series are sometimes used as a source of descriptive data. For example, a review of the medical notes of men with prostate cancer diagnosed between 1949–86 revealed that the survival rates of men with localized prostate cancer who were managed conservatively were similar to the expected survival rate in the general male population of the same age (Warner and Whitmore, Jr 1994). This study suggests that men with low-grade prostate cancer might be safely treated expectantly, without recourse to radical surgery. However for the reasons that follow, it may be difficult to relate the case series to the population at risk. Due to difficulties identifying appropriate denominators, incidence risks and rates cannot be directly calculated and differences between groups in the same population cannot be directly assessed. Since not all patients with the condition will be receiving medical care, there may be a selection bias on the grounds of severity. In specialist hospitals, there may be preferential referral of a particular type of case. Finally the case series may be incomplete.

Individual case reports and case series, however, form the basis of surveillance schemes in many countries for the identification of rare adverse reactions to newly-marketed drugs. They have been successful in providing early leads for potential problems (see Box 6.4). However, case reports and case series can be misleading as a

---

Box 6.4   Early leads provided by case reports of suspected adverse drug reactions

- Phocomelia (the absence of limbs or parts of limbs) due to *in-utero* exposure to thalidomide.
- Oculomucocutaneous syndrome caused by practolol.
- Deaths from liver disease due to benoxaprofen.
- Hepatocellular adenomas in women who had taken oral contraceptives.
- Severe persistent visual field constriction associated with vigabatrin.
  (Eke *et al.* 1997)

---

result of a number of biases, including: (i) reverse causality, where a newly-marketed drug is given to patients with more severe disease, the symptoms of which are mistaken for side-effects; (ii) reporting bias, where adverse publicity or case reports of a possible association between the drug and event leads to a surge in the reporting rates with that particular drug but not to a similar surge in reporting rates with other drugs (also called notoriety bias); (iii) the difficulty of identifying appropriate denominators for the calculation of rates. For example, case reports to the Medicines and Healthcare products Regulatory Agency (MHRA) in the UK suggested an association between sertindol (an anti-psychotic drug) and sudden death. However, cohort studies, which allow a comparison of actual death rates and are less prone to reporting bias, found no association between the drug and sudden death (Moore *et al.* 2003).

Record linkage studies

As well as using routine data for descriptive analyses, routine databases can be used as a source of exposure or outcome data in case-control, cohort or cross-sectional stuides. This is only possible, however, if the registers contain a unique identifier than can be linked to other registers or to unique identifiers within a specific epidemiological study. For example, in Nordic countries everyone is assigned a personal number used for all economic, census and health records – mortality, hospital admissions and cancer incidence data can be readily traced for a census sample and other cohorts (Rasmussen *et al.* 2003); in the UK a national register, the NHS Central Register, is widely used for follow-up studies of exposures related to future risks of cancer, all-cause and cause-specific mortality (Gunnell *et al.* 1998a); in the Avon Longitudinal Study of Pregnancy and Children birth cohort, routinely collected growth data from health visitor records are linked to other questionnaire, physical examination and biochemical data collected longitudinally on each child (Martin *et al.* 2004c).

Morris *et al.* (1997) used a record linkage database to investigate the adverse consequences of poor adherence to insulin treatment among young patients (mean age: 16 years) with Type 1 diabetes resident in Tayside, Scotland. Using a unique patient identifier known as a Community Health Number (CHNo), records were linked between hospital diabetes clinics, pharmacies that dispense prescriptions, hospital discharge databases, community diabetic screening and biochemistry databases. The authors found that non-adherence with recommended insulin therapy among young people was relatively common (28 per cent) and was linked with poor control of diabetes and higher rates of admission for complications.

Epidemiological modelling

Results from epidemiological studies can be applied to population denominators and other routine data sources to estimate the population impact of interventions. For example, Martin *et al.* (2002) estimated the need for coronary revascularization among 45–84-year-olds with stable angina, unstable angina and acute myocardial infarction. Six key steps along the pathway of care from initial diagnosis in primary or secondary care to revascularization were defined and the frequency of indications for coronary revascularization (based on ability to benefit as defined by randomized trials, expert panel ratings or by informal consensus) estimated using routine hospital admissions data and data from studies in the general population, primary and secondary care. Data were applied to the mid-1998 population of England. The study suggested that the UK national target of 1500 revascularization procedures per million population is credibly related to population need.

Ecological studies (synonyms: correlation, aggregate, geographical studies)

An ecological study is one where the unit of observation and analysis is a group rather than an individual. In this type of study, the exposure of individuals is not linked to their outcome. Instead of carrying out individual measurements of study participants (as in cross-sectional, case-control or cohort studies), aggregate measures of both exposure and outcome at the level of entire populations are used. The group is often defined according to a geographic area (ecological studies are sometimes referred to as 'geographic' studies). Groups may also be defined in other ways, such as according to place of birth, occupation, socioeconomic status and so on. Figure 6.4 is an example of an ecological study (Mangtani *et al.* 1995). The

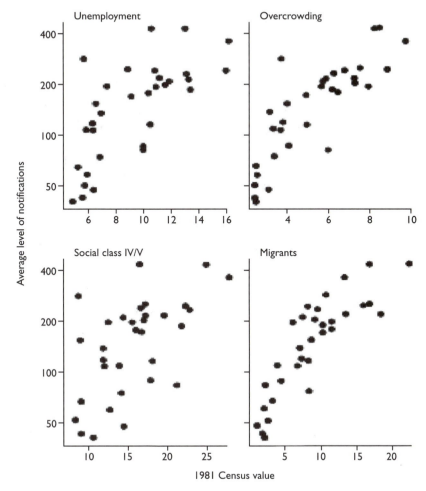

Figure 6.4   Scatter plots of average tuberculosis notification rates from 1982 to 1991 (ten-year average standardized notification ratio) against percentage unemployed, living in overcrowded accommodation, in social class IV/V, and migrated from new Commonwealth countries in 1981 in 32 London boroughs

Source: Mangtani *et al.* BMJ 1995; 310: 963–966. Reproduced with permission from the BMJ Publishing Group.

exposures are the percentage of people unemployed, living in overcrowded accommodation, in social class IV/V, and who migrated from new Commonwealth countries in 32 London boroughs. The outcome is the average tuberculosis notification rate in each of the London boroughs. The data suggest an increase in tuberculosis associated with overcrowding and the proportion of migrants in an area.

Ecological studies are generally based on routinely available data, and are therefore relatively easy to perform and inexpensive. Where data are not available from routine data collection systems, they may be obtained from previously conducted surveys. Furthermore, studies on individuals of any design can be analysed ecologically using data aggregated by geographical area. For example, Yusuf *et al.* (1998) identified 7987 consecutive patients presenting with unstable angina from 95 hospitals in six countries and followed them up for six months. Although the study was based on the follow-up of individuals (cohort study), the data were analysed ecologically by comparing the mean intervention rates in the six countries with mean rates of cardiovascular death, myocardial infarction, stroke, refractory angina and major bleeding. The rates of invasive procedures were highest in Brazil and the USA, intermediate in Canada and Australia, and lowest in Hungary and Poland. There were no differences, however, in rates of cardiovascular death or myocardial infarction among these countries. On the other hand, rates of stroke were higher in Brazil and the USA than in the countries with lower intervention rates (see Figure 6.5).

Uses of ecological studies

Ecological studies have a number of important uses in epidemiology. Firstly, they often provide important *hypothesis-generating evidence*. The above study by Yusuf *et al.*, for example, suggests that a policy of routine invasive procedures in patients with unstable angina may not be beneficial and could even be harmful. Randomized trials should assess the relative impact of conservative and more invasive approaches to the management of patients with unstable angina (Yusuf *et al.* 1998). Ecological comparisons conducted in the 1950s and 1960s gave rise to prevailing ideas on the causes of cancer (e.g. dietary factors and colon cancer, hepatitis B and liver cancer, aflatoxins and liver cancer, human papilloma virus and cervical cancer).

Secondly, some exposures in epidemiology – for example air pollutants, water quality, naturally occurring fluoride levels, ionizing radiation, neighbourhood social characteristics and sunlight – are largely geographic in character and, in the absence of individual exposure measurements on a large number of people, can only be studied ecologically. Thirdly, error in measuring exposure may be greater for individuals than for populations. Such errors tend to increase the apparent similarity between exposed and unexposed groups, leading to the underestimation (attenuation) of the true association (Gardner and Heady 1973). This bias, which may be substantial, is sometimes also called regression dilution bias (MacMahon *et al.* 1990). Fourthly, ecological studies may be useful for monitoring the effectiveness of population interventions such as health education campaigns, mass screening and vaccination programmes (e.g. the Community Intervention Trial for Smoking Cessation – COMMIT investigators 1995). Fifthly, many important individual-level risk factors for disease do not vary enough within populations to enable their effects to be identified or studied. Ecological studies may be useful to investigate the effects of exposures that are relatively homogeneous within populations but show wide variability between populations. For example, the relationship between blood pressure in childhood and sodium levels in drinking water has been investigated ecologically, by comparing mean blood pressure levels in areas with high and low sodium in the public drinking water (Hofman *et al.* 1980).

Lastly, ecological studies can be used to test hypotheses. Investigating the relationship between blood pressure and the sodium content of drinking water is a test of the hypothesis that blood pressure levels are influenced by sodium intake. Recently, investigators tested the hypothesis that the measles, mumps, rubella (MMR) vaccine is associated with the development of autism by comparing age-specific secular trends in uptake of the MMR vaccine with trends in autism (see Figure 6.6). They found a marked increase in the incidence of autism in children's electronic general practice records over 11 years. They concluded that MMR could not be the cause of this observed increase since vaccine coverage remained constant over the same time.

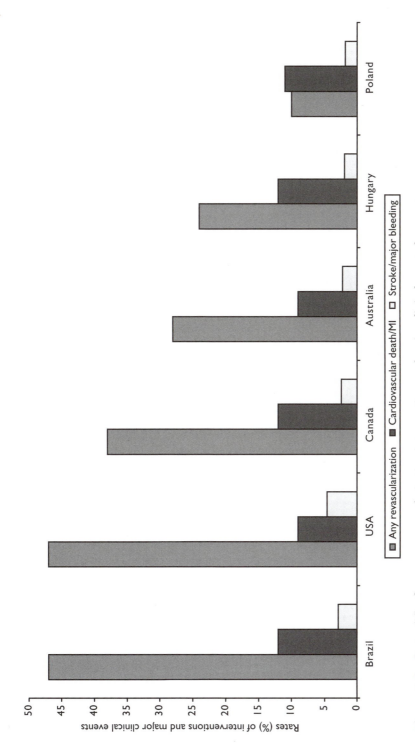

Figure 6.5 Rates (%) of coronary revascularization interventions and major clinical events, by country
Source: Yusuf *et al.* (1998)

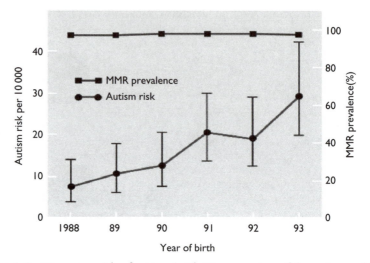

Figure 6.6   Four-year risk of autism (with 95 per cent confidence intervals) among boys aged 2 to 5 years and prevalence of MMR vaccine, by annual birth cohort

Source: Kaye *et al.* BMJ 2001; 322: 460-463. Reproduced with permission from the BMJ Publishing Group.

Limitations of ecological studies

Ecological studies have a number of limitations. First is the assumption that the average characteristics of *populations* are applicable to *individuals* within the population (the *ecological fallacy*). A famous example relates to the association between suicide rates and religion in regions of Prussia. Durkheim ([1897] 1997) found that the rate of suicide was positively correlated with the proportion of Protestants in a region. This finding could be interpreted as evidence that Protestants were more likely to commit suicide than Catholics. Without information on the religion of those who actually commit suicide, however, an equally plausible explanation is that Catholics who live in regions dominated by Protestants have high suicide rates. The implication of this alternative explanation is that living in a Protestant area has a contextual effect on suicide risk among minority Catholics.

Secondly, exposures are often estimated from data collected for another purpose, which generally provide only an indirect or crude measure of the factor of interest. For example, data on smoking, alcohol and prescribed drug use are often based on sales data, which only partly reflect consumption.

Thirdly, ecological studies may be subject to bias introduced by systematic errors in the measurement of exposures. For example, differences in the methodologies used to assess national consumption of dietary fats may to some extent explain the association between the incidence of breast cancer and the apparent consumption of dietary fat (Willett and Stampfer 1990). Similarly, the completeness of ascertainment of cases of a disease may vary across regions and countries.

Fourthly, data on known or potential confounding factors are not generally available in ecological studies, and even if available, would be difficult to control for at an individual level. In the early part of the twentieth century, rates of breast-feeding were highest in those areas which had the highest infant mortality rates (Fildes 1998), but for the individual child, breast-feeding protected against infant mortality (Grulee *et al.* 1935). The ecological association between high rates of breast-feeding and high infant mortality rates is probably confounded by poverty. In a contemporary example, Rowan *et al.* (2004) elegantly demonstrated that case-mix is an important confounding factor when comparing the performance of hospitals, and that the star rating system (zero to three) employed by the English Department of Health may not reflect the quality of clinical care provided by hospitals once case-mix is controlled for (see Figure 6.7).

Fifthly, it may be difficult to decide on, and control for, an appropriate induction or latent period between exposure and the outcome of interest. Finally, non-linear relationships can rarely be identified from ecological analyses as exposures represent the average for the population. Positive or negative linear relationships at the ecological level may mask more complicated relationships at the individual level. An example of different ecological- and individual-level relationships between alcohol consumption and coronary heart disease mortality is given by Hennekens and Buring (1987: 105–6).

Investigating ecological determinants of health

Despite their limitations, ecological studies have a number of advantages (see Table 6.6). They have been useful in describing differences in populations and may generate important hypotheses that can be investigated using individual study designs. The ecological fallacy limits the ability to make inferences about associations at the individual level. On the other hand, exposures such as social capital, social fragmentation, income inequality and the physical environment are ecological in nature and are difficult to measure at the individual level. These exposures are clearly important and indicate that, in many epidemiological studies, factors operating at the individual level and at different levels of aggregation should ideally be taken into account simultaneously (Blakely and Woodward 2000). For example, a study might examine the contextual effects of living in a poor area, controlling for individual poverty level. Individual exposures (e.g. health-related behaviours, diet, alcohol consumption, smoking, psychosocial factors) operate within an ecological context. The ecological context may be an important factor explaining disease rates at the

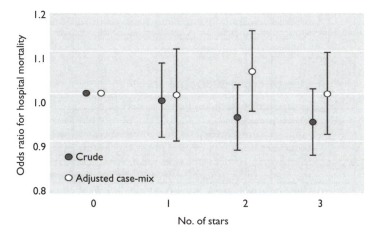

Figure 6.7 Crude and case-mix adjusted odds ratios for hospital mortality by star rating of acute Hospital Trust

Source: Rowan *et al.* BMJ 2004; 328: 924–925. Reproduced with permission from the BMJ Publishing Group.

Table 6.6   Advantages and disadvantages of ecological studies

Advantages	Disadvantages
• Inexpensive and can be relatively quick to perform using routine data	• Results from aggregate level analyses cannot reliably be applied at the individual level (ecological fallacy)
• Logical approach if exposure is environmental or social in nature	• Effects of ecological fallacy are difficult to remove
• Useful to generate hypotheses that can be tested in individual-level studies	• Often heavily confounded
• Useful for studying group exposure like weather, pollution, ionizing radiation	• Systematic bias in measurement may generate spurious associations
• May include populations with very wide ranging levels of exposure – may be the only practical method if exposure is relatively homogeneous within a population but differs between populations (e.g. water quality)	• Routinely collected data may only crudely measure the factors of interest

population level and the purpose of a study may be to understand differences in disease rates between populations (Bobak and Marmot 1996). Similarly, successful interventions to improve the health of populations have to be implemented at individual and societal levels. A methodologic overview of ecological studies is provided by Morgenstern (1998).

Cross-sectional studies (synonym: prevalence survey)

A cross-sectional study describes the frequency (or level) of a particular attribute, such as a specific exposure, disease or other health-related event in a defined population or a sample of a *population at a given point in time*. In a cross-sectional study, participants are contacted at a fixed point in time and the relevant information is obtained from them; they are sometimes described as a 'snapshot' of the health experience of the population.

Use of cross-sectional studies

Cross-sectional studies have a variety of uses (see Box 6.5). They may be established to specifically estimate the distribution of physiologic or biochemical measures (e.g. blood pressure levels); to determine the *prevalence* of health-related exposures and outcomes; and to assess the impact of health experiences (e.g. number of days lost from work). As data are collected for research purposes, cross-sectional studies allow the standardized measurement of the attribute of interest, supplementing routine data with potentially more accurate data. As they are population-based, the information they yield contrasts with clinical case studies, which are restricted to patients under medical care and which lack information on denominators. From a public health perspective, prevalence data are used to describe the burden of disease in a community, to plan health and social services, to design and monitor appropriate public health interventions and to monitor changes or trends in populations.

Cross-sectional studies can be descriptive or analytical (hypothesis testing). For example, the fourth survey of morbidity in England and Wales was a cross-sectional

> **Box 6.5 Applications of cross-sectional studies**
>
> - The measurement of the prevalence (e.g. the prevalence of hypertension in a population) or distribution (e.g. the distribution of systolic blood pressure in a population) of an attribute. In studies of the apparently well, cross-sectional studies discover people with previously unknown disease (i.e. they uncover the iceberg of disease). These data can be used to describe the range of normal variation in a population and to plan for health care utilization and resource allocation.
> - Prevalence rates in different sub-groups within a study may be contrasted to identify high-risk populations and to test hypotheses.
> - Cross-sectional studies conducted at different times, different locations or in different sub-groups can be compared to identify high-risk populations and to test hypotheses.
> - By conducting repeat surveys using the same methods on the same population over time, secular changes or the effect of an intervention can be measured.
> - Cross-sectional surveys have been used as the basis for cohort studies

study carried out between September 1991 and August 1992 to estimate the prevalence of diseases presenting to GPs (descriptive study) (Office of Population Censuses and Surveys, Department of Health and Royal College of General Practitioners 1995). These data have also been used analytically, for example to investigate the variation in consultation patterns by young men for a number of illnesses by social class, housing tenure, employment status, ethnicity, smoking status, marital status and urban/rural residence (Martin *et al.* 2001).

Cross-sectional studies can also be repeated using the same sampling methods to evaluate secular changes in the prevalence of an attribute of interest and evaluate interventions (a *repeat cross-sectional study*). For example, cross-sectional surveys of breast-feeding practices have been conducted in the UK since 1975 (Foster *et al.* 1997). These data have not only been used to document secular trends in the initiation and duration of breast-feeding (descriptive study) but also to estimate associations between maternal characteristics and the prevalence of breastfeeding (analytical study).

Cross-sectional studies can be used as the basis for long-term follow-up (cohort) studies (see section on cohort studies). For example, a cross-sectional survey of the health and diet of 4999 children in England and Scotland was conducted between 1937–9. Data on the children's names, ages and residence were recorded and measurements included the height and weight of the children. In 1988, the demographic data were used to construct a cohort study by linking details about the original participants to their death certificates notified by the NHS Central Register (the Boyd Orr cohort) (Gunnell *et al.* 1996). These data have now been used for a number of studies, such as investigations of the long-term impact of childhood diet on future cancer risk (Frankel *et al.* 1998; Maynard *et al.* 2003).

Timing of a cross-sectional study

Although cross-sectional studies are sometimes characterized as a 'snapshot' of the experience of a population, in reality a study takes some time to conduct; while measurement is simultaneous in an individual, the study is usually conducted over a period of time, varying from days to years. The time period of data collection can affect estimates of prevalence. For example, when the period of data collection is long and if the disease is chronic, the *point prevalence* may be overestimated because incident cases will occur during the period of the fieldwork. The probability of detecting a case of disease is related to its duration, which may bias measures of the point prevalence of acute diseases. Acute events vary greatly by season or where incidence changes rapidly. In such situations, the date on which the study was done is likely to be important and repeat cross-sectional studies may be needed to gain a true understanding of the prevalence of the outcome of interest. In some situations, conducting a study over a year may even out any seasonal differences, giving a more valid annual measure of prevalence. The study of the point prevalence of an infectious disease such as chicken-pox, however, should probably be conducted over a week or two.

Designing and conducting a cross-sectional survey

The ideal cross-sectional study is a geographically defined representative sample of the population of interest. A sample of the population is usually selected for study, as collecting data on every individual in the population would be logistically and financially prohibitive. The target population, the sampling frame, the selected sample and the study sample should all be precisely defined. The target population is the population to which the results will be extrapolated. The sampling frame is the population from which the sample is selected. The selected sample are those people who are randomly selected from the sampling frame and invited to participate in the study. Finally, the study sample comprises those who actually participate. It is important that the study sample is representative of the target population. This allows inferences from the study sample to be generalized to the target population. If a reasonably high response rate is achieved (i.e. the study sample is a high proportion of the selected sample) the results can be generalized to the target population (avoiding the problem of measuring everyone). The adequacy of the response rate depends on the aim of the study and the likelihood of non-response bias. For a rare disease a response rate of 85 per cent might be unacceptable as a handful of cases in the unexamined 15 per cent might greatly alter (bias) the results. In a survey of the distribution of blood pressure in a population, this response might be considered good.

For example, if we wanted to estimate the true prevalence of hypertension among the inhabitants of Bristol, UK (target population), we would need to have a list of potential participants, known as a *sampling frame*. Then, we would measure the blood pressures of a random sample of the inhabitants (the selected sample). This is illustrated in Figure 6.8.

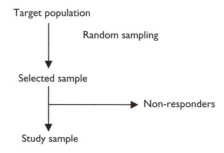

Figure 6.8   Stages in the selection of subjects in cross-sectional studies

Recruitment of sample

The principle of random sampling is that everyone or every sampling unit (e.g. household or school) in the study population should have a predetermined (non-zero) chance, usually an equal chance, of selection. The initial procedure is a complete list of the whole population from which the sample is to be drawn, since only in this way will everyone have a non-zero chance of selection. Examples of lists of populations include up-to-date age/sex registers in general practice, the electoral register, factory payroll (for surveys based on occupational groups), or school registers. In some situations the investigator may restrict the sample by studying a sub-group of the population (e.g. the interest may be in estimating the prevalence of foot ulcers in people with diabetes).

A number of sampling strategies exist which may be more appropriate than simple random sampling, depending on the objectives of the study, the availability of a sampling frame, the size and geographical spread of the source population and costs. These sampling strategies are summarized in Table 6.7. For example, an investigator may wish to ensure a larger sample size for particular groups/strata within a population than would be expected with simple random sampling. This can be achieved by sampling each sub-group separately (stratified sampling). Minority groups are thus sampled with a higher probability than other strata (over-sampled). In the 1999 Health Survey for England, stratified sampling was used to increase the numbers of people who identified themselves to be from an ethnic minority group, ensuring more precise estimates of factors of interest within each sub-group than would have been possible with simple random sampling (Saxena *et al.* 2004).

To correct estimates of prevalence and other epidemiological measures for different sampling strategies, other than simple random sampling, analyses must be weighted according to the sampling strategy (Korn and Graubard 1999).

In general, the estimates of prevalence obtained in a cross-sectional study will not be quite the same as the true prevalence of the population. It may be that the prevalence rates differ because of bias but, even in the absence of any source of bias,

Table 6.7   Sampling methods

Strategy	Description
Simple random sampling	When the population has been enumerated, each individual is assigned a number and a sample of the required size selected by use of a table of random numbers
Systematic sampling	For example, by taking every *n*th person on a list. This may result in a biased sample – to select every *n*th person on an electoral register would lead to an under-representation of members of the same family since they would be grouped together on the list
Multistage sampling	In order to obtain a representative sample of schoolchildren in a large city, first draw a random sample of schools and then within each selected school draw a sample of children
Stratified sampling	Used to achieve an even distribution of people in different groups (e.g. defined on the basis of age, sex or ethnicity). Divide the list into the groups (strata) of interest and then draw equal-sized random samples from each strata (e.g. the Health Survey for England 1999 and the NHANES[1] survey in the USA both over-sampled people from different ethnic backgrounds)

[1] NHANES: National Health and Nutrition Examination Survey

the sample prevalence will generally differ from the true population prevalence simply because it depends on which of the potentially eligible participants happened to be included in the sample. In other words, the sample prevalence will *not* be a perfectly precise estimator for the true population prevalence. If further samples of the same size are taken from the same population, each of these samples are likely to have a different (sample) prevalence, the difference being due to sampling variation. The precision of a prevalence estimate can be quantified by calculating a confidence interval. This is covered in Chapter 21 of this book.

Limitations of cross-sectional studies

Since both exposure and outcome are identified at one time point, costs are small and loss to follow-up is not a problem. However, cross-sectional studies have a number of limitations. Firstly, since both exposure and outcome are measured simultaneously it may be difficult to determine whether (a) exposures changed as a result of the outcome or (b) the outcome resulted in the subject being exposed or caused the suggested exposure. For example, a person who has coronary heart disease may start to smoke less. In this case, there would be an underestimation of the effect of smoking on coronary heart disease if cross-sectional prevalent data were relied upon. If the outcome causes an exposure, associations may arise as a result of reverse causality. For example, in a cross-sectional study showing an increased risk of bowel cancer associated with low cholesterol levels, it would be difficult to determine whether low cholesterol caused bowel cancer or was secondary to the disease. Establishing a temporal relationship, however, is less problematic for fixed exposures, such as sex, birth weight, eye colour, blood group and genotypes, which undoubtedly precede the outcome.

Even if participants are asked to recall their past exposure, this information may be unreliable leading to recall bias, and information on the timing of disease diagnosis would be needed in order to be certain that the exposure preceded the outcome. In some situations current exposure may be a useful proxy for past exposure. For example, in a cross-sectional study to assess the impact of adverse childhood environmental circumstances on the development of insulin resistance and diabetes in adulthood, Lawlor *et al.* (2002) used as their exposure current leg-length, a recognized proxy for nutritional and socioeconomic circumstances in infancy and childhood.

Secondly, cross-sectional studies consider prevalent rather than incident cases; therefore the data will reflect determinants of survival as well as aetiology. The most severely affected cases may die as soon as they get the disease (survivor bias). These are then not represented in the prevalent data of a cross-sectional study. Those with a short duration of illness will also be under-represented. In contrast, cases with a long duration of illness will be over-represented. This can have an influence on both aetiological studies and when relying on prevalence data to plan health services. In aetiological studies, if exposure is related to the duration but not the risk of developing the disease, exposure-disease associations will be biased: if exposure does not alter disease risk but is positively associated with survival/duration, a positive exposure-disease association will be observed: if exposure is inversely associated with survival/duration, an inverse exposure-disease association will be observed. When planning health services, if prevalence data under-represent the most severely affected individuals who die early, they would not be identified and their needs would not be addressed.

Thirdly, selection bias occurs in cross-sectional studies when study participants are not representative of the target population about which conclusions are to be drawn. This arises if excluded participants differ from included participants with respect to the prevalence or distribution of the variable of interest. This bias could arise from at least three sources. First, the choice of study sampling frame may be important. For example, the use of general practice lists as the sampling frame excludes those who are not registered with the NHS, and those who live in the most deprived areas of a practice catchment area are less likely to participate (Smith *et al.* 2004); the electoral register excludes those who are not eligible to vote or who are unwilling to divulge their details; and the telephone directory and the register of licensed drivers (popular sampling frames in the USA) exclude those without a telephone or driver's licence. Second, people with severe disease may be institutionalized and either not on the list from which the study sample was drawn or not available for study. Third, low response rates will bias results if non-responders differ from responders (response bias) with respect to the parameter of interest (prevalence or distribution). It does not matter, however, if responders are atypical in other respects.

Selection bias can be assessed in at least four ways. First, findings can be compared in participants who respond with and without a reminder; if differences are found this suggests that those who respond most readily may be unrepresentative. Second, a small random sample could be drawn from the non-responders and intensive efforts to recruit them could be employed. Findings are then compared with the earlier responders. Third, if there is information on the non-responders (e.g. age, sex, residence), differences in these characteristics between responders and non-responders may suggest the possibility of selection bias. Fourth, sensitivity analyses could be performed to assess the effect on observed prevalence estimates of a range of imputed values in the non-responders.

Finally, for the study of rare events, a very large population would need to be surveyed to identify enough cases. In this situation, it may be better to employ intensive case finding based on all sources of information. For example, in a study to estimate the prevalence and adverse consequences of non-adherence to insulin injection therapy among young people with Type 1 diabetes in Tayside, Scotland, Morris *et al.* (1997) employed a record linkage study to identify all cases in Tayside based on routine records from a number of sources (prescriptions, hospital admissions data, outpatients data) that were linked by a unique identifier. The advantages and limitations of cross-sectional studies are listed in Table 6.8.

Table 6.8 Advantages and disadvantages of cross-sectional studies

Advantages	Disadvantages
• Quick and relatively easy as no follow-up is required	• Problem with direction of causality (reverse causality)
• Can be used to investigate many exposures and outcomes	• In aetiological studies, survival bias a potential problem as the sample is based on prevalent rather than incident cases
• Useful for measuring the true burden of disease in a population	• Not efficient for rare diseases
	• Recall bias
	• Not suitable for diseases of short duration
	• Prevalence estimates are potentially biased by low response rates
	• Migration in and out of population influences prevalence

Case-control studies

In a case-control study, a case group or series of patients who have the outcome of interest and a control (or comparison) group of individuals without the outcome are selected for investigation and the proportions with the exposure of interest in each group are compared.

For example, to investigate socioeconomic factors influencing access to hospital eye services for glaucoma, investigators examined 110 patients who had first presented with advanced glaucoma (cases) and 110 controls who initially presented with early glaucoma (Fraser *et al.* 2001). Both cases and controls were prospectively identified from consecutive patients seen at the eye departments of three hospitals in England and who met strict case definition criteria. After patients gave informed consent, they were telephoned by a trained interviewer blind to case-control status and asked a series of standard questions regarding socioeconomic status, education, ethnic origin, use of general medical services and use of sight testing (optometric) services. The investigators found that adverse socioeconomic circumstances and lower education levels were more commonly found in those with an increased risk of late presentation with glaucoma, suggesting socioeconomic inequalities in accessing NHS services for glaucoma.

This example highlights the key concepts of case-control studies. They involve measuring the frequency of an exposure, both among participants with the disease or condition of interest (cases) and participants without the disease or condition of interest (controls), to test whether an exposure is found more or less commonly among cases than controls. Unlike cohort studies (see section on cohort studies), the starting point is participants who either do (cases) or do not (controls) have the particular disease under study, and the investigation involves looking backward in time to asses antecedent exposures. If the exposure is more common among cases, it is associated with an increased risk of disease/health-related event and may be a causal factor. If it is less common among cases, it may be a protective factor. The key steps in planning a case-control study are: (i) defining objective criteria for the diagnosis of a case; (ii) the selection of cases and controls; and (iii) the estimation of exposure status.

Case definition

The definition of a case requires three distinct considerations: (i) objective criteria for case definition; (ii) eligibility criteria; and (iii) whether to select incident or prevalent cases.

The requirement for objective case definition is to avoid dilution of the case series with some individuals who are not cases and reducing the chances of detecting real differences between cases and controls. The criteria for defining a case may be pathological (e.g. cases with a histological diagnosis of breast cancer), radiological (e.g. cases with a CT scan of a brain tumour), microbiological (e.g. cases with sputum positive for the tuberculosis bacillus), clinical (e.g. cases of Parkinson's disease diagnosed by a neurologist), self-reported (e.g. depression as assessed by a questionnaire), or may be the result of a coding exercise (e.g. death certificate diagnoses). The criteria used will determine to what extent the non-cases are likely to be misclassified as cases, and vice versa. To judge the extent of misclassification, particularly when categorization requires some element of subjectivity, cases can be sub-classified according to whether they are definite, probable or possible cases. If exposure-outcome associations weaken from the definite to the possible category, this suggests increasing misclassification of non-cases to cases with increasing uncertainty.

For example, in a case–control study to determine the association between myocardial infarction and use of different types of oral contraceptive pill (OCP), women were eligible as cases if they were aged 16–44 and had suffered an incident myocardial infarction between 1993–5 (MICA study) (Dunn *et al.* 1999). Cases were identified from hospital episode statistics, the deaths register of the Office for National Statistics for England and Wales and from the Information and Statistics Division of the Department of Health or the Registrar General's Office in Scotland. International classification of diseases, ninth revision (ICD-9) code 410 or tenth revision (ICD-10) code 121 were used as identifiers of acute myocardial infarction. A validation study showed a 33 per cent false negative rate and 0 per cent false positive rate in using only these codes for identifying the cases. Diagnostic information for each potential case was extracted from the hospital notes, and these data were submitted to a panel of three cardiologists, blinded to exposure status, for confirmation of diagnosis. Criteria for diagnosis were according to the World Health Organization, with inclusion of the case depending on a majority decision of the diagnosis as being 'definite' or 'possible'. Cases in which the woman died before reaching hospital or before investigations had been done were validated on the result of the post-mortem findings.

There must be an unambiguous statement of eligibility criteria for the selection of individuals as cases. The same eligibility criteria that were applied to cases must also be applied to controls. Inclusion criteria may include: a minimum age, time period, or area of residence; exclusion criteria may include: mental or terminal illness, not being able to read or speak English (or other relevant language) or other factors which mean that data collection will be problematic or unethical. Cases should be restricted to those whose outcome has a reasonable probability of being induced by the exposure. In the above case-control study to determine the association between myocardial infarction and use of different types of OCP (Dunn *et al.* 1999), women with a history of pregnancy in the six weeks before the date of the myocardial infarction, or a history of menopause, hysterectomy, oophorectomy and breast or ovarian cancer were excluded as it is not likely that such women will have been recently exposed to the OCP. The same exclusion criteria must be applied to the controls, otherwise the study will overestimate any risk associated with the OCP.

Not all eligible individuals will take part in the study as they may refuse, move away or die. In presenting the results of the study, a statement of the total number who met the inclusion criteria, the numbers in the final study sample and reasons for any omissions will allow the extent of selection bias to be assessed (see section on interpretation and sub-sections on bias).

An important distinction is whether only *incident, prevalent* or *dead* cases are included (Breslow and Day 1980). Unlike prevalent cases, incident cases have not been acted upon by the determinants of survival. If prevalent cases are studied, factors may not just be causally related to the disease but may also be factors related to the duration of disease and/or survival. If incidence and survival differ with respect to risk factors, the use of prevalent cases would give a biased estimate of exposure-outcome associations. The possibility of bias as a result of using prevalent cases was first highlighted by Neyman in 1955 using hypothetical data and has been termed 'Neyman's bias' (Neyman 1955; Hill *et al.* 2003).

In a more recent example using real data, investigators tested the hypothesis that smoking exerts a protective effect on Alzheimer's disease and other types of dementia in 668 people aged 75–101 years (Wang *et al.* 1999). In a cross-sectional analysis, smokers had a 40 per cent lower risk of prevalent Alzheimer's disease and dementia than non-smokers (i.e. those with Alzheimer's had a lower prevalence of smoking). However, over a three-year follow-up period, smoking was associated with a 10 per cent and 40 per cent *increased* risk of incident Alzheimer's disease and dementia, respectively. This suggests that smoking does not protect against the *development* of Alzheimer's disease or dementia. The apparent protective association in the cross-sectional analysis might have been due to the fact that smokers who developed Alzheimer's disease had higher death rates (i.e. smoking was also a determinant of survival from Alzheimer's disease). Therefore, smokers who developed Alzheimer's disease would be more likely to have been under-sampled in the original cross-sectional study. This would result in a lower prevalence of smoking among those surviving with Alzheimer's disease versus those without Alzheimer's disease.

Other advantages of using incident rather than prevalent cases are related to the valid assessment of exposure status: (i) in prevalent cases exposure may change subsequent to disease; (ii) the use of incident cases reduces the time period for remembering past events; (iii) recent medical, employment or other records are likely to be available and more informative than older records. A dietary study of fat consumption and heart disease found relatively little difference between cases and controls. However, it was shown that cases reduced their fat consumption after a heart attack and although they were asked about prior diet, their current diet was distorting their recall of past diet. Use of prevalent cases may be unavoidable, such as in studies of congenital malformations (Roodpeyma *et al.* 2002).

Sources of cases

Cases can be obtained from a number of sources: clinical case-series, a population-based register of cases or a disease registry, hospital admissions, primary care records, new cases identified in a cohort study, or occasionally cross-sectional studies (often prevalent cases, but will include incident cases). A number of sources may be used to identify a single case-series. For example, in a case-control study of predictors of severe obstetric morbidity, cases who met the definition for severe morbidity were selected from maternity computer databases, labour ward and postnatal ward diaries, staff reporting and a fortnightly manual review of all medical records (Waterstone *et al.* 2001).

The source of cases needs to be carefully considered. There are a number of advantages to selecting cases from a population register or a cohort study: (i) they are most likely to be incident cases; (ii) they are likely to be representative of all cases in the population of interest; (iii) the source population giving rise to the cases is well defined, so the population from which control participants should be drawn is easy to identify and incidence rates in exposed and non-exposed individuals can be calculated.

It is unnecessary to include all cases from the source population; cases can be randomly selected for inclusion in a case-control study as long as the sampling is *independent of the exposure under study*. Cases identified in a single clinic or treated by a single medical practitioner can be used in a case-control study, even if they are a highly selected group. The corresponding source population for the cases treated in a clinic is all people who would attend that clinic and be recorded with the outcome of interest if they had the event in question (Rothman and Greenland 1998). This source forms the population from which the controls should be sampled (see below). Bias in the selection of cases arises when exposed cases are more (or less) likely to be selected for the study than unexposed cases. This may occur, for example, if having both the exposure and the outcome of interest increases the chance of hospitalization. This bias, which affects the interpretation of hospital-based case-control studies, is sometimes referred to as 'Berkson's bias' after the author who first described it, although it can also be thought of as a form of selection bias.

In an example of case selection bias, several case-control studies conducted in the 1970s suggested a strong association between the use of oestrogen (hormone) replacement therapy by postmenopausal women and their risk of endometrial cancer (cancer of the lining of the uterus/womb). It is argued by others, however, that oestrogen therapy causes uterine bleeding regardless of its association with cancer, and that such bleeding in a postmenopausal woman triggers further investigation of the cause of the bleeding, which in turn reveals cancers that would remain otherwise undetected in women not taking oestrogen. Therefore, the detection rate for endometrial cancer among those exposed is greater than for those who are unexposed (and not subject to invasive gynaecological investigations), leading to an overestimate of the risk of endometrial cancer associated with oestrogen therapy. For a detailed discussion of this controversy, see Rothman and Greenland (1998: Chapter 9).

Control selection

The control group provides an estimate of exposure prevalence in the population giving rise to the cases (Schlesselman 1982). The choice of appropriate controls is the most difficult decision in designing case-control studies, as an inappropriate choice may result in selection bias (leading to a biased estimate of risk). The crucial principle is that the controls should represent the population of persons who would have been included as cases if they had developed the outcome in question during the study period.

Rothman emphasizes that the definition of the source population that gave rise to the cases should determine the population from which the controls are sampled (Rothman and Greenland 1998). For example, the source population for cases identified in a single outpatient clinic is all people who would have attended the clinic had they developed the outcome during the study period. The difficulty is in identifying potential clinic attendees. Failure to exclude controls who would not have attended the clinic, however, could result in a biased estimate of the association between the outcome and exposures that are correlated with factors related to seeking such medical attention. Without a precisely defined source population it may be difficult to select controls in an unbiased fashion (Rothman and Greenland 1998). For example, women who are motivated to participate in breast cancer screening are more likely to have risk factors for breast cancer, such as a family history. If screen-detected cases are compared with general population controls, the magnitude of associations between breast cancer and certain risk factors may be overestimated. This bias is a type of self-selection or referral bias. Unbiased associations might be obtained by selecting both cases and controls from among screened women, thus controlling for the selection forces influencing participation in a screening programme.

To ensure that controls are representative of the source population with respect to exposure, controls must also be sampled independently of their exposure status. Furthermore, the exclusion/inclusion criteria for the identification of cases must apply equally to the controls and vice versa. The degree of diagnostic effort and methods (e.g. questionnaire, review of medical records) required to rule out disease/ outcome in the controls to minimize misclassification will depend on the outcome being investigated and how common it is (greater effort being required to rule out misclassification the more common the outcome).

In some instances, specific case-control studies are conducted (nested) within well-defined cohorts and are referred to as nested case-control studies. In a nested case-control study it is relatively straightforward to ensure that the controls are a representative sample of the population from which the cases are drawn, since both cases and controls arise from the same cohort. Conceptually, all case-control studies may be best understood as nested within a hypothetical cohort (Rothman and Greenland 1998). The source population is the population that that would have been included in a cohort study and which gives rise to the cases. In a cohort study, exposed and unexposed groups are defined and the number of cases in each group identified. In a case-control study the same cases are identified and then classified as to whether they belong to exposed or unexposed groups. In a cohort study, the exposed and unexposed groups provide the denominators for incidence risk or rates. In a case-control study, we do not know the denominators for incidence risk or rates; instead a control group is sampled from the source population that gave rise to the cases. Individuals in the control group are then classified into exposed and unexposed categories. If controls are sampled from the source cohort that gave rise to cases, independent of exposure, the same proportion of controls will be exposed as the proportion of people exposed in the original source population (Rothman and Greenland 1998). In reality, some populations are easily identifiable but in other instances the members of the source population may be hard to identify. A detailed synthesis of the principles of control selection in case-control studies is presented in three companion papers by Wacholder *et al.* (1992a, 1992b, 1992c).

Sources of controls

There are several possible sources of controls, including, among others, population controls, neighbours or relatives of cases, hospital- or clinic-based controls, random digit dialling, people who have died, and friends of cases. Each offers particular advantages and disadvantages that must be considered for any particular study.

Population controls

If cases come from a precisely defined and identified population, and random sampling from the source population of cases is feasible, this is often the best source of controls. In this situation the study is said to be population-based. Random sampling from the source population may be feasible if a population register exists (e.g. electoral registers, general practice lists) or can be compiled (e.g. by canvassing households in targeted neighbourhoods or random-digit telephone dialling). While control selection bias is less likely to occur in population-based case-control studies, it is not always avoided. There may be selection forces involved in the process of people seeking medical care or attention that lead them to be identified as cases. In contrast, controls selected from the general population will include people who would *not* have gone to medical facilities even if they had developed the disease. These people will systematically differ from people who do go to medical facilities.

Another problem in selecting population controls is that the response rate may be lower than among hospital controls, a 'captured' population. If non-response is related to the exposure under study, this may bias associations. Randomly dialling telephone numbers simulates a random sample of the source population and is popular in the USA. However, people who spend more time at home or households with multiple telephone lines will be over-sampled.

Friends, relatives and neighbourhood controls

If the source population cannot be listed, one or more controls who reside in the same neighbourhood as a case can be identified and recruited into the study. The use of friends and relatives is a convenient method of control selection and usually results in good response rates, as these groups have greater motivation to take part than a randomly selected population. This strategy may also offer a degree of control for potential confounding factors, as cases and controls will tend to be similar with respect to socioeconomic and lifestyle factors. For example, Danesh *et al.* (1999) used sibling controls in a case-control study of the chronic stomach infection, *Helicobacter pylori*, and risk of heart attacks. Since both exposure and outcome are strongly socially patterned, this choice may control for confounding by social factors that are otherwise difficult to measure. The danger is that cases and controls will also be inadvertently matched on the very exposure of interest. For example, we tend to marry partners that are similar to us in backgrounds and lifestyle, and will share most early life exposures with siblings. Spouses and siblings will thus be more similar with respect to exposure prevalence than a comparison with the source population would suggest, so that we potentially may reduce the power of a study to detect an effect (see later sub-section on matching).

Hospital- or clinic-based controls

In hospital- or clinic-based case-control studies the source population represents those who would have been treated in a given clinic or hospital if they had developed the disease in question. Hospital controls have advantages. Firstly, they are likely to have been subject to the same intangible selection forces (e.g. socio-economic position, area of residence, ethnicity) that influenced cases to seek medical advice. Secondly, they are easily identified and usually cooperative. Finally, since they have experienced illness and hospitalization the quality of their recall of past events may be similar to cases.

However, the source population may be hard to identify, as the hospital's catchment population is often ill-defined and may differ by specialty. Although other patients treated at the same hospital may constitute a sample of this source population for use as controls, they are by definition a non-random sample, increasing the likelihood of selection bias. For example, hospital controls will over-represent exposures associated with diseases leading to hospitalization (e.g. smoking, heavy alcohol consumption) and the choice of hospital (e.g. private versus public). Thus, determinants of hospitalization (and the choice of hospital) must be carefully considered in studies using hospital controls. To test whether heavy alcohol consumption increases the risk of stroke, it may not be wise to select patients from trauma, orthopaedic or gastroenterology wards as controls. This is because heavy alcohol consumption is associated with conditions giving rise to admissions to these wards (liver disease, peptic ulcers, falls, osteoporosis). Therefore, hospital controls are more likely to be heavy drinkers than the population from which the cases arose, and will bias results towards the null (i.e. not demonstrating an effect where a true effect exists). To avoid control selection bias, anyone who is hospitalized for a disease thought to be related to the exposure of interest should be excluded from the control series. The dilemma is that this approach may lead to the exclusion of many diagnostic categories, making it difficult to find controls. The use of a variety of diagnoses may dilute any bias that might result from using as controls specific diagnostic groups unknowingly related to exposure.

Dead people

In some studies, cases are dead from their disease. The advantage of using dead people as controls is that this may enhance comparability. Using dead controls, however, will misrepresent the exposure distribution in the source population if exposure is related to survival. If interviews are needed to obtain exposure information, proxy respondents for any dead cases will be needed. In the MICA study described earlier (Dunn *et al.* 1999), investigators interviewed the husband or a close relative of the women who had died. Overall, 73 per cent of women who survived a heart attack were interviewed, but interviews were achieved for only 20 per cent of those who died. As the authors accepted, this may have introduced a bias, if for example certain types of OCP were particularly liable to cause sudden death from a heart attack. Rothman suggests that to enhance comparability of exposure information, while avoiding the problem of using dead controls, proxy respondents for live controls who are matched to dead cases can be used (Rothman 2002).

Ascertainment of disease/exposure status

Exposure measurement in case-control studies is performed retrospectively: it is crucial, therefore, that the information gathered about the study participants is not influenced by knowledge of their case-control status. Exposure measurement based on the participants' personal recall is prone to measurement error and *recall bias*. For example, amongst cases previous consideration of factors leading to their diagnosis may influence their response. It is better, if possible, to obtain more objective data on past exposures such as the participants' GP records, or school records or biochemical, immunological and microbiological measures from stored serum. It is unlikely that the subsequent development of disease would have affected the accuracy or completeness of such sources of exposure information. The interviewer (or medical records abstractor) should be blind to the case or control status of the participants to avoid observer bias. In multi-centre studies or studies involving a large number of interviewers or observers, standardization of data collection is important (see section on interpretation, sub-sections on bias).

The basis on which a person should be considered exposed depends on the part of a person's exposure history that is relevant to the aetiology of the outcome under study. This in turn depends on an understanding of the mechanism by which the exposure influences the outcome of interest. If the time period assessed by the measuring instrument is not the true time period of aetiological relevance this will lead to misclassification of the exposure of interest.

For example, the risk of heart attacks with newer (third-generation) OCPs was compared with older (second-generation) OCPs (Dunn *et al.* 1999). Dunn *et al.* ascertained contraceptive history in a case-control study of young women who had and had not suffered a heart attack. It is possible that recall bias may have occurred because interviewees were asked to recall their contraceptive history. The adverse publicity about third generation OCPs generated by a 'Dear doctor' letter from the United Kingdom Committee on Safety of Medicines in October 1995 may have biased responses to the interviews which were conducted between December 1996 and February 1998. In an attempt to overcome recall bias, the interviewees were unaware (blind) of the main objective of the study and the investigators provided photographs of all marketed OCPs to increase the accuracy of recall. Despite these measures, the odds ratio between third and second generation oral contraceptives was 1.41 on the basis of records from GPs but 2.06 when the estimate was based on the women's recall. This suggests that recall bias may have influenced the reporting of type of OCP among cases who had heard about the adverse publicity.

Matching

In some studies controls are recruited to 'match' each case with respect to certain characteristics, such as age, sex, ethnicity, smoking status or social class. In the past, the rationale for matching has often been that cases and controls will be similar to each other apart from the exposure of interest; thus it is argued that associations will not be confounded by the matching factors. However, the methodological and logistical issues raised by matching in case-control studies are much more complicated than they first appear (Rothman and Greenland 1998: Chapter 10). There are two main reasons to match. Firstly (and most importantly), by ensuring that the distributions of a confounder are similar in cases and controls, matching *can* improve the statistical efficiency (information per subject studied) of a study. For example, if the age distribution of cases is shifted strongly towards older ages compared with the source population, matching by age ensures the ratio of controls to cases is constant over age strata, a situation which maximizes the precision of a study. Secondly, individual matching of cases to controls *may* be equivalent to matching for a complex of underlying factors that are difficult to measure. For example, recruiting siblings of cases as controls may help the investigator to control for ill-defined socioeconomic or genetic factors. However, unless there are very strong arguments for matching, such as the presence of known strong confounding factors that are difficult to quantify, matching is not advisable for a number of reasons, described by Wacholder *et al.* (1992c) and summarized below.

- Matching can create a selection bias masking associations between an exposure and an outcome. This situation can arise if matching is based on: (i) an intermediate variable that is part of the pathway through which the exposure influences the outcome; (ii) a factor that is a surrogate for or a consequence of disease; or (iii) a correlate of an imperfectly measured exposure. If this occurs, cases and controls are said to be over-matched.
- Loss of statistical efficiency occurs if the matching factor is correlated with the exposure but is not a risk factor for the outcome of interest (and so cannot be a confounding factor). For example, suppose a study of smoking and lung cancer matched on alcohol intake. Since alcohol intake is strongly associated with smoking, many of the matched case-control groups (known as matched sets) will be identical with respect to smoking status, and will not contribute any information to the analysis. Since the estimation of the effect of the exposure variable is based only on those matched sets that are discordant for exposure, matching on alcohol intake will lead to relatively few informative strata in the analysis, with substantial loss in the efficiency of the study but with no advantage in terms of controlling for confounding. If a factor which is not actually a confounder is matched upon, the study will need to be considerably larger than an unmatched study to have the same power to detect a given association. Conversely, any potential gains in efficiency from matching on a true confounder are likely to be modest.
- If a study is matched at the design stage then this should also be reflected in the method of data analysis, even if the matching factors are not confounders in the source population. If one inappropriately analyses matched data the results can be seriously biased, generally in the direction of the null value of no association. The statistical techniques for the analysis of matched data are found in Chapters 5 and 7 of Breslow and Day (1980).
- Once participants have been matched in a case control study there is little flexibility in the analysis stage. The influence of the matching characteristic on the outcome can no longer be studied and overmatching that occurs by design cannot be corrected in the analysis. Unless there are compelling reasons, a better

strategy could be to control for confounding factors during the analysis using stratification or regression methods.

- Matching adds costs and complexity to a sampling scheme, can result in cases being excluded if no matching control can be found, and may increase the duration of a study in order to obtain the relevant information from the cases and then interview many potential controls to find those that match. As the number of matching variables increases the logistical difficulty of conducting the study is likely to intensify.

Rather than individually pairing a case with one or more controls, frequency matching (a variant of stratified sampling) can be undertaken. This involves choosing cases and controls to have the same overall distribution of the matching factor. For example, to frequency match by age and sex, age could be classified in five- or ten-year bands. Hence if a case is identified as male aged 63 (strata male and age band 60 to 64 years) a control is randomly selected who is also male and aged between 60 to 64 years. The matching factor (e.g. age band) must still be included in statistical models to ensure unbiased estimates of exposure effect. Frequency matching may not control confounding to any great degree, however, and further statistical methods may be needed at the analysis stage.

Advantages and disadvantages of case-control studies

The advantages and disadvantages of case-control studies are given in Table 6.9. One important advantage of case-control studies is that they are much more cost-effective than cohort studies for the study of rare events. This is because there is no need to follow up large numbers of people to ensure that a sufficient number get the outcome to allow meaningful statistical comparisons. For example, if one wanted to study a disease such as multiple sclerosis, one would need data on around 100,000 people to obtain enough participants with the disease. It is much cheaper to find 100 multiple sclerosis patients and 400 controls and carry out a case-control study. Secondly, for outcomes with long induction periods, no lengthy follow-up is

Table 6.9 Advantages and disadvantages of case-control studies

Advantages	Disadvantages
• Relatively quick as the investigator does not need to wait for incident cases	• The temporal sequence between exposure and outcome may be difficult to establish (which came first – exposure or disease?)
• More efficient for rare diseases and diseases with long latency as large sample size and long follow-up not required	• Obtaining valid information about past exposures may be difficult (recall or observer bias)
• Allow testing of multiple exposure hypotheses for a given disease	• Selection of an appropriate control group may be difficult (selection bias)
	• Not suitable for investigating rare exposures (unless a large proportion of cases are attributable to that exposure)
	• Cannot provide direct estimates of the incidence of disease in those exposed and those unexposed (unless a population-based case-control study)

required. Thirdly, many different exposures can be investigated in relation to a single outcome.

Case-control studies, however, are susceptible to two types of bias because exposure and disease have already occurred at the time participants enter a study: (i) differential selection of either cases or controls into the study on the basis of their exposure status (selection bias); and (ii) differential reporting or recording of exposure information based on disease status (recall or observer bias).

To avoid selection bias, it is important to ensure that the selection of cases and controls is independent of exposure status (Breslow and Day 1980), and that the controls are sampled from among those who would have been designated study cases if they had developed the disease in question. The choice of population or hospital controls influences the degree to which selection bias will be an important factor in interpreting the study results, and will depend on the particular issue under investigation. To avoid information bias cases and controls must be similar with respect to the accuracy and completeness of data.

Case-control studies cannot provide direct estimates of the incidence of the outcome in those exposed and those unexposed. Thus it is usually not possible to compute the absolute impact of the exposure on the occurrence of the outcome. However, it is possible to estimate incidence rates in those exposed and those unexposed in population-based case-control studies in which the incidence rate in the total population of interest is known and the distribution of exposure among controls is assumed to be representative of the whole population. Given incidence rates in those exposed and those unexposed, absolute measures of effect can be calculated, such as rate differences (see section on measures of exposure effect). Details of how to calculate incidence rates from population-based case-control studies are given by dos Santos Silva (1999: Appendix 16.1).

Case-control studies are not suitable for rare exposures because few cases will have been exposed. An exception is if a large proportion of cases are attributable to that exposure. Finally, the temporal relation between exposure and disease may be difficult to establish. The possibility that the exposure is the result of the outcome under investigation (reverse causality) should be considered.

Deciding how to recruit controls is the single most important decision when designing a case-control study since this determines both the validity of the estimate and what is estimated (risk ratio, rate ratio or odds ratio). Matching in a case-control study can improve statistical efficiency (the amount of information per subject studied) but has several disadvantages including selection bias, over-matching and the need to control for both the matching variables and unmatched confounders at the analysis stage.

Cohort studies (synonyms: prospective study, follow-up study, incidence study, or longitudinal study/survey)

In ancient history, a cohort was a tenth (about 400 men) of a legion of the Roman army. In modern epidemiology, a cohort study refers to 'any designated group of individuals who are followed or traced over a period of time' (Last 1995). This group (the study population) are measured at *baseline* for particular characteristics or exposures that are suspected of being related to the outcome under investigation. The entire study population is then followed up over time for the development of new events (see Figure 6.9). The incidence of the outcome in the exposed individuals is then compared with the incidence in those not exposed. Cohort studies are analogous to intervention trials in that people are selected on the basis of their

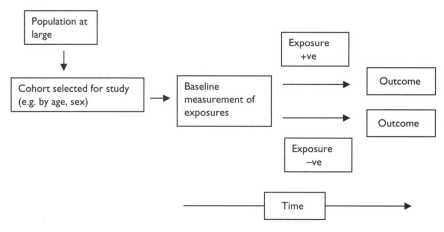

Figure 6.9 Design of a simple cohort study

exposure status and then followed up in time, but differ from them in that the exposure of interest is not under the direct control of the investigators. The construction of the sampling frame and the measurement of exposures occur before the onset of disease, thus avoiding the possibility that disease itself might cause modification of measured exposures – always a concern in case-control studies – and ensuring that causes come before effects in time sequence.

Cohort studies are useful in studying the incidence of health-related events in populations; exploring or generating hypotheses about the causes of health-related events (by calculating incident rate ratios); and for examining the natural history of disease (prognosis) and other outcomes. For example, Hemingway *et al.* (2001) conducted an observational cohort study of consecutive patients undergoing coronary angiography at three London hospitals. Before patients were recruited, a nine-member expert panel independently rated the appropriateness of percutaneous transluminal coronary angioplasty (PTCA) and coronary-artery bypass grafting (CABG) on a nine-point scale (with 1 denoting highly inappropriate and 9 denoting highly appropriate) for specific clinical indications. These ratings were then applied to the participants in the cohort, although the patients were treated without regard to the ratings. A total of 2552 patients were followed for a median of 30 months after angiography. Medical (i.e. drug only) treatment was common among patients with indications for which revascularization had been deemed appropriate by the expert panel. During follow-up, these medically treated patients had higher mortality and a higher prevalence of angina than patients who underwent revascularization. The authors concluded that the findings support the validity of ratings of appropriateness in measuring underuse of revascularization after angiography. Such underuse was common among patients considered appropriate candidates for revascularization and was associated with a poorer prognosis.

Selection of participants

The choice of study population depends on the hypothesis under investigation and on practical constraints. Possible cohorts include a *general population cohort*, a more *narrowly defined population* that can be readily identified and followed up (such as registered doctors or nurses), or a *highly exposed group* of people. Whatever the source of the study population, the aim is to ensure that cohort members are representative of the population from which they are drawn and to which inferences of causation are to be made.

A *general population cohort* can be drawn from a geographically well-defined area which is initially surveyed to establish baseline exposure to a number of factors and then examined periodically to ascertain outcome. This type of cohort study allows a large number of common exposures to be considered in relation to a large number of outcomes. Once a general population cohort is assembled, the cohort members can be classified according to many potential factors of interest. Thus, a cohort study can provide a comprehensive picture of the health effects of a given exposure.

In an example of a more *narrowly-defined population*, all non-industrial civil servants aged 35–55 years working in the London offices of 20 departments were invited to participate in a prospective cohort study (Whitehall II study). The final cohort consisted of 10,308 participants (3413 women) with an overall response rate of 73 per cent. Follow-up of this cohort by means of repeat examinations, questionnaires and linkage with the NHS Central Register has permitted the assessment of the effects of a wide variety of exposures (e.g. employment grade, lifestyle and behavioural factors, economic circumstances, social circumstances at work, social support) on the risk of numerous outcomes in older age (e.g. disease prevalence, chronic disease risk factors, cause-specific mortality, self-perceived health status and symptoms, physical functioning, psychological and cognitive outcomes) (Marmot *et al.* 1991). The study was limited to civil servants, illustrating how the generalizability of cohorts is limited by decisions made at the outset which were designed to improve the feasibility of a study.

Participation in a long-term follow-up study may involve taking a lot of time off work, inconvenience, or concern about detecting unrecognized disease. Participants agreeing to take part in the study may therefore differ from the general population in many ways, including their exposure to risk factors, and hence their disease incidence. For example, participants may tend to be non-smokers or from less deprived areas and therefore healthier (Smith *et al.* 2004). Furthermore, it may be difficult to maintain contact with a general population cohort over a long period of time. It is possible to assess the direction and extent of potential selection bias by obtaining information about non-participants or losses to follow-up from other sources, although this may raise ethical problems. As in Whitehall II, it may be preferable to draw a population cohort from well-defined occupational groups, such as civil servants, registered doctors or nurses. Such professional groups are easy to identify, and are likely to be compliant and willing to participate in the study, resulting in high response rates at baseline and low rates of loss to follow-up. These advantages are likely to reduce selection bias.

In the Whitehall II study, participants completed questionnaires that assessed self-reported angina and formal physician diagnoses of angina five times during follow-up; on three occasions, electrocardiograms were also obtained. Hemingway *et al.* (2003) showed that of the 11 per cent of participants with evidence of angina during follow-up (based on the Rose angina questionnaire and/or an abnormal study electrocardiogram), about 70 per cent had no evidence of a doctor diagnosis of angina. Furthermore, undiagnosed angina was associated with a more than twofold increased risk of impaired physical functioning and, among those who also had an abnormal electrocardiogram, a twofold increased risk of all-cause mortality (compared with people who did not experience angina or myocardial infarction during follow-up).

If the exposure is rare, a study of the general population will have little statistical power to detect an effect unless it is prohibitively large, as very few people would have been exposed to the factor of interest. This problem can be overcome by deliberately selecting a *highly exposed group* (*special exposure cohort studies*). For example, Martin *et al.* (1998) used a cohort design to examine the association between the long acting β_2 agonist bambuterol (a drug used to control the symptoms of asthma) and the occurrence of adverse effects, including coronary heart disease and heart failure. Since exposure to bambuterol is relatively rare, the authors identified all individuals in the UK who had been prescribed the drug (via the UK Prescription Pricing Authority). This group formed the exposed cohort. Individuals prescribed two other similar anti-asthma drugs formed comparator cohorts. Six months and one year after the first prescription was issued, questionnaires were sent to the prescriber asking for details of events occurring after that prescription (prescription event monitoring). This design allowed the full range of adverse effects of exposure to bambuterol on the health of individuals to be studied, including outcomes that are relatively uncommon in the general population (such as heart failure). In this study a threefold increased risk of non-fatal heart failure associated with bambuterol was observed. Other examples of special exposure cohort studies include occupational cohorts heavily exposed to industrial chemicals and populations with special dietary habits (such as Seventh-Day Adventists).

The inclusion/exclusion criteria for a cohort study should be clear and unambiguous. Once a person satisfies the entry criteria and enters a cohort study, they begin to contribute person-time at risk. Since most cohorts involve participants entering the study at different points in time, the exact data of entry of each subject should be recorded.

Choice of comparison group

Many cohorts begin with a single cohort in which people have varied (heterogenous) exposure histories. Comparisons of outcome experience are made within the cohort across sub-groups defined by one or more exposures. This is called an *internal comparison group*. In such cohorts it is possible to examine the effect of more than one exposure (as in Whitehall II described above) and the choice of the group of people in the cohort who will be regarded as unexposed depends on the particular hypothesis under investigation.

Although comparison groups are usually identified within the cohort, sometimes separate cohorts are set up at the outset. If a particular exposure or characteristic of interest is rare then the identification of separate cohorts may be necessary (external comparison groups). The cohort study of bambuterol, described above, uses an external comparison group, namely individuals prescribed other anti-asthma drugs (Martin *et al.* 1998). The advantage of this external group is that it was similar to the bambuterol cohort with respect to asthma history, and individual-level data on potential confounding factors could be included in the analysis (though confounding by the indication for the drug will always be difficult to control for (Blais *et al.* 1996)). Some cohort studies use as the external comparator group the general population in the same geographical area as exposed individuals. Disease rates observed in the cohort are compared with those of the general population at the time the cohort is being followed up. However, the ability to control for important confounding factors is limited using this strategy.

Measurement of exposure

The cohort study begins by establishing baseline data, usually from a cross-sectional study or routine information systems such as health visitor records. Choices have to be made about the range of exposures that will be measured. These may be assessed by abstracting data from routine records (e.g. medical or employment records), asking questions (e.g. dietary and smoking habits), taking measurements (e.g. blood pressure, lung function), performing investigations (e.g. vascular ultrasound scan) or laboratory tests (e.g. coagulation factors) and taking direct measurements of the environment in which the cohort members live.

Obtaining accurate information is essential if exposure–outcome associations are to be credible. Depending on the hypothesis under investigation information may be required on dates and ages when exposure started and stopped, dose and pattern of exposure (intermittent versus constant) and changes over time. The method of exposure measurement will also need to be considered. Smoking histories may be less accurate than urinary cotinine measurement as participants may lie about their habits, under-reporting their true level of smoking. Inaccuracy (misclassification) of this nature will tend to dilute the strength of relationship found with disease (see section on interpretation). In a simple cohort study, baseline measurements may never be repeated which means that changes in exposure cannot be studied. Over time, however, people tend to change their lifestyles and may be exposed to different levels of a risk factor. Cohort studies become much more useful if repeated exposure measurements are performed at regular intervals. For example, plasma insulin levels that are persistently elevated over a period of eight years may be more predictive of future risk of the metabolic syndrome and diabetes than a single measurement performed several years ago (Bao *et al.* 1996). Historical cohorts can be constructed from records made many years previously (e.g. Gunnell *et al.* 1996).

Follow-up and measurement of outcomes

The major challenge for long-term cohort studies is to maintain contact with the cohort to ascertain outcome events. If a large proportion of people are lost to follow-up for reasons that are related to both the exposure and outcome of interest the validity of the study may be threatened by selection bias (see section on interpretation). Therefore it is important that every effort is made to maintain contact or to ascertain the outcomes of those who migrate, move residence or die. It is particularly important to know when outcome events occurred as this enables person-time denominators to be calculated.

The cohort can either be followed up directly with repeated surveys of the same population (e.g. by questionnaires, telephone contact, home or clinic visits) or baseline data can be linked to routine surveillance systems (e.g. cancer registries and registers holding details of death certificates). The use of routine surveillance systems to trace and follow up participants is far less costly than if the investigators have to maintain regular personal contact with them. Routine surveillance systems, however, are limited by the extent and quality of the available data and may be subject to periodic changes in coding and method of ascertainment.

A major advantage of cohort studies is that it is possible to study the effect of an exposure on *multiple outcomes* at different periods of a person's life course. A mortality follow-up can be accomplished just as easily for all causes of death as for any specific cause. Health surveillance for one disease end point can sometimes be expanded to include many other end points without much additional work. As an example, Table 6.10 shows the multiple outcome measures available in the Boyd Orr cohort.

To avoid information bias (see section on interpretation), it is important that defined criteria are established for determining who has and has not experienced a relevant outcome and that the method of ascertainment is the same for exposed and unexposed groups throughout the study. Investigators who assess the outcomes should be kept blind to the exposure status of the study participants so that decisions on how a person should be categorized are not swayed by knowledge of the exposure. This is particularly important when there is a degree of subjectivity in assessing the presence or absence of an outcome. The level of diagnostic work-up

Table 6.10   Outcome measures available in the Boyd Orr cohort

Time period	Data
Childhood	Measured height, leg length, foot length and weight
Adolescence	Self-report date of menarche (age of onset of menstruation)
Early adulthood (at age 19–44 years)	Self-report height, leg length and weight (validated on a sub-sample of 294 subjects)
Late adulthood	Rose angina and self-report coronary heart disease; measured height, leg length and weight; waist, hip and thigh circumferences; blood pressure; ultrasound measures of atherosclerosis; lung function; tests of physical function; blood tests for growth factors, lipid profile, glucose homeostasis, insulin resistance, cortisol and testosterone; *Helicobacter pylori*; death certificates for cause-specific mortality; incident cancer registrations

that is demanded in clinical practice is often unrealistic in epidemiological studies and simpler methods are used. For example, for acute myocardial infarction in clinical practice it is usual to require a history of severe chest pain and the results of serial electrocardiograms and cardiac enzymes. In contrast, a cohort study may rely on self-completed chest pain questionnaires, one-off electrocardiographic evidence of a previous myocardial infarction, hospital activity analysis notifications or death certificates (Yarnell *et al.* 1994). In general, this is acceptable as the point of epidemiological cohort studies is to make comparisons of disease occurrence between exposed and unexposed groups – not to decide on individual treatments.

Analytical considerations

In a cohort study, the population at risk should be free of the outcome of interest at the start of follow-up. The baseline examination of the potential study population should therefore identify all existing cases with the outcome of interest. Selection criteria may either require such participants to be excluded from study participation altogether or to be excluded at the analysis stage. It may, however, be difficult to guarantee that all people are outcome-free at entry to the study. For example, diseases such as cancer, Alzheimer's disease and diabetes have long latent periods (a long interval between disease initiation and onset of clinically identifiable disease). In such situations, a reasonable approach would be to exclude events occurring during some time period immediately following entry into the study (e.g. for cancer, the first two to three years). In some situations the disease or outcome cannot plausibly develop until an induction period has passed. As Rothman states 'the induction period corresponds to the time that it takes for the causal mechanism to be completed by the action of the complementary component causes that act after exposure' (Rothman 2002). In such a situation, events might not be included in the analysis if there was insufficient time for the event to be plausibly related to the exposure.

A date should be specified as the end of the overall follow-up period and the vital status on that date must be specified for all cohort members. All participants whose vital status is known contribute person-time at risk until that date, or until the outcome of interest or death if these events occurred earlier. Those whose vital status is not known at the end of the follow-up period are considered 'lost to follow-up' and the last date for which their vital status was known is taken as the end of their person–time at risk.

Some events might be excluded from the calculation of incidence risks or rates if they are the second occurrence of the outcome of interest (e.g. a second myocardial infarction). This is because distinguishing between a new and recurrent event can be difficult and because second or subsequent events may have different causes. If only the first event is of interest, then any person who develops the event is removed from the population at risk at the time they develop the event – this is consistent with the requirement that members of a population at risk must be eligible to develop the outcome. If the interest is in the total number of events, then a person would remain in the population at risk even after the first event, though it would not be possible to distinguish between first and later events. Alternatively, separate incidence rates could be calculated for first, second, third and all subsequent events. The population at risk for a second event is those who had the first event; upon having a first event the person would leave the population at risk for the first event and enter the population at risk for the second.

If the outcome is a short–term or curable disease, such as a urinary tract infection, the person is no longer at risk during the episode of infection, but could be part of the population at risk again from the time of recovery. If a person who is part of a long–term cohort emigrates and is no longer available for follow-up, they are no longer at risk at the point of embarkation. If they return to the country in which the study is being conducted and can continue to be followed-up, they can become part of the population at risk at the time of re-entry.

Advantages and disadvantages of cohort studies

The advantages of cohort studies include: (i) the time sequence between exposure and outcome is clearly observed; (ii) many different disease outcomes can be studied in relation to a wide range of exposures; (iii) disease rates and risks for each exposure can be estimated, which can then be compared using both absolute or ratio measures of effect (see next section on measures of exposure effect).

In many studies, however, only a small minority of those at risk actually develop the event and/or there is a long introduction period. An important disadvantage of cohort studies, therefore, is the necessity to obtain information on exposures and other variables from large populations and to conduct lengthy follow-up in order to measure event risks or rates. Cohort studies can therefore be expensive and time consuming and not useful for rare diseases. Historical cohorts based on information assembled in the past reduce the need for lengthy follow-up, but are dependent on the quality of the information recorded. Secondly, knowledge of a person's exposure history may influence outcome assessment, introducing information bias. Thirdly, losses to follow-up introduce selection bias if the reasons for the loss are related to both the exposure and outcome. Fourthly, as in all epidemiological studies, it is important that the groups being compared are as similar as possible with respect to all other factors that are related to the outcome. Since the investigator has no control over who is or is not exposed, it is likely that exposure groups will differ in relation to factors other than the ones being investigated. These confounding factors need to be identified, measured and controlled for in the analysis. The advantages and disadvantages of cohort studies are summarised in Table 6.11.

Table 6.11   Advantages and disadvantages of cohort studies

Advantages	Disadvantages
• Direct measurement of incidence of disease in exposed and unexposed groups	• Can to be expensive and time-consuming
• Time relationships between exposure and disease known	• Not useful for rare diseases
• Reduced bias in exposure measurement	• Historical cohorts are very dependent on quality of records
• Multiple outcomes can be studied	• Losses to follow-up can bias findings (selection bias)
• Allows direct calculation of attributable risk	• Outcome assessment can be influenced by knowledge of exposure (information bias)
• Effects of rare exposures can be evaluated by appropriate selection of cohorts	
• Natural history of disease can be evaluated	

Measures of exposure effect, interpretation, design, planning and conduct of epidemiological studies

Measures of exposure effect

Each of the preceding study designs allows the calculation of different measures of the effect of an exposure. Measures of effect compare the frequency of the outcome of interest in exposed and unexposed populations (treated as the baseline). This section describes the calculation and interpretation of relative and absolute measures of effect. It is important to calculate confidence intervals around these summary measures to determine the precision of the effect estimate and the range of values within which it is likely that the true effect lies. For the calculation and interpretation of confidence intervals, the reader is referred to Chapter 21.

Risk and rate ratios

Cohort studies allow the calculation of incidence risks and rates of an outcome of interest, in those who were exposed and those who were not. The strength of the association between an exposure and the outcome of interest is then investigated by calculating a risk or rate ratio:

$$\text{Risk ratio} = \frac{\text{Risk in the exposed group}}{\text{Risk in the unexposed group}}$$

$$\text{Rate ratio} = \frac{\text{Rate in the exposed group}}{\text{Rate in the unexposed group}}$$

These measures indicate how much more likely the exposed group is to develop the outcome compared with the unexposed group:

- If the *risk (rate) ratio* = 1, then there is *no difference* between the exposure groups.
- If the *risk (rate) ratio* = 0.5, then exposure *halves* the risk of death.
- If the *risk (rate) ratio* = 0.75, then exposure *reduces* the risk of death by 25 per cent.

- If the *risk (rate) ratio* = 2.0, then exposure *doubles* the risk of death.
- If the *risk (rate) ratio* = 10.0, then exposure *increases* the risk of death tenfold.

If more than one exposure group is used (e.g. normal weight, mild overweight, obesity and extreme obesity) trends in risk across exposure categories can be assessed.

For example, Table 6.3 (see p. 105) showed the results of a cohort study investigating the risk of VTE in women using OCPs with differing progestagen components (Jick *et al.* 1995). The incidence rates in those on third and second generation pills, respectively, were 28.8 per 100,000 women-years versus 16.1 per 100,000 women-years. This gives a rate ratio of 1.79. The interpretation of this rate ratio is that women had a 1.79-fold (or 79 per cent) increased risk of suffering a VTE while on a third generation OCP compared with women on a second generation OCP.

Another way of analysing cohort data which takes into account different lengths of follow-up is to use survival analysis methods. Kirkwood and Sterne (2003: Ch. 26) provide an excellent introduction to survival analysis.

Risk and rate differences

Risk and rate ratios are *relative* measures of effect. In a cohort study, it is also possible to calculate an *absolute* measure of the effect of the exposure, a risk or rate difference. This is simply the difference in risk (or rate) between exposed participants and non-exposed participants.

Risk difference = risk in exposed − risk in unexposed

or

Rate difference = risk in exposed − risk in unexposed

Absolute measures of effect express the excess number of cases associated with an exposure (a risk difference of 0.00 implies no effect). To illustrate the difference between risk ratios and risk differences, data on the association between cigarette smoking and male mortality from the UK doctor's cohort study is shown in Table 6.12 (Doll and Peto 1976). The risk ratio suggests that smokers are 14 times more likely to get lung cancer than non-smokers, whereas they are at a 62 per cent increased risk of heart disease (risk ratio = 1.62). However, when cigarette smokers are compared to non-smokers using risk differences the risk of lung cancer is increased by 130 cases per 100,000 men, whereas the risk of ischaemic heart disease is increased by 256 cases per 100,000 men. The absolute *impact* of smoking is different for these two diseases. This is because the risk difference reflects the fact that ischaemic heart disease is a more common cause of death than lung cancer. In contrast, the risk ratio (the amount by which an exposure multiplies the risk of an event) is interpretable regardless of the size of the risk. Note that risk differences

Table 6.12 Association between cigarette smoking and male mortality from UK Doctor's cohort study

Disease	Risk of death in smokers/100,000	Risk of death in never smokers/100,000	Risk ratio	Risk difference (per 100,000)
Lung cancer	140	10	14	130
Ischaemic heart disease	669	413	1.62	256

Source: Doll and Peto (1976: data are from Table IV)

have units (risk per 100 or per 1000), while ratio measures are unitless. The magnitude of the risk ratio does not predict the magnitude of the risk difference.

The risk ratio measures the *strength* of the association. The risk difference indicates how many extra cases the exposure is responsible for. In the above example, for every 100,000 cigarette smokers, there will be 130 extra lung cancer deaths and 256 extra heart disease deaths. The risk difference is useful as a measure of the *impact* of an exposure – its value can be translated into the number of cases of the outcome that could be prevented if the exposure were completely eliminated (assuming that the relationship between exposure and disease is causal). In the above example, the importance of smoking as an aetiological factor was given by the risk ratio, and was more important for lung cancer than heart disease. From a public health viewpoint, smoking is much more important for heart disease because more cases of heart disease than lung cancer would be avoided if everyone stopped smoking.

In the study by Jick *et al.* on the risk of VTE associated with the OCP (1995), although the third generation pills nearly doubled the risk of VTE compared with second generation pills, the risk difference was 12.7 per 100,000 women years at risk (28.8 minus 16.1). Thus third generation pills were responsible for an extra 12.7 cases for every 100,000 women-years of treatment compared with second generation pills (assuming that the relationship between exposure and disease is causal). This suggests that the absolute risk of developing a VTE while on a third generation OCP are small. The choice of OCP comes down to weighing up this risk, one that would cause about one death in one million users each year, against the possible benefits of third generation pills (Weiss 1995).

Odds ratios

In cohort studies, the risk ratio measures the association between exposure and outcome. The further away from one (in either direction), the stronger the association. In case-control studies the strength of the association between exposure and outcome is measured using odds ratios.

Since a case-control study starts off with an arbitrary number of cases with the outcome of interest, it is usually not possible to know what proportion of exposed participants had the outcome – we just know what proportion of cases and controls are exposed. Thus the risk ratio and risk difference cannot usually be directly calculated. However, we do know the *odds of exposure* among cases and controls, and hence can calculate an estimate of exposure effect – the odds ratio.

Odds are a way of presenting probability that is familiar among those who bet. The odds is the chance in favour of one side in relation to another side. For example, the odds that a single throw of a die will produce a six are 1 to 5 or 1/5 (the probability of throwing a six is 1/6). In epidemiology, the odds of an event is the probability that an individual experiences the event divided by the probability that they do not. Odds can be compared using odds ratios: the ratio of two odds.

Data on which an odds ratio is based are often presented as a '2-by-2 table' (see Figure 6.10). This classifies participants, by outcome status, into whether or not they are exposed to an hypothesized factor. In Figure 6.10, the odds of exposure to non-exposure for cases is a:c while for controls this is b:d. Therefore the odds ratio is a:c/b:d. This equation is equivalent to (a $\times$ d/b $\times$ c), which is why it is sometimes called the cross–product ratio. An exposure that may have caused an outcome will be more common in cases than controls giving an odds ratio greater than 1, and one that may protect against the outcome will be less common, giving an odds ratio less than 1. If there is no association the odds ratio will be 1.

Comparison of odds ratio and rate ratio

Figure 6.10   2-by-2 table

Table 6.13   2-by-2 table for coronary heart disease (i)

	Coronary heart disease		
	Yes	No	Total
Above average body mass index	$a = 119$	$b = 1357$	$n_1 = 1476$
Average or less than average body mass index	$c = 83$	$d = 1387$	$n_0 = 1470$

To demonstrate the calculation of odds ratios and risk ratios in cohort and case-control studies, data from the Boyd Orr cohort are presented in Table 6.13. In this example, a sample of participants from the Boyd Orr cohort is used to examine the association between body mass index in childhood and development of coronary heart disease in adulthood.* The 2946 eligible individuals were divided into above average body mass index (a measure of body fatness) (n = 1476) and at or below average body mass index (n = 1470). Overall, there were 202 deaths from coronary heart disease. Table 6.13 shows the number of individuals who died from coronary heart disease by body mass index category.

The *risk ratio* is $RR = (a/n_1) \div (c/n_0) = (119/1476) \div (83/1470) = 1.43$

The *odds ratio* is $OR = (a/c) \div (b/d) = (119/83) \div (1357/1387) = 1.47$

In other words, those who are above average for body mass index have a risk of coronary heart disease mortality that is 1.43 times (43 per cent) greater than the risk to those who are at or below average for body mass index. Because the outcome is rare (i.e. the risk of coronary heart disease is low), the risk ratio and odds ratio are almost identical.

Suppose that a case-control study is conducted among the cohort members. All 202 cases of heart disease are found, and their body mass index as a child is ascertained. A total of 202 controls are then randomly sampled from the cohort. Since the exposure prevalence in the non-diseased source population from which the

* The data differ from a previous publication (Gunnell *et al.* 1998b) as the numbers of deaths have been updated and the analysis is highly simplified for illustrative purposes.

Table 6.14   2-by-2 table for coronary heart disease (ii)

	Coronary heart disease	
	Yes	*No*
Above average body mass index	a = 119	b = 101
Average or less than average body mass index	c = 83	d = 101

cases arose was 50 per cent, the exposure prevalence in an unbiased control series should be 50 per cent, which is what was obtained. The resulting 2×2 matrix is shown in Table 6.14.

Since in a case-control study we do not know the total number of individuals, neither the risk of heart disease, nor the risk ratio, can be directly calculated. However we can calculate the odds ratio:

$$OR = (a/c) \div (b/d) = (119/83) \div (101/101) = 1.43$$

This example also shows that the odds ratio can be used to compare cases and controls because the ratio of the odds of exposure (a/c) among cases compared to the odds of exposure among the healthy group (b/d) is equivalent to the odds of disease in exposed compared with unexposed. This is shown algebraically:

$$OR = a/b/c/d = a \times d/b \times c = a/c/b/d$$

The odds ratio is a popular summary measure in epidemiology for the following reasons. Firstly, in several study designs it approximates well to the rate or risk ratio. Secondly, in case-control studies, where the risk or rate ratio cannot be calculated, it provides an alternative measure of this. For a rare disease, the odds is approximately the same as the risk (see above) and so the odds ratio is approximately the same as the risk ratio. It can be shown, however, that depending on the method of control selection the odds ratio can be equivalent to either the relative risk or relative rate, even if the disease is not rare (e.g. if incident cases and controls are recruited concurrently, an analysis matched on time of selection provides an unbiased estimate of the rate ratio). For further information, Rodrigues and Kirkwood (1990) provide a useful discussion of sampling schemes for control selection. Finally, the odds have desirable mathematical properties (in particular the natural log of the odds ratio can take any value from minus infinity to plus infinity and has an approximately normal distribution), permitting easy manipulation in mathematical models, for example in multiple logistic regression. Odds are also used as a summary measure in meta-analysis.

Interpretation of epidemiological studies

The epidemiological literature is littered with conflicting reports and examples of randomized trials which have failed to confirm even apparently robust findings from observational epidemiological studies (Davey Smith and Ebrahim 2002). Thus when interpreting findings from epidemiological studies it is essential to consider the extent to which observed associations between an exposure and an outcome are spurious: i.e. explained by bias or confounding.

Bias

Bias refers to a departure from the *true* value when one observes an association between an exposure and an outcome (Last 1995). Unfortunately, the true value of a parameter that is being estimated, and hence the amount of bias in any given study, can never be known – only the observed study estimate. Nevertheless, steps can be taken in the design, execution and analysis of a study to reduce bias. Some 35 types of bias have been described, but in general bias can be considered to arise as a result of systematic errors in the way sample members are selected and followed up (selection bias) or in the way information was obtained about them (information bias).

Types of bias

Selection bias is 'an error due to systematic differences in characteristics between those who are selected for study and those who are not' (Last 1995). Selection bias may arise as a result of: (i) the methods used by investigators to select participants; (ii) those factors that influence a person's decision to participate; and (iii) losses to follow-up in a cohort study. Selection bias gives an observed result among study participants that differs from the result that would have occurred among those who were eligible for the study but who did not take part. As the result (e.g. a prevalence estimate in a cross-sectional study, or an estimate of the association between an exposure and disease in an analytical study) among non-participants is not observed, the presence of selection bias must usually be inferred.

For example, if volunteers are recruited into a cross-sectional study then it is likely they will differ from the general population in either being more sick (and therefore interested in the disease, or hoping to seek help from the study) or under-representing the sick (as the illness may make participation problematic). Therefore, prevalence rates calculated on the basis of such studies will be misleading (self-selection bias).

Even if participants are randomly selected, it is very rare for cross-sectional studies to achieve 100 per cent response rates. If response probability is related to a factor in the study – such as illness or risk factor status – then prevalence rates will be biased. For example, in studies of recreational drug use it is likely that non-responders will be made up of a disproportionate number of people with the greatest exposure (response rate bias).

Non-participation is also common in case control and cohort studies. However, while this may restrict their generalizability, it does not necessarily bias observed associations in these studies. Selection bias can occur in case-control and cohort studies, however, if correlates of non-participation are associated with both exposure and outcome and this leads to an observed exposure-outcome association in participants that differs from the (unobserved) association in non-participants.

In case-control studies, selection bias occurs if the selection of cases or controls is related to the exposure under study. For example, hospital controls will over-represent risk factors for diseases leading to hospitalization (e.g. heavy alcohol consumption), whereas controls selected from the general population will include people who would not have sought medical help even if they had developed the disease. The selection of cases can be biased if exposed cases are more (or less) likely to be selected for study than unexposed cases. Consider a case-control study of the relationship between use of the OCP and Type 2 diabetes (which is often sub-clinical and goes undetected in a large proportion of people). Since OCP use is related to a higher frequency of medical check-ups, a sub-clinical disease such as diabetes is more likely to be diagnosed in these women than other women (ascertainment bias). As a result, in a study comparing cases of diabetes with controls without diagnosed diabetes, a spurious association with OCP use may ensue.

In cohort studies, information on outcomes is usually not available for those who drop out. People who are lost to follow-up may have different probabilities of the outcome of interest compared with those who remain under observation. This may lead to biased estimates of the incidence of the outcome in those who stay in the study. If the bias on the incidence estimates is the same in exposed and unexposed groups, the rate ratio will be unbiased. If losses to follow-up are related to both the exposure and the outcome, however, the rate ratio estimate will be biased. For example, in a cohort study using mailed questionnaires to assess the relation of smoking and heart attack, if those who both smoke and develop a heart attack are less (or more) likely to respond than non-smokers who develop the disease, a biased estimate of the exposure-outcome relationship will be obtained. As it is difficult to determine whether losses to follow-up were systematically associated with exposure it is essential to keep losses to a minimum and to attempt to evaluate outcome status in those who are lost.

Information bias is 'a flaw in measuring exposure or outcome data that results in different quality (accuracy) of information between comparison groups' (Last 1995). That is, information bias arises from systematic differences in the way that exposure or outcome was measured between comparator groups. Measurement error is the difference between the exposure or outcome measures in the study and the true exposure or outcome. If, as a result of measurement error, inaccurate information is collected about either the exposure or the outcome or both, an individual (or other unit of analysis) may be placed into the wrong category or population sub-group (misclassification). Information bias occurs if measurement error (misclassification) distorts the true association between an exposure and an outcome. It is therefore important to design a study which minimizes misclassification and to assess the likely effect of misclassification.

Nevertheless, misclassification is inevitable because measurements in free-living humans are invariably imperfect. For example, Armstrong *et al.* (1994) tabulate several sources of errors in the measurement of exposure status, including:

- faulty design of the measuring instrument;
- machine imprecision;
- errors or omissions in the study protocol;
- poor execution of the protocol;
- inaccurate observation;
- estimating past circumstances using contemporary measures;
- limitations due to participant characteristics (inaccurate recall; short-term biological variability);
- errors during data entry and analysis.

Variation arising from problems with measurement instruments and observer technique are compounded by biological variation in participants. For example, blood pressure varies continuously in response to activity, anxiety, time of day and ambient temperature. Such biological variation can cause a systematic bias. If, for example, blood pressure measurements in one group (e.g. breast-fed infants) are made in the morning and in another group (e.g. bottle-fed infants) are made in the evening, the observed mean blood pressures will differ (e.g. suggesting a blood pressure difference between breast-fed and bottle-fed infants) even if they are the same when measured under similar conditions.

There are two types of misclassification bias: *non-differential* and *differential*. These terms refer to the fact that the effect of misclassification depends on whether the misclassification with respect to exposure (or outcome) is dependent on the individual's outcome (or exposure) status.

Non-differential misclassification occurs when the degree of misclassification of exposure is independent of outcome, or the degree of misclassification of outcome is independent of exposure. Because such errors will tend to increase the apparent similarity between the exposed and unexposed groups, non-differential misclassification of *exposure* leads to underestimation (dilution) of the true association (Armstrong *et al.* 1994). Thus in case-control and cohort studies, ratio measures of effect are biased towards unity (the null value of 1.0) and in a cohort study the rate difference is reduced towards zero. The effect of non-differential misclassification of *outcome* depends on the type of study. In case-control studies, odds ratios are attenuated towards the null. In cohort studies, under-ascertainment (more likely than over-ascertainment) of outcome does not bias the rate ratio, but the rate difference is biased towards zero (Rothman and Greenland 1998). In a cohort study, over-ascertainment of outcome will bias the rate ratio towards unity, but there is no bias in the rate difference.

Non-differential misclassification is potentially of concern in studies that seem to indicate the *absence* of an effect, where a real effect may have been obscured. On the other hand, if a study reports an association despite non-differential misclassification, an estimate of effect without non-differential misclassification could be even greater.

Differential misclassification occurs when the degree of misclassification of exposure or outcome measurements are not independent of each other. This may occur, for example, if unexposed people are under-diagnosed for disease more often than exposed people. Differential misclassification is more problematic as it can result in either an underestimate, overestimate or no effect on the measure of association, depending on the situation. There are two types of information bias arising from differential misclassification: (i) *recall bias*; and (ii) *observer* (interviewer) *bias*.

Recall bias is a problem in case-control studies and occurs when cases recall or report exposures differently from controls, for example because of their knowledge or feelings about the disease. The direction of the bias depends on which group has less accurate recall: if controls are less likely than cases to recall an exposure this leads to an overestimate of the odds ratio. For example, case-control studies of birth defects often require the reporting of prenatal exposures months or years after the exposure and birth have occurred. Mothers who have given birth to a baby with a serious birth defect may recall past exposures more accurately than mothers of normal babies, as such a major event is likely to encourage people to reflect more carefully on the circumstances leading up to the diagnosis than they would have done otherwise. To reduce recall bias one could use as a control group infants with other malformations, since completeness of recall among mothers of infants with other malformations may approximate that among cases (Lieff *et al.* 1999).

Observer bias is a source of differential misclassification if the interviewer in a case control study knows the participants' outcome status and this influences the information that is obtained about exposures, or if an observer in a cohort study knows the participants' exposure status and this influences the classification of outcome status. Observer bias is more likely to occur the greater the degree of subjective judgement that is required to classify exposure or outcome status. It is important to be aware that errors in the measurement of confounders may attenuate attempts to control for confounding factors, resulting in associations that are incompletely adjusted for the effects of confounding (residual confounding).

Reducing bias

Bias is an issue of study design and can irreparably distort the results of small and large studies alike. Selection bias can be avoided by: (a) maximizing response rates; (b) not allowing self-referrals; (c) ensuring that cases and controls are selected independently of exposure; (d) taking diagnostic (ascertainment) and referral practices into account when designing a study; and (e) reducing losses to follow-up by using multiple methods of contact and surveillance. Information bias can be reduced by the use of repeated measures, standardizing conditions of measurement, automated measurement procedures, training of field workers, using objective measures of data collection and using more than one source of information. Blinding the participants, researchers and statisticians can reduce bias when knowledge of a subject's exposure or outcome status may influence the information obtained. In case-control studies, data should be obtained as far as possible from sources that are independent of the subject's own reporting (e.g. clinical notes, prescription data, stored blood).

Confounding

The studies described in this chapter are all observational studies in which participants' exposure patterns are observed without attempting to change them. A crucial issue in their interpretation is whether there is an association with a third variable that provides an alternative explanation for the observed association between exposure and disease. This is known as confounding. The verb 'confound' stems from a Latin word (*confundo*) meaning to mix up. In epidemiology, confounding occurs when the effects of two associated exposures (or risk factors) have not been separated and it is therefore incorrectly concluded that the effect is due to one, rather than the other, variable. The effect of the exposure under study is mixed with the causal effect of another exposure.

For example, when death rates for lung cancer in lorry drivers are compared with the general population, it appears that there is a significant excess risk of lung cancer for lorry drivers. This might lead to the incorrect inference that lorry driving exposes the worker to an important occupational hazard. However, this inference would not be valid if it was shown that lorry drivers smoked more than the general population. Smoking is an alternative explanation for the excess lung cancer risk in lorry drivers (see Figure 6.11).

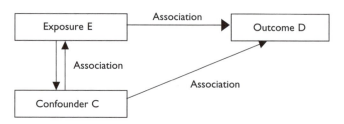

Figure 6.11   A simple representation of confounding

Exposure E (e.g. lorry driving) is associated with outcome D (e.g. lung cancer risk); a confounding factor C (e.g. smoking) is associated with exposure E and the outcome D

Confounding can seriously distort the findings of observational epidemiological studies of all types and it can often be difficult to separate such spurious associations from ones which may be causal (Davey Smith and Ebrahim 2002). For example, the previously described cohort study by Hemingway *et al.* (2001) suggested that patients who would be considered appropriate candidates for revascularization have a poorer prognosis if they are treated medically rather than by revascularization. This association may have been explained by observed differences in the baseline characteristics of the medically and surgically treated patients: there were significantly more patients with heart failure, diabetes and previous myocardial infarction, and fewer treated with beta-blockers in the medically treated group. All these factors are associated with prognosis and may therefore have confounded the observed association between appropriateness rating and outcome. Thus, it is difficult to be sure that the medically treated patients considered appropriate candidates for intervention would indeed have done better had they undergone revascularization.

Factors that are on the causal pathway between an exposure and a disease (intermediate variables) should not be regarded as confounding factors, even if it is believed that they are directly related to disease risk. For example, modest alcohol consumption may lower coronary heart disease risk by increasing the level of high-density lipoprotein (HDL) cholesterol. Using the statistical methods indicted below, it may be tempting to *control* for HDL cholesterol level as it is associated with both alcohol intake and coronary heart disease. However, controlling for a factor that is on the causal pathway leads to an underestimation of the strength of the causal effect of the exposure on the outcome.

The above discussion suggests the following properties of a confounding factor:

1 A confounding factor must be associated with the outcome of interest because it causes, or is a proxy measure of a cause of, the disease.
2 A confounding factor must be associated with the exposure under study in the source population.
3 A confounding factor must not be on the causal pathway between exposure and disease (i.e. a confounder must not be an effect of the exposure).

A factor that is related to the outcome of interest merely because of an association with the exposure of interest cannot be a confounding factor (i.e. a confounding factor must be predictive of the outcome among unexposed individuals).

What can be done about confounding? Firstly, observational studies could be performed in populations in which the exposure of interest and potential confounding factors are not strongly associated with each other. For example, breast-feeding is strongly socially patterned in developed countries, but socioeconomic gradients were less pronounced in pre-Second World War cohorts. Results on the long-term impact of breast-feeding from such cohorts may be less likely to be confounded by socioeconomic factors (Martin *et al.* 2004b). Secondly, the study can be restricted to participants who are similar in relation to the confounder. A researcher interested in causes of lung cancer other than smoking may establish a study only of non-smokers. Thirdly, by measuring confounders better, for example carrying out more and better measurements on a smaller number of participants, a greater degree of statistical control may be possible at the analysis stage by employing standardization, stratified analysis or multi-variable regression models (Davey Smith and Ebrahim 2002).

Many studies only measure a limited range of confounders, often with substantial measurement error. Even after 'controlling' for confounding using standard statistical techniques, *residual confounding* may remain and lead to spurious associations being reported in the literature (Davey Smith and Phillips 1992). Since confounding represents a serious potential threat to the validity of interpretations of epidemiological studies the possibility that confounding accounts for the findings of studies should always be considered in detail.

Designing, planning and conducting an epidemiological fieldwork study

The above section describes the theoretical principles underlying the major study designs, their analysis and interpretation. The practical issues in conducting an epidemiological study are clearly unique to each project, but some general issues can be highlighted.

Designing, planning and conducting an epidemiological study starts with the development of answerable research questions that justify (in terms of the originality and significance of their findings) the resources that will be expended in carrying the study out. The study design, population and methods of recruitment then need to be defined, and a sample size calculated to ensure that the proposed study will have enough power to detect an important minimum effect.

At the development stage of a study, database requirements can be easily underestimated, leading to unanticipated problems during the conduct of fieldwork and when data are being analysed. It is therefore worth discussing the database with your database manager early on in the project, to ensure that adequate resources are applied for. A good database should fulfil a number of tasks, including for example:

- administration of invitations to participate with a clear audit trail;
- follow-up of non-responders;
- logging changes of address and surnames;
- logging variable names, sources of data, units and how data items are coded;
- logging of consent items;
- logging the location of blood aliquots;
- providing a user-friendly data entry interface, with semi-automated features where feasible;
- automated production of letters, outstanding administrative task lists and interim reports;
- monitoring the quality of data collection by individual fieldworkers;
- rapid communication of results with GPs;
- the manageable collection of data on multiple events per person in long (events per person recorded in multiple rows) as well as wide (events coded in multiple columns) format (e.g. the coding of multiple drugs per person is manageable in long format but becomes unwieldy in wide format).

Planning the conduct of the study will be greatly helped by the preparation of a detailed organizational timetable. This should cover key tasks such as:

- securing ethical approval;
- designing and testing study instruments;
- developing job descriptions;
- recruitment, training and appraisal of staff;
- ordering of equipment and consumables;
- obtaining insurance and clinical liability cover;
- preparation of patient and GP information sheets, consent forms and questionnaires;
- development of a database to cover the administration of the study as well as data entry of questionnaire responses, measurements etc.;
- preparation of a detailed risk assessment for clinical studies;

- conducting a pilot study and subsequent protocol revisions;
- recruitment of study participants;
- the collection of data (interviews, clinics, blood sampling);
- conducting a reliability study (see below);
- analysis of bloods and other physiologic variables;
- data entry, merging of electronic results files with the master database and data checking;
- data analysis;
- preparation of reports, conference abstracts and scientific papers.

A *study manual* should be prepared which provides a step-by-step guide for all aspects of the administration, data collection and data processing of the study. Laboratories will need a detailed protocol for the collection, processing, transport and storage of blood samples. This also applies if third parties are to conduct analyses of other physiological data, such as Minnesota coding of electrocardiographs or image analyses of X-rays and ultrasound scans. A *coding manual* with all coding values and rules will be required and given to fieldworkers and data entry clerks. Aspects that could be covered by the study manual are listed in Box 6.6. It is worth keeping a contemporaneous list of people who should be acknowledged when the results are disseminated.

Inviting participants

Improving response rates can be aided by providing detailed information sheets for participants. These should cover the overall purpose of the study, why the person has been asked to participate, what will happen if they agree to take part, what they will get out of it, who is organizing the study, who is funding the study, who provided ethical approval, who to contact for further information and the address (if available) of the study website. It might help to provide transport for participants who may have difficulty getting to clinics and, for those who can travel, to provide details of parking and public transport and to offer to refund transport costs. Home visits and weekend appointments might need to be arranged. Every effort should be made to contact non-responders, including second reminders and telephone calls. Sometimes studies offer breakfasts (e.g. if participants had been asked to fast) or provide participants with the results of clinically relevant findings (e.g. ECG findings, blood cholesterol profile, blood pressure, height and weight readings). A participant's consent will be required to transfer such data to their GP.

The administrative database should have the subject's unique study ID, followed by sufficient personal identification to permit any planned follow-up: an address for postal contact, full name, date of birth and national health/social security number for later tracing of mortality or cancer. If GP or hospital follow-up is envisaged, the subject's consent to this should be recorded.

Questionnaires and other data-collection instruments

Epidemiological data are often obtained by means of questionnaires, which may be self-administered or administered at interview. Good design of questionnaires and other data-collection instruments requires skill and the reader is referred to a number of textbooks on the issue for more detailed information (e.g. see Armstrong *et al.*, 1994: Chapters 6 and 8). Self-reported data based on simple questions may provide valuable epidemiological information when face-to-face follow-up of participants is not possible because of logistical or financial reasons. However, it is worth considering a validation study on a small sub-set of participants. In a questionnaire

Box 6.6   Aspects that can be included in the study manual

Method for contacting and inviting subjects
  Who to approach
  Inclusion/exclusion criteria
  What information the study sample and participants will receive (sample information sheets and invitation letters)
  Administrative procedures for responders and non-responders
  Reminder intervals
  Making and confirming appointments (including provision of maps, details of parking and local public transport, contact telephone numbers)
  Special instructions (e.g. wear clothing that is easily adjustable, fast from midnight)

Research clinic
  Reception procedures
  Consent forms
  Framework of assessments being made
  Setting up and calibrating measurement equipment
  Examination, questionnaire and venepuncture protocol
  Guide to completing data entry sheets
  Processing, transporting, labelling and storing blood
  Protocol for feedback of results and for informing GP of any markedly abnormal results
  Subject departure procedures
  Protocol violations/departures from plan
  Answering questions about the study
  Health and safety
  Identifying and inviting subjects for repeatability studies
  Inventory of equipment required at the field station
  Useful telephone numbers/emails

Data processing
  Coding values and rules
  Dealing with anomalies
  Valid data ranges
  Logic checks

Financial procedures
  Petty cash
  Claiming travel expenses
  Administering participant expenses
  Travel and medical insurance

follow-up of the Boyd Orr study in 1997–8, participants were asked to report their birthweight (and to consult parents, sisters or someone else if they did not know). A validation study on a sub-sample of participants with both a recorded and self-report birthweight indicated moderate validity, though low birthweight people tended to under-report their birthweight (Kemp *et al.* 2000). There was no evidence that accuracy of recall was related to the participants' age, sex or childhood socioeconomic position.

The data recording form

This should be laid out with a clear idea of exactly how the information is later to be extracted and analysed. The statistician, database manager and an experienced data clerk should be involved at this stage. The design of the form should aim to help standardization, speed and accuracy in recording under field conditions, and coding and retrieval of results afterwards. Non-numerical information should be ringed or ticked, rather than written out. The layout should facilitate subsequent numerical coding and data extraction, with one answer box for each item of information. Transcription errors are reduced if non-numerical information is 'precoded' (i.e. assigning numbers to non-numerical information – e.g. 1 for men, 2 for women). The results can then be entered straight into the database.

An orderly and uncluttered layout results in fewer mistakes in the field and in data entry. Observers should be trained to complete forms accurately, completely and legibly (including instructions for confusing numbers and letters, such as I and 1, 4 and 9, 1 and 7). A training session should be devoted to explaining why the project is dependent on the quality of data recording. The data entry forms should be tested both in the field on representative participants and in the office for subsequent coding and data extraction. During the study, the observers' performance can be reviewed by sitting in on an interview/physical examination. Units of measurement should be specified on the form (e.g. height in metres or feet).

Each observer should initial the data they were responsible for checking. As soon as possible after each subject has been seen, the data recording forms should be checked for completeness and accuracy. Each observer's performance should be monitored and constructive feedback given. Tabulations and scatter plots of the data at regular intervals throughout data collection are useful to detect systematic patterns in the data, for example, refusal levels, missing data, or measurement drift.

The computer database should include in its tables a unique variable name for each piece of information, a specification of the data type and a description of the variable (e.g. where the information came from, its questionnaire number, units of measurement, coding values etc.). This will facilitate transfer to a statistical database and, in the long term, helps to ensure that future researchers will not be baffled by any of the variables contained in the database.

Quality control

Standardization and quality control are essential in epidemiological studies. A primary concern is to reduce measurement error and its effects (see section on interpretation, and sub-sections on bias), but other issues such as the safety of researchers and participants and the possibility of fraudulent data also need to be considered. Measurement error can influence a study at any stage of its development, and quality control procedures are required during the entire study period from instrument development to data collection, coding, derivation of variables and analysis. A comprehensive summary of quality control procedures is provided by Armstrong *et al.* (1994: Chapter 5, Table 5.3). Some of the key issues are listed below.

- Measurement techniques need to be standardized and observers trained and regularly tested. The study manual can serve as a major training tool.
- A pilot study can identify practical difficulties before the start of the main study.
- Monitor initial data collection closely (e.g. for fraud, measurement technique and data recording) and solve problems early.

- Blind observers to the main hypotheses to reduce differential information bias.
- Randomly allocate observers to participants to avoid systematic bias.
- Reliability studies of multiple observers (data collectors) who each collect data on the same participants can identify those who need additional training. By identifying sources of disagreements in repeated measures for a subject, an instrument can be improved.
- It may be possible to avoid the problem of inter-observer variability by using a single observer.
- A comparison of the distribution of variables among data collectors and analysis of trends in the variables over time can identify systematic differences between observers and measurement drift over time.
- Shortly after data collection procedures on a participant have been completed the forms should be reviewed for missing items, illegible handwriting, inadequate answers, inadmissible codes and ranges, and logical inconsistencies among responses. Errors identified by this review should be resolved by checking back with the subject, observer or original records. They may suggest a need for improving study procedures and for further training by some observers.
- Consistency, range and logic checks (e.g. ranges of dates of birth, height, blood pressure, categorical responses) can be built into the computerized data entry forms/tables to prevent data entry mistakes.
- Data entry errors can be identified by duplicate data entry.
- It is important to establish and maintain close contact with blood and other analytical laboratories so that standard criteria for collecting, storing and analysing specimens are established at the outset.
- For quality control of laboratory assays, a random sample of specimens can be sent to the laboratory and tested twice, using different identification numbers so that the laboratory staff are unaware that they are duplicates.
- At the analysis stage, range and consistency checks should be run for each variable to identify incorrect, unusual or illogical values. The distribution of each variable should be plotted to identify unlikely outliers. These data should be checked against the original data recording form as it may be possible to correct the error.
- Errors can arise during the derivation of variables from raw material or during the analysis. In the database, the original raw data should be kept separate from tables of derived variables. The method of deriving variables from the raw data should be logged. All programs, calculations, commands and outputs by which each of the study results are obtained should be documented for future reference. This is easily done in some statistical packages, such as Stata. This facilitates later checking and audit.
- Computers can fail, be damaged or be stolen and backup copies should be taken regularly.

Conclusions

Each study design has strengths and weaknesses and no one design is unreservedly superior (see Box 6.7). RCTs can provide unbiased estimates of treatment efficacy (MacMahon and Collins 2001), but the epidemiological study designs outlined in this chapter may be needed to investigate other hypotheses. Data from routine data sources are used to describe trends (time, place, person), for health care planning, to generate hypotheses and in record-linkage analytical studies. Ecological studies look for associations between exposures and outcomes in populations rather than in individuals. Cross-sectional (prevalence) studies describe the health of populations.

Box 6.7   Overview of epidemiological study designs

- Cohort studies: subjects are selected on the basis of their exposure status and then followed up over time. In contrast with intervention studies, the allocation of exposure is not determined by the investigator. An historical cohort is assembled from past records on exposure status; in a prospective cohort, exposure status is measured in the present.
- Case-control studies: a group of people with the condition of interest ('cases') and a group without that condition ('controls') are identified and the prevalence of the relevant exposure is measured in the two groups and compared.
- Cross-sectional studies: a group of subjects (sample) is selected from a defined population (study population) and contacted at a single point in time. On the basis of information obtained from the subjects at that point in time they are classified as having or not having the attribute of interest.
- Ecological studies: where the unit of observation and analysis is a group rather than an individual. Instead of observing individual measurements in study participants, aggregate measures that represent an entire population are used.
- Studies based on routine data: routine surveillance systems are used to obtain data on the exposure(s) and outcome(s) of interest. This type of study can be conducted without establishing contact with any of the subjects. Such studies can be carried out at the individual or ecological (aggregated) level.

Source: adapted from dos Santos Silva (1999)

In case-control studies participants are selected according to the presence or absence of the outcome and their exposure status assessed. In a cohort study, participants are selected who are initially free of the outcome event of interest, classified according to exposure status and then followed up over time to determine the incidence of the outcome according to exposure. Thus cohort studies involve complete enumeration of the denominator (people or person-time). As a result, cohort studies provide estimates of event rates and risks for each exposure, which can then be compared using rate/risk differences or ratios; case-control studies provide estimates of ratio measures of effect. Ratio measures of effect indicate the strength of an association while absolute measures indicate the public health importance of an exposure (assuming causality).

When interpreting the results of a study, it is important to consider alternative explanations for an observed association, including chance, bias, confounding and reverse causality. The avoidance of bias requires the careful design and conduct of a study. When evaluating a study for bias it is important to assess its source, strength and likely direction. Confounding is a mixing of effects that can seriously distort the interpretation of observational epidemiological studies. Attempts to control for confounding can be made at the design and/or analysis stage of a study but it is important to remember that residual or persistent confounding may be present even after many factors have been controlled for. If epidemiological study designs in health services are to improve population health and the delivery of services, and inform future research, an appreciation of their strengths, weaknesses and interpretation is required by clinicians, managers and health service organizations, as well as by researchers.

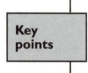

Key points

- Epidemiological study designs have been increasingly used in the evaluation of interventions and in assessing the provision and impact of health services.

- The results of RCTs are considered to provide evidence of the highest grade, while observational studies are often viewed as having less validity due to their potential biases.

- Observational studies provide an important, and possibly sole, source of evidence where experimentation is unethical, difficult to implement, unnecessary, inappropriate or difficult to generalize, and are useful for generating hypotheses, identifying rare, serious adverse effects, and for evaluating complex systems.

- The principal observational methods in epidemiology are cohort, case-control, cross-sectional and ecological studies. Routine databases are also major sources of information.

- Measures of the occurrence of health-related events are prevalence, incidence risks and incidence rates. As crude rates mask differences between age and sex groups, age and/or sex specific rates are often presented; when comparing populations, age and/or sex standardized rates may need to be calculated.

- Each study design allows the calculation of different measures of the effect of an exposure. Measures of relative and absolute effect compare the frequency of the outcome of interest in exposed and unexposed populations (risk and rate ratios, risk and rate differences, odds ratios).

- Selection bias can be avoided by maximizing response rates, ensuring that cases and controls are selected independently of exposure, taking diagnostic and referral practices into account when designing a study and reducing losses to follow-up by using multiple methods of contact and surveillance.

- Information bias can be reduced by using repeated measures, standardizing conditions of measurement, using automated measurement procedures, training fieldworkers, limiting the number of observers and employing specific techniques such as 'blinding'.

- Confounding represents a serious potential threat to the validity of data interpretation, and the possibility that study results are due to unmeasured or residual confounding always requires consideration.

- Conducting epidemiological fieldwork requires meticulous organization and preparation, a detailed study manual with clear fieldwork protocols, a well-designed database and quality-control procedures in place at each stage of the process.

References

Albertsen, P.C., Hanley, J.A., Gleason, D.F. and Barry, M.J. (1998) Competing risk analysis of men aged 55 to 74 years at diagnosis managed conservatively for clinically localized prostate cancer, *Journal of the American Medical Association*, 280: 975–80.

Anand, S.S., Yusuf, S., Jacobs, R. *et al.* (2001) Risk factors, atherosclerosis, and cardiovascular disease among Aboriginal people in Canada: the Study of Health Assessment and Risk Evaluation in Aboriginal Peoples (SHARE-AP), *Lancet*, 358: 1147–53.

Armstrong, B.K., White, E. and Saracci, R. (1994) *Principles of Exposure Measurement in Epidemiology*. Oxford: Oxford University Press.

Aylin, P., Bunting, J., De Stavola, B., *et al.* (1999) Mortality from dementia in occupations at risk of exposure to bovine spongiform encephalopathy: analysis of death registration, *British Medical Journal*, 318: 1044–45.

Bao, W., Srinivasan, S.R. and Berenson, G.S. (1996) Persistent elevation of plasma insulin levels is associated with increased cardiovascular risk in children and young adults: the Bogalusa Heart Study, *Circulation*, 93: 54–59.

Bay-Nielsen, M., Kehlet, H., Strand, L. *et al.* (2001) Quality assessment of 26304 herniorrhaphies in Denmark: a prospective nationwide study, *Lancet*, 358: 1124–28.

Beasley, R., Smith, K., Pearce, N. *et al.* (1990) Trends in asthma mortality in New Zealand, 1908–1986, *Medical Journal of Australia*, 152: 570–3.

Bhopal, R. (2002) *Concepts of Epidemiology: An Integrated Introduction to the Ideas, Theories, Principles and Methods of Epidemiology*. Oxford: Oxford University Press.

Black, N. (1996) Why we need observational studies to evaluate the effectiveness of health care, *British Medical Journal*, 312: 1215–8.

Blais, L., Ernst, P. and Suissa, S. (1996) Confounding by indication and channeling over time: the risks of beta 2- agonists, *American Journal of Epidemiology*, 144: 1161–9.

Blakely, T.A. and Woodward, A.J. (2000) Ecological effects in multi-level studies, *Journal of Epidemiology and Community Health*, 54: 367–74.

Bloor, K., Freemantle, N., Khadjesari, Z. and Maynard, A. (2003) Impact of NICE guidance on laparoscopic surgery for inguinal hernias: analysis of interrupted time series, *British Medical Journal*, 326: 578.

Bobak, M. and Marmot, M. (1996) East-West mortality divide and its potential explanations: proposed research agenda, *British Medical Journal*, 312: 421–5.

Boston, N.K., Boynton, P.M. and Hood, S. (2001) An inner city GP unit versus conventional care for elderly patients: prospective comparison of health functioning, use of services and patient satisfaction, *Family Practice*, 18: 141–8.

Breslow, N.E. and Day, N.E. (1980) *Statistical Methods in Cancer Research, Volume 1: The Analysis of Case-control Studies*. Lyon: IARC.

Brown, L.M., Pottern, L.M., Hoover, R.N. *et al.* (1986) Testicular cancer in the United States: trends in incidence and mortality, *International Journal of Epidemiology*, 15: 164–70.

Coldman, A.J., Phillips, N. and Pickles, T.A. (2003) Trends in prostate cancer incidence and mortality: an analysis of mortality change by screening intensity, *Canadian Medical Association Journal*, 168: 31–5.

COMMIT investigators (1995) Community intervention trial for smoking cessation (COMMIT): II. Changes in adult cigarette smoking prevalence, *American Journal of Public Health*, 85: 193–200.

Concato, J., Shah, N. and Horwitz, R.I. (2000) Randomized, controlled trials, observational studies, and the hierarchy of research designs, *New England Journal of Medicine*, 342: 1887–92.

Danesh, J., Youngman, L., Clark, S. *et al.* (1999) Helicobacter pylori infection and early onset myocardial infarction: case-control and sibling pairs study, *British Medical Journal*, 319: 1157–62.

Davey Smith, G. and Ebrahim, S. (2002) Data dredging, bias, or confounding, *British Medical Journal*, 325: 1437–8.

Davey Smith, G. and Phillips, A.N. (1992) Confounding in epidemiological studies: why 'independent' effects may not be all they seem, *British Medical Journal*, 305: 757–9.

de Lusignan, S., Hague, N., Brown, A. and Majeed, A. (2004) An educational initiative to improve data recording in the management of ischaemic heart disease in primary care, *Journal of Public Health*, 26: 34–7.

Doll, R. and Peto, R. (1976) Mortality in relation to smoking: 20 years' observations on male British doctors, *British Medical Journal*, 2: 1525–36.

dos Santos Silva, I. (1999) *Cancer Epidemiology: Principles and Methods*. Lyon: IARC.

Dunn, N., Thorogood, M., Faragher, B. *et al.* (1999) Oral contraceptives and myocardial infarction: results of the MICA case-control study, *British Medical Journal*, 318: 1579–84.

Dunn, N.R., Arscott, A., Thorogood, M. *et al.* (2000) Regional variation in incidence and case fatality of myocardial infarction among young women in England, Scotland and Wales, *Journal of Epidemiology and Community Health*, 54: 293–8.

Durkheim, E. ([1897] 1997) *Suicide: A Study in Sociology*, ed. G. Stimpson, trans. J.A. Spaulding and G. Stimpson. New York: Free Press.

Ebrahim, S., Ben-Shlomo, Y., Ho, D. *et al.* (2002) *Coronary Revascularisation in the South West Region, 1991–2000: Equity in the Use of CABG and PTCA by Gender, Age, Deprivation and Geography*. Bristol: South West Public Health Observatory.

Eke, T., Talbot, J.F. and Lawden, M.C. (1997) Severe persistent visual field constriction associated with vigabatrin, *British Medical Journal*, 314: 180.

Fildes, V. (1998) Infant feeding practices and infant mortality in England, 1900–1919, *Continuity and Change*, 13: 251–80.

Foster, K., Lader, D. and Cheesborough, S. (1997) *Infant Feeding 1995: A Survey of Infant Feeding Practices in the United Kingdom Carried out by the Social Survey Division of ONS on Behalf of the Department of Health, the Scottish Office Department of Health, the Welsh Office and the Department of Health and Social Services in Northern Ireland*. London: The Stationery Office.

Frankel, S., Gunnell, D.J., Peters, T.J. *et al.* (1998) Childhood energy intake and adult cancer – The Boyd Orr cohort study, *British Medical Journal*, 316: 499–504.

Frankel, S., Eachus, J., Pearson, N. *et al.* (1999) Population requirement for primary hip replacement surgery: a cross-sectional study, *Lancet*, 353: 1304–9.

Fraser, S., Bunce, C., Wormald, R. and Brunner, E. (2001) Deprivation and late presentation of glaucoma: case-control study, *British Medical Journal*, 322: 639–43.

Gardner, M.J. and Heady, J.A. (1973) Some effects of within-person variability in epidemiological studies, *Journal of Chronic Disease*, 26: 781–95.

Grimes, D.A. and Schulz, K.F. (2002) Descriptive studies: what they can and cannot do, *Lancet*, 359: 145–9.

Grulee, C.G., Sanford, H.N. and Schwartz, H. (1935) Breast and artificially fed infants: a study of the age incidence in the morbidity and mortality in twenty thousand cases, *Journal of the American Medical Association*, 104: 1986–8.

Gunnell, D.J., Frankel, S., Nanchahal, K. *et al.* (1996) Lifecourse exposure and later disease: a follow-up study based on a survey of family diet and health in pre-war Britain (1937–1939), *Public Health*, 110: 85–94.

Gunnell, D.J., Davey Smith, G., Frankel, S. *et al.* (1998a) Childhood leg length and adult mortality: follow-up study of the Carnegie (Boyd Orr) survey of diet and health in pre-war Britain, *Journal of Epidemiology Community Health*, 52: 142–52.

Gunnell, D.J., Frankel, S., Nanchahal, K. *et al.* (1998b) Childhood obesity and adult cardiovascular mortality: a 57-y follow-up study based on the Boyd-Orr cohort, *American Journal of Clinical Nutrition*, 67: 1111–18.

Hemingway, H., Crook, A.M., Feder, G. *et al.* (2001) Underuse of coronary revascularization procedures in patients considered appropriate candidates for revascularization, *New England Journal of Medicine*, 344: 645–54.

Hemingway, H., Shipley, M., Britton, A. *et al.* (2003) Prognosis of angina with and without a diagnosis: 11-year follow up in the Whitehall II prospective cohort study, *British Medical Journal*, 327: 895–900.

Hennekens, C.H. and Buring, J.E. (1987) *Epidemiology in Medicine*. Boston, MA: Little, Brown.

Hill, G., Connelly, J., Hebert, R., Lindsay, J. and Millar, W. (2003) Neyman's bias revisited, *Journal of Clinical Epidemiology*, 56: 293–96.

Hofman, A., Valkenburg, H.A. and Vaandrager, G.J. (1980) Increased blood pressure in schoolchildren related to high sodium levels in drinking water, *Journal of Epidemiology and Community Health*, 34: 179–81.

Jha, A.K., Perlin, J.B., Kizer, K.W. and Dudley, R.A. (2003) Effect of the transformation of the Veterans Affairs health care system on the quality of care, *New England Journal of Medicine*, 348: 2218–27.

Jick, H., Jick, S.S., Myers, M.W. *et al.* (1995) Risk of idiopathic cardiovascular death and nonfatal venous thromboembolism in women using oral contraceptives with differing progestagen components, *Lancet*, 346: 1589–93.

Jick, H., Rodriguez, L.A.G. and Perez-Gutthann, S. (1998) Principles of epidemiological research on adverse and beneficial drug effects, *Lancet*, 352: 1767–70.

Jones, J.K., Gorkin, L., Lian, J.F. *et al.* (1995) Discontinuation of and changes in treatment after start of new courses of antihypertensive drugs: a study of a United Kingdom population, *British Medical Journal*, 311: 293–5.

Kaye, J.A., Melero-Montes, M.d.M. and Jick, H. (2001) Mumps, measles and rubella vaccine and the incidence of autism recorded by general practitioners: a time trend analysis, *British Medical Journal*, 322: 460–3.

Kemp, M., Gunnell, D., Maynard, M. *et al.* (2000) How accurate is self-reported birth weight among the elderly? *Journal of Epidemiology and Community Health*, 54: 639.

Kirkwood, B.R. and Sterne, J.A.C. (2003) *Essential Medical Statistics*, 2nd edn. Oxford: Blackwell Science.

Korn, E.L. and Graubard, B.I. (1999) *Analysis of Health Surveys*. New York: Wiley.

Last, J.M. (1995) *A Dictionary of Epidemiology*, 3rd edn. New York: Oxford University Press.

Lawlor, D.A., Ebrahim, S. and Davey Smith, G. (2001) Sex matters: secular and geographical trends in sex differences in coronary heart disease mortality, *British Medical Journal*, 323: 541–5.

Lawlor, D.A., Ebrahim, S. and Davey Smith, G. (2002) The association between components of adult height and Type II diabetes and insulin resistance: British Women's Heart and Health Study, *Diabetologia*, 45: 1097–106.

Lieff, S., Olshan, A.F., Werler, M., Savitz, D.A. and Mitchell, A.A. (1999) Selection bias and the use of controls with malformations in case-control studies of birth defects, *Epidemiology*, 10: 238–41.

MacMahon, S. and Collins, R. (2001) Reliable assessment of the effects of treatment on mortality and major morbidity, II: observational studies, *Lancet*, 357: 455–62.

MacMahon, S., Peto, R., Cutler, J. *et al.* (1990) Blood pressure, stroke and coronary heart disease. Part 1, prolonged differences in blood pressure: prospective observational studies corrected for the regression dilution bias, *Lancet*, 335: 765–74.

Majeed, A. (2004) Sources, uses, strengths and limitations of data collected in primary care in England, *Health Statistics Quarterly*, 21: 5–14.

Mangtani, P., Jolley, D.J., Watson, J.M. and Rodrigues, L.C. (1995) Socioeconomic deprivation and notification rates for tuberculosis in London during 1982–91, *British Medical Journal*, 310: 963–6.

Marmot, M.G., Stansfeld, S., Patel, C. *et al.* (1991) Health inequalities among British civil servants: the Whitehall II study, *Lancet*, 337: 1387–93.

Martin, R.M., Dunn, N.R., Freemantle, S.N. and Mann, R.D. (1998) Risk of non-fatal cardiac failure and ischaemic heart disease with long acting beta2 agonists, *Thorax*, 53: 558–62.

Martin, R.M., Sterne, J.A.C., Mangtani, P. and Majeed, A. (2001) Social and economic variation in general practice consultation rates amongst men aged 16–39, *Health Statistics Quarterly*, 9: 29–36.

Martin, R.M., Hemingway, H., Gunnell, D. *et al.* (2002) Population need for coronary revascularisation: are national targets for England credible? *Heart*, 88: 627–33.

Martin, R.M., Sterne, J.A.C., Gunnell, D. *et al.* (2003) NHS waiting lists and evidence of national or local failure: Analysis of health service data, *British Medical Journal*, 326: 188–92.

Martin, R.M., Davey Smith, G., Frankel, S. and Gunnell, D. (2004a) Parents' growth in childhood and the birth weight of their offspring, *Epidemiology*, 15: 308–16.

Martin, R.M., Davey Smith, G., Tilling, K. *et al.* (2004b) Breastfeeding and cardiovascular mortality: the Boyd Orr cohort and a systematic review with meta-analysis, *European Heart Journal*, 25: 778–86.

Martin, R.M., Ness, A.R., Gunnell, D. *et al.* (2004c) Does breastfeeding in infancy lower blood pressure in childhood? The Avon Longitudinal Study of Parents and Children, *Circulation*, 109: 1259–66.

Maynard, M., Gunnell, D., Emmett, P. *et al.* (2003) Fruit, vegetables, and antioxidants in childhood and risk of adult cancer: the Boyd Orr cohort, *Journal of Epidemiology and Community Health*, 57, 218–25.

McCarron, P., Okasha, M., McEwen, J. and Davey Smith, G. (2001) Changes in blood pressure among students attending Glasgow University between 1948 and 1968: analyses of cross sectional surveys, *British Medical Journal*, 322: 885–9.

Merlo, J., Lynch, J.W., Yang, M. *et al.* (2003) Effect of neighborhood social participation on individual use of hormone replacement therapy and antihypertensive medication: A multilevel analysis, *American Journal of Epidemiology*, 157: 774–83.

Moore, N., Hall, G., Sturkenboom, M. *et al.* (2003) Biases affecting the proportional reporting ratio (PPR), in spontaneous reports pharmacovigilance databases: the example of sertindole, *Pharmacoepidemiology and Drug Safety*, 12: 271–81.

Morgenstern, H. (1998) Ecologic studies, in K.J. Rothman and S. Greenland (eds) *Modern Epidemiology*, 2nd edn, pp. 459–80. Philadelphia, PA: Lippincott-Raven.

Morris, A.D., Boyle, D.I.R., McMahon, A.D. *et al.* (1997) Adherence to insulin treatment, glycaemic control, and ketoacidosis in insulin-dependent diabetes mellitus, *Lancet*, 350: 1505–10.

Neyman, J. (1955) Statistics – servant of all sciences, *Science*, 122: 401–6.

Office of Population Censuses and Surveys, Department of Health and Royal College of General Practitioners (1995) *Morbidity Statistics from General Practice: Fourth National Study 1991–1992*. London: HMSO.

Padkin, A., Rowan, K. and Black, N. (2001) Using high quality clinical databases to complement the results of randomised controlled trials: the case of recombinant human activated protein C, *British Medical Journal*, 323: 923–6.

Rasmussen, F., Gunnell, D., Ekbom, A. *et al.* (2003) Birth weight, adult height, and testicular cancer: cohort study of 337,249 Swedish young men, *Cancer Causes and Control*, 14, 595–8.

Rodrigues, L. and Kirkwood, B.R. (1990) Case-control designs in the study of common disease: updates on the demise of the rare disease assumption and the choice of sampling scheme for controls, *International Journal of Epidemiology*, 19: 205–13.

Roodpeyma, S., Kamali, Z., Afshar, F. and Naraghi, S. (2002) Risk factors in congenital heart disease, *Clinical Pediatrics*, 41: 653–8.

Rothman, K.J. (2002) *Epidemiology: An Introduction*. New York: Oxford University Press.

Rothman, K.J. and Greenland, S. (eds) (1998) *Modern Epidemiology*, 2nd edn. Philadelphia, PA: Lippincott–Raven.

Rowan, K., Harrison, D., Brady, A. and Black, N. (2004) Hospitals' star ratings and clinical outcomes: ecological study, *British Medical Journal*, 328: 924–5.

Rychetnik, L., Frommer, M., Hawe, P. and Shiell, A. (2002) Criteria for evaluating evidence on public health interventions, *Journal of Epidemiology and Community Health*, 56: 119–27.

Saxena, S., Ambler, G., Cole, T.J. and Majeed, A. (2004) Ethnic group differences in overweight and obese children and young people in England: cross-sectional survey, *Archives of Disease in Childhood*, 89: 30–6.

Schlesselman, J.J. (1982) *Case-control Studies: Design, Conduct, Analysis*. New York: Oxford University Press.

Skegg, D.C.G. (2000) Pitfalls of pharmacoepidemiology, *British Medical Journal*, 321: 1171–2.

Smith, A.G., Fear, N.T., Law, G.R. and Roman, E. (2004) Representativeness of samples from general practice lists in epidemiological studies: case-control study, *British Medical Journal*, 328: 932.

Thomas, J., Paranjothy, S. and James, D. (2004) National cross-sectional survey to determine whether the decision to delivery interval is critical in emergency caesarean section, *British Medical Journal*, 328: 665–8.

Thomson, H., Hoskins, R. and Petticrew, M. (2004) Evaluating the health effects of social interventions, *British Medical Journal*, 328: 282–5.

Tunstall-Pedoe, H., Kuulasmaa, K., Mahonen, M. *et al.* (1999) Contribution of trends in survival and coronary-event rates to changes in coronary heart disease mortality: 10-year results from 37 WHO MONICA project populations. Monitoring trends and determinants in cardiovascular disease, *Lancet*, 353: 1547–57.

Tunstall-Pedoe, H., Vanuzzo, D., Hobbs, M. *et al.* (2000) Estimation of contribution of changes in coronary care to improving survival, event rates, and coronary heart disease mortality across the WHO MONICA Project populations, *Lancet*, 355: 688–700.

Vainio, H. and Morgan, G. (1998) Cyclo-oxygenase 2 and breast cancer prevention, *British Medical Journal*, 317: 828–30.

Wacholder, S., McLaughlin, J.K., Silverman, D.T. and Mandel, J.S. (1992a) Selection of controls in case-control studies: I. Principles, *American Journal of Epidemiology*, 135: 1019–28.

Wacholder, S., Silverman, D.T., McLaughlin, J.K. and Mandel, J.S. (1992b) Selection of controls in case-control studies: II. Types of controls, *American Journal of Epidemiology*, 135: 1029–41.

Wacholder, S., Silverman, D.T., McLaughlin, J.K. and Mandel, J.S. (1992c) Selection of controls in case-control studies: III. Design options, *American Journal of Epidemiology*, 135: 1042–50.

Wang, H.X., Fratiglioni, L., Frisoni, G.B. *et al.* (1999) Smoking and the occurrence of Alzheimer's disease: cross-sectional and longitudinal data in a population-based study, *American Journal of Epidemiology*, 149: 640–4.

Warner, J. and Whitmore, W.F. Jr (1994) Expectant management of clinically localized prostatic cancer, *Journal of Urology*, 152: 1761–5.

Waterstone, M., Bewley, S., Wolfe, C. and Murphy, D.J. (2001) Incidence and predictors of severe obstetric morbidity: case-control study commentary: obstetric morbidity data and the need to evaluate thromboembolic disease, *British Medical Journal*, 322: 1089–94.

Weiss, N. (1995) Third-generation oral contraceptives: how risky? *Lancet*, 346: 1570.

Willett, W.C. and Stampfer, M.J. (1990) Dietary fat and cancer: another view, *Cancer Causes and Control*, 1: 103–9.

Yarnell, J.W., Sweetnam, P.M., Marks, V. *et al.* (1994) Insulin in ischaemic heart disease: are associations explained by triglyceride concentrations? The Caerphilly prospective study, *British Heart Journal*, 71: 293–6.

Yusuf, S., Flather, M., Pogue, J. *et al.* (1998) Variations between countries in invasive cardiac procedures and outcomes in patients with suspected unstable angina or myocardial infarction without initial ST elevation, *Lancet*, 352: 507–14.

Acknowledgements: Thanks are due to all the teachers on the Department of Social Medicine undergraduate and short courses. In particular Yoav Ben Shlomo, David Gunnell, Matthias Egger, Shah Ebrahim, Una Fallon, Jonathan Sterne and Andy Ness. David Gunnell commented on an earlier draft of this chapter.

7 | Finding and using secondary data on the health and health care of populations

Mary Shaw

Introduction

This chapter considers secondary, or existing, sources of data that can be used to understand population health and to contribute to health services research. 'Secondary sources of data' refers to data that have been collected and published by others – such as routine statistics collected through the census and mortality statistics, hospital episodes statistics, or government-funded surveys such as the Health Survey for England. These sources of data offer great potential to the health researcher. They bypass the huge cost and effort involved in primary data collection (someone else will already have forked out for that). Moreover, they often have very large samples, and sometimes include the entirety (or a great proportion) of the population of interest. Access to data through the internet has opened up the possibility of using secondary sources to anyone with a personal computer and a reasonable modem. A vast range of data are thus at the fingertips of any keen and curious researcher.

However, there are also limitations and difficulties associated with the use of existing data. Constraints are imposed by the questions and sample that have been formulated by other researchers – often for purposes different from those of the secondary researcher. Moreover, a profusion of readily available data does not preclude the importance of having a predefined research question and following a rigorous analytical method. This chapter thus addresses the topic of secondary data for health research, with the aim of achieving some balance between highlighting its potential and acknowledging its pitfalls.

To begin with, data from patient records are considered, first in a historical context, and then with reference to primary care. Then data from secondary care are covered as well as disease registers. Following this, record linkage is covered, and some of the key surveys that are available as secondary data. Finally, data from surveys are considered. The aim is not to provide a comprehensive list of resources, but to highlight some key sources which are generally available, and to show the type of research questions that they have been used to address.

Data from patient records: historical documents

Looking at the records kept about an individual from when they have been a patient has always been a first point of call for epidemiological data and this method has been used to answer a range of research questions. Medical records can continue to tell a story long after the deaths of the individuals concerned – historians of medicine and historical demographers make great use of the patient records of times past. A paper by Haines and Shlomowitz (2003) is an example of the exploration of the records of a particular group of people, in this case emigrants from Britain on voyages to South Australia between 1848 and 1885, following a long tradition of the study of maritime mortality. Haines and Shlomowitz argue that the voyages, which were highly scrutinized by the government, can be seen as 'a laboratory for epidemiologists to trace the progression of infectious disease in a closed environment'. They report 323 voyages using the records kept by the surgeons who accompanied such journeys and who were required by the government to submit logs and journals for auditing purposes. These can be used to understand the nature of disease and death on board ship. The findings show that on the majority of voyages – which had an average duration of 95 days – there were less than six deaths, although for some this was considerably higher, with infants and young children accounting for three-quarters of the total. Table 7.1 shows this information by cause

Table 7.1 Data from patient records: government-assisted voyages to South Australia 1848–85

Cause of death				Age				
	Infants	1	2	3–5	6–10	11–20	21+	Total
Non-infectious								
Accidental death	15	3	2	1	3	5	3	35
Kidney, liver, bowel, abdominal	14	23	6	8	1	3	19	74
Heart, cancer, natural causes	7	1				3	13	24
Brain-cerebral	60	31	11	11	5	5	7	130
Wasting and deficiency	106	36	6	9	3	5	14	179
Maternal mortality (non-infectious)						3	6	9
Premature birth (and stillborn)	57							57
Perinatal	13							13
Unknown/unclassified	62	31	12	11	3	7	27	153
Infectious								
Diarrhoea related	136	124	20	12	7	11	27	337
Fevers: water/lice borne	28	22	8	13	12	14	41	138
Fevers low, inflammatory	8	4	4	5	6	19	30	76
Measles and measles related	25	53	30	24	3	1		136
Upper respiratory	78	60	19	24	9	5	17	212
Whooping cough	19	23	6	3		1		52
Tuberculosis related	17	24	5	10	2	9	30	97
Fevers, infantile incl. remittent	4	8	3	2	1			18
Chicken-pox		1					2	3
Scarlatina/scarlet fever	7	18	9	18	7	2	1	62
Skin infections	1						2	3
Maternal mortality (infectious)						1	10	11
Sexually transmitted	1							1
TOTAL: ALL CAUSES	**658**	**462**	**141**	**151**	**62**	**94**	**252**	**1,820**

Source: Haines and Shlomowitz (2003)

of death. As in England and Wales at the time, the major causes of death for infants and 1-year-olds were diarrhoeal disease, wasting and deficiency disorders, premature births and upper respiratory infection (including whooping cough, measles and brain-cerebral causes including convulsions). Interestingly, the proportion of deaths with unknown causes was lower for maritime deaths than for those on land, reflecting the greater completeness of the record-keeping of ships' surgeons. Among older passengers, deaths due to causes such as tuberculosis were lower on land, due to the selection of only (apparently) healthy individuals for emigration. Maternal deaths (those resulting from childbirth) were also markedly lower at sea. Haines and Shlomowitz suggest that this may be due to the fact that on land much streptococcal infection was spread by doctors. This historical example shows how records originally kept for another purpose can prove to be a rich source of information for the secondary researcher.

Patient records from primary care: from paper to electronic records

In a contemporary context, information about patients can be used in a number of ways. The main purpose of such records is to inform the effective clinical management of the individual patient. For example, Simpson (2003) has reported that a patient record system designed to assist multidisciplinary teamworking in a palliative care setting improved the clarity of information exchanged, enhanced communication, avoided duplication and maintained the continuity of the patient's journey. Beyond clinical management, (electronic) patient records can also be used to inform a range of questions, such as the health needs assessment of populations, health service use and planning, as well as the explorations of epidemiological hypotheses. Here we consider data collected in the context of primary care – see Box 7.1 for a list of the sources covered.

The computerization of patient records introduces huge potential for the collation, linkage and analysis of primary care data. However, information that is entered

---

Box 7.1   Sources of data collected in primary care

- Data from computerized general practice records.
- General practice audits and needs assessments.
- Data derived from projects such as PRIMIS using MIQUEST (PRIMIS took over from the pilot CHDGP – Collection of Health Data from General Practice project).
- Data derived and collated from general practice databases such as the General Practice Research Database.
- Data derived from surveys such as the Fourth National Survey of Morbidity in General Practice.
- (Local) disease registers.
- Routine National Health Service (NHS) activity such as the General Medical Services (GMS) statistics database and the Royal College of General Practitioners' weekly returns.
- Prescribing Analysis and Cost (PACT) data.

Source: adapted from Majeed (2004)

onto electronic databases needs to be standardized, and often the detail and nuance of individual paper records is lost – electronic data thus tend to be somewhat pithier. Often what are essentially qualitative data are funnelled into quantitative categories. Walsh (2004) considers this essentially sociological process of the formation of electronic records, and points to the process of the reduction of the patient's narrative from a story metaphor into 'information' that can be easily managed. Some aspects of the patient's story are necessarily lost, others are emphasized, and the clinician's concept of the patient's illness is altered. However, not everyone is so pessimistic about electronic records. In a study comparing paperless and paper-based records in 25 general practices in the Trent region, Hippisley-Cox *et al.* (2003) found that paperless records compared favourably with manual records – they were more fully understandable, legible, more likely to have at least one diagnosis recorded, to have recorded advice given, the specialty of any referral made, and the dose of any prescription. Preferences for data – whether standardized data which are suitable for quantitative data analysis, or the richer and less structured prose of hand-written notes – will depend upon the perspective of the researcher and their research question. However, the transition from paper to electronic records is underway and inevitable, although there may be some teething problems which may relate to way that data are coded by doctors and to the marrying of different computer systems.

Another issue made even more apparent by the electronic collation of patient information, which should be of central concern to researchers, is that of data protection. Patient records are held by an institution (in this case the general practice) and contain data pertaining to the patient, practitioner and institution. Any such database will contain some sensitive data, and so must be protected, particularly as informed consent is not usually practicable (although it is becomingly increasingly expected for data used in research). Electronic data are open to abuse on a scale not previously possible with paper records – they can be copied and shared in a matter of seconds (at least theoretically). Any research using electronic patient records thus needs to consider patients' rights as well as the requirements of research; the Data Protection Act of 1998 has wide-ranging implications in this respect and is an essential element to good research practice (see Box 7.2).

Box 7.2   Data Protection 1998: principles

The Act states that personal data shall be:

* collected and processed fairly and lawfully;
* held for only the specific and lawful purposes described in the register entry;
* only disclosed to those people described in the register entry concerned;
* adequate, relevant and not excessive in relation to the purpose for which they are held;
* accurate and, where necessary, kept up to date;
* held no longer than is necessary for the registered purpose;
* held under secure conditions;
* accessible to the individual concerned who, where appropriate, shall be allowed to have data corrected or erased.

Source: adapted from the University of Bristol website

Some caution is necessary when using and interpreting patient records. Such records will always be dependent on the individual patients presenting to a health service professional. There may be a host of reasons why people do or do not seek medical help. This phenomenon – that not all symptoms experienced by individuals are presented to medical professionals – is known as the 'illness iceberg', with most symptoms remaining hidden and unreported (Last 1963). Other forms of help other than the professional sector may be consulted instead – the popular and folk, as well alternative or complementary therapies (see Box 7.3) – in preference to consulting a general practitioner (GP). Little is known about help-seeking within these other sectors. Conditions which are associated with acquiring stigma (e.g. sexually transmitted infections) may mean that people are especially reluctant to seek help. Inclination to seek help will thus vary according to factors such as ethnicity, cultural group and beliefs, age, gender, social class and so on, as well as according to the nature of the condition itself (a patient is more likely to present to services with a broken leg than with depression). It is important to keep these sociological factors in mind when using and interpreting statistics from secondary sources. For a more extensive discussion of these issues, see Scambler (2003).

Box 7.3   Sectors in the health care system

'In every culture, illness, the responses to it, individuals experiencing it and treating it, and the social institutions relating to it are all systematically interconnected. The totality of these interrelationships is the health care system . . . In our model, health care is described as a local cultural system of three overlapping parts: the popular, professional, and folk sectors'.

- **Popular sector:** includes immediate family, social and kinship networks and self-medication.
- **Folk sector:** includes non-professional but specialist therapists and healers.
- **Professional sector:** includes professionally organized systems of medicine with formal and standardized modes of recruitment, training and qualifications.

Source: Kleinman (1980)

Using data derived from primary care

With these shortcomings and restrictions (but also huge potential) in mind, what can (electronic) patient records be used for in a research context? Small-scale studies can be conducted (i.e. studies which collect, analyse or audit data from a single or selected group of general practices, usually for the purposes of addressing a specific research question). For example, Kam *et al.* (2002) reviewed 116 patient records from general practice in an audit of the effectiveness of acupuncture on musculo-skeletal pain. They found that 69 per cent of patients had a 'good or excellent' response to the treatment. A Dutch study (van der Weijden *et al.* 1996) analysed over 3500 patient records randomly sampled from 20 general practices to investigate the prevalence and targeting of cholesterol testing in general practice. They found low rates of testing among those most likely to benefit. As these two examples indicate, the analysis of patient records from general practice has the potential to inform our understanding of issues (either as outcomes or causes) that are not currently measured in a routine or systematic way (e.g. use of complementary and alternative medicines, lifestyle factors such as smoking, alcohol and illicit drug use) and to provide information about the needs of specific patient groups (e.g. prisoners, people with diabetes, recipients of joint replacement, people resident in a certain area).

The National Health Service (NHS) report *Information for Health* (NHS Executive 1998) reported the variable quality of primary care data and noted a lack of expertise in information management and analytic skills: 'The most valuable repository about the current health of the population may well be GPs' records and it is ironic that these are virtually unused for local health surveillance and service audit'. In response, the NHS Information Authority launched a training and support service to help primary care organizations take full advantage of their clinical computer systems. This service – PRIMIS (Primary Care Information Services) – provides free training and assistance to information facilitators employed by Primary Care Trusts (PCTs), who then cascade knowledge and skills to GPs and practice staff. Part of this training includes the use of MIQUEST, which is a query manager – a methodology for extracting data from different types of general practice systems, adopted as a standard for this purpose in the NHS. An example of analysis using PRIMIS and MIQUEST can be found in a paper by Horsfield and Teasdale (2003). They interrogated data from 317 general practices in 23 PCTs on the topic of clinical data related to coronary heart disease (CHD), its management, co-morbidity and interventions. They reported significant and systematic gender inequalities in the monitoring and treatment of CHD.

Whereas PRIMIS is primarily for use by PCTs and GPs, and is most suited to answering questions concerning the health of local populations, the General Practice Research Database (GPRD) is a more general resource. This database is the world's largest computerized record of anonymized patient data from general practice (see www.gprd.com for full details). It has been collecting patient records in the UK continuously since 1987 and now contains over 35 million patient years of data. The GPRD currently collects information on approximately 3 million patients, equivalent to about 5 per cent of the UK population. Data are provided by contributing general practices from all around the UK. The database includes:

- demographics, including age and gender of patient (information on ethnicity is not collected);
- medical diagnosis, including comments;
- all prescriptions;
- events leading to withdrawal of a drug or treatment;
- referrals to hospitals;
- treatment outcomes, including hospital discharge reports where patients are referred to hospital for treatment;
- miscellaneous patient care information (e.g. smoking status, height, weight, immunizations, lab results).

Who can access the GPRD? The database is operated on a self-financing, non-profit basis and the data are licensed for use exclusively for medical and health research purposes on a non-profit making basis. A scientific and advisory group reviews the protocols for studies. GPRD is used by a range of researchers based in academic institutions, as well as by government and health service researchers and research staff in the pharmaceutical industry. Uses of the data are restricted to medical and health research purposes in areas such as clinical research planning, drug utilization studies, studies of treatment patterns, clinical epidemiology, drug safety studies, health outcomes, pharmacoeconomics and health service planning.

For example, Kaye *et al.* (2003) used the GPRD to look at changes in antipsychotic drug prescribing over a ten-year period – they reported an increase, primarily due to increased average annual duration of use rather than higher rates of new use. Soriano *et al.* (2003) looked at the prevalence of doctor-diagnosed asthma using GPRD data, showing an increase over the 1990s. In a rather different vein, Smith *et al.* (2003) note that the GPRD can be used to look at the prevalence of head lice and prescriptions for parasiticidal agents, noting that the GPRD provides data not available from other sources. Published reports also utilize and make accessible these data, and many can be found via the National Statistics website (www.statistics.gov.uk) which published *Key Health Statistics* (Series MB6) from this source. For instance, the report *Social Focus on Men* (ONS 1998) used GRPD data on CHD, as shown in Table 7.2.

Table 7.2   Prevalence of treated CHD among men by age, 1998

England & Wales	*Rates per 1000 male patients*
35–44	4.9
45–54	30.2
55–64	94.5
65–74	184.0
75 and over	229.2
All men aged 35 and over	78.5

Source: ONS (1998)

GPRD data can also be used to support more complex analyses. Hoare (2003) used GPRD data to look at the prevalence of ten treated diseases and their relationship with two different measures of deprivation (the Townsend Index and the Index of Multiple Deprivation 2000), finding that both resulted in very similar patterns of health inequalities.

In terms of the quality of GPRD data, Hollowell (1997) considered this issue and reported that this is likely to be adequate for many purposes. However, 'because the GPRD data recording protocol does not require all consultations to be recorded, prevalence estimates for some chronic conditions are likely to be more valid where both diagnostic and treatment data can be used to identify prevalent cases'. Also, the GPRD data were found to slightly under-represent smaller practices and practices in Inner London. Nonetheless, Hollowell described the GPRD as a 'unique and valuable resource of national public health information'.

Data derived from a series of surveys of morbidity in general practice, run by the Office for National Statistics (ONS) (formerly OPCS, the Office of Population Censuses and Surveys) in conjunction with the Royal College of General Practitioners and the Department of Health, have also been a key resource for understanding patterns of primary care. The series is carried out approximately every ten years, with the first conducted in 1955–6. The Fourth National Survey of Morbidity in General Practice (NSGP4) is the most recent; data were collected in 1991/2.

The 1991/2 survey consists of a nationally representative sample of GPs' and practice nurses' recorded details of every face-to-face contact with their patients over the course of a year, in order to examine the pattern of disease seen in general practice. Data from all face-to-face contacts over one year in 60 general practices with half a million patients in England and Wales were collated (with an average of 3.8 contacts per person). Additional socioeconomic data were collected from 83 per cent of patients by interviewers. In general, the study sample was representative of the population enumerated in the census by age, sex, marital status, housing tenure, economic position, occupation and whether they lived in an urban or rural area; the proportion who smoked was similar to that recorded in the General Household Survey. There were small differences in the proportions of people by social class, and ethnic minority groups, people living alone and residents of inner-city areas were under-represented in the study sample.

No decision has been made as to whether there will be another NSGP. However, as with the census, such large studies have a relatively long shelf-life. The data are available on CD-ROM, and researchers continue to make use of them. For example, a recent paper by Martin and Gunnell (2004) considered the prevalence of mental illness among young adults aged 16–39, looking specifically at rural/urban differences. They sought to uncover whether lower consultation rates in rural areas could be explained by socioeconomic circumstances but found that large differences remained even after adjusting for social class, housing tenure and marital status. The authors suggested that a possible explanation for this may be the greater stigma attached to mental illness in rural areas, particularly for males.

Box 7.4   Four characteristics of disease registers

- Registers are based on people not events.
- People registered have a feature in common.
- Information held about these people is updated in a defined and systematic manner.
- The register is based on a geographically-defined population.

Source: Donaldson (1992) cited in Newton and Garner (2002)

Other sources of information on primary care are (local) disease registers, which gather information on chronic diseases (see Box 7.4). The source of data for registers can include, but is not limited to, primary care. Many registers are locally based, and attempt to collect information on all occurrences of a specific disease in a defined population. They vary in size, quality, coverage, completeness, purpose, funding and accessibility (see Box 7.5 for some examples of the topics and populations covered). Registers have tended to be run differently in different areas, although the NHS Plan and various National Service Frameworks are moving this situation towards greater integration; PCTs hold the responsibility for taking this forward. The White Paper, *Saving Lives: Our Healthier Nation* (Department of Health 1999), was particularly strong on the point of moving forward the potential of such registers.

Cancer registries are an exception to the tendency for localization in that they are part of a national network. Cancer registration is the process of recording all relevant details concerning cancer, including diagnosis, treatment and death. Prior to 1993 the collection of data in cancer by registries, and its transmission to the ONS, was voluntary. However, in 1990 the working party on the National Cancer Registration System (based at the ONS) recommended that registries collect a standard core minimum data set (CMDS). Some registries were also encouraged to collect data in addition to the minimum requirements with the objective being to promote comparability and standardization of information collected. The data collected are used to produce the National Cancer Registration Dataset, and are also used for:

- management of resources for prevention, diagnosis and treatment;
- commissioning and evaluating services, including screening programmes;
- planning and evaluating clinical management and treatment (including clinical audit);
- research into causes of, and survival from, cancer;
- education of professionals and public.

An example of some of the trend data that are quickly and easily downloadable from cancer registries is shown in Figure 7.1, where a decline in the age-standardized mortality rate from breast cancer in the southwest region of England can be seen over two decades.

Box 7.5   Some examples of disease/treatment registers, old and new

- National Leprosy Register, Norway. Set up in 1856 and maintained until 1973.
- Blind Persons Act 1920 led to case definition and the registration of all those who qualified for grants.
- Diabetes – as most people who have diabetes have it for life and have continuing health problems, diabetes registers are now seen as key to the provision and monitoring of effective care.
- Mental Health Register – covers people with severe long-term mental health problems who require and have agreed to regular follow-up.
- National Pacemaker Database – set up in 1976 and run by the Royal Brompton Hospital in London. Registration is voluntary and thought to be about 85 per cent complete.
- Twin registers – not registers of disease as such, but of the diseases experienced by twins, allowing for the investigation at the relative importance of genetic and environmental influences. The largest twin register is held in Sweden, made up of more than 140,000 cases.

Source: adapted, with additions, from Newton and Garner (2002)

Disease registers can be used for epidemiological research, needs and technology assessment, and to monitor clinical care and service quality: 'Disease registers evoke strong feelings. Epidemiologists enthuse about their potential to generate fundamental knowledge. Clinicians see them as a direct route to rational clinical practice. To public health practitioners they provide a "window" on the population. Registry staff often feel parental about "their" registers. To some patients, however, registers seem unnecessarily intrusive, an affront to their autonomy and liberty' (Newton and Garner 2002). Hence, again, issues related to the management of personal, identifiable information and data protection are a central concern. The data held on registers are rarely useful if they are anonymized – personal and identifiable information is needed in order to link individuals in four ways: to avoid double-counting; to construct longitudinal records to follow patient trajectories; to validate the register against external datasets; and to make linkages with other datasets on different topics for the purposes of exploring epidemiological hypotheses (Newton and Garner 2002).

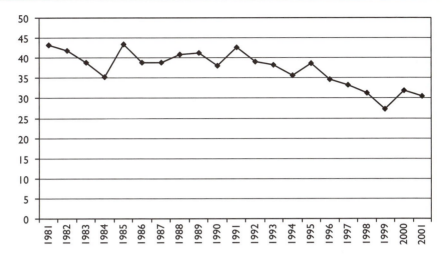

Figure 7.1 Age-standardized mortality rate per 100,000, females, South West, 1981–2001

Source: South West Cancer Intelligence Service (swcis.org.uk)

It has been suggested that the first example of a disease register was the Domesday Book (Weddell 1973), produced in 1086 to document the extent and value of royal land. The information collected for the Domesday Book was used as a basis for the collection of tax, and totalitarian regimes in more recent times have misused population registers. This chequered history is echoed to some degree in the cautiousness that people still feel today regarding the use of information that is held about them – the process of registration thus needs to be justified and overt (Newton and Garner 2002).

A range of research questions (in addition to the monitoring of disease trends) have been investigated using disease registers. For example, Davenport *et al.* (1996) looked at the occurrence of false positive in the Scottish Motor Neurone Disease Register. Nevitt and Hutchinson (1996) investigated the prevalence of psoriasis in a semi-urban general practice population. Meara *et al.* (1999) created a community-based disease register for Parkinson's disease using computerized prescribing records from general practice, and investigated difficulties in diagnosis.

Other sources of data derived from primary care include general medical services (GMS) statistics (http://www.primary-care-db.org.uk/indexmenu/gms_desc.html). These are a summary of data relating to general medical practitioners, their patients, partnerships and services. The GMS statistics division of the National Health Service Executive (NHSE) collects twice-yearly statistical returns from health authorities for each registered general practice in England and Wales. A wide range of information is collected including the age and sex breakdown for each registered practice population in the country, details of practice organization such as staffing, list size and GP characteristics, and details of service provision such as asthma and diabetes services and immunization. Using this information, it is possible to profile primary care provision and registered practice populations in particular areas. The data are currently available to the academic community and NHS staff only and the GMS database covers the categories shown in Table 7.3.

The Royal College of General Practitioners' Weekly Returns Service is also a source of information about services in primary care. It is run by the Royal

Table 7.3   Information collected in GMS (GMS) statistics

GP characteristics	Practice activity	Practice characteristics	Patient characteristics
GPs by country of qualification	Number of practices	Total patients	Patients by age and sex
GPs by age group	Total number of GPs	Female patients	Fringe patients
Female GPs	GPs offering asthma services	Male patients	Deprivation claims
Part-time GPs	GPs offering diabetes services	Rural patients	Patients for whom drugs are dispensed
Female part-time GPs	GPs offering minor surgery	Personal Medical Services pilots	Patients in rural areas
Salaried GPs	GPs offering child health surveillance services		
Female salaried GPs	GPs using deputising services		
Restricted GPs	Health promotion services		
Female Restricted GPs	Out of hours cover		
Course organizers	Contraceptive services provision		
Approved trainers	Maternity services provision		
Seniority allowance entitlements (1997)	Small-share partners Dispensing GPs Postgraduate education allowances Basic pay allowances Deprived patient claims MMR2 provision Telephone treatment for temporary residents Practice quality service payments Claims for minor surgery (1997) Claims for night visits (1997)		

Source: http://www.primary-care-db.org.uk/indexmenu/gms_desc.html

College's Birmingham Research Unit, and collects data from 73 practices spread across England and Wales. Participating GPs summarize diagnoses and consultation/episode type (first/new episodes/ongoing consultations) for their registered population and data are extracted to provide a weekly return, which includes age-specific weekly incidence of diseases. Hence these data are continuous in terms of data collection. Data collection started in 1967 using paper records, collecting information on a limited number of conditions. The system was computerized in 1994 and now collects data on all diagnoses made by GPs during a consultation. This source is particularly useful for examining seasonal trends. Figure 7.2 shows the weekly incidence (per 100,000 all ages) for 'influenza-like illness' in regions North, Central and South for 2004 compared with a five-year average (1999–2003).

It is also possible to get some information on prescriptions. The Prescribing Analysis and Cost (PACT) database contains information on prescriptions that are dispensed by pharmacists. This information is made available through the NHS Prescription Pricing Authority, but only for those working within PCTs. They can

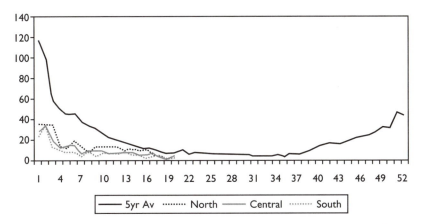

Figure 7.2 Weekly incidence (per 100,000, all ages) for 'influenza-like illness' in regions North, Central and South for 2004 (Jan–May) compared with a five-year average (1999–2003)

Note: Horizontal scale shows week number.
Source: http://www.rcgp.org.uk/bru/a4-influenza.asp. Last update: 19 May 2004. Access this website for updated version of this figure.

access two systems through the NHS net – the 'Prescribing Toolkit' or 'ePACT.net'. The Prescribing Toolkit system can be used to make comparisons between different PCTs, as well as for monitoring trends, whereas in ePACT.net users can select the specific areas (to presentation level) and time period (last three years of available data) they require, and how they wish the information to be displayed. PACT data are also available to GPs and nurse prescribers to provide them with information, at GP and practice level, on prescribing habits and costs.

For the health researcher, PACT data are limited in their availability (the primary purpose is to monitor costs, as the name implies) and also in their applicability. Data recorded include the quantity prescribed, but not dose or duration, and there is no information on indications – i.e. why a drug has been prescribed. Hence the data from PACT have to be combined with information on standard doses for the purposes of interpretation. In some circumstances, however, the information can be used as a proxy measure for morbidity.

Some examples of research using PACT data include Smith *et al.* (2003), who validated the data from the GPRD on prescriptions for head lice using data from PACT (noting additional insights from GPRD). One of the main uses of PACT data is to look at variations and trends in prescribing. For example, Baxter *et al.* (1998) have looked at prescriptions for lipid lowering drugs in four health author-ities. They found that prescribing for these drugs increased exponentially following research evidence showing their efficacy. However, the prescribing patterns of indi-vidual practices were highly variable and the extent to which this reflected differ-ences in clinical need necessitated further investigation (reflecting one of the main weaknesses of PACT data). Wathen and Dean (2004) used PACT data to look at the impact of the National Institute for Clinical Excellence (NICE) guidelines on prescribing decisions. They looked at prescribing in one PCT (North Devon) before and after the publication of five different technology assessments. They found that for four of these appraisals there was an increase in prescribing immedi-ately after NICE guidance was issued, but that information from other sources and personal experience were also important factors. Interestingly, for the fifth issue (zanamivir inhalers) NICE guidelines were universally rejected. In this study the use of PACT data was enhanced considerably by additional data collected from GPs, which gave information on the context and decisions behind prescribing choices.

Patient records and other data derived from secondary care

The preceding section considered various sources of information about the health and health care of populations that are derived from primary care. In this section we consider some of the main sources of data derived from secondary care – i.e. when a patient has been referred or transferred from the care of a GP in a primary care setting to another provider of care, usually a specialist in a hospital setting. There are two main sources of information about the activity that goes on in hospitals: hospital activity statistics, which are mainly concerned with the capacity of services (number of beds, staffing, waiting lists, etc.) and hospital episodes statistics, where the focus is more on patients, containing administrative, admission and clinical data for individuals.

Hospital activity statistics

A wide range of measures are available that monitor hospital activity (see Table 7.4). These are mainly used within the NHS for the purposes of monitoring hospital activity and for performance management. They are available from the Department of Health website, at Trust and PCT level and by data type. Data are collected annually after the end of the financial year with the exception of critical care where data are collated biannually.

Hospital episodes statistics

Information about hospital activity can also be derived from hospital episodes statistics. These form a database, compiled by the Department of Health, which contains all patient-based records of 'finished consultant episodes' (FCEs) for ordinary admissions and day cases by diagnosis, operation and speciality from NHS hospitals in England. An FCE is a continuous period of inpatient care administered by a particular consultant within a single hospital provider (normally an NHS Trust). If responsibility for an admitted patient is passed to another consultant, or if the patient is transferred to another Trust, a new FCE will commence. The information held in the hospital episodes statistics database can be used to answer a wide range of questions about topics such as: variations by age, sex and ethnicity; diagnoses; operations and procedures performed (including day-case surgery); information relating

Table 7.4 Hospital activity data in England

Beds	A & E	Outpatients	Misc.
Beds open overnight Critical care beds Day-only beds Residential care beds	A & E attendances Admissions from A & E Total time in A & E	Outpatient attendances Waiting in outpatients Ward attendances	Cancelled operations NHS written complaints Imaging and radiodiagnostics Supporting facilities Day care attendances

Source: http://www.performance.doh.gov.uk/hospitalactivity

to costs from Healthcare Resource Groups (HRGs); variations by NHS Trust, health authority areas or area-level deprivation; waiting time before treatment and length of stay in hospital; and admission method (e.g. elective or emergency).

Episodes data can be accessed through published 'annual reference volumes'. From 1994/5 these have used a 100 per cent sample of data (25 per cent before then) and the data are grossed to take into account variations in coverage and completeness of diagnostic coding (Hansell *et al.* 2001). Data are also available through the Department of Health Enquiry Point, and through the 'Safe Haven' service based in Public Health Observatories (see Box 7.6).

Box 7.6   Public Health Observatories and the HES Safe Haven service

Public Health Observatories were launched in 2000 and there are currently nine regional Observatories. Their main tasks are to support local bodies by:

- monitoring health and disease trends and highlighting areas for action;
- identifying gaps in health information;
- advising on methods for health and health inequality impact assessments;
- drawing together information from different sources in new ways to improve health;
- carrying out projects to highlight particular health issues;
- evaluating progress by local agencies in improving health and cutting inequality;
- looking ahead to give early warning of future public health problems.

The Observatories operate Safe Havens (the classification refers to strict operating protocols) whereby they have access to a regional extract of hospital episodes statistics data covering ten years. Requests for bespoke analyses can be made to each Observatory from those working within that region.

Source: adapted from www.pho.org.uk

Because episodes data are so comprehensive they form a powerful epidemiological dataset and can be used to investigate a range of issues. For example, Shaw *et al.* (2004) considered revascularization procedures (coronary artery bypass grafting (CABG) and percutaneous transluminal coronary angioplasty (PTCA)) carried out in England between 1991 and 1999. They looked at trends over time, and variations by gender in order to investigate the issue of equitable provision. Using a proxy measure of need in the form of admissions for acute myocardial infarction they found that although men over 40 were approximately twice as likely to be admitted to hospital with a diagnosis of acute myocardial infarction in each of the three time periods studied (1991–3, 1994–6, 1997–9), they were between three and five times more likely than women to have a CABG or PTCA operation (see Figure 7.3). This imbalance was more marked for CABG than for PTCA. Thus if the rate of admission due to acute myocardial infarction is taken to be a reasonable proxy for the ratio of need for revascularization in women compared to men (in the absence of direct indicators of need), and assuming that women and men do not differ markedly in their ability to benefit from revascularization, a twofold sex difference in CABG and PTCA procedures would be predicted, making it unlikely that the observed three- to fivefold sex difference in revascularization rates could be attributed to differences in clinical need or better response to medical treatments.

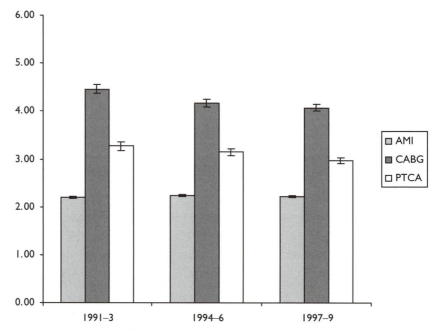

Figure 7.3   Male : female ratio (age-standardized) for acute myocardial infarction and revascularization (CABG or PTCA), with 95 per cent confidence intervals for ages 40+ years, England, 1991–3, 1994–6, 1997–9

Source: Shaw *et al.* (2004)

Although it is a powerful dataset due to its (intended) completeness, one of the main deficits of the current hospital episodes statistics system is that it does not collect data from the private sector. Hence a large proportion of information about the health care of a section of the population is missing. This will be particularly apparent for certain procedures which are more likely to take place in the private sector (e.g. hip replacements). Also excluded are outpatients and non-surgical interventions, which may be an issue depending on the research question. There are also some concerns with the consistency, completeness and accuracy of coding in the statistics dataset which are particularly pertinent for data fields such as ethnicity. As with any secondary data set, then, caution should be taken to be fully aware of the state of the data which are being used.

Record linkage

There are a number of ways that 'linking' is referred to in health and health services research and these are set out in Box 7.7.

Most often the term 'record linkage' is used to refer to the integration of data from two (or more) separate sources. A prime example of a study using record linkage is the Oxford Record Linkage Study. This consists of a continuous set of linked hospital admission records and birth and death records for 5 million people resident and/or treated in the former Oxford Regional Health Authority area from 1963 to 1999 (when data collection ceased) and is used for preparing health service

Box 7.7   Linking records

• **Linking data on individuals over time:** linking data on the same individual from the same data source at different time points (e.g. linking GP records to see how many times an individual consults their GP in a given time period). The unit of analysis does not have to be individuals, but could be households or organizations.
• **Linking data on individuals from different sources:** this refers to, for examples, linking data on illicit drug users and hospital and mortality records (see e.g. Bartu *et al.* 2004).
• **Probabilistic linkage:** ideally, unique personal identifiers are used to link data from different sources. However, often these do not exist, or are not in a format so as to be useful for electronic linking (e.g. an individual's name may be spelt differently in different datasets). Probabilistic linkage is based on a computed calculation of the probability that the records relate to the same person; a threshold of likelihood is set, above which the match is accepted, below which it is rejected (Gill 1997).
• **Ecological linkage:** when data are not held (or made available) at an individual level but are available at an area level, then different data sources can be matched. For example, comparing the mortality rates and levels of deprivation of areas. Such analyses are prone to the ecological fallacy, which refers to the inference of group or area characteristics as individual (e.g. assuming that in an area of high levels of illness containing many teenage mothers, that teenage mothers in that area will necessarily have high levels of illness) (Tunstall *et al.* 2004).

statistics as well as epidemiological and health service research (Gill 1997). The data linked in this study have been used to address a wide range of research questions. For example, Goldacre *et al.* (2004) looked at the prevalence of skin cancer in people with multiple sclerosis (MS) in order to investigate the relationship between solar radiation and MS; the results supported the hypothesis that solar radiation had some protective influence on the development of MS.

Another study which has been based on record linkage and has proved to be a valuable research resource for understanding health and its determinants is the ONS Longitudinal Study (ONS-LS). The ONS-LS is a representative 1 per cent sample of the population of England and Wales containing linked census and vital events data (Hattersley 1997). The study started in 1974 when the sample was taken from the 1971 census using four dates of birth as the criterion for membership. This sample has been added to using the 1981, 1991 and 2001 censuses using the same four dates of birth. The addition of new sample members born on LS dates and the recording of exits via emigration and death are used to reflect population change. Routinely collected data on the mortality, fertility, cancer registrations, infant mortality of children born to LS sample mothers, widow(er)hoods and migration are linked into the sample using the NHS Central Register (see Box 7.8). Figure 7.4 shows the hypothetical event history of an ONS-LS member.

The dataset produced by the linkage in the ONS-LS has produced a wide range of studies (a full range of publications can be found on the Centre for Longitudinal Study Information and User Support (CeLSIUS) website (www.celsius.lshtm.ac.uk)). For example, it has been particularly useful for examining migration in relation to other sociodemographic (and health) factors. Glaser and

> ## Box 7.8   The NHS Central Register (England and Wales)
>
> The NHS Central Register exists in order to maintain a central record of all patients registered in England and Wales for NHS purposes and to ensure that medical records are passed between health authorities effectively and GPs are paid correctly.
>
> Information is passed to the Register electronically from health authorities who are given information via GPs. Health authorities advise when patients register with GPs in their area. The local registration service advises the Register on a weekly basis of all births and deaths registered in England and Wales in order that the Register can be updated.
>
> Main topics covered are name and surname, date of birth, sex and the health authority to which a person is registered. These are held with previous values of these factors (i.e. previous health authority or name). Medical information is not held.
>
> *Source:* www.statistics.gov.uk

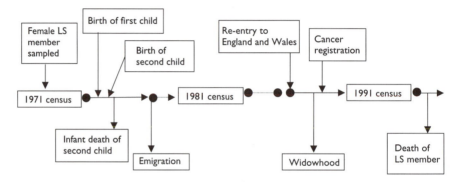

Figure 7.4   Event history and linkage of an ONS–LS member

Source: adapted from Hattersley (1997)

Grundy (1998) looked at changes in living arrangements by region in England and Wales between 1971 and 1991. They found dramatic changes in the living arrangements of older people – by 1991 the majority of individuals over 75 were in solitary households, even in Wales where as recently as 1971 a larger proportion of people in this age group were living with relatives, such as married children, than were living alone. The ONS–LS has also been extensively used to examine health outcomes by ethnic group. For example, Harding (1998) found that the incidence of ovarian, cervical, lung and prostatic cancer was higher in second generation Irish living in England and Wales than in all other persons in England and Wales and that differences in socioeconomic status did not explain these patterns. In addition, the ONS–LS has been an important source of information on social class patterns in mortality, as it overcomes numerator–denominator bias (see Chapter 6). For example, White *et al.* (2003) have recently published analyses of mortality by social class through the 1990s, reporting widening inequalities for men (mainly accounted for by an increasing social class gap in ischaemic heart disease, cerebrovascular disease and respiratory disease), but decreasing inequalities among women (accounted for by an inverse social class gradient in breast cancer).

A key way in which record linkage is used in epidemiological studies is through the 'flagging' of individuals on the NHS Central Register to see if they have died and to undertake survival analysis. The subjects of a study (e.g. people employed in a particular industry, or resident in a certain area) can be identified on the Register. Their records are flagged with a cipher representing the study so that when deaths notified to the Register are found to relate to such entries, researchers can be informed of the deaths and supplied with copies of the death certicificates. For approved medical research projects with the appropriate informed consent, data on the following can also be supplied: cancer registration information, name of the health area in the UK in which the patient is currently registered, notification of change of name, or the fact a person is no longer registered with a UK NHS doctor.

The flagging of records has been used to investigate a diverse range of study populations, many of which would not otherwise be possible. For example, Macfarlane *et al.* (2003) used flagging of cancer registration to determine whether UK service personnel who served in the Gulf War of 1990/1 had a higher incidence of cancer than those who were not deployed; they found no evidence of an excess risk of cancer for service personnel. In a rather different study, McCarron *et al.* (2003) compared former students of Glasgow University according to the subjects they had studied as undergraduates. Almost 10,000 alumni were traced on the NHS Central Register, 939 of whom had died. Compared with former medical students, former arts and law students had excess all-cause and cardiovascular disease mortality. Former medical students had lower lung cancer mortality than other alumni but higher mortality from alcohol-related causes including accidents, suicide and violence. The authors concluded that the lower mortality risks observed among former medical students may be due to their better employment prospects and healthier lifestyle behaviours, although the high mortality from alcohol-related causes underscores the complexity of choice of health behaviour.

Record linkage thus provides the potential for a wider range of research questions to be addressed than can be usually tackled from a single data source. It is particularly useful for research topics which require detailed clinical/medical and also sociodemographic data, and for research questions which emerge some time after events have already taken place (such as the health effects of the Gulf War example cited above). However, record linkage is also a hugely time-consuming and costly task. While information technology has made linkage a real possibility, and in many cases a reality, data protection and confidentiality issues loom large. Individuals are becoming increasingly concerned about who has access to their personal and medical information, and for what purposes; record linkage is intrinsically intrusive and opens up a Pandora's box of issues related to privacy and the role of the state.

Surveys as a source of information on the health of the population

In addition to routinely collected data sources, which collate information relating to entire populations, data collected through surveys is an important source of information about the health and health care of the population. Surveys are particularly useful for collecting information about specific groups of people, or about specific topics, when routine data sources may not be sufficiently detailed to be useful for research purposes. Such surveys may be conducted just once, they may be continuous (i.e. repeated over time with different samples each time) or they may follow a sample of people longitudinally/prospectively (forming a panel or cohort study). Box 7.9 lists some of the key surveys which are available to researchers. The UK Data Archive is a useful place to start searching for and finding out about these sources.

> **Box 7.9   Some major surveys available to researchers**
>
> • **Health Survey for England (HSE):** The HSE is a series of annual surveys
>   about the health of people living in England. It began in 1991 and has been carried
>   out annually since then. A number of core questions are included every year but
>   each year's survey also has a particular focus on a disease, condition or
>   population group. Topics are brought back at appropriate intervals in order to
>   monitor change. The survey is sponsored by the Department of Health to
>   provide better and more reliable information about various aspects of people's
>   health and to monitor selected health targets.
> • **National Child Development Study (NCDS):** The NCDS, conducted by
>   the Centre for Longitudinal Studies at the Institute of Education in London, is a
>   continuing longitudinal study which is seeking to follow the lives of all those living
>   in Great Britain who were born between 3 and 9 March 1958. The aim of the
>   study is to improve understanding of the factors affecting human development
>   over the whole lifespan. To date there have been six survey sweeps in 1965, 1969,
>   1974, 1981, 1985 and 1999–2000 (age 41–2).
> • **British Household Panel Survey (BHPS):** The BHPS is carried out by the
>   Institute for Social and Economic Research (ISER), incorporating the Economic
>   and Social Research Council (ESRC) Research Centre on Micro-Social Change at
>   the University of Essex. The main objective of the survey is to further
>   understanding of social and economic change at the individual and household
>   level in Britain (the UK from Wave 11 onwards), to identify, model and forecast
>   such changes and their causes and consequences in relation to a range of
>   socioeconomic variables. The BHPS is designed as a research resource for a wide
>   range of social science disciplines and to support interdisciplinary research in
>   many areas.
> • **Millennium Cohort Study (MCS):** The ESRC-funded MCS offers large-scale
>   information about the new century's babies, and the families who are bringing
>   them up, for the four countries of the UK. Its first sweep, carried out during
>   2001–2 laid the foundations for a major new longitudinal research resource. The
>   MCS will follow the lives of a sample of nearly 19,000 babies born between 1
>   September 2000 and 31 August 2001 in England and Wales, and between 22
>   November 2000 and 11 January 2002 in Scotland and Northern Ireland. The
>   study's broad objective was to create a new multi-purpose longitudinal dataset,
>   describing the diversity of backgrounds from which children born in the new
>   century are setting out in life.

Population data: demographics and deprivation

The most important survey of all is the decennial population census, being in effect
a survey of the whole population. The census is a count of the number of people
normally resident in the UK on a particular night (Shaw *et al.* 2000). It is thus a
'snapshot' of the population and its social and economic conditions, providing vital
information on the number of people in the population and its sub-groups. These
data are subsequently used as the denominators in the calculation of (age-
standardized) rates or morbidity and mortality in countless studies. This enables
meaningful comparisons to be made across groups and areas as well as over time.
    The census is a hugely expensive exercise and as a result is only carried out every

ten years. In between censuses, mid-year population estimates are derived from the preceding census, birth and death registration data, data about internal and international migration as well as claims for political asylum (Shaw *et al.* 2000).

Information relating to the health of the population was first collected in the 1851 census which included a question on 'infirmities' which was used until 1911. In 1971, the only information on illness was recorded as temporary sickness from work. In 1981, the category 'permanently sick or disabled' was added as a residual category for economic activity, but children or retired people could not be included. In 1991, everyone was asked the question: 'Do you have any long-term illness, health problem or handicap which limits your daily activities or the work you can do? Include problems which are due to old age'. This item is known as 'limiting long-term illness' (LLTI). In 2001, the census for the first time also included a question on general health, asking: 'Over the last 12 months would you say your health has been: Good? Fairly good? Not good?' Table 7.5 shows the responses to this general health question, by age and sex, in 2001.

As the census is the key source of information about the number of people in the population, there are few studies which *don't* make use of census data, either directly or indirectly. However, many studies make use of the census as their sole source of data. Doran *et al.* (2004) looked at the general health question referred to above in relation to social class by region of residence in order to address the issue of whether there is a north-south divide in social class inequalities in health. They found a north-west/south-east divide in social class inequalities, with each of the seven social classes having higher rates of poor health in Wales, the North East and the North West regions of England than elsewhere, the widest health gap being between social classes in Scotland and London.

While it is only recently that census data have been used as a direct source of information about the self-reported health status of the population, the combination of census data with mortality data has a long history. In 1837, William Farr

Table 7.5 Data from the 2001 census: self-reported general health by age and sex (England and Wales)

	Good (%)	Fairly good (%)	Not good (%)	All (%)
Males				
0–15	91	8	1	100
16–24	86	12	2	100
25–44	77	17	5	100
45–64	60	27	14	100
65–74	42	39	19	100
75+	31	43	26	100
All ages	71	20	8	100
Females				
0–15	91	8	1	100
16–24	80	17	3	100
25–44	73	21	6	100
45–64	56	30	14	100
65–74	39	42	19	100
75+	28	44	29	100
All ages	66	24	10	100

Note: figures may not sum to 100 due to rounding error.
Source: Social Trends 34 (2004) (Table 7.3)

was the first to combine census data with figures on births, deaths and marriages (see Davey Smith *et al.* 2001). Census data have since that time continued to provide the denominators which when combined with mortality data (and also birth data) form information on mortality rates. Table 7.6 lists some routine statistical publications from the ONS which include this mortality data, as well as data on birth and populations.

The census has also been used as a key source of information about the extent of deprivation in the population. Deprivation has been described as a state of 'observable and demonstrable disadvantage relative to the local community or the wider society or nation to which an individual, family or group belong' (Townsend 1987). The Townsend Deprivation Index is a measure of multiple deprivation for areas which is derived from four variables from the 1991 census: percentage unemployment of those aged 16–64; percentage households with no car; percentage households not owner-occupied; and percentage overcrowding (> 1 person per room). Based on this, areas are assigned a Townsend deprivation score, and this has been widely used in studies of health (as well as in resource allocation) to investigate the ecological relationship between deprivation and health. For example, Payne and Saul (1997) looked at the relationship between the prevalence of angina, rates of coronary revascularization and Townsend score for electoral ward of residence. They found that while angina and deprivation were positively associated, rates of revascularization and deprivation were not associated, suggesting that the use of interventional cardiology services is not commensurate with need.

Table 7.6   Population, births and deaths: some routine statistical publications produced by the ONS

Series	Topic
Population data	
PP1	Mid-year population estimates
PP2	National population projections
PP3	Sub-national population projections
Vital statistics	
VS1	Vital statistics summary (population, births, deaths, fertility and mortality rates)
VS2	Birth statistics (births by age of mother, number of previous children, type of establishment where birth occurred and birth weight)
VS3	Mortality statistics (deaths by cause, age and sex)
VS4	Vital statistics for wards (births and deaths)
VS4D	Deaths from selected causes by wards
VS5	Infant mortality
FM1	Birth statistics
Death data	
DH1	Mortality statistics: general
DH2	Mortality statistics: cause
DH3	Mortality statistics: childhood, infant and perinatal
DH4	Mortality statistics: injury and poisoning
DH5	Mortality statistics: area
DH6	Mortality statistics: childhood
DS	Decennial supplements

Source: adapted from Moon *et al.* (2000)

Conclusions

Secondary and routine data can be a relatively fast and cheap source of information for the researcher interested in the health and health care of the population (although extensive costs in terms of time and money are involved in establishing and maintaining datasets). They are thus attractive for the researcher who likes to be adventurous without having to venture into the complicated world of data collection and who prefers a desk and computer to being 'in the field'.

Routine data sources tend to consist of very large sample sizes, if not the population as a whole, and can thus confer a great deal of statistical power. While the lack of depth and detail limits their application, they are useful for conveying a population context and for understanding the use of and requirement for services, and can be used for hypothesis generation; many researchers have used routine and secondary sources with imagination. However, when using routine and secondary data it is necessary to exercise caution regarding accuracy, completeness, timeliness and fitness for purpose (Moon *et al.* 2000). Close attention should be paid to the details of sampling, response, and the wording of original items collected.

Information technology and online access make the collection, storage, linkage and analysis of many datasets widely available but this is not without its pitfalls: websites and links come and go, they can be difficult to navigate, and ease and speed of availability should not detract from considered attention to detail. Moreover, even when data are held anonymously, the personal information in routine and secondary datasets is often effectively identifiable. Patient records, for example, that are rich in detail, can never be truly anonymous (Behlen and Johnson 1999). Researchers must act as responsible stewards of data. In sum, routine and secondary data sources can be considered a necessary, but not necessarily sufficient, approach to understanding population health.

Key points

- Secondary sources of data are sources of information that have been collected by others.

- These data sources bypass the cost and effort involved in primary data collection, and tend to consist of very large samples, conferring a great deal of statistical power.

- Constraints on the use of large datasets are imposed by the research questions and samples formulated by others.

- Caution must be exercised when using secondary data to ensure that it is suitable for the purpose intended, the adequacy of its design, its accuracy and completeness.

- Data protection is of central concern when using electronic records of patient information held by an institution. The data are sensitive and must be protected. Patients' rights and issues of confidentiality are essential elements of good research practice.

- Record linkage refers to the integration of data from two or more separate sources. A well-known example is the ONS-LS which represents a 1 per cent sample of the population of Britain, and links census and vital events data.

Acknowledgements

Thanks to Debbie Lawlor for access to her extensive notes from her short course on 'Sources of routinely collected data for research' held in the Department of Social Medicine at the University of Bristol. Mary Shaw is funded by the South West Public Health Observatory.

Further reading

Charlton, J. and Murphy, M. (eds) (1997) *The Health of Adult Britain 1841–1994*. London: The Stationery Office. A good example of the use and presentation of routine data on health including mortality, life expectancy, use of health services and changes in factors which have influenced health. Also useful as a resource for the documentation of secular trends.

Dorling, D. and Simpson, S. (eds) (1999) *Statistics in Society*. London: Arnold. This book takes an incisive and critical look at official statistics in Britain. How they are funded, how they are collected, and how they are presented – each stage of the process is addressed. The values they represent, what is measured and what is not (e.g. income, disabled children) and how they change over time (e.g. the measurement of 'unemployment') are laid bare. This book will change forever how you think about official statistics.

Health Statistics Quarterly. A journal published four times a year and available free online, *Health Statistics Quarterly* is an invaluable resource covering the latest trends in the UK's health. It contains an overview of the latest news, a review of related publications for release, commentary on the latest health findings, topical articles illustrated with colour charts and diagrams, and regularly updated statistical graphs and tables. It also highlights trends in health and details the latest quarterly information on deaths, childhood mortality, cancer survival, abortions, congenital anomalies and morbidity.

Kerrison, S. and Macfarlane, A. (1999) *Official Health Statistics: An Unofficial Guide*. London: Arnold. This book is a publication by the Radical Statistics Health Group and takes a meticulous and informative look specifically at official statistics relating to health. The book is organized into sections covering the measurement of ill health in the population, social inequalities and the environment, and official sources of information on the NHS and local authorities.

Levitas, R. and Guy, W. (1996) *Interpreting Official Statistics*. London: Routledge. This book takes a sociological slant on official statistics in Britain, looking at what information is produced (and what is not) as well as how that information is produced. Examples of how official statistics have been suppressed, manipulated and misinterpreted since 1979 are presented.

ONS (1996) *Medical Research at the Office for National Statistics: A Review*. Studies on Medical and Population Subjects No. 65. London: The Stationery Office. This review presents a brief account of more than 450 diverse medical research projects and programmes that have been assisted by the ONS (and its predecessors) up to June 1996. Includes studies using data derived from the linkage of study subjects with the NHS Central Register over the last 50 years.

Population Trends. A sister publication to *Health Statistics Quarterly*, *Population Trends* covers population and demographic information. It contains commentary on the latest findings, topical articles on relevant subjects such as one-parent families, cohabitation, fertility differences, international demography, population estimates and projections for different groups, regularly updated statistical tables and graphs, showing trends and the latest quarterly information on conceptions, births, marriages, divorces, internal and international migration, population estimates and projections, and so on.

Social Trends. A reference source which draws together social and economic data from a wide range of government departments and other organizations; it paints a broad picture of British society today, and how it has been changing.

Resources

Some key websites are listed here.

Name	Website/email	Data
Office for National Statistics (ONS)	www.statistics.gov.uk	Large amount of health-related data including much ONS data (births, deaths, marriages, migration, census etc) links to Hospital Episodes Statistics (HES) data, primary care data, neighbourhood statistics etc. Good first point of contact for any routine data.
National Assembly for Wales	www.wales.gov.uk/keypubstatis-ticsforwales/index.htm	First point of contact for statistics on Wales.
Scottish Executive Central Statistics Unit	www.scotland.gov.uk	Source of statistics on Scotland.
Northern Ireland Statistics and Research Agency	www.nisra.gov.uk	Northern Ireland's official statistics organization.
UK Data Archive	www.data-archive.ac.uk	Curator of the largest collection of digital data in the social sciences and humanities in the UK. Free access to registered academic users.
Centre for Longitudinal Study Information and User Support	www.celsius.lshtm.ac.uk	Researchers can apply to CeLSIUS with research proposals, to gain access to the ONS-LS dataset.
Association of Public Health Observatories	www.pho.org.uk	Sources of routine data for England at regional and PCT level.
The Wellcome Trust – History of Medicine Library	http://library.wellcome.ac.uk/doc_WTL038911.html	A starting point for finding mortality statistics for England and Wales in printed sources.

References

Bartu, A., Freeman, N.C., Gawthorne, G.S. *et al.* (2004) Mortality in a cohort of opiate and amphetamine users in Perth, Western Australia, *Addiction*, 99(1): 53–60.

Baxter, C., Jones, R. and Corr, L. (1998) Time trend analysis and variations in prescribing lipid lowering drugs in general practice, *BMJ*, 317: 1134–5.

Behlen, F. and Johnson, S. (1999) Multicenter patient records research: security policies and tools, *Journal of the American Medical Informatics Association*, 6(6): 435–43.

Davenport, R., Swingler, R., Chancellor, A. and Warlow C. (1996) Avoiding false positive diagnoses of motor neuron disease: lessons from the Scottish Motor Neuron Disease Register, *Journal of Neurology, Neurosurgery & Psychiatry*, 60(2): 147–51.

Davey Smith, G., Dorling, D. and Shaw, M. (2001) *Poverty, Inequality and Health in Britain: 1800–2000 – A Reader.* Bristol: The Policy Press.

Department of Health (1999) *Saving Lives: Our Healthier Nation*. London: The Stationery Office.

Donaldson, L. (1992) Registering a need, *British Medical Journal*, 305: 587–8.

Doran, T., Drever, F. and Whitehead, M. (2004) Is there a north-south divide in social class inequalities in health in Great Britain? Cross-sectional study using data from the 2001 census, *British Medical Journal*, 328: 1043–5.

Gill, L. (1997) OX-LINK: the Oxford Medical Record Linkage System, in *Record Linkage Techniques – 1997: Proceedings of an International Workshop and Exposition*, Arlington, VA, 20–1 March (http://www.fcsm.gov/working-papers/gill.pdf).

Glaser, K. and Grundy, E. (1998) Migration and household change in the population aged 65 and over, 1971–1991, *International Journal of Population Geography*, 4: 323–39.

Goldacre, M., Seagroatt, V., Yeates, D. and Acheson, E. (2004) Skin cancer in people with multiple sclerosis: a record linkage study, *Journal of Epidemiology and Community Health*, 58(2): 142–4.

Haines, R. and Shlomowitz, R. (2003) Causes of death of British emigrants on voyages to South Australia, 1848–1885, *The Journal of the Society for the Social History of Medicine*, 16(2): 193–208.

Hansell, A., Bottle, A., Shurlock, L. and Aylin, P. (2001) Accessing and using hospital activity data, *Journal of Public Health Medicine*, 23(1): 51–6.

Harding, S. (1998) The incidence of cancers among second generation Irish living in England and Wales, *British Journal of Cancer*, 78(7): 958–61.

Hattersley, L. (1997) Record linkage of census and routinely collected vital events data in the ONS Longitudinal Study, in *Record Linkage Techniques – 1997: Proceedings of an International Workshop and Exposition*, Arlington, VA, 20–21 March (http://www.fcsm.gov/working-papers/hattersley.pdf).

Hippisley-Cox, J., Pringle, M., Cater, R. *et al.* (2003) The electronic patient record in primary care – regression or progression? A cross sectional study, *British Medical Journal*, 326: 1439–43.

Hoare, J. (2003) Comparison of area-based inequality measures and disease morbidity in England, 1994–1998, *Health Statistics Quarterly*, 18: 18–24.

Hollowell, J. (1997) The general practice research database: quality of morbidity data, *Population Trends*, 87: 36–40.

Horsfield, P. and Teasdale, S. (2003) Generating information from electronic patient records in general practice: a description of clinical care and gender inequalities in coronary heart disease using data from over two million patient records, *Informatics in Primary Care*, 11(3): 137–44.

Kam, E., Eslick, G. and Campbell, I. (2002) An audit of the effectiveness of acupuncture on musculoskeletal pain in primary health care, *Acupuncture in Medicine*, 20(1): 35–8.

Kaye, J., Bradbury, B. and Jick, H. (2003) Changes in antipsychotic drug prescribing by general practitioners in the United Kingdom from 1991 to 2000: a population-based observational study, *British Journal of Clinical Pharmacology*, 56(5): 569–75.

Kleinman, A. (1980) *Patients and Healers in the Context of Culture*. Berkeley, CA: University of California Press.

Last, J. (1963) The iceberg: 'Completing the clinical picture' in general practice, *Lancet*, 6: 28–31.

MacFarlane, G., Biggs, A-M., Maconochie, N., Hotopf, M., Doyle, P. and Lunt M. (2003) Incidence of cancer among UK Gulf War veterans: cohort study, *British Medical Journal*, 327: 1373–5.

Majeed, A. (2004) Source, uses, strengths and limitations of data collected in primary care in England, *Health Statistics Quarterly*, 21: 5–11.

Martin, R. and Gunnell, D. (2004) Patterns of general practitioner consultation for mental illness by young people in rural areas: a cross-sectional study, *Health Statistics Quarterly*, 21: 30–3.

McCarron, P., Okasha, M., McEwen, J. and Davey Smith, G. (2003) Association between course of study at university and cause-specific mortality, *Journal of the Royal Society of Medicine*, 96(8): 384–8.

Meara, J., Bhowmick, B. and Hobson, P. (1999) Accuracy of diagnosis in patients with presumed Parkinson's disease, *Age & Ageing*, 28(2): 99–102.

Moon, G., Gould, M. and colleagues (2000) *Epidemiology: An Introduction.* Buckingham: Open University Press.

Nevitt, G. and Hutchinson, P. (1996) Psoriasis in the community: prevalence, severity and patients' beliefs and attitudes towards the disease, *British Journal of Dermatology*, 135(4): 533–7.

Newton, J. and Garner, S. (2002) *Disease Registers in England: A Report Commissioned by the Department of Health Policy Research Programme in Support of the White Paper Entitled Saving Lives: Our Healthier Nation.* Oxford: Institute of Health Sciences.

NHS Executive (1998) *Information for Health.* http://www.nhsia.nhs.uk/def/pages/info-4health/contents.asp.

ONS (Office for National Statistics) (1998) *Social Focus on Men.* London: The Stationery Office.

Payne, N. and Saul, C. (1997) Variations in use of cardiology services in a health authority: comparison of coronary artery revascularisation rates with prevalence of angina and coronary mortality, *British Medical Journal*, 314: 257.

Scambler, G. (ed.) (2003) *Sociology as Applied to Medicine.* London: Saunders.

Shaw, M., Dorling, D. and Grundy, J. (2000) Surveying the population: health topics in the census of population and other surveys, in S. Kerrison and A. Macfarlane (eds) *Official Health Statistics: An Unofficial Guide*, pp. 14–38. London: Arnold.

Shaw, M., Maxwell, R., Rees, K. *et al.* (2004) Gender and age inequity in the provision of coronary revascularisation in England in the 1990s: is it getting better? *Social Science & Medicine*, 59: 2499–2507.

Simpson, M. (2003) Multidisciplinary patient records in a palliative care setting, *Nursing Times*, 99(3): 33–4.

Smith S., Smith, G., Heatlie, H. *et al.* (2003) Head lice diagnosed in general practice in the West Midlands between 1993 and 2000: a survey using the General Practice Research Database, *Communicable Disease & Public Health*, 6(2): 139–43.

Social Trends (2004) No. 34 London: The Stationery Office. Eds. Carol Summerfield and Penny Babb. Office for National Statistics.

Soriano, J., Kiri, V., Maier, W. and Strachan, D. (2003) Increasing prevalence of asthma in UK primary care during the 1990s, *International Journal of Tuberculosis & Lung Disease*, 7(5): 415–21.

Townsend P. (1987) Deprivation, *Journal of Social Policy*, 16(2): 125–46.

Tunstall, H., Shaw, M. and Dorling, D. (2004) Glossary: places and health, *Journal of Epidemiology and Community Health*, 58: 6–10.

van der Weijden, T., Dansen, A., Schouten, B. *et al.* (1996) Comparison of appropriateness of cholesterol testing in general practice with the recommendations of national guidelines: an audit of patient records in 20 general practices, *Quality in Health Care*, 5(4): 218–22.

Walsh, S. (2004) The clinician's perspective in electronic health records and how they can affect patient care, *British Medical Journal*, 328: 1184–7.

Wathen, B. and Dean, T. (2004) An evaluation of the impact of NICE guidance on GP prescribing, *British Journal of General Practice*, 54(499): 103–7.

Weddell, J. (1973) Registers and registries: a review, *International Journal of Epidemiology*, 2(3): 221–8.

White, C., van Galen, F. and Chow, Y. (2003) Trends in social class differences in morality by cause, 1986 to 2000, *Health Statistics Quarterly*, 20: 25–37.

8 Quantitative social science: the survey

Ann Bowling

Introduction

Quantitative research focuses on measuring quantities and relationships between attributes, following a set of scientifically rigorous procedures. It collects highly structured data and is deductive in approach – i.e. the investigator starts with ideas, develops a theory and testable hypotheses from them, and tests them with data. Quantitative research is appropriate in situations where there is pre-existing knowledge about the phenomenon of interest which permits the use of standardized methods of data collection, such as the survey. Many quantitative methods exist for measuring people's psychological attitudes (e.g. preferences for type of clinical treatment), self-perceptions (e.g. of their health) and behaviour (e.g. smoking, exercise). These range from experimental studies based in psychology laboratories to interview and self-administered questionnaire surveys. The survey is the most common quantitative method which is used to describe social phenomena.

The survey is a method of collecting information, from a *sample* of the population of interest. As such, the survey is different from a census, which is a complete enumeration and gathering of information, as distinct from partial enumeration associated with a sample. The unit of analysis in a survey is usually the individual, although it can also be an organization (e.g. medical clinic), or both of these in multilevel studies. While most surveys are based on questioning people, they can also take documents as their focus for research (e.g. surveys of historical documents, media outputs, medical records), or be based on direct observation (e.g. as in traffic surveys). The modern social survey originated in Victorian Britain, with the Victorians' enthusiasm for data collection, and the work of social reformers concerned with poverty and its enumeration. Most notable among these were Booth's (1889–1902) surveys of poverty, which were based on interviewing school attendance officers about the living conditions of schoolchildren's parents, and Rowntree's research on poverty, using interviewers to collect information about housing, occupation and earnings directly from families, which was published in 1902.

Descriptive surveys are carried out in order to describe populations (e.g. knowledge, attitudes, perceptions, health, behaviour or other phenomena of interest) to study associations between variables and to establish trends. Surveys aim to collect information as accurately and precisely as possible, and try to do this in such a way that if they were repeated at another time or in another area the results would be comparable. Their distinguishing feature is that the same information is collected from each member of the survey sample. They can also cover large samples of people. A major advantage of surveys is that they are carried out in natural settings, and random probability sampling is often easier to conduct than for experimental studies. This allows statistical inferences to be made in relation to the broader population of interest and thus allows generalizations to be made. This increases the external validity of the study.

Surveys which are carried out at one point in time are known as *cross-sectional* or *descriptive surveys*, and they aim to collect information about current and past phenonema, and to explore associations between variables. *Longitudinal surveys* are conducted at more than one point in time, either prospectively (e.g. surveying people at several points over the future course of time) or retrospectively (e.g. going back in time analysing records), and aim to explore cause and effect relationships. Thus, they are sometimes referred to as *analytical surveys*.

The survey method is also used in epidemiology (see cross-sectional, case-control and cohort studies (i.e. surveys) in Chapter 6). Whatever the label, the basic principles of the survey method are similar. The methodological difference is in the way in which study members are selected for inclusion (see Moon *et al.* 2000).

Sampling for surveys

Sampling

In statistical terms, a population is an aggregate of people or objects. Since the population of interest may contain too many members (e.g. people) to study conveniently, samples of the population from a complete and accurate listing of members are drawn. Sampling is cheaper in time, staff and resources. Statistical sampling is recommended because when the estimates of the characteristics of the population are calculated at the analysis stage, the precision of the estimates can be determined from the results. Since all sample results are liable to be affected by sampling errors, the estimates should be accompanied by information about their precision. This is known as the *standard error*.

Statements based on randomly selected samples are probability statements, based on inference because of sample non-response and potential bias in measurements. Sampling theory and estimation does not apply to samples selected by non-random methods. To enable inferences to be made about a study population, the relation between the sample and the population must be known. The selection procedure must be random and depend on chance, such as tossing a coin or the use of random number tables (see Armitage and Berry 1987 for an example of a random number table). A small sample, however random in selection, is likely to be less accurate in its representation of the total population than a large sample.

Sampling error

All survey results are called estimates because they are subject to a range of errors (see Bowling 2002 for types). In addition, any sample is just one of an almost infinite number that might have been selected, all of which can produce slightly different estimates. It is relatively unlikely that the mean of a sample, for example, will be exactly the same as the total population mean. The difference between the two is the error. Sampling error is the probability that any one sample is not completely representative of the population from which it was drawn.

Sampling errors show the amount by which a sample estimate can be expected to differ from the true value of that variable in the population. Sampling error is determined by the proportion of units (e.g. people) who possess the characteristic of interest, the distribution of this variable in the population, the sample design and the sample size. Sampling error cannot be eliminated but it should be reduced to an acceptable level. The existence of sampling error means that whenever a hypothesis is tested there is a finite possibility of either rejecting a true hypothesis (Type I error) or accepting it when it is false (Type II error) (see Box 8.1).

Box 8.1   Type I and II errors

- **A Type I error** (or *alpha error*) is the error of rejecting a true null hypothesis that there is no difference between the variables tested (and, by corollary, acceptance of a hypothesis that there are differences which is actually false).
- **A type II error** (or *beta error*) is the failure to reject a null hypothesis when it is actually false (i.e. the acceptance of no differences when they do exist).

Errors can occur for two reasons. One is that the sampling is not carried out properly, resulting in a biased sample. This is called *systematic error*. The other reason is the chance factors that influence the sampling process. For example, an unusually unrepresentative sample could be chosen. This is called *random error*. Just as the means of all possible samples have their own distribution, so do the errors of the samples. Theoretically the errors are normally distributed with a mean of zero, so the errors balance out over all samples.

The sampling frame

In order to be able to draw a sample, a *sampling frame* is needed. The sampling frame for a survey is the list of population members (units) from which the survey sample is drawn. Surveys depend on it containing a complete and accurate listing of every element in the target population, and every element should be included only once. Commonly used sampling frames for national surveys in Britain include the register of electors, from which individuals can be sampled, and the postcode address file (for 'small users', which includes all private household addresses). Where the latter is used the entire household can be included in the survey or members within the household unit can be randomly sampled for inclusion in the study (often on the doorstep by the interviewer using a predefined formula).

Many lists include the problem of blanks (e.g. electors who no longer reside at the listed address in the electoral roll, empty properties in the postcode file). There are methods of substitution which are available in this case, in order that target sample size is not adversely affected. Lists can also be incomplete. For example, the electoral register may be incomplete (e.g. people who do not register to vote will not be listed on it) and biased (e.g. people in ethnic minority groups and inner-city populations may be less likely to register). This is a more serious problem as it will lead to a biased study. Many investigators use lists of clients or consumers, which can suffer from duplicated entries, incomplete coverage of the population of interest and bias among those on the list, all of which can threaten external validity (generalizability of the data). This can lead to coverage error. Given that lists are rarely perfect, investigators should make checks of their lists against any other available lists of the study population where possible.

Studies focusing on specific diseases or organizational populations (e.g. hospitals, primary care centres) will generally take the lists of patients in the relevant sections as the sampling frame, but even these can be out of date, incomplete and unrepresentative of the population of interest (e.g. not everyone with a disease or medical condition consults a doctor about it, or is referred to a specialist). Investigators need to be aware of all the limitations of their sampling frames and attempt to address them in order to enhance the external validity of their results. *External validity* relates to the generalizability of the research results to the wider population of interest. This is in contrast to *internal validity* which refers to the psychometric properties of the measurement instrument. Sampling is concerned with sample selection in a manner that enhances the external generalizability of the results.

The sampling unit

A member of the sample population is known as a *sampling unit*. The sampling unit may be an individual, a household, an organization (e.g. hospital) or a geographical area, or all of these (i.e. multilevel). The sampling procedures are based on the units of study. If the study is multilevel (comprising more than one of these units) then calculations have to be made of the number of units at each level to be included in the sample (see Mok 1995), and multilevel techniques of analysis are required.

Sample size

It is important to calculate the required *sample size* as accurately as possible in order to be able to generalize the survey findings to the whole population of interest. When the survey results are analysed, estimates of the population parameters are calculated (e.g. mean values, proportions, percentages), and statistical tests can be used to estimate differences in predefined outcome variables between groups (e.g. men and women; older and younger age groups; people with a disease of interest and those without). The survey needs to be designed at the outset so that the sample size is sufficiently large to have a good chance of detecting significant differences between the groups studied where they exist. Investigators should also consider the need for sub-group analysis, issues of item and total non-response, and sample attrition in the case of longitudinal designs, all of which will increase desired sample sizes. The calculation of statistical power varies with study design (e.g. follow-up studies require different power calculations from cross-sectional studies in order to allow for sample attrition). Sample size in relation to experimental design has been discussed in detail by Pocock (1983).

The size of the sample aimed for should be calculated at the design stage of the study using a power calculation. The probability that a statistical test will produce a difference between the groups tested at a given level of significance is called the *power* of the test. The 0.05 level of significance is usually selected, and the power should be greater than 0.8 (Crichton 1993). For a given test, the achieved statistical significance of the results will depend on the true difference between the populations that are being compared by the investigator, the sample size and the level of significance selected (Bland 1995). If the statistical power of a study is too low, then the study results will be questionable because the study might have been too small to detect any differences. As stated earlier, the erroneous rejection or acceptance of the null hypothesis (the *null hypothesis* is a statistical artifice and always predicts the absence of a relationship between the variables) is known as a Type I or Type II error (see also Chapter 21).

Decisions about sample size also require a decision to be made about whether the study will conduct one-sided or two-sided hypothesis tests of statistical significance. One-tailed (sided) tests examine a difference in one specified direction only, whereas two-tailed tests examine relationships in both directions. If a test is significant with a two-tailed test it inevitably is with a one-tailed test. For example, in clinical research, a one-sided hypothesis only allows for the possibility that the new treatment is better than the standard treatment. A two-sided hypothesis allows assessment of whether the new treatment is simply different (better or worse) from the standard treatment. Although one-sided testing reduces the required sample size, it is sensible always to use two-sided tests, as one-sided testing rests on a subjective judgement that an observed difference in the opposite direction would be of no interest.

It should also be noted when selecting statistical tests that many of them require certain assumptions to be fulfilled, one being that the sample distribution of the characteristic of interest (e.g. scores on a measurement scale) should be normally distributed (e.g. in a symmetrical, bell-shaped curve, which has the greatest distributions of the characteristic in the middle, and the smallest distributions towards each extreme). Variables are usually normally distributed (e.g. the heights of adult men and women, with most people having medium heights, and falling across the middle bulk of the curve, and shorter and taller people at the extreme ends) (see also Chapter 21).

The normal curve is simple in that there are only two constants in its formula: the mean and the standard deviation (the *standard deviation* is a measure of dispersion, based on the difference of values from the mean value: the square root of the arithmetic mean of the squared deviations from the mean). If the mean and standard deviation are specified by the investigators then the complete normal curve can be drawn (see Chapter 21 and Bowling 2002 for formula). Variables which produce skewed distributions require statistical manipulation in order to transform them to normal distributions before most statistical techniques can be applied (e.g. some less sensitive health status measures which, instead of producing a reasonable spread of responses across categories, score most members of a general population at the positive end of the health continuum).

With a very large sample it is almost always possible to reject any null hypothesis (Type I error), as statistics are sensitive to sample size; therefore the investigator must be careful not to report findings as highly significant (e.g. $P < 0.001$) with large sample sizes. A factor that is large enough to produce statistically significant differences in a small sample is more worthy of attention than a factor that produces small differences that can be shown to be statistically significant with a very large sample. The implication is that statistical significance does not necessarily imply differences that are of social or clinical importance. There are many statistical packages available for the calculation of sample size, based on calculations of statistical power. All depend on some estimation of the likely differences between the groups within the sample. Investigators should use as few tests of significance as possible in order to minimize the risk of a Type I error being made (i.e. the risk of obtaining chance significance is increased with multiple testing). Statisticians encourage investigators to report the actual significant *and* non-significant P values, rather than refer to arbitrary levels (e.g. $P < 0.05$), and to present the magnitude of observed differences and the confidence intervals of their data (Pocock 1985). The *confidence intervals* express the uncertainty inherent in the data by presenting the upper and lower limits for the true difference.

Probability theory

Statistical tests of significance apply probability theory to work out the chances of obtaining the observed result (see Chapter 21). The significance levels of $P < 0.05$, 0.01 and 0.001 are commonly used as indicators of statistically significant differences between variables. For example, if the P value for a test is less than 0.05, then one can state that the difference is statistically significant at the 5 per cent level. This means that there are less than 5 chances in 100 that the result is a false positive (Type I error). This 5 per cent level is conventionally taken as the level required to declare a positive result (i.e. a difference between groups) and to accept or reject the null hypothesis. The smaller the value of P (e.g. $P < 0.05$, $P < 0.01$, $P < 0.001$, $P < 0.0001$), the less likelihood there is of the observed inferential statistic having occurred by chance. The choice of 0.05 is arbitrary, although selecting a higher level will give too high a chance of a false positive result.

Bayesian and frequentist theory

There are alternative inductive and deductive approaches to drawing inferences from statistical data, known as Bayesian theory and the more predominant frequentist approach (see Chapter 21). Bayesian theory is based on a principle which states that information arising from research should be based only on the actual data observed, and on induction of the probability of the true observation given the data. The Bayesian approach starts with the probability distribution of the existing data, and adds the new evidence (in a model) to produce a 'posterior probability distribution' (Lilford and Braunholtz 1996). Frequentist theory involves the calculation of P values which take into account the probability of observations more extreme than the actual observations, and the deduction of the probability of the observation. Interested readers are referred to Berry (1996), Freedman (1996) and Lilford and Braunholtz (1996). The last have called for a shift to Bayesian analysis and sensitivity analyses (a method of making plausible assumptions about the margins of errors in the results) in relation to public policy.

Non-response bias

All surveys are subject to non-response (e.g. people refusing to take part, being uncontactable and so on). Bias from this is due to differences in the characteristics between the responders and non-responders to the study. Non-response is a major source of potential bias, as it reduces the effective sample size, resulting in loss of precision of the survey estimates. In addition, to the extent that differences in the characteristics of responders and non-responders are not properly accounted for in estimates, it may introduce bias into the results. Research results on the characteristics of non-responders are inconsistent. Non-response among successive waves of a study can be a particular problem in longitudinal research (known as *withdrawal bias*).

Methods of drawing a sample

There are several techniques for sampling the units to be included in a survey, and their principles are described in this section.

Random sampling

Sampling theory assumes the use of the method of *random sampling*. Random sampling gives each of the units in the population targeted a calculable (and non-zero) probability of being selected for inclusion in the study. Random sampling relates to the method of sampling – not to the resulting sample. While the representativeness of the study population is enhanced by the use of methods of random sampling, a random method of selection can still, by chance, lead to an unrepresentative sample. The methods of random sampling are described below. Random samples are *not* necessarily equal probability samples whereby each unit has an equal chance of selection. Both *simple* and *unrestricted random sampling* give each unit an *equal chance* of being selected.

Unrestricted random sampling

Statistical theory generally relates to *unrestricted random sampling*. The members of the population (N) of interest are numbered and a number (n) of them are selected using random numbers. The sample units are *replaced* in the population before the next draw. Each unit can therefore be selected more than once. With this method, sampling is random and each population member has an *equal* chance of selection.

Simple random sampling

The members of the population (N) of interest are numbered and a number (n) of them are selected using random numbers *without replacing them*. Therefore each sample unit can only appear once in the sample. With this method, sampling is random and each population member has an *equal* chance of selection. As this method results in more precise population estimates, it is preferred over unrestricted random sampling.

At its most basic, names can be pulled out of a hat at random, although computer programs are usually designed to sample randomly, or to generate random number tables to facilitate manual random sampling. For example, with random number tables, the members of the population (N) are assigned a number and n numbers are selected from the tables, with a random starting point, in a way that is independent of human judgement. Random number tables are preferable to mixing numbered discs or cards in a 'hat', as with the latter it is difficult to ensure that they are adequately mixed to satisfy a random order.

In sampling without replacement, the assumption underlying statistical methods of the independence of the sample has been violated, and a correction factor should, strictly, be applied to the formula to take account of this (see Blalock (1972 for method).

Systematic random sampling

Selection from lists is called *systematic random sampling*, as opposed to simple random sampling, as it does *not* give each sample member an equal chance of selection. Instead, the selection of one sample member is dependent on the selection of the previous one. With systematic random sampling there is a system to the sampling in order to select a smaller sample from a larger population. For example, if the target sample size is 100 and the total eligible population for inclusion totals 1000, then a 1 in 10 sampling ratio (sampling fraction) would be selected. The sampling would start at a random point between 1 and 10. Thus once the sampling fraction has been calculated, the random starting point determines the rest of the sample to be selected. If it is *certain* that the list is, in effect, arranged randomly then the method is known as *quasi-random sampling*.

Systematic random sampling leads to a more even spread of the sample across the list of units than simple random sampling, except if the list really is randomly ordered (then the precision of the sample is the same). It is rare for lists of sampling units (e.g. names) to be in purely random order (e.g. they may be organized in alphabetical order, which means they are organized in a systematic way), so it is rare that the selection from such a list equates with simple random sampling. The method can lead to serious biases if the list is ordered so that a trend occurs, in which case the random starting position can affect the results (such as with lists ordered by seniority of employment grade in an organization). Such lists need reshuffling.

Stratified random sampling

A commonly used method of guarding against obtaining, by chance, an unrepresentative sample which under- or over-represents certain groups of the population is the use of *stratified random sampling*, which is a method of increasing the precision of the sample. With this method, the population of interest is divided into layers (strata) (e.g. adults aged 55–65, 65–75 and 75+) and a sample is drawn from each stratum, using simple or systematic random sampling.

If the sampling fraction is the same for each stratum it is known as *proportionate stratified sampling*, and this method is an improvement on simple random sampling as it will ensure that the different groups in the population (strata) (e.g. age, sex, geographical area) are correctly represented in the sample in the proportions in which they appear in the total population.

If the sampling fractions vary for each stratum the sampling procedure is known as *disproportionate stratified sampling*. A disproportionate stratified sample would be taken if some population strata are more heterogeneous than others, making them more difficult to represent in the sample (particularly in a smaller sample). Therefore a larger sampling fraction is taken for the heterogeneous strata in order to provide results for special sub-groups of the population. For example, it is common to take a larger sampling fraction in areas where a range of ethnic minority groups reside in order to ensure that they are represented in the sample in sufficient numbers for analysis. This may lead to lower precision than a simple random sample, unlike proportionate stratified sampling. There are different methods for calculating the standard error for proportionate and disproportionate stratified sampling.

Cluster sampling

The process of sampling complete groups of units is called *cluster sampling*. With this method, the population of interest can be divided into sub-populations. The units of interest are grouped together in clusters and the clusters are sampled randomly, using simple or systematic random sampling; the units within the sampled clusters are then included in the study. The reasons for doing this are economic. For example, for an interview survey, rather than randomly sampling 200 individual households from a list of 200,000 in a particular city (which would lead to a sample spread across the city, with high travelling costs for interviewers), it would be more economical to select randomly a number of areas (clusters) in the city and then include all the households in those areas. The areas can be naturally occurring or artificially created by placing grids on maps. The same procedure can be used in many situations: for example, for sampling patients in clinics. The overall probability of selection has not changed. This method is also advantageous when there is no sampling list.

Multistage sampling

The selection of clusters can be multistage. For example, one can select geographical districts (the primary sampling units, PSUs) within a region, and within these sample electoral wards, and finally within these sample households). This is known as *multistage sampling* and can be more economical, as it results in a concentration of fieldwork for interview surveys.

Sampling with probability proportional to size

Sampling with *probability proportional to size* (PPS) is common in multistage samples, as they generally have different size units. If one PSU has a larger population than another it should be given twice the chance of being selected. Equal probability sampling is inappropriate because if the units are selected with equal probability (i.e. the same sampling fraction) then a large unit may yield too many sample members and a small unit may yield too few. Instead, one could stratify the units by size and select a sample of them within each size group, with variable sampling fractions. Or one could sample the units with PPS: then the probability of selection for each person will be the same and the larger units cannot exert too great an effect on the total sample. The sizes of the primary sampling units must be known in order to carry out this method.

Sampling for telephone interview surveys

In order to conduct telephone interviews with the target population, the interviewer has to be able to access their telephone numbers. If the study is one of a specific population, such as people aged 65 years and over in a particular area, this can be problematic. Even if the rate of telephone ownership is high, people may not be listed in telephone directories ('ex-directory'). For some target populations (e.g. hospital outpatients) telephone numbers may be accessed through medical records, although ethical committees are likely to request that the investigator offer sample members the chance to decline to participate by post first.

Random digit dialling is a method which overcomes the problem of telephone owners not being listed in telephone directories. This is only suitable for general population and market research surveys. The method involves a prior formula and requires study of the distribution of exchanges and area codes. It requires the identification of all active telephone exchanges in the study area. A potential telephone number is created by randomly selecting an exchange followed by a random number between 0001 and 9999 (non-working and non-residential numbers are excluded from the sample). This method can substantially increase the cost. There is also the issue of who to select for interview: the interviewer will have to list all household members and randomly select the person to be sampled and interviewed; not an easy task over the telephone, especially if the required sample member is not the person who answered the telephone. Kingery (1989) compared different methods of sampling for telephone surveys of older people, and reported that random digit dialling was a very time-consuming method. For example, in the state of Georgia, USA, it took about 500 hours of calling to provide a maximum of 80 respondents aged over 65 who were willing to take part in a 20-minute telephone interview. It also took twice as long to contact eligible respondents aged over 55 as younger respondents, and response rates among older sample members were lower than with younger members. Techniques of sampling for telephone interviews, and discussion of issues of non-reponse, can be found in Groves *et al.* (1988).

Non-random sampling: quota sampling

Quota sampling is a method favoured by market researchers and opinion pollsters for its convenience and speed of sample recruitment. It is a method of stratified sampling in which the selection within geographical strata is non-random, and it is this non-random element which is its weakness. The geographical areas of the study are usually sampled randomly, after stratification (e.g. for type of region, parliamentary constituencies, sociodemographic characteristics of the area), and the quotas of types of people for interview are calculated from available data (numbers (quota) of males, females, people in different age bands and so on), in order to sample – and represent – these groups in the correct proportions, according to their distribution in the population. The choice of the sample members is left to the interviewers.

Interviewers are allocated an assignment of interviews, with instructions on how many interviews are to be in each group (e.g. with men, women, specific age groups). They then usually stand in the street(s) allocated to them until they have reached their quota of passers-by willing to answer their questions.

It is unlikely that quota sampling, however large the sample, results in truly representative samples of the population. There is potential for interviewer bias in the unconscious selection of specific types of respondent (such as people who appear to be in less of a hurry, or people who look friendlier). If street sampling is used then people who are in work, ill or frail have less likelihood of inclusion and people who are housebound have no chance of inclusion. It is not possible to estimate sampling errors with quota sampling, because the method does not meet the basic requirement of randomness. Not all people within a stratum have an equal chance of being selected because not all have an equal chance of coming face to face with the interviewer.

The advantages of the different sampling methods are summarized in Box 8.2.

Box 8.2   Techniques of sampling

- **Random sampling** gives each of the units in the population targeted a calculable (and non-zero) probability of being selected.
- **Simple and unrestricted random sampling** give each population member an equal chance of selection.
- **Systematic sampling** leads to a more even spread of the sample across a list than simple random sampling.
- **Stratified random sampling** increases the precision of the sample by guarding against the chance of under- or over-representation of certain groups in the population.
- **Cluster sampling** is economical, and the method is advantageous when there is no sampling list for the units within the clusters (e.g. households within geographical areas). Cluster sampling can be multistage, which is more economical.
- **Sampling with probability proportional to size** gives the sampling unit with the larger population a proportionally greater chance of being selected.
- **Sampling for telephone interviews** involves the use of specialized formulae, and even random digit dialling can be relatively time-consuming and complex.
- **Quota sampling** is preferred by market researchers for practical reasons; but the non-random element is a major weakness.

Types of survey

It was pointed out earlier that surveys can be designed to measure phenomena such as events, behaviour, perceptions and attitudes in the population of interest (e.g. the prevalence of symptoms or diseases, reported use of, and attitudes towards, health services). These types of survey are called *descriptive surveys* because the information is collected from a sample of the population of interest and descriptive statistics are calculated. They are also known as *cross-sectional surveys* because the data are collected from the population of interest at one point in time. Respondents are generally asked to report on current or recent (e.g. within the last month) events, feelings and behaviour, thus these surveys are called *retrospective*.

Statisticians often refer to descriptive, cross-sectional surveys as *observational research* because phenomena are observed rather than tested. This is a misleading description because direct observational and participant observational methods are specific methods used by social scientists. Descriptive surveys are also sometimes casually referred to as *correlation studies* because it is not generally possible to draw conclusions about cause and effect from them. A different type of survey aims to investigate *causal associations* between variables. These analytic surveys are known as *longitudinal surveys* and are carried out at more than one point in time over a period which is usually prospective (e.g. interviewing people over the forward passage of time), but can be retrospective (e.g. going back in time, as in using records).

Descriptive surveys: retrospective (ex post facto), cross-sectional surveys

The retrospective cross-sectional survey is a survey of a defined, random cross-section of the population at one particular point in time. Cross-sectional studies are labelled as retrospective because they involve questioning respondents about past as well as current behaviour, attitudes and events. Examples are the British General Household Survey (see Walker *et al.* 2001) and the US General Social Survey (see Schieman and Van Gundy 2000).

Descriptive studies literally describe the phenomenon of interest and observed associations in order to estimate certain population parameters (e.g. the prevalence of falls among elderly people), to *test hypotheses* (e.g. that falls are more common among people who live in homes that are poorly lit) and to *generate hypotheses* about possible cause and effect associations between variables. They can, in theory, range from the analysis of routine statistics to a cross-sectional, retrospective survey which describes the phenomenon of interest in the population and examines associations between the variables of interest. Descriptive studies can provide valuable information about characteristics of populations of interest, and about the speed of social or attitudinal change, and influencing factors.

Cross-sectional surveys, using standardized methods, are a relatively economical method in relation to time and resources, as large numbers of people can be surveyed relatively quickly, and standardized data are easily coded. The method is popularly used in the social sciences (e.g. psychology, sociology, economics) to investigate social phenomena, and in epidemiology (see Chapter 6) to investigate the prevalence (but not incidence) of disease (e.g. the population is surveyed at one point in time and the characteristics of those with disease are compared to those without disease in relation to their past exposure to a potential causative agent).

Retrospective studies are frequently criticized because they involve retrospective questioning (e.g. respondents may be asked questions about past diet and other lifestyle factors), and there is the potential for selectivity in recall and hence recall bias. Great care is needed with questionnaire design and the time reference periods asked about in order to minimize bias. However, even prospective studies involve questions about the past (i.e. between waves of the study), although the time references are shorter, and retrospective studies can provide useful indications for future investigation.

As with all descriptive studies, because it is difficult to establish the direction of an association (cause and effect), cross-sectional surveys cannot be used to impute such causality. For example, an association found between being overweight and breast cancer could be interpreted either as that being overweight might cause breast cancer, or that having breast cancer might lead to being overweight; or some third unknown variable may lead to both. Cross-sectional studies can only point to statistical associations between variables; they cannot alone establish causality. However, while descriptive studies cannot provide robust evidence about the direction of cause and effect relationships, the increasing sophistication of statistical techniques can help to minimize this limitation. In addition, generated hypotheses can, if appropriate and ethical, be tested later on in longitudinal or experimental studies.

Analytic surveys: prospective longitudinal surveys

Longitudinal surveys are analytic, rather than descriptive, because they analyse events at more than one point in time rather than cross-sectionally and, if the data collection points have been carefully timed, they can suggest the *direction* of cause and effect associations. Most longitudinal surveys collect data prospectively – over the forward passage of time. Longitudinal surveys can also be carried out retrospectively: for example, by collecting data about respondents from more than one time period in the past (e.g. from medical or other historic records).

The prospective, longitudinal survey, then, takes place over the forward passage of time (prospectively), i.e. with more than one period of data collection. It tends to be either panel (follow-up of the same population) or trend (different samples at each data collection period) in design. These types of study are also known as *follow-up studies*. If the sample to be followed up has a common characteristic, such as year of birth, it is called a prospective, longitudinal *cohort study* (see p. 135). This is a method which has been commonly employed by social scientists, and also by epidemiologists, for example to measure the incidence and aetiology of disease (see Chapter 6).

Prospective, longitudinal studies require careful definitions of the groups for study and careful selection of variables for measurement. Data have to be collected at frequent time intervals (or they have the same disadvantages of memory bias as retrospective studies), and response rates need to be high. Results can be biased if there is high sample attrition through natural loss (such as death), geographical mobility or refusals over time. There should be a clear rationale to support the timing of repeated survey points (e.g. at periods when changes are anticipated), as well as the use of sensitive instruments with relevant items which will detect changes. These surveys are sometimes referred to as 'natural experiments' – as interventions occurring in the course of events can be observed (with frequent and careful timing of follow-up periods), and the sample is then 'naturally' divided into cases and controls. Thus, incidence rates can be calculated in exposed and unexposed groups, and possible causal factors can be documented.

Prospective longitudinal surveys are expensive, take a long time and need a great amount of administration (e.g. to update and trace addresses, deaths or other losses of sample members), computing (e.g. merging of databases for different follow-up waves) and effort in order to minimize sample attrition. However well conducted the survey, it is often difficult, in practice, to use longitudinal data to suggest a causal relationship between a variable (e.g. an exposure) and an outcome (e.g. a disease) for a number of reasons. These include the difficulties in timing the successive follow-up waves and the long period of follow-up often required. In addition, the detection of any change in people as a result of an intervention, once intervening extraneous variables and any sampling biases have been ruled out, can always be due to *regression to the mean*. A regression artefact occurs when participants have an extreme measurement on a variable of interest which is short-lived and may simply be due to an unusual and temporary distraction. Longitudinal studies are often justified when cheaper, and less complex, cross-sectional data have suggested the appropriate variables to be measured.

Members of longitudinal samples can also become conditioned to the study, and even learn the responses that they believe are expected of them (as they become familiar with the questionnaire); they may remember, and repeat, their previous responses; they can become sensitized to the research topic and hence altered (biased) in some way; there can be a reactive effect of the research arrangements.

Trend, panel and prospective cohort surveys are all types of longitudinal survey, and are described next.

Trend surveys

A *trend survey* aims to sample a representative portion of the population of interest at the outset of the study and, in order to take account of changes in the wider population over time, to draw a new sample at each future measurement point. This method is popular in market research and polling (e.g. surveys of political attitudes over time). It is also used by epidemiologists in order to identify sample members with differing levels of exposure to a potential disease and to enable incidence rates to be calculated (the number of new cases of disease occurring in a defined time period). Disease incidence rates are compared in the exposed and unexposed groups. Epidemiologists often call this a method of surveying a *dynamic population*, as opposed to a *fixed population* survey. The sample members should be derived from a random sample of the population. Information is sought from the members by post or by interview.

Panel surveys

A *panel survey* is the traditional form of longitudinal design. A sample of a defined population is followed up at more than one point in time (e.g. repeated questionnaires at intervals over time), and changes are recorded at intervals. Although the wider population may change over time, the same sample is interviewed repeatedly until the study terminates or the sample naturally dwindles as sample members have left (e.g. they have moved, dropped out of the study or died). Each person accumulates a number of units of months or years (known as 'person-time') of observation. The aim is to study the sample's experiences and characteristics (e.g. attitudes, behaviours, illnesses) as they enter successive time periods and age groups, in order to study changes.

Again, the sample members should be derived from a random sample of the population, and this can be based on a cohort sample. Information is sought from the members by post or by interview. Bowling and Gabriel's (2004) longitudinal survey of the quality of life of older people is an example of a panel survey. This was based on a national random sample of people aged 65 and over living at home in Britain. Respondents were followed up over time, with the aim of examining the factors associated with positive ageing and having a good or bad quality of later life.

Responses to the same question on successive occasions in panel surveys will generally be positively correlated, and in such cases the variance of the change will be lower for a longitudinal survey than for surveys of independent samples. A further advantage of this method is that not only can trends be assessed, but the method can identify people who change their behaviour or attitudes, as well as other characteristics (e.g. health status).

Cross-sectional and longitudinal cohort studies

It was pointed out earlier that if the population to be sampled has a common experience or characteristic which defines the sampling (e.g. all born in the same year), this is known as a cohort study (e.g. the British birth cohort surveys – see Wadsworth 1991). The key defining feature of a cohort is this sharing of the common characteristic. A cohort study can be based on analyses of routine data, and/or on assessments and data collected for the study.

Technically, *cohort studies* can be *cross-sectional* and retrospective (collection of data at one point in time about the past), *longitudinal* and retrospective (collection of data at more than one point in time over the past) or longitudinal and prospective (collection of data at more than one point over the forward passage of time). However, even prospective studies include retrospective questioning about events that have occurred between waves of interviews. The prospective cohort study is one of the main methods used in epidemiological research (see Chapter 6) to investigate aetiology (causes of disease).

Cohort sequential studies

Some longitudinal cohort designs involve taking cohorts at different points in time (e.g. a sample of 18–25-year-olds in different years) in order to allow for cohort effects (the sharing of common experiences which can lead to the unrepresentativeness of the cohort). These are known as *cohort sequential studies*, and cross-sectional, cohort and cohort sequential analyses can be carried out. However, they cannot properly control for period effects (e.g. changing economic, social or political circumstances over time which explain differing results). A well-known example of this method is the longitudinal study of people aged 70 years in Gothenberg, Sweden. The study commenced with one cohort born in 1901–2, which has been followed up for more than 20 years. The analyses indicated that there was some impact of the environment on health and functioning and so two more cohorts (born five and ten years after the first cohort) were added. In addition, in order to test hypotheses about the influence of lifestyle, environmental factors and the availability of health care on ageing and health, a broad sociomedical intervention was added to the third age cohort (Svanborg 1996).

As with longitudinal studies, cohort samples must be complete and the response rates at each wave of the study need to be high in order to avoid sample bias. In addition, a main problem with analysing data from cohort studies is the 'cohort effect'. This refers to the problem that each cohort experiences its society under unique historical conditions, and contributes to social change by reinterpreting cultural values, attitudes and beliefs and adjusting accordingly. For example, a cohort that grows up during times of economic depression or war may develop different socioeconomic values from cohorts brought up in times of economic boom or peace.

Case-control studies

Epidemiologists also commonly undertake case-control studies (see Chapter 6) in which the cases are selected who already have the outcome or exposure of interest (e.g. people with the disease of interest, the cases). This is in contrast to longitudinal cohort surveys where sample members are selected before they experience the outcome of interest. Thus case-control studies work backwards to detect potential causes (e.g. by using retrospective surveys, historical and medical records), making comparisons with a group without the disease but with the same opportunities for exposure to the risk factors (the controls) in order to identify the factors which occur more or less often in the cases in comparison with the controls. The aim is to indicate the factors which might elevate or reduce the risk of the disease under investigation (these studies can provide estimates of relative risk, but they cannot measure incidence or prevalence; see Moon *et al.* 2000 for clear examples of methods of selection of cases and controls).

Questionnaire methods of data collection in surveys

Interview and self-completion (e.g. mailed) structured questionnaire methods are the most common vehicles of data collection in surveys. If an interview method is preferred, the issue of whether to use structured or semi-structured questionnaires needs to be addressed, as well as whether the interview is to be face to face or by telephone (either personal interviewer-led or automated). If the self-administered questionnaire is preferred, it has to be decided whether it should be given to sample members personally (e.g. in clinic settings), with a prepaid envelope to return it in once completed, or whether it is to be sent directly to sample members by post, or even posted electronically on the internet or distributed by email (the latter two methods are less common in Europe than the USA because of lower levels on access to the internet (especially among low income and very elderly communities), as well as lack of sampling frames (e.g. email address lists)). Each method has its advantages and disadvantages, and each has implications for bias.

Structured questionnaires involve the use of fixed (standardized) questions, batteries of questions, tests (e.g. psychological) and/or scales which are presented to respondents in the same way, with no variation in question wording, and with mainly precoded response choices. Semi-structured questionnaires include mainly fixed questions but with no, or few, response codes, and are used flexibly to allow interviewers to probe, and to enable respondents to raise other relevant issues.

The strength of structured questionnaires is the ability to collect unambiguous and easy to count answers, leading to quantitative data for analysis. Because the method leads to greater ease of data collection and analysis, it is relatively economical and large samples of people can be included. The weakness of structured questionnaires is that the pre-coded response choices may not be sufficiently comprehensive and not all answers may be easily accommodated. Some respondents may therefore be 'forced' to choose inappropriate precoded answers that might not fully represent people's views.

Structured interview and self-administered questionnaire methods rest on the assumption, then, that questions can be worded and ordered in a way that will be understood by all respondents. This may not always be justified, as respondents may not all share the same perspective and the same words, terms and concepts may not elicit the same response from different respondents. And there is always scope for bias: for example, interviewer bias in interview studies, recall (memory) bias and framing, in which respondents' replies are influenced by the design (frame) of the question and the precoded response choices. Many questions are about socially desirable attitudes, states and behaviour leading to potential social desirability bias (the respondent's desire to present a positive image).

Box 8.3   Paper and pencil, and electronic modes

Questionnaires can be administered to respondents on paper or electronically.

- **The traditional 'paper and pencil' modes of questionnaire administration are:** verbal face-to-face interviewing, verbal telephone interviewing, postal questionnaires and other methods of self-administration such as handing paper questionnaires to people in person and asking them to complete them in ink and return them to the researcher.
- **Electronic methods include:** computer assisted personal (face-to-face) interviewing (CAPI) and computer assisted telephone interviewing (CATI). With these, the questionnaire is in the form of a computer program that displays the items to the interviewer on a computer screen (on a laptop in the case of personal interviewing). The interviewer reads the prompted questions to the respondent and enters their responses by pressing the appropriate keys on the keyboard. Respondents themselves can also complete questionnaires electronically using a computer mouse/keyboard, either at a computer within an organizational facility (e.g. psychology laboratory, clinical setting), on the internet or via email (either a questionnaire is emailed to a respondent to complete or the respondent connects to a website where a programme administers the questionnaire). With audio computer-assisted self-administered interviewing (ACASI) the programme displays questions on the computer screen and instructs the respondents audibly (e.g. via headphones). Interactive voice response methods with automated telephone lines are also well developed, in which a computer plays a recording of the questions over the telephone and respondents indicate their responses by pressing indicated handset keys. The range of electronic methods has been described by Tourangeau *et al.* (2000).

Different questionnaire methods, then, can involve either paper and pencil, electronic (computer mouse/keyboard) and telephone keypad vehicles for collecting the data (see Box 8.3). They can also be conducted in different settings (e.g. home, office, clinic). Modes of data collection also differ from each other at different levels (see Box 8.4). Because of these differences between levels, it is difficult to separate out the potential biasing effects of each of the different modes of data collection on the quality of the data obtained. It is well established from experimental studies that minor changes in question wording, question order or response format can result in major differences in type of response (Schuman and Presser 1981; see also Chapter 17). For example, analyses of responses to a question on disability in five large-scale population surveys concluded that the effects of mode of administration were difficult to separate out from the effects of variations in question wording and order effects (position in the questionnaire), question framing effects and the context effects of different surveys (Bajekal *et al.* 2004).

> ### Box 8.4   Differences between modes of survey data collection
>
> Modes of data collection differ at different levels:
>
> - **The method of contacting the respondents:** ranging from an initial letter of introduction, giving notice of the study to personal face-to-face, email or telephone contact at the same time as the provision of, or administration of, the questionnaire, depending on its mode of administration.
> - **The medium of delivering the questionnaire to respondents:** in person, by telephone, by post or electronically (e.g. by email).
> - **The administration of the questions:** by interviewers using either an electronic or paper questionnaire (face-to-face or by telephone), by self-administration via automated electronic or telephone programmes or by traditional self-administration methods in which respondents present/read the questions and record responses on a paper copy of the questionnaire (e.g. postal questionnaires).

Burden of questionnaires on respondents

There are at least four steps involved in answering questionnaires, which place cognitive demands on respondents:

- comprehension of the question;
- recall of requested information from memory;
- evaluation of the link between the retrieved information and the question;
- communication of the response (Tourangeau 1984; Bajekal *et al.* 2004).

It is likely, then, that the channel of questionnaire presentation (e.g. auditory, oral, visual) affects the cognitive burden placed on respondents, especially the demand for literacy in the case of visual self-administration methods. And as each mode inevitably imposes different cognitive requirements on respondents, and varies in the amount of privacy and anonymity they afford respondents, these can affect the process of responding to questions. Thus they have a potential influence on the quality of the data obtained.

Probably the least burdensome method is the personal, face-to-face interview (*auditory channel*) as this only requires the respondent to speak the same language in which the questions are asked, and to have basic verbal and listening skills. No reading skills are required (unless written materials for the respondent are contained within the interview). The presence of a friendly, motivating interviewer can increase response and item response rates, and maintain motivation with longer questionnaires. The interviewer can probe for responses, clarify ambiguous questions, be trained to follow complex question-skipping and routing instructions, can help respondents with enlarged show cards of response choice options, can use memory jogging techniques for aiding recall of events and behaviour and can control the order of the questions.

Telephone interviews, however, makes greater auditory demands and may be burdensome to respondents. In addition, very elderly people may have problems with recall, hearing and finger/wrist dexterity. Telephone interviews require basic verbal and language skills, and also require access to, or ownership of, a telephone.

The most burdensome modes are likely to be self-administered *visual* and *written* methods, as these demand that respondents are literate in reading the language(s) of the survey, that they do not have visual impairments and that they have the dexterity (e.g. of wrist, fingers) to complete the questions. They require respondents to tick a box on a paper questionnaire or press an electronic key or a key on a touchtone telephone handset to indicate their response. Respondents are required to read or listen, recognize numbers and key answers accurately. With visual and written methods respondents also need the ability to follow instructions. The significant minorities of people with limited literacy skills in western populations, including those not fluent in the main language of the country of residence, means that these demands need to be considered seriously by researchers.

Electronic methods require access to a computer and internet facilities, basic computer literacy and also familiarity with numbers and keyboards, which excludes a large proportion of the population. They have literacy requirements regarding reading the questions and replying, and can also have auditory requirements (ACASI). However, they do have more complete item response rates than the various paper and pencil methods (Tourangeau *et al*. 1997).

Effects of mode of administration on data quality

So, what are the effects of the different modes of questionnaire administration on the data that are ultimately obtained? Much of the research on the effect of mode of questionnaire administration on data quality is to be found in specialized books, internal reports (e.g. of large survey organizations) and in specialized social science journals. Most research comparing mode of questionnaire administration was conducted in the USA and is based on comparisons of separate samples, rather than controlled, experimental designs. The most notable reviews include those by Tourangeau *et al*. (2000) and De Leeuw and van der Zouwen (1988), based on their analysis of data quality in telephone and face-to-face surveys.

Data quality is a vague concept, especially when there is no 'gold standard' of the correct answer (e.g. as in research on attitudes, perceived health, quality of life etc.). It could be defined in terms of survey response rates, questionnaire item response rates, the accuracy of responses, absence of bias (e.g. social desirability bias, interviewer bias, acquiescence bias) and completeness of the information obtained. De Leeuw and van der Zouwen (1988) conducted a comparative meta-analysis of data quality in telephone and face-to-face surveys, and listed the following indicators for data quality:

- **Response rate:** the number of completed interviews divided by the total number of eligible sample units.
- **Accuracy of response (validity):** checks can be made against a 'true value' only when validating information is available.
- **Absence of social desirability bias:** when the answer is determined by socially acceptable norms, rather than the true situation. This is inversely proportional to the number of socially desirable answers on a particular question.
- **Item response:** this is inversely proportional to the number of missing responses in the questionnaire.
- **Amount of information:** this is indicated by the number of responses to open-ended questions or checklists.
- **Similarity of response distributions obtained by different modes of questionnaire administration:** this is indicated by lack of significant differences between the estimates obtained using different modes of administration.

More broadly, sources of error in surveys relate to (i) survey design, the sampling frame and sampling, non-response and item non-response (*non-measurement errors*) and (ii) survey instrument and data collection processes (*measurement errors*). Mode of questionnaire administration has effects on elements of both these sources.

The most common methods of administering questionnaires in surveys are described next (postal and self-administered paper questionnaires, face-to-face and telephone interviews).

Postal and self-administered questionnaires

A common method of covering a large, geographically spread population relatively quickly and more economically than interview methods is to mail respondents a questionnaire to complete at home, with a reply-paid envelope for its return. A variation is to give the sample members a questionnaire in person and ask them to complete it at home, and return it to the investigator in a reply-paid envelope (e.g. patients in clinics can be approached in this way).

The self-administered or postal questionnaire is less of a social encounter than interview methods and can be posted to people to minimize social desirability and interviewer bias. It is useful for sensitive topics, as there is more anonymity. However, the method is only suitable when the issues and questions are straightforward and simple, when the population is 100 per cent literate in a common language(s), and when a sampling frame of addresses exists. It is less suitable for complex issues and long questionnaires, and it is inappropriate if spontaneous replies are required. The data obtained are generally less reliable than with face-to-face interviews, as interviewers are not present to clarify questions or to probe. The replies also have to be accepted as final. There is no control over who completes the questionnaire even if respondents are instructed not to pass the questionnaire on, or over the influence of other people on the participants' replies. Respondents can read all the questions before answering any one of them, and they can answer the questions in any order they wish – and question order, which can be controlled in interview situations, can affect the type of response. There is also no opportunity to supplement the postal questionnaire with observational data, unlike in interviews (brief descriptions by the interviewer at the end of the interview can be valuable, e.g. of the respondent and the setting, interruptions and how the interview went). Response rates are generally lower for postal questionnaires than for personal interviews. However, there are well-established methods of enhancing response rates to postal questionnaires.

A systematic review of methods to influence response to postal questionnaires by Edwards *et al.* (2001) found that the odds of response were substantially higher with the use of financial incentives, the use of shorter questionnaires, providing a second copy of the questionnaire with follow-up reminder letters to non-responders (repeat mailings are usually carried out at three and six weeks after initial mailings), 'user friendly' questionnaires and university sponsorship (and also if a well-known or senior person sends the questionnaire – i.e. signs the accompanying letter). Other factors which also increased response were pre-notification of the survey (McColl *et al.* 2001), non-monetary incentives (e.g. a key ring), providing personalized questionnaires, the use of coloured ink (i.e. not blue or black), the use of stamped as opposed to franked envelopes and first-class outward mailing. Response was considerably lowered if sensitive questions were included, when the questionnaire started with general questions and when people were offered the opportunity to opt out of the study.

Face-to-face interviews

Face-to-face interview methods vary from in–depth, unstructured or semi-structured (i.e. structured questions without response codes) methods to highly structured, pre-coded response questionnaires, or they can involve a combination of the two (a structured, pre-coded questionnaire, but with open-ended questions to allow the respondent to reply in his or her own words, where the range of responses is unknown or cannot be easily categorized). Sometimes, measurement instruments are handed to the respondents (self-completion or self-administration scales) to complete themselves during face-to-face interviews (e.g. scales of depression where it is thought that the interviewer recording of the response may lead to social desirability bias).

The *advantages* of face-to-face interviews are: interviewers can probe fully for responses and clarify any ambiguities; more complicated and detailed questions can be asked; more information, of greater depth, can be obtained; inconsistencies and misinterpretations can be checked; there are no literacy requirements for respondents; and questions in structured schedules can be asked in a predetermined order, minimizing any question order bias. With a well-trained interviewer, open-ended questions can be included in the questionnaire to enable respondents to give their opinions in full on more complex topics. They also provide rich and quotable material which enlivens research reports. Open-ended questions are used for topics which are largely unknown or complex, and for pilot studies.

The potential errors made by interviewers (e.g. by making incorrect skips of applicable questions and sub-questions) can be minimized by CAPI (use of laptop computers which display a menu-driven questionnaire, which enable respondents' replies to be directly keyed in and which automatically display the next question, skips, errors and so on). The *disadvantages* are that interviews can be expensive and time-consuming, and there is the potential for interviewer bias and additional bias if interpreters are used for some participants. Techniques for reducing potential bias include good interviewer training in methods of establishing rapport with people, putting them at ease and appearing non-judgemental. Structured and semi-structured interview questionnaires, if carefully designed for the topic, can yield highly accurate data.

Response rates are generally higher with surveys using interviewers than for self-completion questionnaire surveys (e.g. postal) or telephone interviews (McColl *et al.* 2001). Methods of increasing response rates to interviews include the appearance of a presentable interviewer with a friendly, neutral demeanour and the sponsorship of the survey by a bone fide organization. The relevance of the topic to the individual is also important (e.g. health surveys generally appeal to people because they tend to be interested in their health) (McColl *et al.* 2001).

Telephone interviews

Interviews conducted by telephone (land-lines) appear to have equal accuracy rates as face-to-face interviews in relation to the collection of data on general health status and the prevalence of depressive symptoms. Their main *advantage* is that, in theory, the method is economic in relation to time (i.e. no travelling is involved for the interviewer) and resources (i.e. travelling and associated costs are not incurred). However, telephone interviewing is not necessarily a cheap option. At least three call backs will be required, given estimates that 50 per cent of diallings are met with the engaged tone or there is no reply, and an increasing number of telephones have answering machines. The latter tend to be owned by younger, unmarried people in higher socioeconomic groups (Mishra *et al.* 1993). This necessitates repeated call backs, which can be time-consuming, if sampling bias is to be minimized. There is the potential bias of over-representing people who are most likely to be at home (and who answer the telephone), who may be unrepresentative of the wider population.

One technique in telephone interviewing is CATI. The interviewer asks the questions from a computer screen and respondents' answers are typed and coded directly onto a disk. The advantage is speed, and minimization of interviewer error when asking questions (e.g. the computer prompts the interviewer to ask the next question and only when the answer has been keyed in does the computer move on to the next question, skips are displayed, out of range codes keyed in error are displayed).

Surveys using telephone interviews have been popular for many years in the USA, where levels of telephone ownership are high, and also among market researchers (e.g. random digit dialling or sampling from telephone directories or lists). They are slowly becoming more popular among social researchers in Europe, although they have the disadvantage that people in the lowest socioeconomic groups have lower rates of telephone ownership, and consequently there is potential for sample bias owing to their being under-represented in the sample.

Apart from potential sample bias, the main *disadvantage* of the method is that it is only suitable for use with brief questionnaires and on non-sensitive topics, and results in less complete information and more 'don't knows'. Telephone interviews also tend to suffer from a high rate of premature termination (the respondent does not wish to continue with the interview) (Frankfort-Nachmias and Nachmias 1992). A systematic review comparing response rates of telephone and postal surveys on health-related topics was inconclusive (McColl *et al.* 2001). An overview by Oksenberg and Cannell (1988) reported that individual response rates for telephone interviewers ranged from 6–42 per cent. These were associated with interviewers' style of speech, with interviewers who spoke rapidly, loudly and with variability of speech having the highest response rates.

The main advantages and disadvantages of the most common methods of administering questionnaires are summarized in Box 8.5.

Box 8.5   Main advantages and disadvantages of survey questionnaire methods

- **The advantage of postal questionnaires** (i.e. mailing respondents a questionnaire to complete at home, with a reply-paid envelope for its return) is that they can cover large populations relatively quickly and economically. But postal and other self-completion methods are only suitable when the issues and questions are straightforward and simple, and the population is 100 per cent literate in a common language(s).
- **The main advantages of face-to-face interviews** are that the interviewers can probe fully for responses and clarify any ambiguities, and can control the sequence of questions. More complicated and detailed questions can be asked and there is no literacy requirement (although there is a language requirement). But interviews are expensive, time-consuming and have the potential for interviewer bias.
- **Interviews conducted by telephone** are economic, and appear to have equal accuracy rates to face-to-face interviews in relation to the collection of data on health. But they are only suitable for use with short, straightforward questionnaires, mainly on non-sensitive topics, and are limited to people with telephones, and who are in to answer them.

Non-response and response rates

Non-response is important because it reduces the effective sample size (which results in the loss of precision of the survey estimates) by potentially introducing bias if the non-respondents differ in some way from the respondents (non-response error). For example, if a study of patients' experiences of treatment for angina receives responses from 60 per cent of patients receiving medication only and from just 20 per cent of those who have undergone surgery, then the survey estimates are biased away from surgical patients' experiences.

In telephone interviews, some telephones may be engaged, be linked to answering machines which screen calls, or remain unanswered. In postal surveys some sample members will not return postal questionnaires because they may not be able to complete them (due to poor eyesight, stiff fingers, frailty, illiteracy, or literacy in a language other than that of the questionnaire). In interview surveys, some people will not be at home when the interviewer calls, or not speak the same language as the interviewer (in such cases a decision has to be made about the use of translators or translated questionnaires). In all types of study, some sample members will directly refuse to participate (this is the most common source of non-response in well-planned and conducted surveys), will be away, will have moved, died, been admitted to hospital or are too ill/frail to take part at the time of the study. These are all sources of non-response. In addition, non-coverage of the unit (e.g. where a household or person or clinic is missing from the sampling frame) is also a type of non-response. People who have died before the start of the study ('blanks') can be excluded from the sampling frame and from the calculation of the non-response rate.

The response rate is calculated out of the number of eligible respondents successfully included in the study, as a percentage of the total eligible study population. There is no agreed standard for an acceptable minimum response rate, although it appears to be generally accepted that a response rate of 75 per cent and above is good. This still leaves up to 25 per cent of a sample population who have not responded and who may differ in some important way from the responders (e.g. they may be older and iller), and thus the survey results will still be biased.

Weighting for non-response

There are weighting procedures which can be used in the analyses to compensate for unit non-response (e.g. weighting of the replies of males aged 16–24 if they have a particularly high non-response, on the assumption that the non-responders and responders in this group do not differ). If the survey estimates differ for respondents and non-respondents, then the survey results will consistently produce results which under- or overestimate the true population values (response bias). If some information can be obtained about the non-respondents, and the survey estimates are different for the respondents and the non-respondents, then it may be possible to use statistical weighting methods which attach weight to the responding units in order to compensate for units not being included in the final sample.

The most commonly used weighting method is population-based weighting (which requires that the sample be divided into weighting classes where the population total within each class is known, e.g. from census data). Less commonly used, because investigators do not have the required information, is sample-based weighting (which requires that information in relation to key study variables is available for both responding and non-responding units). Thus the possibility of weighting for non-response depends on the availability of some data about the non-respondents directly or about the respondents and the whole population. The principles and procedures for weighting for non-response have been outlined briefly by Barton (1996), and in detail by Kalton (1983) and Elliot (1991). However, weighting does make assumptions about the non-responders and it is preferable to minimize non-response rather than to compensate for it by weighting sample results (see methods of improving response in Bowling 2002).

Conclusions

This chapter has covered the main principles of sampling for surveys, methods of reducing non-response, the different types of cross-sectional and longitudinal survey methods and the different approaches to administering survey questionnaires. In sum, surveys aim to collect information as accurately and precisely as possible, and to collect the same information from each member of the survey sample. The use of random probability sampling in survey designs allows statistical inferences to be made in relation to the broader population of interest and thus allow generalizations to be made. The main methods of data collection are face-to-face interviews, self-administered questionnaires (e.g. postal) and telephone interviews. Internet and email questionnaires are relatively uncommon in Europe, although increasing in the USA. The best-quality data is obtained in face-to-face interview surveys, although these are expensive and there is always potential for interviewer and social desirability bias. Less common survey methods include surveys of documents (e.g. of medical records) and direct observation (e.g. as in traffic surveys). All methods require effort and skill to minimize non-response and any sample bias.

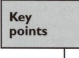

Key points

- The distinguishing feature of a survey is that the same information is collected from each member of the survey sample. They can also cover large samples of people.

- Surveys aim to collect information as accurately and precisely as possible, in such a way that if they were repeated at another time or in another area the results would be comparable.

- Sampling theory assumes the use of the method of random sampling. The use of random probability sampling allows statistical inferences to be made in relation to the broader population of interest and thus allow generalizations to be made.

- It is important to calculate the sample size required at the design stage of the study as accurately as possible, using a power calculation, in order to be able to generalize the survey findings to the whole population of interest.

- Random sampling gives each of the units in the population targeted a calculable (and non-zero) probability of being selected for inclusion in the study. Random sampling relates to the *method* of sampling, not to the resulting sample.

- Statements based on randomly selected samples are probability statements, based on inference because of sample non-response and potential measurement bias.

- Surveys can be carried out at one point in time (descriptive, cross-sectional surveys), collecting information about past and current phenomena, or at more than one point in time ('longitudinal'), either retrospectively or prospectively.

- Structured interview and self-administered questionnaire methods assume that questions can be worded and ordered in a way that will be understood by all respondents. This may not always be justified as respondents may not all share the same perspective.

- The channel of questionnaire presentation (e.g. auditory, oral, visual) affects the cognitive burden placed on respondents, especially the demand for literacy in the case of visual self-administration methods.

- Sources of error in surveys relate to (i) survey design, the sampling frame and sampling, non-response and item non-response (*non-measurement errors*) and (ii) survey instrument and data collection processes (*measurement errors*). The mode of questionnaire administration has an effect on elements of both these sources.

References

Armitage, P. and Berry, G. (1987) *Statistical Methods in Medical Research*, 2nd edn. Oxford: Blackwell Scientific Publications.

Bajekal, M., Harries, T., Breman, R. and Woodfield, K. (2004) *Review of Disability Estimates and Definitions*, in-house report no. 128. London: Department of Work and Pensions.

Barton, J. (1996) *Weighting for Non-response – An Overview*, briefing, 4, 14–16, NHS Health Survey Advice Centre. London: Office of Population Censuses and Surveys.

Berry, D.A. (1996) *Statistics: a Bayesian Perspective*. Belmont, CA: Duxbury Press.

Blalock, H.M. (1972) Social Statistics, 2nd edn. London: McGraw-Hill.

Bland, M. (1995) *An Introduction to Medical Statistics*. Oxford: Oxford University Press.

Booth, C. (ed.) (1889–1902) *Labour and Life of the People of London*, 17 vols. Basingstoke: Macmillan.

Bowling, A. (2002) *Research Methods in Health*, 2nd edn. Buckingham: Open University Press.

Bowling, A. and Gabriel, Z. (2004) An integrational model of quality of life in older age: a comparison of analytic and lay models of quality of life, *Social Indicators Research*, 69: 1–36.

Crichton, N.J. (1993) The importance of statistics in research design, in G.T. Lewith and D. Aldridge (eds) *Clinical Research Methodology for Complementary Therapies*. London: Hodder & Stoughton.

De Leeuw, E.D. and van der Zouwen, J. (1988) Data quality in telephone and face-to-face surveys: a comparative meta-analysis, in R.M. Groves, P.P. Biemer, L.E. Lyberg. *et al.* (eds) *Telephone Survey Methodology*. New York: Wiley.

Edwards, P., Roberts, I., Clarke, M. *et al.* (2001) *Methods to Influence Response to Postal Questionnaires (Cochrane Methodology Group)*, the Cochrane Library, Issue 1. Chichester: Wiley.

Elliot, D. (1991) *Weighting for Non-response: A Survey Researcher's Guide*. London: Office of Population Censuses and Surveys.

Frankfort-Nachmias, C. and Nachmias, D. (1992) *Research Methods in the Social Sciences*, 4th edn. London: Edward Arnold.

Freedman, L. (1996) Bayesian statistical methods: a natural way to assess clinical evidence, *British Medical Journal*, 313: 569–70.

Groves, R.M., Biemer, P.P. and Lyberg, L.E. (eds) (1988) *Telephone Survey Methodology*. New York: Wiley.

Kalton, G. (1983) *Compensating for Missing Survey Data*. Ann Arbor, MI: Institute for Social Research, University of Michigan.

Kingery, D.W. (1989) Sampling strategies for surveys of older adults, in F.J. Fowler (ed.) *Health Survey Research Methods*. Rockville, MD: National Center for Health Services Research and Health Care Technology Assessment.

Lilford, R.J. and Braunholtz, D. (1996) The statistical basis of public policy: a paradigm shift is overdue, *British Medical Journal*, 313: 603–7.

McColl, E., Jacoby, A., Thomas, L. *et al.* (2001) Design and use of questionnaires: a review of best practice applicable to surveys of health service staff and patients, *Health Technology Assessment*, 5(31).

Mishra, S.I., Dooley, D., Catalano, R. and Serxner, S. (1993) Telephone health surveys: potential bias from non-completion, *American Journal of Public Health*, 83: 94–9.

Mok, M. (1995) Sample size requirements for 2-level designs in educational research, Institute of Education, University of London, *Multilevel Modelling Newsletter*, 7: 11–15.

Moon, G., Gould, M. and colleagues (2000) *Epidemiology: An Introduction*. Buckingham: Open University Press.

Oksenberg, L. and Cannel, C. (1988) Effects of interviewer vocal characteristics on response, in R.M. Groves, P.P. Biemer and L.E. Lyberg (eds) *Telephone Survey Methodology*. New York: Wiley.

Pocock, S.J. (1983) *Clinical Trials: A Practical Approach*. Chichester: Wiley.

Rowntree, B.S. (1902) *Poverty: A Study of Town Life*. London: Longman.

Schieman, S. and Van Gundy, K. (2000) The personal and social links between age and self-reported empathy, *Social Psychology Quarterly*, 63: 152–74.

Schuman, H. and Presser, S. (1981) *Questions and Answers in Attitude Surveys*. New York: Academic Press.

Svanborg, A. (1996) Conduct of long-term cohort sequential studies, in S. Ebrahim and A. Kalache (eds) *Epidemiology in Old Age*. London: BMJ Publishing Group.

Tourangeau, R. (1984) Cognitive sciences and survey methods, in T. Jabine, M. Straf, J. Tanur and R. Tourangeau (eds) *Cognitive Aspects of Survey Methodology: Building a Bridge Between Disciplines*. Washington, DC: National Academy Press.

Tourangeau, R., Rasinski, K., Jobe, J.B. *et al.* (1997) Sources of error in a survey of sexual behaviour, *Journal of Official Statistics*, 13: 341–65.

Tourangeau, R., Rips, L.J. and Rasinski, K. (2000) Mode of data collection, in R. Tourangeau, L.J. Rips and K. Rasinski (eds) *The Psychology of Survey Response*. Cambridge: Cambridge University Press.

Wadsworth, M.E.J. (1991) *The Imprint of Time: Childhood, History and Adult Life*. Oxford: Oxford University Press.

Walker, A., Maher, J., Voulthard, M. *et al.* (2001) *Living in Britain: Results from the 2000 General Household Survey*. London: The Stationery Office.

9 Approaches to qualitative data collection in social science

Simon Carter and Lesley Henderson

Introduction

There are many forms of data collection in qualitative research and these are under-pinned by a variety of different methodological and theoretical approaches. Thus qualitative data collection methods can include: in-depth structured or unstructured interviews including oral and life histories; group discussions and interviews; participant and non-participant observational studies; and analysis of textual and narrative sources such as reports, diaries, letters and film or television. In turn these qualitative methods are made sense of in different ways by contrasting theoretical approaches, such as symbolic interactionism, feminism, Marxism, ethnomethodology and structuralism/post-structuralism.

Despite the diversity of methods and approaches involved in qualitative data gathering it is important that newcomers to this form of research should not feel intimidated. Indeed, the necessary skills to become a qualitative researcher are those required for everyday social life. For example, we all have experience of interviews, either because we have directly taken part in them (e.g. job interviews), or because we have indirectly witnessed them (e.g. politicians being interviewed on radio or television). Most of us are skilled at making observations of daily life either as participants or non-participants and we all critically consume textual and narrative artefacts on a regular basis. To become a successful qualitative researcher simply requires that these same basic skills are applied in a systematic and rigorous manner to the subject or issue being studied.

Put simply, qualitative research is any form of data collection that generates narrative or non-numeric information. However, at a slightly deeper level, most qualitative research would seek to adopt an *emic perspective* (see Box 9.1). In other words, qualitative research attempts to gain access to the insider's view of his or her own social world without, at the stage when data is being collected, making any value judgements. This is research that focuses on the experiences and meanings of individuals or groups in order to analyse how and why people form associations with other people, with things and with their immediate environments. Its ultimate goal is to use *ethnographic* and *ethnomethodological* approaches in order to connect social theory to the very fabric of the lived and everyday world.

Throughout this chapter we intend to illustrate some of the broad principles of qualitative data gathering involved with two specific methods, namely: interviewing and focus groups. Where possible we use examples and case studies to illustrate how

---

Box 9.1   Some definitions

- **Emic perspective:** idea from ethnography that research should try and find the insider's view of his or her social world.
- **Ethnography:** a methodology associated with anthropology and European sociology that seeks to systematically describe the culture of the individuals or group under investigation. The goal is to adopt an emic perspective.
- **Ethnomethodology:** studies the ways that local social interactions are used by people to make sense of their social worlds. Focuses on how everyday activities are understood and how social 'reality' is produced.

---

these techniques may be applied practically. First, however it is important to consider some underlying assumptions about qualitative research.

Many researchers may come to qualitative research from one of the disciplines where quantitative methods more commonly predominate. Within these disciplines most people will be more familiar with research that seeks to test hypotheses. In other words, an existing body of knowledge or literature will suggest a statement predicting a relationship between variables (e.g. between exposure to the sun and skin cancer) and this relationship can then be tested using traditional quantitative methods. In contrast, qualitative research cannot be used to test a hypothesis. Often, for those people coming from a quantitative discipline and who may have internalized a hypothesis-testing approach, this aspect of qualitative research can be difficult to 'unlearn'.

For the most part, qualitative research is about the emergence of new social theory or the development of existing social theory. This means that qualitative research can be complementary to quantitative research in two ways: before carrying out quantitative research the use of qualitative research can suggest theories that can then form hypotheses to be tested; and, after quantitative surveys have been carried out, qualitative research can be used to provide a deeper exploration of the mechanisms that may link variables. For example, in the 1980s much quantitative research suggested that while overall rates of smoking among women were declining this change was not uniform, with lower socioeconomic groups having higher rates of women smokers. In addition, women's rates of smoking cessation were lower than for men. Hilary Graham (1987, 1993), using qualitative methods, explored the relationship between smoking cessation and women's experiences. This suggested that women largely smoke for dissimilar reasons and in different situations to men. Women's smoking is often used to cope with disadvantage, stress and the multiple demands made of their time. In addition, when trying to give up smoking, women were shown to have less confidence and to perceive more barriers than men.

Thus we can begin to see that there are a number of strengths to a qualitative research approach: it is *interpretative* in form, and follows a *naturalistic paradigm*; it allows for multiple perspectives; and it focuses on *processes* (see Box 9.2). Hence in the study of health and health services the value of qualitative approaches are that they can address research questions that are not always directly amenable to quantitative work, such as how do beliefs about health or illness influence behaviour? How do patients use prescription drugs and artefacts (e.g. metered asthma dose inhalers) in 'real life' rather than as specified in the instructions? How do various actors (e.g. patients, physicians, families, health services) understand and produce differing realities in terms of central policies relating to health care?

Box 9.2   Interpretive, naturalistic and process approaches

- **Interpretative research:** any style of research relying for explanation on the interpretations people themselves place on the reasons behind their actions.
- **Naturalistic paradigm:** assumes that there are multiple interpretations of reality and the goal for the researcher is to understand how individuals produce their own reality within their own social worlds. Considers how the artefacts of everyday life (e.g. talk, beliefs, objects) contribute to the fabric of social reality.
- **Process:** considers how social worlds are built up in the context of biographies, life cycles, environments, artefacts and social change.

We can also begin to identify situations in which qualitative research methods may be particularly useful:

- to allow the emergence of new *social theories* on topics or issues about which little is known; this may in turn allow for the generation of hypotheses that can then be tested;
- to explore more fully any insights suggested by quantitative surveys or experiments, for example, by investigating the *social context* of findings;
- as a way of extending and developing existing *social theory* or *theoretical frameworks* (see Box 9.3).

Box 9.3   Social theory and theoretical frameworks

- **Social theory:** in its simplest sense social theory is an explanation of something and can just be an answer to 'what', 'when' or 'why' questions. However, social theory also refers to more developed bodies of structured knowledge that may have developed over years and even decades (e.g. feminism, Marxism, phenomenology, symbolic interactionism).
- **Theoretical frameworks:** the conceptual underpinning(s) of a research study. May be based on an emergent theory or a specific conceptual model.

The following sections explore the key issues concerning in-depth interviews and focus groups.

In-depth interviews

An in-depth interview is simply a structured encounter between researcher and research participant with the aim of eliciting information. Interviews offer a practical, flexible and relatively economical way of gathering research data. There are a number of advantages to this research method, such as: making it possible for the researcher to directly intervene in the research process; allowing the researcher to guide participants to talk about specific issues; and allowing the researcher to ask a number of participants the same broad questions on a particular theme. There are three main types of interview, namely structured interviews, unstructured interviews and semi-structured interviews.

Structured or standardized interviews are normally used in quantitative or survey research and involve asking the same set of specific questions in precisely the same way to every research participant. The most familiar form of the structured interview is its use by market researchers who typically work from a predesigned script and pose a number of 'closed' questions (e.g. 'Is the reputation of your local hospital good, average or poor?'). This approach is a way of attempting to generalize beyond the immediate sample and to test hypotheses. It is not, however, an appropriate approach within qualitative research where the aim is to *generate hypotheses* and uncover the meanings of events in the lives of research participants. Indeed, to use a structured or standardized interview script within a qualitative interview would remove many of the strengths of this approach.

By contrast, *unstructured interviews* are entirely participant-led. In other words, research participants are allowed to tell their own stories, at length, in their own words with little direction or intervention from the researcher. This is a method commonly used within oral history projects and the researcher may return to the same interviewee over a period of several weeks to build up a vivid picture and record people's lifetime memories. This is a very powerful method of gathering rich data, while at the same time allowing those who may have been hidden from traditional histories to be heard. This is important because traditional approaches to history cannot tell us every aspect of the past because they tend to concentrate on 'public' events, important people and official documents. In contrast, unstructured oral histories may reveal equally important 'private' issues such as changing attitudes to disability, sexuality or unplanned pregnancies. Even though this method of interview is described as 'unstructured' the researcher is likely to have some basic issues and topics that they wish to cover, but questions will tend to be open in order to invite opinion and description. A good researcher will not ask too many questions and will allow the interviewee to largely set their own agenda. Within this type of interview the researcher should not be uncomfortable with pauses, gaps and silences. As well as seeking descriptions of events there will be an attempt to explore emotions and feelings.

Despite the rich data that unstructured oral histories can provide, the method has some disadvantages: it is time-consuming; it generates large amounts of data that then need to be analysed (e.g. just one subject may generate five to ten hours of taped interview which could translate into 150–300 pages of transcript); and the method requires a particular set of skills and approaches. Thus for many qualitative health-related research projects (e.g. exploring patient experiences or lay public understandings of genetic risk) it is more likely that semi-structured interviews will be the most efficient way of gathering research data.

Semi-structured interviews involve a mix of 'open' and 'closed' questions. The questions are planned but flexible. Interview sessions are designed typically with three stages which should be paced appropriately. The first stage involves introducing the topic and the broad aim of the research to the respondent. At this point interviewers would normally reiterate the confidential nature of the session and outline how the data will be used (e.g. 'Your comments may appear in published work but you will not be named or identified'). Formal written consent along these lines is sought before the interview commences. (For particularly sensitive issues, it may be decided to only seek verbal consent. For example, if conducting research on sexual behaviour some people may decline to be interviewed if they have to sign a consent form.) This should be done without overly focusing on details which may either intimidate the interviewee or prejudice their responses. Initial questions are designed to establish research participants' biographical details (e.g. age, number of children and length of time with current GP). This stage fulfils two purposes. Firstly, this information may be very useful in building up a picture of the respondent and contextualizing their later responses. Secondly, and just as importantly, it creates a comfortable atmosphere for the interviewee because these questions are relatively easy to answer and will not be overly sensitive.

After this initial stage, the interviewer would typically move on to ask more open-ended questions (e.g. 'Tell me about the last time you visited your GP?', 'How do you feel when you are sitting in the waiting room at your surgery?'). Questions can progressively become more personal or sensitive if necessary, such as asking about more psychosocial aspects of health (e.g. the impact of illness on personal relationships). Although the researcher works from a pre-planned topic guide it is likely that supplementary questions and analytical themes will be generated during the session. In this way the session and line of questioning is guided by the interviewee's responses with the interviewer adopting a receptive approach (e.g. 'Can you tell me a little more about that?'). Interviews often conclude with open-ended 'rounding off' questions (e.g. 'Is there anything else that you would like to add?', 'Is there anything about your local GP practice that you would like to change?'). At the end of the interview participants are usually given a written contact name and address in case they have any questions about the research later.

Semi-structured interviews allow the participant the opportunity to expand on areas which they feel are important, to uncover their 'framework of meanings' (Britten 1995). The researcher may probe for more detail or return to the same topic for clarification as the interview progresses. The key to running successful interview sessions is to quickly establish rapport with the interviewee who is never asked leading questions (e.g. 'I think that, do you?') or provided with judgements on expressed views (e.g. 'I think you may be wrong there!'). The goal is to allow the respondent to develop their own narratives while the researcher maintains overall control of the interview via a structured topic guide which covers areas that are considered important to the research question. Interview questions should be simple and unambiguous (e.g. avoid double-barrelled questions or overly scientific/medical jargon). Interviewers should not dominate the session and it is crucial that participants are allowed to explain their perspectives and ideas in detail without interruption or being hurried.

Interviewers should be very careful not to come across as judgemental and the aim should always be to build rapport and to create a 'safe' space in which lay participants can reveal their own views and opinions. It is sometimes the case with health-related research that participants initially give an account which responds to what they assume the researcher would *wish* to hear (e.g. participants may overstate 'healthy' behaviour and understate 'unhealthy' behaviour or disclose only views which are likely to be professionally approved). Distinguishing between 'public' and 'private' accounts is therefore crucial both at the data collection stage and at the point of analysis. The aim for the qualitative researcher is not to make judgements about the 'truth' or otherwise of statements but rather to understand how these make sense within a particular social world (Potter and Wetherell 1994).

The interviewer should also guard against making unwarranted assumptions and this may be particularly difficult where research is motivated by the desire to 'improve' health. For example, many researchers examining smoking behaviour may have clear views on the damaging effects of this practice on health but these views need to be strongly *bracketed* during data collection (see Box 9.4). Respondents need to be asked to fully explain their responses as this will be necessary to avoid ambiguity and differences over the use and meanings of common words.

Interview responses can be elicited from respondents by devices other than simple direct questions. With careful consideration a variety of prompts and probes

> **Box 9.4   Bracketing and phenomenology**
>
> - **Bracketing:** a process used by researchers working from a phenomenological tradition to identify their own preconceived beliefs about a phenomenon in order to minimize personal biases.
> - **Phenomenology:** a research methodology which has its roots in philosophy and which focuses on the lived experiences of individuals.

can be usefully employed during semi-structured interviews. One of the most common devices is the vignette – a short illustrative narrative or story connected with the topic under investigation. For example, in research on attitudes to genetic screening a story may be told (or given to respondents to read) involving a couple with particular characteristics seeking information about inherited disorders. At the end of the story the respondent may be asked how they would advise the couple if they were close friends. Another common prompt may be to ask respondents to comment on official leaflets (e.g. health education material). Finally, it can sometimes be helpful to have respondents engage in some practical activity. For example, if one was conducting research into attitudes to risk and health it may be possible to prepare cards with various activities (e.g. smoking, drinking, dangerous sports, driving) and then ask respondents to sort the cards according to risk and explain their reasoning as they carry out the task (Carter 1998). The important point about all these prompts and probes is that they should be directed towards generating a narrative on the part of the respondent. They should *not* be used as a 'test' of knowledge or comprehension.

Focus groups

This section outlines some key issues concerning the use of focus groups as a research tool. Focus groups have grown in popularity over the past decade. Indeed, it is likely that this qualitative method is now one of the most widely known social research methodologies. For example, the term has moved from the provinces of market research into social currency with newspaper reports and political sketch writers frequently citing 'focus groups' as a term of abuse – particularly due to their use by political parties (e.g. 'New Labour' in Britain) as a means of public consultation. The assumption which characterizes these pejorative assessments of the method is that focus groups work against creativity and difference and that the group process may override the 'dissenting' voice. In short, that the public may be fickle and the use of this method as a tool of public consultation leads to a 'rudderless' form of government without either conviction or ideological belief.

While some of the criticisms of the use of this method by political elites may be worthy of further consideration and debate, the focus group, if used systematically, can still be a powerful research tool. It may be used in a variety of ways to access the views of men, women and young people who are rarely asked their opinion; to discuss difficult or sensitive topics; and to produce rich data very quickly in ways which may not be possible with other qualitative or quantitative research methods.

Despite the recent popularity of this method, focus groups are not a new form of research. They were used by the social scientist Robert Merton to examine public reactions to wartime propaganda (Merton and Kendall 1946; Merton *et al.* 1956).

The method has also been most associated with market research (Lazarsfeld 1972) and used to examine consumer motivations – here of course research is funded by paying clients who have clear vested interests in the outcome of such studies. Focus groups have also been used as a method for both academic and commercial research on mass communications and audiences. Here television or film extracts are used as stimulus materials to engage participants in discussion.

More recently, however, focus groups have been increasingly used within the field of health research. Indeed, it could be argued that focus groups are a particularly appropriate method to study health-related topics for a number of reasons:

- Most health-related decisions are made within a social context rather than in isolation. For example, first-time mothers are more likely to select the same method of infant feeding as their friends and family; young people who take recreational drugs tend to do so with their friends. Information from health educators is thus mediated culturally by peers and family. A focus group study therefore allows the researcher to tap into ways in which health behaviour may be simply considered 'normal' or 'aberrant'.
- Focus groups can replicate the cultural context in which people discuss and 'make sense of' ideas concerning risk and danger. For example, lay understandings about specific diseases and their causes.
- Focus groups allow the 'safe' discussion of topics which may prove embarrassing or difficult to talk about on a one-to-one basis. For example, acute mental distress or sexual health issues.
- Focus groups may draw together those who are considered difficult to access such as groups who may be more typically disenfranchized from research agendas due to literacy problems or lack of social confidence. For example, low-income young males or unemployed middle-aged men.
- Focus groups allow the researcher to explore gaps which may exist between policy-makers and service users. For example, identifying local colloquialisms and 'slang' that relate to sexual matters or drug-related topics can help develop more appropriate health education material.

What is a focus group?

Focus groups are discussions organized to explore a specific set of issues. They are focused in the sense that the group is involved in a collective activity – for example, watching a film or examining a single health education message. The aim of a focus group in a research setting is not to change opinions or to test 'correct' knowledge. In addition, focus groups are distinguished from 'group interviews' by the 'explicit use of the group *interaction* as research data' (Morgan 1988). Thus focus groups should not alternate between researchers posing questions and research participants responding in turn to these questions (as with group interviews). Rather, the aim should be to set up the conditions where interaction within the group can take place in order to explore both similarities and differences within a group and across a set of group sessions. The focus group session will be based on topics provided by the researcher who may also take on the role of moderator or facilitator.

Research questions and study design

As with all qualitative research, focus groups cannot be used to quantify findings and they should not be conducted if the research aims to examine 'how many?' type questions. Focus groups can however allow you to explore 'how' people make sense of information and 'why' they may respond in particular ways by allowing an exploration of 'how' health-related information, from all sources, is socially mediated. Focus groups can also be a powerful tool in the exploration of people's 'frameworks of understanding'. The method is also appropriate for 'difficult to access' research participants where literacy and confidence problems may exclude them from other more individually-focused research studies. In addition, with the appropriate care and attention, focus groups can be suitable for tackling sensitive topics in a supportive environment where a one-to-one approach may become too 'loaded'. For example, the potential ethical and logistical difficulties of exploring the perspectives of young women who had been sexually abused were overcome by convening a focus group with survivors of teenage abuse. The session took place at the premises of a support organization where the young women regularly met (Henderson 1996).

Focus groups can be usefully deployed as a research tool in their own right but they can also be used in connection with other research methods in order to develop or complement questionnaire/survey data. For example, a series of focus groups on recreational drug use could allow the researcher to access the language, thoughts, feelings and emotions of those who take drugs together and thus develop a more appropriate questionnaire for use with a larger group of recreational drug users by using locally relevant language. Focus groups could also complement large-scale survey data by revealing unexpected or ambiguous findings (e.g. why people 'know' that using condoms protects them against HIV/AIDS but may not use them; why people understand that sunbathing is linked to skin cancer but still seek a suntan on holiday).

As has been mentioned above, the key feature of focus group research is the explicit use of interaction as research data, which allows the researcher to explore the participants' attitudes and priorities in ways which may not be possible via traditional interviews. Group participants can be encouraged to generate and explore their own questions and develop their own analysis of common experiences. Focus groups can generate unexpected findings which give valuable additional insights into a research topic. A focus group study designed to examine possible links between the 'glamour' and 'fantasy' of television medical dramas and inappropriate use of accident and emergency hospital departments found that 'real life' casualty departments were perceived as dirty and frightening places to be avoided. However, it emerged within these sessions that many people, particularly those with children, felt increasingly anxious about health matters (due to the increased volume of health information, from leaflets in the local GP surgery to media campaigns about meningitis). The study identified how concerned parents would bring children to casualty departments for reassurance (Philo and Henderson 1999).

Focus groups can elicit other forms of communication such as jokes and storytelling which may be far less likely to occur in one-to-one sessions and which are crucial to ways of understanding. For example, focus groups which were conducted on public understandings of HIV/AIDS highlighted the importance of gossip and storytelling, particularly in relation to urban myths concerning the 'vengeful AIDS carrier' (Kitzinger 1998).

Focus groups provide the opportunity to identify group norms and cultural values – for example, what information is freely discussed? Are some issues 'off limits' for discussion within particular groups? Group settings can be empowering and may allow participants to be more critical than in academic research settings. This may be particularly apparent if the group is 'naturally occurring' and participants know each other prior to the research session.

Conflict and debates within a focus group are just as important as similarities and consensus. Thus the focus group can allow the researcher to observe how people react to each other's different experiences within a controlled setting. Debates between group participants can allow the researcher to explore how people 'make up their minds' about differing perspectives and which sources are most salient. This is a very important aspect of focus group research that is often overlooked. Focus groups allow the researcher, albeit in contrived circumstances, to follow the social processes involved in people reaching an opinion about an issue. In this respect focus groups can be used to explore issues about which people may not have any fixed views prior to the group session. Thus focus groups can explore how attitudes and opinions are formed, for example in relation to emerging and new health technologies (e.g. genetics, stem cell research, nanotechnology). Focus groups can also be a useful measure of how attitudes and beliefs change over time. A study which investigated public understandings of food safety and BSE (commonly termed 'Mad Cow Disease') initially conducted 26 focus groups with members of the public between 1992 and 1993 and subsequently reconvened half of these groups in 1996 to explore whether beliefs had changed in light of new government information on the links between BSE and Creutzfeldt-Jakob disease (Reilly 1999).

Protocol and practical conduct of focus group sessions

The focus group method requires a number of issues to be considered beforehand and careful preparation is necessary to ensure the smooth running of a group session. One of the first issues to consider is who will take part in the focus group and whether the group will be 'naturally occurring' or will be strangers at the outset of the group session (e.g. recruited for their demographic characteristics via an agency). There are advantages and disadvantages for both these compositions. If a naturally occurring group is used they will already have information about each other and so the gap between what people 'express' and what they 'really' do in practice may be picked up by other respondents. In addition, a naturally occurring group will already be familiar with each other and this can allow an 'animated' discussion to develop more easily. A study of lay understandings of breast cancer found that while women often had no idea that a breast cancer 'gene' had been discovered, the idea of 'breast cancer families' and inherited risk was already subject to everyday debate before the research session (Henderson and Kitzinger 1999). However, the same familiarity may also be inhibiting for some discussions. For example, the existing power dynamics between respondents who work together may inhibit discussion about topics such as 'bullying at work'.

Group sessions can be intensive and demanding on the researcher. The ideal number of participants is between six and eight as group interaction can become more difficult to generate with fewer participants. Conversely, where focus groups are run with more than eight participants it can be difficult for the facilitator to manage the session and ensure that all members are fully participating. The gender composition of a group is crucial and requires forethought. Some health topics are more appropriately discussed within a same-sex setting and mixed-sex groups may exclude those who cannot take part for cultural reasons. However, for some topics a mixed group may be better placed to generate research insights.

The environment in which the group takes place may influence the ability of participants to freely exchange information and sessions should be adapted to suit the participants. For example, school students tend to respond differently within a classroom as compared with the more relaxed setting of a local youth club. Ideally the sessions will take place in a warm, comfortable and quiet room and will last for between one and two hours. In practice, group sessions may conclude within 45 minutes or run on for three hours depending on the level of discussion generated. Sessions may take place in a noisy community centre or busy workplace and facilitators may struggle to maintain control of the group against background distractions and interruptions.

The stages of the focus group session are likely to echo those of the semi-structured interview with initial ground-setting introductions followed by topic-related predefined open questions, the possible use of an exercise, visual prompts and other materials and any final rounding-off comments. Every focus group is fully tape-recorded and when considering the use of recording equipment it is necessary to use a multi-directional microphone. Of course just as in interviews it may sometimes be appropriate to switch the tape off when or if requested by respondents. For transcription purposes it is important to be able to identify speakers and it is worth asking each speaker to identify themselves at the beginning for the tape (they do not have to give their own name). A rough sketch of the seating plan can help the researcher to recall who said what and to follow up any responses which require clarification in an individual interview.

Facilitating approaches are no different to those of other qualitative research sessions in that a receptive and sensitive style is likely to engender confidence in the participants. As with other forms of qualitative research it is important that the researcher does not display personal judgements or knowledge. Researchers may at different points take a 'fly on the wall' approach by allowing the group discussion to unfold with little intervention. Alternatively the facilitator may become more directive by occasionally playing 'devil's advocate' to prompt debate. Prompts can include such tactics as: 'echoing back' or summarizing and repeating what has been said; asking the entire group if they agree with a point which has been made by an individual (e.g. 'Does everyone agree with what X has just said?'); or explicitly inviting those who are less vocal to respond to a particular issue. It is important that the facilitator does not assume that they 'know' what people mean. For example, a study which used focus groups to examine people's motivations for sun exposure identified the numerous ways in which people understand the concept of 'good health' (Carter 1997). In particular, health was understood as the avoidance of danger (e.g. likely to lead to sun avoidance) but was also seen as connected to feelings of attractiveness and confidence (likely to lead to sun exposure).

Although this approach may be more participant-led than other forms of data collection it is important that the facilitator maintains control of the session. Researchers typically have a checklist of topics or questions to be covered which will be supplemented by the group priorities. It is valuable to note when an issue is raised spontaneously as compared with the group simply responding to the facilitator prompting debate. Facilitators sometimes have a research assistant to take notes on non-verbal communication (e.g. participants withdrawing from the group), the use of jokes, laughter, personal anecdotes and gender issues.

The distinctive characteristic of focus groups is the use of 'interaction' and it is vital to consider ways in which this can be maximized. Stimulus exercises which can be adapted for those lacking in literacy skills can generate debate and operate as a point of continuity across the groups. A form of exercise can be a useful 'ice breaker' and will focus the group on the topic under investigation. Full participation is difficult to achieve and an exercise can help with this. Exercisces might involve the use of statement cards, writing straplines for health promotion materials, using images from magazines or designing a poster. A focus group study of infant feeding and first-time mothers used an exercise where women were shown a health education poster for breast-feeding and invited to generate ideas for completing the strapline 'Breastfeeding is . . .' (Henderson *et al.* 2000). Group members could be invited to write dialogue for photographs taken from television news stories (Kitzinger 1990) or develop scripts for soap opera storylines (Philo 1996). The important point about any exercise is that it is appropriate to the research question and the research setting and all exercises should be piloted prior to use in fieldwork.

Disadvantages of focus groups

Many of the potential disadvantages to using focus groups as a research tool can be overcome by careful and sensitive planning beforehand. However, it is the case that the relatively public setting of a group may operate to inhibit the exchange of sensitive information. For example, individuals who may not have told their friends about experiencing a stigmatizing illness are likely to be equally reluctant to reveal such information within a research session. Those participants who do not 'fit' with the group norms (e.g. being gay within a homophobic community) may be silenced within the group setting and facilitators will have to manage the expression of homophobic, sexist or racist views. By complementing the focus group sessions with individual interviews it is possible to conduct follow-up research sessions with participants who appear reluctant to communicate within the group. At the close of each group session all members should be allowed the opportunity to give additional information in confidence to the facilitator (either verbally or written). Focus group studies also produce 'messy' data in comparison to other data collection methods. It may be time-consuming to analyse many transcripts and each group will naturally differ in terms of the order in which they address specific issues and how they are discussed.

Sampling in qualitative work

Unlike a lot of quantitative research there are no hard and fast rules to aid sampling while conducting qualitative research. Sampling may depend on a range of factors including the aims of the study; the specific issues or questions that will be addressed; what may have credibility, especially for the eventual audience of the research; and simply what is practical within the project resources and time constraints. However, the lack of any formal formulas or devices to aid decisions about sampling does not mean that the process should be unsystematic. At the very least all choices concerning sampling strategies and sample size need to be made transparent and explicit (see Table 9.1).

One of the main difficulties may be for those researchers coming from a more quantitative discipline or background and it may be necessary for them to unlearn some of their internalized tenets. While quantitative research uses a statistical framework in order to guide sampling, qualitative research often favours a more theoretical conceptualization of sampling. This approach is in keeping with the

Table 9.1 Sampling strategies

Statistical sampling	*Theoretical sampling*
Categories tend to be predetermined (e.g. female under 30)	Relevant categories emerge from the research process
Decisions about sampling (e.g. how many, who, where and when) happen at start of project	Decisions about sampling (e.g. who, when, and where) are an ongoing process and changes will occur as a result of initial findings
Every case investigated until sample size reached	Stop when 'theoretical saturation' happens

---

Box 9.5   Selection of respondents

- **Convenience sample:** a sample that is fortuitously gathered or found in one place, setting or source (e.g. drinkers in a pub, patients in a health centre), assumed to be typical of the population of interest.
- **Purposive sample:** a sample in which respondents, subjects, or settings are deliberately chosen to reflect some features or characteristics of interest (e.g. patients with terminal cancer).
- **Quota sample:** a sampling technique which takes account of characteristics of the wider population, making sure that their distribution is replicated in the composition of the study sample (e.g. ethnic background, gender, income distribution) or that particular sub-populations are well represented in the study (e.g. people with disabilities). Representative in terms of characteristics on the basis of which selection has been made.
- **Snowball sample:** starting with an initial contact, the researcher asks this contact for referrals to other respondents who may be able to contribute to the research topic. Particularly effective with difficult to reach groups (e.g. recreational drug users).

---

general ethos of qualitative methodologies and allows sampling categories to emerge from the research process. In addition, decisions about which individuals, groups and environments to sample will also come out of the research process and may well change as research progresses. Finally, sampling will stop when 'theoretical saturation' is reached – in other words, when no new insights are gained from conducting more interviews, focus groups or observations.

Within qualitative research the actual selection of respondents may be based on a variety of established techniques such as *convenience*, *purposive*, *quota* or *snowball sampling* (see Box 9.5). The eventual decision about which of these approaches may be ultimately linked to the aims of the research. However, as with all aspects of qualitative research, the most important factor here is that the researcher should constantly display *reflexivity* (see Box 9.6) about the research processes and be prepared to explicitly justify their choices. The overall goal of the reflexive researcher in qualitative research is not to create a neutral, impersonal and objective report of the issue being investigated. Qualitative research cannot bring about standardized results of this type, because:

> at the heart of the qualitative approach is the assumption that a piece of qualitative research is very much influenced by the researcher's individual

---

Box 9.6   Reflexivity

- **Reflexivity:** refers to the researcher's active and constant reflection on all aspects of the research process. In other words, the researcher should always try to maintain a sceptical approach to the evidence provided by respondents and other data sources (e.g. 'Am I being told what I want to hear?'), and to the development of social theory.

attributes and perspectives. The goal is not to produce a standardised set of results that any other careful researcher in the same situation or studying the same issues would have produced. Rather it is to produce a coherent and illuminating description of and perspective on a situation that is based on and consistent with detailed study of the situation.

(Ward-Schofield 1993)

Conclusions

In this chapter we have outlined some of the basic uses of qualitative research methods and the main issues which should be addressed in relation to in-depth interviews and focus groups. Of course, there are many other forms of qualitative data-gathering such as participant and non-participant observation, textual analysis and conversational analysis. We have chosen to concentrate on interviews and focus groups because they are the methods that many researchers will attempt as their first foray into qualitative methodologies. The aim of this chapter has been to emphasize the strengths of qualitative research; how this form of research may offer insights into how and why people behave as they do and why qualitative research may be appropriate to reveal the sociocultural context in which health decisions are made. Examining the everyday 'lived' world of the social subject demands an equally rigorous approach to that required for quantitative research. The 'rules' of qualitative research may differ to those required for quantitative research but there are still some basic principles which should guide any successful study. We have emphasized reflexivity, transparency and the local contexts of research. We have also highlighted the ways in which qualitative research focuses on 'processes' and how these are made 'visible' in research studies.

We have also sought to show that qualitative research is very different to quantitative research but also how it can be complementary to more statistically-orientated research studies. It can illuminate the unexpected finding or help develop more appropriate research materials. The focus on the research participant, whether within the individual interview or the focus group setting, can allow social researchers to access the psychosocial aspects of health decisions or health services policies. We can identify new 'ways of seeing' and generate, rather than test, hypotheses. Qualitative research may be more time-consuming than quantitative research in terms of data collection and analysis – interview and focus group transcripts may not fall neatly into coding categories and software packages – yet the principles of good qualitative research involve an equally rigorous attention to detail. Approaching qualitative research with an open mind, and refraining from judgement and assumptions can allow the researcher to develop fascinating insights into the social world of the research participant. This in turn can allow more specialist materials to be developed in health education in order to gain a richer, more in-depth understanding of contradictory health behaviour and make sense of the priorities, values and conflicting decisions which operate within the everyday social world.

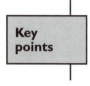

- Qualitative research refers to data collection that generates narrative or non-numeric information. It focuses on the experiences and meanings of individuals.

- The different qualitative methods of data collection are underpinned by a variety of different methodological and theoretical approaches.

- Qualitative data collection methods include in-depth structured or unstructured interviews, including oral and life histories, group discussion and interviews, participant and non-participant observation, and analysis of textual and narrative sources.

- Qualitative research is an interpretive form of research which relies on the interpretations of people themselves for explanations; the process needs to be transparent and reflexive.

- The approach is also naturalistic, and assumes that there are multiple interpretations of reality. The goal for the researcher is to understand how individuals produce their own reality within their own social worlds.

- The methods of qualitative research are particularly useful for allowing the emergence or development of social theories, and for exploring more fully any insights generated by quantitative methods.

- Unstructured interviews are participant-led, and people are permitted to set the agenda, to tell their own stories at length, and in their own words. These methods are time-consuming and generate large amounts of data.

- Semi-structured interviews include a mix of 'open' and 'closed' questions, which are administered flexibly and are unhurried. They allow participants the opportunity to expand on areas which they feel are important and to reveal their perspectives and meanings.

- Focus groups are discussions organized to explore specific issues. They are useful for discussing difficult or sensitive topics, to target groups who are rarely asked their opinion and to produce rich data relatively quickly.

- Qualitative methods demand an equally rigorous approach to that required by quantitative methods.

Further reading

General

Atkinson, P. et al. (2003) *Key Themes in Qualitative Research: Continuities and Changes*. London: AltaMira Press.

Berg, B. (2000) *Qualitative Research Methods for the Social Sciences*, 4th edn. Boston, MA: Allyn and Bacon.

Denzin, N. (1997) *Interpretive Ethnography: Ethnographic Practices for the 21st Century*. Thousand Oaks, CA: Sage Publications.

Denzin, N. K. and Lincoln, Y. S. (2000) *Handbook of Qualitative Research*. London: Sage.

Green, J. and Thorogood, N. (2004) *Qualitative Methods for Health Research*. London: Sage.

Hammersley, M. and Atkinson, P. (1983) *Ethnography: Principles in Practice*. London: Tavistock Publications.

Lincoln, Y. and Denzin, N. (2003) *Turning Points in Qualitative Research: Tying Knots in the Handkerchief*. London: AltaMira Press.

Marshall, C. and Rossman, G. (1999) *Designing Qualitative Research*. Thousand Oaks, CA: Sage.

Silverman, D. (1999) *Doing Qualitative Research: A Practical Handbook*. London: Sage.

Interviews

Bradburn, N.M. and Sudman, S. (1979) *Improving Interview Method and Questionnaire Design*. San Francisco: Jossey Bass.

Breakwell, G. (1990) *Interviewing*. Leicester: British Psychological Society in Association with Routledge.

Finnegan, R. (1992) *Oral Traditions and the Verbal Arts: A Guide to Research Practices*. London, Routledge.

Perks, R. and Thomson, A. (1998) *The Oral History Reader*. London: Routledge.

Samuel, R. and Thompson, P. (1990) *The Myths We Live By*. London: Routledge.

Thompson, P. (2000) *The Voice of the Past: Oral History*. Oxford: Oxford University Press.

Focus groups

Bloor, M., Frankland, J., Thomas, M. and Robson, K. (2001) *Focus Groups in Social Research*. London: Sage

Morgan, D.L. (1998) *The Focus Group Guidebook*. Thousand Oaks, CA: Sage.

References

Britten, N. (1995), Qualitative research: qualitative interviews in medical research, *British Medical Journal*, 311: 251–3.

Carter, S. (1997) Who wants to be 'peelie wally'? Glaswegian tourists' attitudes to suntans and sun exposure, in S. Clift and P. Grabowski (eds) *Tourism and Health: Risks, Responses and Research*. London: Pinter.

Carter, S. (1998) Tourists' and travellers' social construction of Africa and Asia as risky locations, *Tourism Management*, 19(4): 349–58.

Graham, H. (1987) Women's smoking and family health, *Social Science and Medicine*, 25(1): 47–56.

Graham, H. (1993) *When Life's a Drag: Women, Smoking and Disadvantage*. London: Department of Health.

Henderson, L. (1996) *Incest in Brookside: Audience Responses to the Jordache Story*. London: Channel Four Television.

Henderson, L. and Kitzinger, J. (1999) The human drama of genetics: 'hard' and 'soft' media representations of inherited breast cancer, *Sociology of Health and Illness*, 21(5): 560–78.

Henderson, L., Kitzinger, J. and Green, J. (2000) Representing infant feeding: content analysis of British media portrayals of bottle feeding and breast feeding, *British Medical Journal*, 321: 1196–8.

Kitzinger, J. (1990) Audience Understandings of AIDS media messages: a discussion of methods, *Sociology of Health and Illness*, 12(3): 319–35.

Lazarsfeld, P. (1972) *Qualitative Analysis: Historical and Critical Essays*. Boston, MA: Allyn & Bacon.

Merton, R. and Kendall, P. (1946) The focused interview, *American Journal of Sociology*, 51: 541–57.

Merton, R., Fiske, M. and Kendall, P. (1956) *The Focused Interview*. Glencoe, IL: Free Press.

Morgan, D. (1988) *Focus Groups as Qualitative Research*. London: Sage.

Philo, G. (1996) The media and public belief, in G. Philo (ed.) *Media and Mental Distress*. Harlow: Longman.

Philo, G. and Henderson, L. (1999) Why go to casualty? Health fears and fictional television, in G. Philo (ed.) *Message Received*. Harlow: Longman.

Potter, J. and Wetherell, M. (1994) Analyzing discourse, in A. Bryman and B. Burgess (eds) *Analyzing Qualitative Data*. London: Routledge.

Reilly, J. (1999) 'Just another food scare?': public understanding and the BSE crisis, in G. Philo (ed.) *Message Received*. Harlow: Longman.

Ward-Schofield, J. (1993) Increasing the generalisability of qualitative research in M. Hammersley (ed.) *Social Research: Philosophy, Politics and Practice*. London: Sage.

Combined qualitative and quantitative designs

Joy Adamson

Introduction

Combined qualitative and quantitative designs, or what is often termed 'mixed methods research' can be defined as the use of qualitative and quantitative techniques together in either parallel or sequential phases. Mixing methods has a relatively long history. As Hammersley and Atkinson (1995) observe, many nineteenth-century investigators treated qualitative and quantitative techniques as complementary. It was only with the rapid development of statistical methods that these two strands diverged. However, more recently the concept of merging qualitative and quantitative methods has re-entered the arena, in particular in the context of health services research. For example, one of the cross-cutting methodological themes in the Medical Research Council Health Services Research Collaboration is the 'integration of qualitative and quantitative research methods'. The contemporary fashion for the topic is reflected in the recent publication of a rather large handbook of research dedicated to the mixed method approach (Teddlie and Tashakkori 2003). In fact, some go as far as to say that mixed methods have come of age and 'to include only quantitative [or] qualitative methods falls short of the major approaches being used today' (Creswell 2003).

The literature has raised several important issues to consider regarding the use of mixed methods techniques in health research. In a sense, the very existence of this chapter does imply that it is a valid thing to do. However, there is still the fundamental question: should we be mixing methods at all? If we decide that combining methods is an appropriate activity, how should this best be done? Teddlie and Tashakkori (2003) outline several areas which they feel remain unanswered, which will be discussed in this chapter: the utility of mixed methods research, the paradigmatic foundations for this type of approach, design issues, what inferences can be drawn and the actual logistics of the approach. This chapter will provide insights into the current debates surrounding these points in the context of health services research.

As will become apparent in the course of the chapter, one of the difficulties in navigating the current literature relating to combined designs is that of terminology. Authors use different terms interchangeably and use different expressions to refer to the same phenomenon. Where appropriate, such differences in terminology will be highlighted.

This chapter will start by giving a brief overview of some of the philosophical perspectives relating to combined designs, highlighting the pragmatic and critical theory paradigms as particularly important for mixed methods research. This is followed by a discussion of the ways in which we can mix methods, examining important issues including triangulation and complementarity as well as outlining some of the suggested 'typologies' of combined designs. Some examples of the use of mixed methods within health research are then provided and the chapter finally presents some of the more practical issues concerning combined projects.

Philosophical perspectives relating to combined designs

Most researchers are familiar with what can be broadly termed quantitative and qualitative methods and while there is some debate concerning the nature of these two paradigms (if they can be referred to as such), there is a general understanding of the basic premises of each. According to conventional views, each has largely differing theoretical underpinnings and very different approaches relating to the nature of social reality and how this can be examined. Hammersley (1992a) summarizes the distinctions that are commonly made between qualitative and quantitative approaches including: words versus numbers, natural settings versus artificial settings, meanings versus behaviour, idealism versus realism – this list can be extended to include constructivism versus positivism, inductive versus deductive, collectivism versus individualism and researcher control versus participatory (e.g. see Bryman 1992; Baum 1995). It is such epistemological approaches that essentially determine opinions relating to whether qualitative and quantitative techniques can genuinely be combined or should remain as distinct methodological options.

Such basic dichotomies have been challenged. Several reviews of the literature have drawn similar conclusions – that both qualitative and quantitative techniques are not in fact characterized by such polar philosophical assumptions (e.g. Brannen 1992; Hammersley 1992a; Mason 1994; Murphy *et al.* 1998; Maxwell and Loomis 2003). As other authors have laid out the arguments for these conclusions elsewhere, it is unnecessary to rehearse these debates again – suffice to draw upon their conclusions. For example, as Brannen (1992) states, there is no necessary link between choice of method and logic of enquiry, type of inference and sampling strategy. As Maxwell and Loomis (2003) suggest, there are probably no uniform, generic qualitative and quantitative research paradigms, rather resonances and clusterings of perspectives. Bryman (1992) summarized his position that qualitative and quantitative research represent distinctive approaches to social research and that each is associated with a certain cluster of methods of data collection – for example, quantitative research includes survey techniques, experiments and structured observation compared to qualitative research which is typically associated with unstructured or semi-structured interviewing, focus groups, participatory or non-participatory observation and conversation analysis. While each of the two schools may have started out within very different epistemological positions, this is not to argue that they must stay rooted forever within these positions, and they have actually moved to achieve some independence from these foundations. In fact, it is the different strengths and weaknesses of both approaches which lie behind the rationale for their integration (Bryman 1992).

Combined designs have been linked to philosophical positions such as Hammersley's 'subtle realism' (1992b), which he sees as equally appropriate for qualitative and quantitative research. Here Hammersley offers a position which falls somewhere between naïve realism and naïve idealism, maintaining that phenomena do exist independently of the investigator's claims about them and that any claims may be more or less accurate. Within this movement, the researcher represents reality, accepting that any representations are always coming from a particular point of view. Therefore, there may be several different and valid descriptions of the same phenomenon. Qualitative and quantitative techniques would merely provide differing but non-competing representations.

Among those working within the quantitative domain (using techniques which are rooted in positivistic or post-positivistic traditions),[1] there is often less of a sense of the importance of the premises (or theoretical position) within which they are working. This is partly due to the dominant position of quantitative methods over the decades since the 1930s; those who have used qualitative methods have been forced to justify their position – as they are representing 'the other' or the alternative in a way that those within the quantitative domain have not. Coupled with the much broader scope of paradigms underlying qualitative techniques (see Silverman 2001; Guba and Lincoln 1994) and the greater emphasis given to the theoretical standpoint, it is therefore not surprising that some working within the qualitative domain have become 'purists'. Silverman (2001) summarizes this: 'since the 1960s, a story has got about that no good sociologist should dirty their hands with numbers'. The incompatibility of the paradigms underlying the research methods, according to this view, makes attempts to combine these methods nonsensical. In fact, whether they are seen as being capable of 'collaborative coexistence' is a very contested issue (Murphy *et al.* 1998). However, it has been argued that such a position has now been largely discredited and is 'subordinate' to the view being held by most researchers – that qualitative and quantitative methods can be used in a complementary way (Teddlie and Tashakkori 2003).

In a sense, it could now be argued that there has been an emergence of a 'third way', that of the mixed methodologist, which has evolved largely from what is referred to as the *integrationist approach* (Teddlie and Tashakkori 2003). In fact, the whole of a recent textbook on research design (Creswell 2003) is based around qualitative, quantitative and mixed method approaches. The epistemological standpoint that accompanies this 'third way' has been dominated by two approaches – the pragmatic and critical theorist perspectives. Several authors have suggested pragmatism as the most appropriate justification for a mixed method approach. For example, Teddlie and Tashakkori (2003) reiterate their view that it is the research question that is of the utmost importance, over and above either the method that is used or the paradigm that underlies the method. Pragmatism may have greater resonance with more applied areas of research, including health services research.

Alternatively, some have argued in favour of a 'transformative-emancipatory' or 'critical theorist' paradigm, suggesting that the goal of any research should be the creation of a more just and democratic society, and therefore the choice of methods should be determined on ideological grounds. This might include movements such as neo-Marxism, feminism and materialism (Murphy *et al.* 1998). If the aims of research are to emphasize the experiences of those who suffer from oppression and who are aware of the power differentials present in the context of research, then a mixed method approach may hold promising ways of doing so (e.g. Mertens 2003).

Ways in which we can mix methods

There are a number of different ways in which research methods may be combined, including triangulation and complementarity. They are discussed below.

Triangulation

Method triangulation has been among one of the most cited reasons for bringing together qualitative and quantitative techniques. The general premise is that the findings from one type of study can be checked against the findings of the other, therefore enhancing their validity. However, this has not gone unchallenged. On a very basic level there is the issue of whether health researchers can afford the effort required to simply find the same thing twice (Morgan 1998). On a different point, Mason (1994) suggests that as the qualitative and quantitative components of a study tend to yield data on different phenomena, they cannot be compared to check the 'validity' of each other. Bryman (1992) takes up this point, remarking that the data from qualitative and quantitative projects may not be as comparable as those advocating triangulation would imply. Even when exploring the same topic, it is questionable whether the same elements are exposed.

As Mason found when using both qualitative and quantitative methods to investigate patterns of family obligation, researchers would often ask if the findings from different elements of the study contradicted one another (Mason 1994). This raises the issue of how to judge whether the material from two datasets are in fact inconsistent or not (Bryman 1992). Also, how do we respond if our findings are contradictory? Researchers may be unclear about how to resolve discrepancies that may arise (Creswell 2003). There are two explanations for divergent findings: either they are the result of mistakes made when applying one (or both methods) or both are correct and the initial theoretical assumptions have to be modified or revised (Erzberger and Kelle 2003).

Debates concerning the issue of triangulation are leading to a new definition of the term, referring to different viewpoints providing different pictures of the phenomenon under investigation and therefore yielding a more complete picture if brought together (Erzberger and Kelle 2003). However, this has more commonly been thought of as 'complementarity'.

Complementarity

In discussions of the issue of complementarity, the general goal is that the strengths of one method are used in some way to enhance the performance of the other (Morgan 1998). In their review, Murphy et al. (1998) use the term 'instrumental' to refer to decisions made on pragmatic grounds for selection of methods. This is based on the premise that the usefulness of qualitative and quantitative data depends on their appropriateness for a given task. However, within this category of complementarity, researchers tend to consider the issue in one of two ways. Some see the role of qualitative methods as restricted to the exploratory and pilot phases of a research project. In a sense, qualitative methods are reduced to a 'handmaiden' role. An alternative to this position is the more 'horses for courses' approach, whereby the hierarchy between the two methods is eliminated and the researcher selects the method that is best for the task at hand. As Baum (1995) describes in the context of public health research, questions tend to be based on 'here and now' problems and are less concerned with theoretical issues, and it is more appropriate in such settings to integrate different methods. Baum suggests that methodologies for health research should be diverse and selected to suit the problem under investigation – provided we accept that there is no right or wrong way to view the world. He describes selecting methods as choosing from an 'enlarged tool kit' (Baum 1995).

Combined qualitative and quantitative designs

Cresswell (2003) lists four questions that are useful in the selection of a mixed methods strategy: what is the sequence of qualitative and quantitative data collection? What priority will be given to the qualitative and quantitative data collection and analysis? At what stage will the data and findings be integrated? Will an overall theoretical perspective be used?

Many attempts have been made to describe a typology of mixed method research designs. Teddlie and Tashakkori (2003) outline several reasons why such typologies have been used to classify combined designs and these include: to provide a developing field with an organizational structure; to help to legitimize the field of mixed methods and make it distinct from either qualitative and quantitative designs; to establish a common language; and to help researchers to design mixed methods studies.

Typologies

Several authors have attempted to set out different 'typologies' suggesting how a mixed method approach can be used in actual research. These have generally involved issues relating to the priority given to each method and the sequence (e.g. Morgan 1998; Barbour 1999). Cresswell *et al.* (2003) suggest one of the most coherent typologies, advocating six major mixed method approaches, as follows:

- **Sequential explanatory strategy:** priority would typically be given to the quantitative data and the two methods are integrated during the interpretation phase of the study. Generally the findings from the qualitative work would assist in explaining and interpreting the findings from the quantitative study.
- **Sequential exploratory strategy:** an initial phase of qualitative data collection, followed by quantitative data collection and analysis. The findings are integrated in the interpretation phase. This would be useful for the development of a new quantitative instrument.
- **Sequential transformative strategy:** has two distinct data collection phases, but either method may be used first and the findings are integrated at the interpretation phase. The thrust of this type of study is that there is a strong theoretical perspective guiding the research.
- **Concurrent triangulation strategy:** the researcher attempts to confirm or cross-validate the findings from qualitative and quantitative methods within a single study. Creswell also states that this is to offset the weaknesses with the strength of the other method. Integration usually happens at the interpretation phase.
- **Concurrent nested strategy:** both quantitative and qualitative data are collected simultaneously but there is a dominant method to the project. The less dominant method is nested within the main method, but may serve to answer a different question or seek information from a different level. The two types of data are mixed in the analysis phase of the project, which would have to involve the data being transformed so that they can be integrated.
- **Concurrent transformative strategy:** this is guided by theoretical perspective and may take the form of triangulation or nested strategies with the integration most likely to occur in the interpretation phase.

However, this is only one typology of the 40 types of mixed method designs identified by Tashakkori and Teddlie (2003).[2] Such typologies do not necessarily provide any new insights into a mixed method approach – rather they reflect the ways in which qualitative and quantitative methods have been brought together in practical research situations. Such tools do provide researchers with a framework to see where their own research designs are sitting compared to others and can guide efforts to combine qualitative and quantitative methods. However, a problem arises when several competing typologies exist, using different nomenclature and definitions. Therefore, Tashakkori and Teddlie have called for a new simple typology that meets the needs of researchers from many disciplines. Whether this is possible, or necessary, is another issue.

In general it would appear that the process of 'combining' qualitative and quantitative methods can take place at two main stages of the research process – either in the actual data collection/analysis phase or at the interpretation phase. These are discussed further below.

Combination at the data collection/data analysis phase

The distinction needs to be made between intra-method mixing and inter-method mixing. Intra-method refers to concurrent or sequential use of one single method that includes both qualitative and quantitative components. This is contrasted with inter-method mixing which is the concurrent or sequential mixing of two or more methods (Johnson and Turner 2003). Morse (2003) uses different terminology again and refers to the former as mixed methods and the latter as multi-method. This distinction is pertinent to the discussion here. Those for whom integration of qualitative and quantitative methods begins at the data collection phase have the choice of conducting the two components individually or actually bringing them together within the same method (intra-method mixing). Johnson and Turner (2003) discuss major methods of data collection including questionnaires, focus groups, tests (e.g. psychometrics), observation and secondary data, which they argue can all be viewed as within a continuum of purely qualitative and purely quantitative. They suggest that at the centre of this continuum is the mixed approach. The authors go on to suggest ways in which intra-mixing can be achieved: for example, questionnaires with a mixture of open and closed questions; interviews using open-ended questions but where the wording of the questions remains the same and the questions are asked in the same sequence; and mixed focus groups with both open and closed questions posed by the moderator. These echo some of the suggestions by Barbour (1999) and Creswell (2003). However, Bryman (1992) does not agree, claiming that such techniques are unlikely to deliver the relative strengths of qualitative and quantitative methods.

Onwuegbuzie and Teddlie (2003) provide a model for the intra-method data analysis process. The first stage is data reduction, which the authors claim should conform to the techniques that are usually used for qualitative and quantitative data alone (e.g. for quantitative data the production of descriptive statistics, and for qualitative data, coding of themes emerging from the materials). This is followed by displaying the data in the usual ways for both qualitative and quantitative materials individually. The next, and perhaps more controversial, suggestion is that the data are 'transformed' – that is, they are either 'quantitized' or 'qualitized' accordingly. This process may involve counting themes in qualitative data or 'binarizing' themes to calculate effect sizes; or, for quantitative data, producing narrative descriptions of the data. Once this process has been completed, if both qualitative and quantitative information have been collected on the same individuals then the quantitative data can be correlated with the quantitized qualitative data or the two types of data can be consolidated or compared. The authors do say that this last stage may be omitted in preference to moving directly to data integration, where all data are integrated into a coherent whole. The integration stage may lead to the collection of more data and then further analysis and integration.

Morse (2003), however, makes the point that while much of the data produced in this way (e.g. using open-ended questions in the context of a quantitative survey) may help to provide additional information, such data would not stand alone as a robust piece of qualitative work. These data would be incomplete by qualitative standards and would not be publishable apart from the survey data.

Combining at the interpretation phase

Rather than attempting to 'transform' qualitative data into quantitative and vice versa, each component project (qualitative and quantitative) is planned and conduced to answer a particular sub-question on the research topic at hand. Each project stands alone and would be subject to the usual scrutiny of its own methodological standards for validity and reliability. This approach would be referred to as 'multi-method' (Morse 2003) or 'inter-method mixing' (Johnson and Turner 2003).

When referring to the use of qualitative and quantitative methods in a complementary way, we still tend to think of this in terms of each of the qualitative and quantitative components representing different blocks of data collection. However, Bryman (1992) suggests that it may be more beneficial to see the two as more interwoven, in that one element stimulates new ideas for data collection for the other. Bryman likens this to the process of grounded theory which, while more commonly associated with qualitative methods, was intended by the original authors to be used with both kinds of data (Glaser and Strauss 1967). Respecting the time and resource constraints many researchers are under, Bryman does say that this may be easier to achieve if we think of the combination of research methods across research projects rather than just within them.

As Morgan (1998) describes it, there is the effort of completing both a qualitative and quantitative piece of work, and then there is the 'third effort' that is connecting what was learned from each. There is little information relating to how researchers can actually achieve this third effort, but some attempts have been made. For example, Mason (1994) describes the process by which she attempted to integrate the data from the qualitative and quantitative components of her study. She discusses this process at two different levels – at an intellectual level and at a practical level. Intellectually, the researchers had to formulate an account of how they thought the two strands were connected, which was linked to their theoretical position relating to what they saw the data from the two sources as representing and how they saw those parts fitting together. This was accompanied by gluing the pieces together that had been produced from the different methods with different logical principles. By following up similar conceptual themes in the different datasets the researchers were able to explore themes across a representative sample and how people made sense of the experiences in their own lives. They then looked at how the different datasets could be used to address a particular topic (differing from the themes discussed above). For both of these techniques the researchers tended to look at the data side by side to explore the relationships between them. However, this was after they had thought through what types of question could be asked of one or both of the datasets and when it might be appropriate to mix these. Of course, for many of the issues they could only find relevant data in one of the datasets.

While using qualitative methods to test the face validity of standardized measures is not a new concept (e.g. Donovan *et al.* 1993; Mallinson 2002), it has been suggested that they can prompt further data collection within the contexts of a qualitative interview (McMurray *et al.* 1999). Recently, Adamson *et al.* (2004) took this a step further by suggesting the use of structured questions within the context of qualitative data collection as a means of attempting to integrate the findings from a combined qualitative and quantitative approach. The integrity of each method is kept intact, as the quantitative survey using a structured questionnaire is carried out appropriately, by ensuring sufficient sample size and so on; similarly the complementary qualitative study is conducted in the normal way but with elements of the structured questionnaire as part of the topic guide. Overlapping the topics covered in both the qualitative and quantitative components in this way forges a path to integration at the interpretation phase.

Sampling strategies for mixed methods studies

In their chapter on mixed methods sampling, Kemper *et al.* (2003) discuss the view that sampling techniques can be divided into two types: probability sampling and purposive sampling. Within mixed methods studies the authors claim that this generally requires a need for two types of sample and that this is appropriate for situations in which mixed methods studies are linked to two distinct goals. Therefore, if the researcher wishes to use quantitative data within a qualitative framework, they will have to ensure an appropriate sample to be able to make claims from the quantitative data collection and vice versa (Morse 2003).

The quality of mixed methods research

Morse (2003) does warn of the potential threat to validity if we partake in ad hoc mixing of strategies whereby the methodological assumptions of each of the component methods are violated. When she refers to mixed method designs she does not adhere to the viewpoint of what she calls 'mix and match' research.

Teddlie and Tashakkori (2003) attempt to make the distinction between assessment of the quality of how the data are collected and the quality of inferences made from the data. Both qualitative and quantitative methods have techniques to attempt to reduce errors in inferences made from the research, some of which can be applied to both methods.

Examples of mixed methods approaches

In the context of a study considering the use of mixed methods in health services research, O'Cathain (2003) conducted a pilot to examine the most appropriate technique for finding published mixed methods studies. She identified several difficulties with using search terms in both MEDLINE and CINAHL, including a lack of specificity of terms including 'mixed method' and 'qualitative and quantitative'. Using such terms to search standard electronic databases it was particularly difficult to identify studies where the qualitative and quantitative components had been published in separate papers and journals. Attempts at hand-searching and searching of funding bodies' archives of ongoing studies elicited similar problems.

Despite these difficulties, in order to achieve an overview of the publication of mixed methods studies, attempts were made here to identify this type of research using three of the most popular databases in health research. Searches of abstracts were conducted within CINAHL, EMBASE and MEDLINE from 1982 to 2004, using the terms 'mixed methods' and 'multi-method'. Searching started from 1982 because this was the year from which the CINAHL database was available. After duplicates had been removed the term 'multi-method' generated 195 references and 'mixed methods' 91. All abstracts were reviewed and 205 were excluded as not being true mixed methods studies by the definition being used here. The most common reasons for exclusion were that the term mixed or multi-method was referring to the technique or intervention being examined in the paper rather than the study design (84 abstracts), or that the search terms referred to mixing only quantitative techniques (31) or, equally as common, it was not possible to tell from the abstract whether the paper referred to a true mixed methods study (31). Seventeen abstracts referred to mixed qualitative methods only and others were excluded as they referred to unpublished Ph.D. work (17) or literature reviews (14). Twenty-one of the abstracts were from more discursive papers on the topic of mixing methods in the context of health research.

The review process left 63 abstracts which appeared to refer to studies using a combined qualitative and quantitative design. From these only one mixed method study occurred before 1994 and hence it would appear that the increase in publication of this type of study has occurred over the last decade, in particular during and after 1997. The spread is shown in Table 10.1.

The most common location for the publication of mixed methods was the UK (25 abstracts), followed by the USA (16), Australia (8) and Canada (5). The most frequently mentioned study design was questionnaires (survey) together with qualitative interviews (16), however 23 of the abstracts described mixing three or more methods, including combinations of questionnaires, qualitative interviews, focus groups, observations and diaries. Several of the abstracts did not specify the actual methods used, simply mentioning they used both qualitative and quantitative techniques. Only three abstracts reported mixed methods as involving both closed and open-ended questions in a survey.

The disciplines within which the mixed methods studies were taking place could broadly be categorized into three groups: nursing research (23), service/training evaluation (15) and the experience of health and health care (24). Not many of the abstracts provided justification for the study design selected, however, some did make small comments, including triangulation (5), complementarity (3) and 'to receive further insight into the topic' (8).

Four of the abstracts presented findings from only one (either quantitative or qualitative) element of a larger study, mentioning that this was part of a mixed method design and other data were presented elsewhere.

As O'Cathain (2003) pointed out, the publication of qualitative and quantitative components separately is a barrier to the identification of mixed methods researchers using electronic databases. Few of the combined qualitative and quantitative studies known to the author were identified in this review process. Therefore, for the remainder of this section, both studies from the review and those known to the author will be drawn on as examples of combined qualitative and quantitative designs.

Table 10.1 Number of abstracts presenting findings from mixed methods studies, by year of publication

Year of publication	Number of abstracts
2002–3	30
2000–1	13
1998–9	9
1996–7	8
Before 1996	2

Using qualitative methods within trial research

The UK Medical Research Council (MRC) in its document providing guidance relating to the development and evaluation of randomized controlled trials for complex health interventions, highlights qualitative methods as an important feature, in particular in the theoretical and modelling stages of designing a complex intervention. This document emphasizes the usefulness of qualitative techniques in, for example, testing the underlying assumptions in relation to an intervention, identifying which are the 'active ingredients' of a complex intervention and determining which groups of participants are more likely to respond to the intervention (MRC 2000).

Qualitative methods have often been used to help understand issues in randomized controlled trials in several different ways. For example, Featherstone and Donovan (1999) looked at patient understanding of randomization and other common trial terms. Roberts *et al.* (2004) used a combination of qualitative methods (focus groups and individual interviews with adults and children) to consider barriers to the continued use of smoke alarms identified in a trial of the installation of fire alarms in disadvantaged inner-city housing (see also Rowland *et al.* 2002). They make the point that by developing appropriate method linkages between trials and qualitative work, better outcomes may result. They introduced the concept of 'methodological triage' where perhaps a more appropriate design would have started with qualitative work which may have improved take-up of smoke alarms and maintenance instructions. This idea is taken a stage further by Donovan *et al.* (2002) who introduce the concept of embedding the randomized trial within a qualitative study. Using this technique helped to understand the recruitment process and to elucidate the changes needed in the communication of information about the trial (of prostate cancer screening) to enhance recruitment and the conduct of the trial.

Seeking health care

There are several examples of combined designs in research examining sociodemographic determinants of health care seeking behaviour. For example, Richards *et al.* (2000, 2002) have published both quantitative and qualitative elements of a study of chest pain, in particular relating to gender and socioeconomic position. The quantitative study described patterns of help-seeking in a population of 1107 men and women. The qualitative study, which took its sample from the survey respondents, attempted to explore and explain socioeconomic variations in perceptions of, and behavioural responses to, chest pain. While the epidemiological report of the study did not make reference to the qualitative component, the qualitative study did refer to the quantitative element. This may have been due to the fact that the epidemiological study was published first. However, disappointingly there was no attempt in the qualitative paper to integrate the findings from the two publications. While the authors did state in the discussion that the epidemiological work had provided a context for the study, it was not obvious how this had been done or if any further insight had been gained from using both methods.

Rogers and Nicolaas (1998) published in a single paper the findings of a study examining patterns of primary care use through a combined qualitative and quantitative approach. The quantitative element consisted of a survey and diary study to ascertain frequency of health care utilization. The qualitative work was a linked interview study, the sample identified from the survey work. The authors argued that the approach of selecting deviant cases identified from the quantitative analysis provided greater insights into the nature, processes and determinants of help-seeking actions. Again, as would be the case in two separate papers, the findings from the qualitative and quantitative elements were presented separately and the authors did not describe the process of bringing the two strands of data together. However, the paper was able to show evidence that the findings from both types of data had been integrated at a more theoretical level, indicating that health care use is more appropriately viewed as an interplay of structure and agency. The authors do acknowledge that the interviews were, to an extent, driven and constrained by the fact that they followed the survey and diary study.

Health care evaluation

Mixed methods approaches have been utilized in the evaluation of complex health care systems. In the early 1990s this approach was used in the evaluation of nursing home and long-stay geriatric ward care for older people. This was done through both a randomized controlled trial (Bowling *et al.* 1991) and qualitative observational study (Clark and Bowling 1990). While these components were written up separately, the published papers did cross-refer to the results contained in each. From the combination of these two approaches the authors were able to observe that the measurement scales of mental and physical impairment and life satisfaction, used in the trial, were inadequate in terms of discriminating between hospital and nursing home settings. While no differences in outcome were found between settings, relying on the survey data, the observational data support the conclusion that a different quality of life was apparent between settings, indicating that quality of life should be viewed more broadly than by outcomes alone (Clark and Bowling 1990).

Quantitative and qualitative methods have also been combined to answer different research questions relating to health care evaluation. For example, Gompertz *et al.* (1995) compared two health districts, one with no special stroke service compared with another, which had a stroke unit, in terms of patient outcomes. Another researcher on the team took a lead role in the qualitative assessment of patients' views on their admission to hospital (Pound *et al.* 1995).

Tools required to conduct mixed method research

Funding of mixed method studies

Barbour (1999) highlights that it is important to appreciate the stand-alone benefits of both qualitative and quantitative methods and not be driven solely by perceived preference of funders, who do now appear to be supportive of combined qualitative and quantitative approaches. This confirms Bryman's (1992) warning against the 'tactical' use of either qualitative, quantitative or a mixed method approach if this is solely to improve the chances of funding; rather, the research design should be tailored to the question at hand.

The issue of funding has been raised as potentially challenging (Mason 1994), for both researchers and for the funding bodies themselves. For example, mixed method studies by their nature are more time-consuming and are likely to be more complex, especially given the 'meta-interpretation' required to bring together different strands of the findings produced. Such factors would need to be taken account when planning research budgets (Forthofer 2003).

Expertise in mixed methods

Morse (2003) comments that one of the most restricting factors in the way that researchers are able to understand human behaviour is the methodological repertoire of the researcher and his or her knowledge and skill in using these research methods. According to Creswell (2003) a mixed method design requires mixed methods personnel who have a sophisticated knowledge of both paradigms, or, as Mason (1994) suggests, at least for researchers to move comfortably between different parts of the study and to be using a common language. Brannen (1992) claims that it is quite rare that the mixed method research or indeed the individual researcher is likely to put equal emphasis on qualitative *and* quantitative methods. However, is this really the case? As someone who feels equally happy within both qualitative and quantitative frameworks, I could easily name several other researchers who share these skills. Other examples are available in the literature of individuals who do not appear to hold a preference for either method (e.g. Johnstone 2004). However, whether training in both qualitative and quantitative techniques provides insights into the process of integrating these different types of data is another question.

There is also the argument, of course, that in cases for which one of the methods is being used in a complementary fashion, complete mastery of that method may not be necessary (Morgan 1998). It is often the case that researchers are working in multidisciplinary teams and different members take the lead on the qualitative and quantitative components accordingly. It may be more important at a department or research group level to provide a supportive environment for mixed methods research, rather than at the level of the individual researcher.

Texts on how we actually perform the integration

We are starting to become equipped with tools to help us take a mixed method approach to our research studies. For example, Creswell (2003) provides us with checklists for designing a mixed methods procedure, for determining the kinds of information we might think about including in a mixed methods research proposal, and how we might think about the process of mixing methods. However, in many papers purporting to be based on a mixed methods approach there is still a distinct lack of information which explains in a transparent way how the qualitative and quantitative components have been brought together. Some authors are now attempting to address this shortfall by charting the process of their mixed methods approach, even describing the process of report writing (see Johnstone 2004).

Publication of mixed methods studies

Within academic circles there is the well-known pressure to publish. This may lead authors to split combined qualitative and quantitative designs along methodological lines and may be the main reason why quite often these components are published separately. There is also the issue of the different components answering different kinds of question, which will be of interest to different audiences and which lends itself to distinct papers outlining qualitative and quantitative findings. On a more practical level, if the work has been produced within a multidisciplinary team, members of the research group may have different strengths and it makes sense to divide up the work along methodological lines. Finally, journals have different aims and styles that may be more suitable for qualitative and quantitative material (e.g. permitted word count).

Conclusions

While the title of this chapter represents in many ways what appears to be a straight-forward concept, it has been shown that there remains much ambiguity in terms of how such research is to be operationalized in the domain of health.

Since the end of the nineteenth century, when qualitative and quantitative methods were used hand in hand, we have come full circle and there is no doubt that mixing methods has become an increasingly common approach. However, whether this is a 'new discipline' or a 'third paradigm' does not go unquestioned – is it in fact a reinvention of the wheel with a contemporary twist?

Traditionally several distinctions have been made between qualitative and quantitative methods, mainly along epistemological lines. For some these differences have been sufficient to discount the notion of using combined designs. However, these dichotomies have been challenged and it seems unlikely that it is possible to clearly establish one-to-one relationships between theoretical perspective, methodology and technique. Perspectives including subtle realism, pragmatism and critical theory have underpinned much of the movement towards a mixed method approach.

In terms of the ways in which we can conduct combined qualitative and quantitative research, should it be, as Barbour (1999) suggests, more than blotting together techniques developed by different disciplines? Several typologies have been suggested, however it appears that attitudes towards what is a mixed method approach fall along a continuum which ranges from a programme of research with qualitative and quantitative components largely conducted separately, to studies within which qualitative data are quantitized and quantitative data are qualitized. At the start of this continuum it is difficult to distinguish the point at which two separate projects (one qualitatively orientated, one quantitatively) become mixed methods. This threshold remains blurred. It is particularly so when the two components are published separately and in many cases do not refer to the other – is this truly mixed methods research? The end of this continuum has its own, and perhaps more difficult, challenges. For example, how are we to judge the quality of these methods and justify the sample size? As Bryman (1992) suggests, by conducting research in this way, are we losing what we are attempting to gain by no longer experiencing the strengths of qualitative and quantitative methods? Debates continue concerning the basic definitions and nomenclature of combined qualitative and quantitative designs, both within and between disciplines (see Teddlie and Tashakkori 2003).

Bryman (1992) asks if we are to believe some of the arguments for using qualitative and quantitative methods together, does this mean that mixed methods studies will always be superior *per se*? He thinks not necessarily so, bringing us back to perhaps the most important point: that we should be driven by the nature of the research question and use the most robust methods to attempt to address it. A combined qualitative and quantitative design will not be appropriate for all health-related research and we should not be tempted to use either qualitative or quantitative methods in a tokenistic way to accommodate contemporary fashions. Producing good quality research to answer important questions using appropriately selected methods is the ultimate objective.

The field of health research does seem particularly keen on combining qualitative and quantitative research methods, given the pragmatic nature of the discipline, coupled with the complexity of the many factors that influence health and health care. While some of the actual methods of combined designs remain in a developmental stage, the act of applying both types of technique within the same research project or programme has been embraced to fruitful ends.

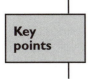

Key points

- Qualitative and quantitative methods of research began with different epistemological positions.
- The use of mixed methods has been defined as the use of qualitative and quantitative methods in parallel or sequential phases.
- The epistemological differences between the methods have often militated against combined designs, but these dichotomies have been challenged.
- Triangulation of research methods has been one of the most cited reasons for using combined approaches, although inconsistent results can be difficult to interpret.
- With complementarity, the general goal is that the strengths of one method are used to enhance the performance of the other.
- There is ambiguity in terms of how qualitative and quantitative designs are operationalized.
- Attitudes to mixed method approaches range from research with both elements, which are conducted separately, to studies that use a single method but with components of each included; each approach produces challenges.
- Ultimately, the researcher should be driven by the research question and the most appropriate methods for addressing it.

Notes

1 Associated with naïve or critical realism, objectivity and truth. From the experimental tradition of testing a hypothesis (Guba and Lincoln 1994).
2 Including, triangulatory, transformative, integrated, component, sequential, parallel, concurrent, simultaneous, branching, nested, explanatory, exploratory, confirmatory, developmental, embedded, hierarchical, equivalent-status, dominant-less dominant, multilevel and two-phase.

Further reading

Brannen, J. (ed.) (1992) *Mixing Methods: Qualitative and Quantitative Research*. Aldershot: Ashgate.
Cresswell, J.W. (2003) *Research Design: Qualitative, Quantitative, and Mixed Methods Approaches*, 2nd edn. Thousand Oaks, CA: Sage.
Tashakkori, A. and Teddlie, C. (eds) (2003) *Handbook of Mixed Methods in Social and Behavioural Research*. Thousand Oaks, CA: Sage.

References

Adamson, J., Gooberman-Hill, R., Woolhead, G. and Donovan, J. (2004) 'Questerviews': using questionnaires in qualitative interviews as a method of integrating qualitative and quantitative health services research, *Journal of Health Services Research and Policy*, 9(3): 139–145.
Barbour, R.S. (1999) The case for combining qualitative and quantitative approaches in health services research, *Journal of Health Services Research and Policy*, 4(1): 39–43.

Baum, F. (1995) Researching public health: behind the qualitative-quantitative methodological debate, *Social Science and Medicine*, 40(4): 459–68.

Bowling, A., Formby, J., Grant, K. and Ebrahim, S. (1991) A randomised controlled trial of nursing home and long-stay geriatric ward care for elderly people, *Age and Ageing*, 20: 316–24.

Brannen, J. (1992) Combining qualitative and quantitative approaches: an overview, in J. Brannen (ed.) *Mixing Methods: Qualitative and Quantitative Research*. Aldershot: Ashgate.

Bryman, A. (1992) Quantitative and qualitative research: further reflections on their integration, in J. Brannen (ed.) *Mixing Methods: Qualitative and Quantitative Research*. Aldershot: Ashgate.

Clark, P. and Bowling, A. (1990) Quality of everyday life in long stay institutions for the elderly: an observational study of long-stay hospital and nursing home care, *Social Science and Medicine*, 30(11): 1201–10.

Cresswell, J.W. (2003) *Research Design: Qualitative, Quantitative, and Mixed Methods Approaches*, 2nd edn. Thousand Oaks, CA: Sage.

Cresswell, J.W., Plano Clark, V.L. *et al.* (2003) Advanced mixed methods research designs, in A. Tashakkori and C. Teddlie (eds) *Handbook of Mixed Methods in Social and Behavioural Research*. Thousand Oaks, CA: Sage.

Donovan, J., Frankel, S.J. and Eyles, J.D. (1993) Assessing the need for health status measures, *Journal of Epidemiology and Community Health*, 47: 158–62.

Donovan, J., Mills, N., Smith, M. *et al.* (2002) Improving design and conduct of randomised trials by embedding them in qualitative research: ProtecT (prostate testing for cancer and treatment) study, *British Medical Journal*, 325: 766–70.

Erzberger, C. and Kelle, U. (2003) Making inferences in mixed methods: the rules of integration, in A. Tashakkori and C. Teddlie (eds) *Handbook of Mixed Methods in Social and Behavioural Research*. Thousand Oaks, CA: Sage.

Featherstone, K. and Donovan, J. (1999) Random allocation or allocation at random? Patients' perspectives of participation in a randomised controlled trial, *British Medical Journal*, 317: 1177–80.

Forthofer, M.S. (2003) Status of mixed methods in the health sciences, in A. Tashakkori and C. Teddlie (eds) *Handbook of Mixed Methods in Social and Behavioural Research*. Thousand Oaks, CA: Sage.

Glaser, B.G. and Strauss, A.L. (1967) *The Discovery of Grounded Theory*. Chicago: Aldine.

Gompertz, P., Pound, P., Briffa, J. and Ebrahim, S. (1995) How useful are non-random comparisons of outcomes and quality of care in purchasing hospital stroke services? *Age and Ageing*, 24: 137–41.

Guba, E.G. and Lincoln, Y.S. (1994) Competing paradigms in qualitative research, in N.K. Denzin (ed.) *Handbook of Qualitative Research*. Thousand Oaks, CA: Sage.

Hammersley, M. (1992a) Deconstructing the qualitative-quantitative divide, in J. Brannen (ed.) *Mixing Methods: Qualitative and Quantitative Research*. Aldershot: Ashgate.

Hammersley, M. (1992b) *What's Wrong with Ethnography? Methodological Explorations*. London: Routledge.

Hammersley, M. and Atkinson, P. (1995) *Ethnography Principles in Practice*, 2nd edn. London: Routledge.

Johnson, B. and Turner, L.A. (2003) Data collection strategies in mixed methods research, in A. Tashakkori and C. Teddlie (eds) *Handbook of Mixed Methods in Social and Behavioural Research*. Thousand Oaks, CA: Sage.

Johnstone, P.L. (2004) Mixed methods, mixed methodology health services research in practice, *Qualitative Health Research*, 14(2): 259–71.

Kemper, E.A., Stringfield, S. and Teddlie, C. (2003) Mixed methods sampling strategies in social science research, in A. Tashakkori and C. Teddlie (eds) *Handbook of Mixed Methods in Social and Behavioural Research*. Thousand Oaks, CA: Sage.

Mallinson, S. (2002) Listening to respondents: a qualitative assessment of the Short-Form 36 Health Status Questionnaire, *Social Science and Medicine*, 54: 11–21.

Mason, J. (1994) Linking qualitative and quantitative data analysis, in A. Bryman and R.G. Burgess (eds) *Analysing Qualitative Data*. London: Routledge.

Maxwell, J.A. and Loomis, D.M. (2003) Mixed methods design: an alternative approach, in

A. Tashakkori and C. Teddlie (eds) *Handbook of Mixed Methods in Social and Behavioural Research*. Thousand Oaks, CA: Sage.

McMurray, R., Heaton, J., Sloper, P. and Nettleton, S. (1999) Measurement of patient perceptions of pain and disability in relation to total hip and knee replacement: the place of the Oxford hip score in mixed methods, *Quality in Health Care*, 8(4): 228–33.

Mertens, D. (2003) Mixed methods and the politics of human research: the transformative-emancipatory perspective, in A. Tashakkori and C. Teddlie (eds) *Handbook of Mixed Methods in Social and Behavioural Research*. Thousand Oaks, CA: Sage.

Morgan, D. (1998) Practical strategies for combining qualitative and quantitative methods: applications to health research, *Qualitative Health Research*, 8(3): 362–76.

Morse, J.M. (2003) Principles of mixed methods and multimethod research design, in A. Tashakkori and C. Teddlie (eds) *Handbook of Mixed Methods in Social and Behavioural Research*. Thousand Oaks, CA: Sage.

MRC (Medical Research Council) (2000) *A Framework for the Development and Evaluation of RCTs for Complex Interventions to Improve Health*. London: MRC.

Murphy, E., Dingwall, R., Greatbatch, D. *et al.* (1998) Qualitative research methods in health technology assessment: a review of the literature, *Health Technology Assessment*, 2(16).

O'Cathain, A. (2003) Developing mixed methods in health services research. Unpublished MA Dissertation, University of Nottingham.

Onwuegbuzie, A.J. and Teddlie, C. (2003) A framework for analyzing data in mixed methods research, in A. Tashakkori and C. Teddlie (eds) *Handbook of Mixed Methods in Social and Behavioural Research*. Thousand Oaks, CA: Sage.

Pound, P., Bury, M., Gompertz, P. and Ebrahim, S. (1995) Stroke patients' views on their admission to hospital, *British Medical Journal*, 311: 18–22.

Richards, H., McConnachie, A., Morrison, C. *et al.* (2000) Social and gender variation in the prevalence, presentation and general practitioner provisional diagnosis of chest pain, *Journal of Epidemiology and Community Health*, 54: 714–18.

Richards, H., Reid, M. and Watt, G. (2002) Socioeconomic variations in responses to chest pain: qualitative study, *British Medical Journal*, 324: 1308–12.

Roberts, H., Curtis, K., Liabo, K. *et al.* I. (2004) Putting public health evidence into practice: increasing the prevalence of working smoke alarms in disadvantaged inner city housing, *Journal of Epidemiology and Community Health*, 58(4): 280–5.

Rogers, A. and Nicolaas, G. (1998) Understanding the patterns and processes of primary care use: a combined quantitative and qualitative approach, *Sociological Research Online*, 3(4).

Rowland, D., DiGuisepi, C., Roberts, I. *et al.* (2002) Prevalence of working smoke alarms in local authority inner city housing: randomised controlled trial, *British Medical Journal*, 325: 998–1001.

Silverman, D. (2001) *Interpreting Qualitative Data*, 2nd edn. London: Sage.

Tashakkori, A. and Teddlie, C. (2003) The past and future of mixed methods research: from data triangulation to mixed model designs, in A. Tashakkori and C. Teddlie (eds) *Handbook of Mixed Methods in Social and Behavioural Research*. Thousand Oaks, CA: Sage.

Teddlie, C. and Tashakkori, A. (2003) Major issues and controversies in the use of mixed methods in the social and behavioural sciences, in A. Tashakkori and C. Teddlie (eds) *Handbook of Mixed Methods in Social and Behavioural Research*. Thousand Oaks, CA: Sage.

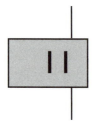

Design and analysis of social intervention studies in health research

Ann Oakley

Introduction

Increasing attention has been paid in recent years both in the UK and internationally to the issue of social intervention evaluation (Oakley 1992, 1998a, 2000a; Boruch 1997; Davies *et al.* 2000; Mosteller and Boruch 2002). While it is a topic of great importance in health research, the scope of social intervention research is broad, encompassing education, social welfare, crime and justice, transport and public policy generally. The relevance of social intervention research in the health field is twofold. Firstly, many health care interventions aimed at improving health or preventing disease and disability are trialling approaches to organizing or providing care, methods of giving information or advice, or other strategies that are not concerned with the provision of clinical care. Secondly, many health care interventions, whatever their nature, have a large social component. For example, the relationship between health professionals and health service users is a crucial element in the effectiveness (or otherwise) of many therapeutic endeavours. Patients who are treated positively by their doctors are more likely than those who are not to feel better as a consequence of seeing them (Thomas 1987; Tudor Hart and Dieppe 1996; Crow *et al.* 1999). In a different guise, the importance of social relationships appears as the 'placebo' effect, which can loosely be described as improved well-being due to the belief that something efficacious has been done (Guess *et al.* 2002). The existence of the placebo effect has to be taken into account in the design and analysis of all research; it also underlies the design of the classical double-blind randomized controlled trial (RCT). This design theoretically discounts the social influence effect because neither patients nor doctors know whether the intervention being evaluated, for example a drug, is likely to be capable of working or not.

The science of placebo therapy is one among many pieces of evidence alerting us to the fact that all interventions have a social component, and all take place in a social context of interactions, relationships, expectations, values and understandings. This fact is disguised by the current fashion for discussing what are called 'complex' interventions as somehow different from 'simple' interventions (a term that is, interestingly, never used). 'Complex' interventions, defined as those 'made up of various interconnecting parts' (Campbell *et al.* 2000) are seen to offer all sorts of unique and often poorly specified challenges. An alternative, overlapping label here is 'behavioural'; again, these kinds of intervention are supposedly much more difficult to evaluate (Stephenson and Imrie 1998). Certain types of intervention are particularly likely to be classified as 'complex' or 'behavioural'. These include those based in community settings or dependent on community mobilization; many health promotion and public health interventions; environmental initiatives; interventions aimed at individual behavioural change; counselling, support or empowerment interventions; and broad public policy programmes.

Aims of the chapter

This chapter considers the challenges of designing and analysing social intervention research in health. The chapter draws particularly on a series of recent systematic reviews of the evidence base in health promotion, and on three recent examples of RCTs of social interventions in the fields of school-based sex education, day care for young children, and support for socially disadvantaged families. These examples are used as case studies to highlight issues related to the importance and feasibility of prospective experimental designs with control groups; the ethics and practicality of randomization; the need to develop and implement process as well as outcome evaluation; the development of a range of outcome measures; the importance of standardizing multicomponent interventions; and the use of multiple methods of data collection.

Different types of social intervention research in health

Some social intervention studies in health do not call for an evaluation design; they are primarily descriptive, and/or are aimed at assessing need, or developing interventions, or examining aspects of the contexts in which interventions are, or may be, implemented. For example, in two recent systematic reviews of the evidence base for promoting children's healthy eating and physical activity, 17 per cent of the studies found in the literature-mapping stage of the reviews were 'non-intervention' studies. These included cross-sectional surveys of children's physical activity or studies of children's beliefs about diet (Brunton *et al.* 2003; Thomas *et al.* 2003) (see Table 11.1). Such studies are necessary to inform the development of effective efforts to promote health, but they do not in themselves provide evaluated

Table 11.1 Studies included in the mapping stages of two systematic reviews of barriers and facilitators research relating to children's healthy eating and physical activity (N = 283)

	%	*N*
Non-intervention studies	17	48
Process–only evaluations	4	12
Outcome evaluations	73	207
RCTs	*38*	*78*
Non-randomized CTs	*37*	*76*
Other design/not stated	*26*	*53*
Systematic reviews	6	16

Source: Brunton *et al.* (2003); Thomas *et al.* (2003)

evidence of effectiveness. In these two reviews, a small proportion of studies – 4 per cent – were also classified as 'process-only evaluations', meaning that they described the implementation of interventions without gathering information about the impact of these on measured outcomes related to children's participation in healthy eating or physical activity. This is a common pattern in systematic reviews of social intervention research in health.

However, questions about the effectiveness of social interventions to promote health are major drivers of research in this area. To continue the above example, 73 per cent of the studies in the two reviews of children's healthy eating and physical activity evaluated the impact of interventions on particular health or behavioural outcomes. The design of these varied: 38 per cent were RCTs; 37 per cent were non-randomized controlled trials, and 26 per cent used some other design (normally pre-and post-test), or the design of the study was unclear. Many outcome evaluation studies measured the impact of interventions on multiple outcomes: the 207 studies reported measuring a total of 666 outcomes. Most – 65 per cent (430/666) – of these were physiological measures or measures of behaviour; 28 per cent (185/666) were measures of knowledge, attitudes or beliefs and 5 per cent (32/666) were concerned with the hard-to-define issue of self-esteem or self-efficacy. Many of these studies also evaluated multicomponent interventions; for example, the 54 outcome evaluations included in the in-depth stage of the two reviews examined 11 different types of intervention, and each study evaluated interventions with an average of over three distinct components (e.g. advice combined with biofeedback and increased access to resources, or financial incentives combined with environmental modification and information).

Evaluating social interventions: which design?

As the above examples show, controlled trials, whether randomized or not, are a common evaluation design in the area of social intervention research in health. Despite such evidence, the view that trials are inappropriate tools for evaluating social interventions continues to hold sway in some quarters (see e.g. Greene and Kreuter 1991; Speller *et al.* 1997; Morrison 2001; Kippax 2003). RCTs are said to oversimplify causation, be inappropriate in complex social settings, ignore the role of theory in understanding intervention effectiveness, be politically unacceptable and too expensive, be unethical and incapable of illuminating processes, and lack feasibility in circumstances where 'blinding' is impossible. The 'inherent complexity' of public health interventions in particular also features in this literature (Rychetnik *et al.* 2002). While each of these points may carry some weight in particular cases, the general argument for RCTs as the prototype for well-designed evaluations of social interventions in health is well made by the many that have successfully been done (Oakley and Fullerton 1996; Boruch 1997; Oakley 2000a).

Scientifically speaking, the design issues relating to social intervention evaluation are exactly the same as for the evaluation of clinical interventions. As in all research, study design needs to address questions of internal and external validity: are differences attributable to the intervention or a product of bias; and to what extent are the results of the study generalizable to a wider population? If the question is 'Does this intervention promote health?' then the appropriate design should incorporate one or more control groups of people not exposed to the intervention under test. It is important that such control groups should be prospectively chosen, i.e. before the intervention is implemented, and should be made up of people who are socially similar to those receiving the intervention; if they are not, then characteristics of the individuals exposed to the intervention may explain its impact (or lack of impact). Random allocation has been shown to be the most efficient way of generating socially similar groups (Kunz *et al.* 2003); an alternative name for RCTs might thus be SECTs – socially equitable comparison tests (Oakley 1998b). Randomization is simply an elegant technical device for improving the science of evaluation design, and its usefulness as a device for minimizing bias in the creation of comparison groups is the only 'special claim' to be made for it (Kleijnen *et al.* 1997).

Three basic points underlie the case for RCTs in evaluating social interventions (Bonell *et al.* 2003; Sheldon and Oakley 2002):

- The first is that the counterfactual is rarely known: we do not know what would have happened had that particular intervention not been introduced; we cannot guess the effects of time, or of the placebo factor, and interpreting the effects of interventions must also tangle with the possible impact of regression to the mean. For example, when a health care Trust is doing badly and a new manager is hired, her or his arrival may be followed by a period of improvement which would have happened anyway, but is interpreted as proof of managerial efficiency.
- A second reason for using RCTs is that most interventions, whether social or clinical, have very modest effects (Berge and Sandercock 2002). It is because of this that good comparison groups are needed in order to reduce the bias and confounding which could mask the existence of such effects.
- The third rationale for the RCT design has to do with complexity. Social systems are always complex, so only the simplicity of a well-designed evaluation can measure the effects of a change to that system. We can only control for those factors whose influence we know about; we cannot control for those of which we are ignorant, and there are many such factors. This is probably the most poorly understood aspect of RCTs. While people argue that in this or that situation RCTs are not possible because of complexity (see e.g. Hunter 1993), it is really the other way around: complexity *demands* the use of RCTs.

Examples abound of biased conclusions being drawn about the effectiveness of social interventions on the basis of poorly designed evaluations. For example, Guyatt *et al.* (2000) have shown that observational studies of adolescent pregnancy prevention initiatives systematically overestimate 'treatment' effects compared with RCTs. By 'observational studies', they mean 'study designs in which patients' preferences, or the judgement of health care workers, determine whether study participants receive an experimental or control intervention'. Their review of 13 RCTs and 17 observational studies examined, for males and females separately, the reported effects of primary prevention interventions on the four outcomes of sexual intercourse, contraceptive use, responsible sexual behaviour and pregnancy. For six of the eight outcomes the summary odds ratio for the observational studies showed a significant intervention benefit ($p < 0.05$), while the RCTs failed to show a benefit for any outcome. In a further analysis, the same team went on to demonstrate how the use of RCTs to evaluate social interventions in health may significantly alter received wisdom about what works to promote health. Meta-analysis of 26 RCTs of interventions designed to prevent adolescent pregnancy did not find any beneficial effects, and there was evidence that five interventions actually increased pregnancy rates (DiCenso *et al.* 2002).

A second example of differences between different evaluation methods comes from a different area of health promotion: workplace health promotion. Studies of workplace interventions aimed at lowering cholesterol level were most likely to show effectiveness when no control group was used in the design; the lowest estimates of effectiveness were found in well-designed trials (see Table 11.2).

Table 11.2   Workplace health promotion programmes aimed at lowering cholesterol level

	Effective interventions according to authors (%)
All studies (N = 52)	81
Studies with no control group* (N = 22)	95
All trials (N = 30)	70
Well-designed trials** (N = 12)	58

* Including those which used 'qualitative' methods to examine effectiveness
** Comparable intervention and control groups, pre- and post-intervention data, reporting on all outcomes
Source: Oakley (2001)

The importance of 'good' RCTs

The hallmarks of a 'good' RCT have been described by Ross and Wight (2003) as:

- trialling a high-quality intervention;
- answering important, relevant questions;
- deploying an ethical control group;
- measuring outcomes with proven high validity;
- having adequate sample size and power;
- including adequate evaluation of the intervention and its delivery;
- documenting external factors that could influence trial outcomes; and
- using culturally sensitive intervention and evaluation designs.

Though this model is recommended for the evaluation of sexual health promotion interventions, it seems a reasonable prescription for all intervention evaluation. Two additional recommendations relate to pilot work and reporting standards. An example of the need for trials to be based on careful pilot work is a recent community trial of smoke alarms in London which found no evidence of impact on fire-related injuries, mostly because few of the free alarms given out had been installed or maintained (DiGiuseppi *et al.* 2002). A study conducted *after* the trial found that only about half of the households given smoke alarms actually used these properly (Rowland *et al.* 2002); it would have been better to have known that such problems were likely in advance of implementing the intervention.

The way in which the design and findings of trials is reported is an area in which many social intervention trials fall down. (Clinical trials are not exempt from these problems, either.) For example, many of the 48 outcome evaluations included in the in-depth stage of three health promotion reviews relating to young people's healthy eating, mental health and physical activity were inadequately reported: 21 per cent failed to give numbers assigned to intervention and control groups, 77 per cent did not present pre-intervention data for all the outcomes measured, 79 per cent failed to report attrition rates and 33 per cent gave insufficient detail about the intervention to allow replicability (see Table 11.3).

The next section describes three social intervention trials in more detail to illustrate some of the challenges relating to social intervention studies in health.

Table 11.3 Reporting of basic methodological data in outcome evaluations in barriers and facilitators research relating to young people's healthy eating, mental health and physical activity (N = 48)

	Reported	*Not reported (%)*
Numbers assigned to intervention and control groups	38	10 (21)
Pre-intervention data for all outcomes	14	34 (77)
Attrition rates	10	38 (79)
Sufficient information given for intervention to be replicable	32	16 (33)

Source: Harden *et al.* (2001b); Rees *et al.* (2001); Shepherd *et al.* (2001)

Three case studies

The Hackney Daycare (HD) and the Social Support and Family Health (SSFH) studies were carried out between 1998 and 2002; the Randomised Intervention of Pupil Peer-Led sex Education (RIPPLE) study began in 1997 and follow-up is ongoing. All three trials were designed primarily to answer questions of effectiveness: do day care, social support and peer-led sex education 'work' in improving health and other outcomes?

The HD study

The HD study is an RCT of high-quality day care provided in the Mapledene Early Years Centre on the disadvantaged Holly Street estate in Hackney, North London. The background to the study is the prevalence of child poverty, the importance of day care in increasing the opportunity for parents to have paid work, and research showing a large unmet need among parents of young children for flexible, high-quality day care. A previous systematic review of eight RCTs of day care (all carried out in North America) showed that this approach to family support improves child development, behaviour and school performance, and reduces some of the long-term adverse effects of poverty (Zoritch *et al.* 1998).

Families eligible to take part in the HD study were those on the admissions list for the Mapledene Early Years Centre. One hundred and twenty mothers and 143 children aged between 6 months and 3.5 years were recruited to the study. Families were randomly allocated either to receive places at the Mapledene Centre or not; places were full- or part-time to suit parental needs within a ten-hour working day, for 48 weeks a year. The trial aimed to examine the effects of Mapledene Centre day care on a range of child, maternal and family outcomes. Postal questionnaires were used after recruitment and at 18 months to collect outcome data; interim questionnaires covering similar areas were administered by a researcher at 9 months to maintain contact with study families. Child development and health was assessed at baseline and 18 months by community paediatricians. Interviews, questionnaires and observations were used to collect process data. A pilot study was carried out to test the acceptability to parents of the proposed design and obtain their views on the kind of day care to be evaluated (Oakley *et al.* 2002), and the trial included an economic evaluation to assess the relative cost effectiveness of Mapledene Centre day care compared to other services used by control group families. Full details of the study can be found elsewhere (Toroyan *et al.* 2003).

The RIPPLE study

The RIPPLE study is an RCT involving 27 coeducational comprehensive schools in England in the evaluation of the effectiveness of peer-led sex education. Questions about the effectiveness of sex education are poorly answered by the existing research evidence due to problems with evaluation design (Oakley *et al.* 1995; Guyatt *et al.* 2000), and this applies also to peer-led methods, which have become increasingly fashionable (Harden *et al.* 2001a). Fourteen mixed sex, non-selective state schools in England were randomly assigned to implement a programme of peer-led sex education and 13 to act as control schools. Training was provided by an external training team to Year 12 students (aged 16/17 years) who volunteered to become peer educators and deliver a short programme of sex education to students in Year 9 (13/14-year-olds). This was given by, and to, two successive year cohorts of students. Follow-ups, using self-administered questionnaires, were carried out in both intervention and control schools when students were in Year 10 and Year 11 (6 and 18 months post-intervention).

The RIPPLE study is designed to answer the question of whether peer-led sex education is effective in decreasing risky sexual behaviour, defined as unprotected sexual intercourse before the age of 16 and regretted sexual relationships (Stephenson *et al.* 2003b). A total of 8766 students took part in the study. Focus groups, interviews and observations were used to collect a wide range of data about the implementation and acceptability of the intervention, and about the provision of sex education in the control schools (Strange *et al.* 2001, 2002a, 2002b). The study was preceded by a pilot study which examined feasibility and developed study instruments in four schools (Stephenson *et al.* 1998).

The SSFH study

The SSFH study is an RCT which aimed to measure the impact and cost effectiveness of two alternative strategies for providing support to mothers in disadvantaged inner-city areas: a programme of visits from health visitors trained in supportive listening (support health visitors – SHVs) and the services of local community support organizations (community group support – CGS). Maternal and child health outcomes for families offered either of the support interventions were compared with those for control women receiving standard services only. This trial built on substantial evidence about the health-promoting capacity of social support (Dean and Hancock 1992; Oakley 1992; Hodnett and Roberts 1996; Ray and Hodnett 2001; Barlow and Coren 2002).

Women living in deprived enumeration districts in the London boroughs of Camden and Islington were eligible for the trial if they gave birth between 1 January and 30 September 1999. A total of 731 families took part. The SHV intervention consisted of the offer of a year of monthly supportive listening visits. The CGS intervention entailed being assigned to one of eight community groups offering drop-in sessions, home visiting and/or telephone support. Outcome data were collected using questionnaires distributed 12 and 18 months post-randomization. A range of process data were also collected, and there was an integral economic evaluation. The study is described in detail elsewhere (Wiggins *et al.* 2004).

Common features of the three social intervention trials

These three trials have a number of design features in common, and these factors are shared with many social intervention trials in health:

- the use of cluster randomization;
- the development and testing of multicomponent interventions;
- the collection of process as well as outcome data;
- the use of multiple measures of outcome.

The next section examines these issues in more detail.

Cluster randomization, equipoise and consent

In cluster RCTs randomization is of groups of individuals, rather than individuals themselves. Reasons for using a cluster design include: the nature of the intervention (which has to be given to groups rather than individuals, a typical feature in much health promotion research); logistic convenience (it is simpler to test the intervention at group level); avoidance of contamination (randomization of groups or communities will generally reduce the chances of individuals in experimental and control groups 'contaminating' one another); and the need to test the 'mass effect' of an intervention (including on individuals not directly exposed to it) (Hayes 2003). Cluster randomization is a common research design in health care, but the randomization of groups of individuals rather than individuals themselves is especially likely in settings such as schools or the community where many social interventions are implemented. The focus on clusters in the design of such trials needs to be matched at the analysis stage, where allowance must be made for the fact that people in the same cluster are more likely to be like one another than those in different clusters. Many cluster RCTs of social interventions in health pay insufficient attention to this issue (MRC 2002).

The clusters randomized in the HD and SSFH studies were families; in the RIPPLE study, schools were randomized either to implement the intervention or not. Cluster randomization raises specific issues about the consent of research participants, as does the use of randomization more generally. A traditional rationale for using random allocation in trials is *equipoise* – uncertainty as to the impact of the intervention(s) under test, such that a rational informed person would have no preference between the 'treatments' (Lilford and Jackson 1995). Two of the three trials could be considered to have fulfilled this criterion: neither the evidence available about the value of peer-led compared with teacher-led education (the RIPPLE study), nor that relating to the relative merits of different forms of family support (the SSFH study) suggested a clear direction for policy. The arguments for using random allocation in the HD study were somewhat different. Firstly, there was the need to quantify more precisely than do existing studies the value of day care in improving children's and families' health and well-being; secondly, a rigorous evaluation of day care in a UK context was needed since this had never been done; thirdly, there was a strong argument for using random allocation as a device for rationing the scarce resource of day care (Toroyan *et al.* 2000). This function of random allocation has been important in the historical development of RCTs, and has a long history as a popular approach to the management of human affairs (Goodwin 1992).

Randomization is often said to be an unethical obstacle in social intervention design, but the objections are usually political, having to do with a resistance among policy-makers rather than trial participants. A recent report on the role of pilots in policy-making in the UK noted that many civil servants and some ministers 'regard random assignment with deep suspicion, and only partly for practical reasons' (Jowell 2003). A key issue is that, where uncertainty exists about the health benefits of the intervention in question, it is not unethical to withhold the intervention from a control group, though this may be cited (by both policy-makers and researchers) as a reason for rejecting an RCT design (see also Thomson *et al.* 2004).

The 'simple' model of randomization and consent specifies that eligible participants are told about the trial and invited to take part; those who say yes are then randomized. (Variations include randomizing first, then seeking consent, and also only seeking consent from people randomized to the intervention group.) However, assent to random allocation in the three trials involved two issues: agreement to the use of random allocation as a policy, and agreement to being randomized. All three trials were approved by the relevant ethics committees, though not without some difficulties, which partly related to the lack of familiarity of health research ethics committees with the challenges of social intervention studies (see Oakley *et al.* 2003). The policy of randomization then needed to be discussed with various stakeholder groups. While this is also a necessary stage in clinical intervention research, the range of stakeholder groups will often be larger in the field of social interventions. In the three trials discussed in this chapter, the relevant stakeholder groups included members of the public as trial participants – mothers and children in the HD and SSFH studies; parents, students and teachers in the RIPPLE study; and service providers – teachers and education authorities in the RIPPLE and HD studies, and local health authority and voluntary organizations in the SSFH study.

Randomization and consent in the HD study

In the HD study the key discussions were with local early years service providers, who needed to be convinced about the need for random allocation of day care places in order best to assess effectiveness. Prevailing admissions policies for local authority early years centres in the UK used a mixture of length of time on the waiting list and 'merit' or 'need' in order to determine which families would be offered places. After a number of meetings with local service representatives, it was agreed that the admission policy would be changed to random allocation for the newly-built centre which already had a substantial waiting list of local families. One key factor in negotiating this was the fact that a senior staff member was familiar with the evaluation literature relating to day care and had earlier in her career worked on one of the large American trials. A second aid to the trial negotiations was a degree of shared acceptance that establishing the effectiveness of day care was a priority in the current UK policy context, since it might help to secure greater funding for this 'Cinderella' component of the education system. The result of all these discussions was an unusually close partnership between the research team and key service providers. This included agreement to randomization of places at the trial centre being carried out in one of the university departments involved in the trial. Families in the HD study were randomized to be offered or not offered places in the centre *whether or not* they agreed to take part in the trial. The status of randomization was as a normal way of allocating services. In agreeing to take part in the research, families did not have to agree to randomization, only to providing questionnaire and interview data and bringing their children for paediatric examination.

Randomization and consent in the RIPPLE study

In the case of the RIPPLE study, the challenge in setting up the trial involved explaining and justifying the design to headteachers and other senior staff. Local education authority school yearbooks were used to identify potential schools. The heads of 343 schools were sent a letter of invitation to take part in the study. The letter contained a description of the study design, including the use of random allocation 'to avoid the possibility of bias which could affect the results of the study'. The 49 schools which responded positively were contacted for further discussion by a researcher or by the health promotion practitioner responsible for developing the peer-led sex intervention; 29 schools were subsequently randomized (two dropped out after randomization but not because they objected to their randomized status).

In the RIPPLE trial consent for schools to be randomized was given by school heads. Post-randomisation, parents in intervention and control schools were sent the same letters requesting consent for their children to take part in the study. These letters referred to the design of the study, but only requested consent for students to complete two questionnaires, explaining that they would still receive sex education even if parental consent to take part in the research was not given. Where students were given the questionnaires to fill in (normally in school time) they were told that they did not have to answer any question if they did not want to, and that they should leave the questionnaire blank if they did not want to take part in the study.

Randomization and consent in the SSFH study

In the SSFH study the proposal to evaluate the effectiveness of supportive health visiting worried some local service providers, who felt that implied in the trial design was the view that statutory health visitors were not supportive, and who were concerned that omitting clinical care from the trial health visitors' practice could raise ethical questions about safety. While these issues did not focus directly on random allocation, implicit in all of them was that the SHV intervention the research team wished to test should not be the subject of a trial because it was self-evidently beneficial and should become part of routine practice. As in the HD study, there was an implicit consensus among local service decision-makers that 'hard' outcome data from the trial (provided, of course, these favoured the SHV intervention) could be used to argue the case for improving and better resourcing routine services, and this consensus eventually helped to secure local service agreement to the conduct of the trial. Unlike the HD study, however, these discussions resulted in a divorce between the service and research aspects of supportive health visiting. The trial health visitors were recruited and employed by one of the university departments involved in the research.

The second intervention evaluated in the SSFH study involved the provision of support by local community groups. The issues here were different again. The research team contacted local councils, the health authority, the community health council and voluntary sector organizations to explain the design of the trial and the need for random allocation of women to both SHV and CGS arms. In agreeing to work on the SSFH study, these community groups needed to understand the design of the trial, but their agreement to the principle of random allocation was limited to accepting that the women referred to them as part of the trial would be referred because they had been randomized to the CGS arm of the trial, and not for the usual reason that they needed or had requested community group support. Consent to randomization in the SSFH study was closest to the 'simple' model referred to above: individual women were told about the trial and their consent was requested.

It is clear from these examples that negotiating the use of random allocation for evaluating social interventions in health is feasible, but it may be a lengthier and generally trickier business than, for example, when setting up a drug trial in a health care setting. The lack of blinding is a generic issue in many social intervention trials: participants cannot be prevented from knowing which group they are in, and the impact on trial outcomes of 'patient preferences' cannot be discounted, although it is hard to measure (MRC 2000).

Multicomponent interventions

Many social interventions defy simple categorization because they are made up of a number of elements. For example, a school-based intervention aimed at promoting young people's mental health may have components of information, the teaching of practical skills, peer support and parental involvement. An intervention designed to reduce obesity by increasing cycling in cities is likely to involve education, information, community mobilization and environmental initiatives such as road redesign. It is easy to exaggerate the differences between social and clinical interventions here; for example, 'compliance' and outcome in drug trials is affected by the way in which drugs are prescribed, who prescribes them, the information that is given, and the colour and appearance of the drugs, among other factors (de Craen *et al.* 1996).

The issue of standardization is important in all intervention evaluation. Where interventions are made up of different components, the challenge of standardization is often greater. The issues in the three trials used as case studies in this chapter were somewhat different. In the HD study, all the intervention children received an intervention provided by the same group of staff in the same setting – though there were differences in staff and provision over time of the kind that would be expected in any day care centre. In the RIPPLE study, standardization was much more of a problem, since the intervention involved a programme of sex education provided by different groups of students to different classes of younger students in two cohorts in 14 different schools. The SSFH study fell in between these two extremes: there were five different research health visitors providing the home visiting intervention, and eight different community groups providing support in the second intervention arm.

The trials were designed in such a way as to ensure that the intervention was as standard as possible. For example, in the RIPPLE study the same team of external trainers was used to train the peer educators in the 14 experimental schools, and the structure and content of the three sessions the peer educators provided to younger students were pre-specified in considerable detail. In the SSFH study similarly, a team of external trainers was engaged to help the five research health visitors develop appropriate supportive and listening skills. On the other hand, no attempt was made to standardize the community support intervention, because the aim here was to evaluate the impact on outcomes for mothers and children of the kind of support normally provided by such groups.

The experience of these three trials suggests that the real issue is not standardization *per se* but the importance of building methods into the trial which make it possible to describe *how the intervention was actually implemented in practice*.

Evaluating processes

The case for undertaking a process evaluation as an integral part of any social intervention trial is a strong one, because there may be a particular premium attached to understanding why something worked, or failed to work, when the intervention is multifaceted and the links with social context may be complex (Gueron 2002). Embedding process evaluations within trials has also been recommended as a way of addressing some of the criticism made of RCTs for evaluating social interventions (Pope and Mays 1995; Pawson and Tilley 1997; Wight and Obasi 2003; Oakley *et al.* 2004). Wight and Obasi list six arguments for collecting process data as an integral part of experimental evaluation as applied to social interventions: to prevent poorly designed and developed interventions; to avoid the false conclusions that can be drawn from intention-to-treat analyses; to study the mechanisms by which interventions work; to distinguish between the different components of a complex intervention; to investigate crucial contextual factors that might facilitate or obstruct the success of the intervention; and to look at differential effects within the target group.

Many social intervention trials in health focus on outcome evaluation only. In the three reviews of young people's health promotion referred to earlier, only 17 per cent (51/302) of the outcome evaluations included in the in-depth stage of the three reviews included integral process evaluations (Harden *et al.* 2001b; Rees *et al.* 2001; Shepherd *et al.* 2001). Process evaluations can study a range of processes, as recommended by Wight and Obasi. For example, the 14 of the 19 studies included in the meta-analysis of the review of children and healthy eating which undertook process evaluation documented a range of aspects, including intervention content, the quality of materials used and the skills of intervention providers (see Table 11.4). Process data can be collected using a range of methods. In the outcome evaluations included in the young people's health reviews mentioned above, methods of collecting data were classified as 'qualitative' in 18 per cent (9/51) of the process evaluations, and as 'quantitative' in 65 per cent (33/51), with the remainder (18 per cent – 9/51) using both approaches. The relatively small proportion focusing on qualitative data may seem surprising in view of the common equation that is made between process questions and qualitative research.

The design of the HD, RIPPLE and SSFH trials included detailed process evaluations. The main objectives were to: document how the interventions were implemented in practice; explore the experiences of control group participants; collect information about participants' views; and document key aspects of the social contexts in which the research was undertaken. Many of these data have value in their own right, but they also have a role to play in explaining the results of the outcome evaluation: if the intervention worked, why did it do so, and if there was no

Table 11.4   Processes evaluated in 14 studies included in the meta-analysis of a review of barriers and facilitators research in the area of children and healthy eating

Process	*Number of studies*
Intervention content	11
Quality of programme materials	3
Perceptions/understanding/acceptability of the intervention	7
Implementation of the intervention	13
Skills/training of intervention providers	1
Consultation/collaboration partnerships	2
Other (design and development; participation and response rates)	2
Total	**39**

Source: Thomas *et al.* (2003)

evidence that it worked, or there was evidence of harm, can the process data throw light on these findings? In the HD, RIPPLE and SSFH studies, a variety of methods were used to collect data relating to the process evaluation questions. All three studies used in-depth interviews and structured questionnaires with intervention recipients, researcher fieldnotes and interviews and questionnaires with staff and/or intervention providers. Researcher observations were used to collect data about the intervention in the HD and RIPPLE studies; taped interactions were used in the RIPPLE and SSFH studies; and in the RIPPLE study focus groups were also carried out with intervention providers and recipients (the peer educators and those receiving the peer-led intervention).

Collecting these types of data provided important information about the progress of the trial. For example, it was clear that, despite our best efforts, the training of the peer educators in the RIPPLE trial had been variable, and when the intervention was delivered some key topics were missed in some schools. In the SSFH study, a major problem was the low uptake of the CGS intervention – only 19 per cent of the women allocated to this arm of the trial used any CGS. Without the process data it would have been difficult to understand why this was so. The process data were also key to understanding what happened to control group participants. Assumptions underlying the design of the three trials had been: for the RIPPLE study, that all students would get some sex education; for the SSFH study, that many families would find community services useful; and for the HD study that some families in the control group would find alternative forms of day care. The process data showed that the first two of these assumptions were false. In the case of the control group in the day care study, the proportion finding other forms of day care was much higher (63 per cent) than expected.

The ability of a process evaluation to explain the outcomes of a trial is demonstrated by a study of peer-led HIV prevention among gay men in London. A controlled trial of an intervention deployed in five London gyms with a large gay membership found no evidence of a significant impact on gay men's risk behaviour (Elford *et al.* 2001). Process evaluation data collected through interviews with peer educators, gym managers and the health promotion team identified attrition and barriers to communication within gyms as the important factors explaining outcome. For example, only one in five potential peer educators remained identified with the project throughout its life, thus limiting the diffusion model on which the trial was based (Elford *et al.* 2002).

Choosing and measuring outcomes

Restriction to a narrow range of 'quantitative' outcomes is a common objection to the use of RCTs to evaluate social interventions. The choice of outcomes in any study clearly has to relate to the research question; in trials there are also issues of statistical power and sample size to consider. There is no point in selecting an outcome which, though important, is likely to be so rare that impractically large numbers of people will need to be recruited to the trial. But the ability of the trial to answer questions that are widely perceived to be relevant and important will partly depend on who has a stake in specifying the outcomes to be measured. An appropriate outcome measure has been defined as 'one that is robust, valid, acceptable, affordable, feasible to measure, and seen as relevant by affected communities, policy-makers and funders. It should also be an outcome in which there is likely to be detectable rate of change as a result of correct intervention delivery' (Cowan and Plummer 2003).

This is an area where qualitative research and pilot work have an important role to play (Davies 2000). An example from the RIPPLE study is the inclusion as key trial outcomes of measures relating to young people's satisfaction with their sexual relationships and ability to control their sexual health, as well as more traditional measures of contraceptive use, sexually transmitted infections (STIs) and pregnancy rates. The importance of these 'subjective' measures emerged during the feasibility study and also from systematic reviews of young people's attitudes to sexual health promotion.

Data analysis

Analysing the data collected in social intervention trials should follow good practice for clinical trials, but there may be additional challenges. Where the study design has specified the inclusion of multiple perspectives, for example in the choice of outcome measures, there may be difficult issues to resolve when the direction of effect appears to be different for different outcomes. In such cases, answering the question as to whether the intervention has 'worked' or not may require the privileging of one set of perspectives over another. Where uptake of an intervention is low, the convention of 'intention-to-treat' analysis may be challenged, and 'on treatment' analysis may also give different answers.

Process data can be analysed using the methods appropriate for each type of data, but the major challenge in social intervention trials with process evaluations is to carry out the analysis in such a way that process data have an integral role, rather than simply being used for illustrative purposes. As Wight and Obasi (2003) note, 'unless [process findings] are analysed in conjunction with outcome findings of a trial they are of no greater value than those generated from smaller scale, exclusively process evaluations'. This is a relatively new area methodologically, and few 'how to do it' guidelines exist.

An example from the RIPPLE study relates to one aim of the process evaluation, which was to examine the process by which the intervention might affect outcomes. Analysis of the questionnaire and focus group data showed that characteristics of sex educators and their ways of interacting with students were perceived by students as crucial. Peer educators were seen as providing more relevant, detailed information, having greater expertise and respect for students than teachers, as being more empathetic, less moralistic and making the sessions more fun. Students also liked the skills-based activities used in the peer-led intervention.

A qualitative analysis was carried out of the data gathered through observation of sex education sessions, and these data were narratively synthesized with the outcome data. Focus group and questionnaire data were used to identify factors that students considered most important in terms of the acceptability of sex education and relevant questions relating to these factors were identified in the questionnaires. These included: the use of participative/active methods; being provided with key information; having practised key skills; feeling positive about the sex educator; and feeling satisfied with the coverage of key topics. There were differences between experimental and control school students on all these dimensions of sex education (see Table 11.5).

Regression analyses were then carried out to examine the relationship between these key dimensions of sex education, intervention or control group status, and outcomes. These analyses indicated that the impact of peer-led sex education on sexual health outcomes was most consistently 'mediated' by students' participation in participative/active methods and practising key skills. Further analyses were

Table 11.5   Key aspects of sex education reported by students in control and experimental schools in the RIPPLE study

Numbers of students reporting:	Control (N = 3559) (%)	Experimental (N = 4211) (%)
Participatory/active methods	892 (25)	2611 (62)
Practising key skills	1270 (43)	3012 (81)
Receiving key information	2329 (80)	3357 (90)
Positive re. sex educator	2070 (58)	2700 (64)
Satisfaction with coverage of key topics	728 (20)	1243 (41)

Source: Strange *et al.* (in press)

carried out to explore whether these dimensions of sex education impacted on sex education differently depending on whether the sex education was delivered by peers or teachers. Significant interactions were found between trial arm and participatory/active methods and practising key skills for some outcomes: knowledge of STI prevention; knowledge of STIs; using a condom at last sex; and using contraception at last sex. Significant interactions between trial arm and participatory/active methods were also found for the outcome using a condom at first sex; between trial arm and receiving key information for the outcomes knowledge of STI prevention and using contraception at last sex; and between trial arm and satisfaction with coverage of key topics for the outcomes knowledge of timing of the emergency contraceptive pill, using a condom at last sex and using contraception at last sex. These findings suggest that, when peers deliver the peer-led sex education using participative and skill-based approaches, the sex education is more effective than when teachers employ similar methods. However, when peers and teachers do not employ these approaches, then sex education is more effective if delivered by teachers.

Conclusions

Many of the design and analysis issues confronting social intervention researchers are the same as those in the area of clinical interventions. Some important research questions in both areas do not call for an evaluation methodology: for example, questions about the extent of need, or the perspectives of health-service users. Where evaluation methods are needed, well-designed prospective experimental studies with random allocation to intervention and control groups are the method of choice, because these offer the best chance of answering questions about the impact of different interventions. It has been noted that the area of 'complex' social and clinical interventions in health care tends to be marked by a paucity of high quality literature (MRC 2000). Different traditions of, and skills in, evaluation methodology among social and health scientists are one important reason for divergent practices relating to the evaluation of social and clinical interventions in health care research, with evaluation methodology being generally stronger in clinical research. Evaluation methodology in health and social policy research in the USA has been notably stronger than in the UK, a factor attributed to different political systems as well as to better training of social scientists in quantitative methods (Jowell 2003). As planks of evidence-based policy and practice, intervention evaluation, experimental methods and systematic research synthesis are methodological skills missing from the research training of many social scientists in the

UK (OECD 2003; Commission on the Social Sciences 2003). 'Paradigm' warfare about the relative merits of 'quantitative' and 'qualitative' methods is another reason for the neglect of well-designed evaluation in the social field (Oakley 1998c, 2000b, 2001).

There are, nonetheless, some particular challenges in social intervention research in health. Social intervention evaluation, more often than clinical intervention evaluation, involves the testing of multicomponent interventions offered to groups of people rather than individuals in situations where blinding is not possible. Increasing experience with such trials is highlighting a number of features of 'good' trial design which apply throughout health research. Prime among these are the need for careful pilot work; the selection of research questions and outcome measures which reflect the concerns of trial participants; the collection of detailed process data; and procedures for analysis which combine a focus on both process and outcome.

Key points

- Many health care interventions have a large social component.

- Some social intervention studies in health do not call for an evaluation design; they are primarily descriptive, aimed at assessing need, delivering interventions or examining aspects of the context in which interventions may be implemented.

- Scientifically, the design issues relating to social intervention evaluation are the same as for the evaluation of clinical interventions.

- An appropriate outcome measure should be robust, valid, acceptable, affordable, feasible to measure and relevant.

- Three basic points underline the case for RCTs in evaluating social interventions: the counterfactual is rarely known (i.e. what would have happened had an intervention not been introduced); most social and clinical interventions have only modest effects, thus good comparison groups are needed to reduce bias and confounding; social systems are complex, so only the simplicity of a well-designed evaluation can measure the effects of a change to that system – complexity demands the use of RCTs.

- The major challenge of process evaluations in social intervention trials is to conduct the analysis in such a way that the process data have an integral role, rather than simply being used in illustration.

- Many social intervention trials in health share common design features, including the use of cluster randomization, the development and testing of multicomponent intervention, the collection of both process and outcome data, and the use of multiple measures of outcome.

- Evaluations of social interventions often involve the testing of multicomponent interventions offered to groups of people in situations where blinding is not possible. This highlights the need for 'good' trial design.

References

Barlow, J. and Coren, E. (2002) Parent-training programmes for improving maternal psycho-social health (Cochrane Review), in *The Cochrane Library*, Issue 1. Oxford: Update Software.

Berge, E. and Sandercock, P. (2002) The nuts and bolts of doing a clinical trial, in L. Duley and B. Farrell (eds) *Clinical Trials*. London: BMJ Publishing.

Bonell, C., Bennett, R. and Oakley, A. (2003) Sexual health interventions should be subject to experimental evaluation, in J. Stephenson, J. Imrie and C. Bonell (eds) *Effective Sexual Health Interventions: Issues in Experimental Evaluation*. Oxford: Oxford University Press.

Boruch, R.F. (1997) *Randomized Experiments for Planning and Evaluation: A Practical Guide*. Thousand Oaks, CA: Sage.

Brunton, G., Harden, A., Rees, R. *et al.* (2003) *Children and Physical Activity: A Systematic Review of Barriers and Facilitators*. London: EPPI-Centre, Social Science Research Unit, Institute of Education, University of London.

Campbell, M., Fitzpatrick, R., Haines, A. *et al.* (2000) Framework for design and evaluation of complex interventions to improve health, *British Medical Journal*, 321: 694–6.

Commission on the Social Sciences (2003) *Great Expectations: The Social Sciences in Britain*. London: Commission on the Social Sciences.

Cowan, F.M. and Plummer, M. (2003) Biological, behavioural and psychological outcome measures, in J. Stephenson, J. Imrie and C. Bonell (eds) *Effective Sexual Health Interventions: Issues in Experimental Evaluation*. Oxford: Oxford University Press.

Crow, R., Gage, H., Hampson, S., Hart, J., Kimber, A. and Thomas, H. (1999) The role of expectancies in the placebo effect and their use in the delivery of health care: a systematic review, *Health Technology Assessment*, 3(3): 1–96.

Davies, H.T.O., Nutley, S.M. and Smith, P.C. (2000) *What Works? Evidence-based Policy and Practice in Public Services*. Bristol: The Policy Press.

Davies, P. (2000) Contributions from qualitative research. In H.T.O. Davies, S.M. Nutley and P.C. Smith (eds) *What Works? Evidence-based Policy and Practice in Public Services*. Bristol: The Policy Press.

Dean, K. and Hancock, T. (1992) *Supportive Environments for Health*. Copenhagen: WHO.

De Craen, A.J., Roos, P.J., de Vries, A.L. and Kleijnen, J. (1996) Effect of colour of drugs: systematic review of perceived effect of drugs and of their effectiveness, *British Medical Journal*, 313: 1624–6.

DiCenso, A., Guyatt, G., Willan, A. and Griffith, L. (2002) Interventions to reduce unintended pregnancies among adolescents: systematic review of randomised controlled trials, *British Medical Journal*, 324: 1426–34.

DiGiuseppi, C., Roberts, I., Wade, A. *et al.* (2002) Incidence of fires and related injuries after giving out free smoke alarms: cluster randomised controlled trial, *British Medical Journal*, 325: 995–7.

Elford, J., Bolding, G. and Sherr, L. (2001) Peer education has no significant impact on HIV risk behaviours among gay men in London, *AIDS*, 15: 1409–15.

Elford, J., Sherr, L., Bolding, G. *et al.* (2002) Peer-led HIV prevention among gay men in London: process evaluation, *AIDS Care*, 14(3): 351–60.

Goodwin, B. (1992) *Justice by Lottery*. Hemel Hempstead: Harvester Wheatsheaf.

Greene, L.W. and Kreuter, M.W. (1991) *Health Promotion Planning: An Educational and Environmental Approach*. Toronto: Mayfield Publishing Company.

Gueron, J. (2002) The politics of random assignment: implementing studies and affecting policy, in F. Mosteller and R. Boruch (eds) *Evidence Matters: Randomized Trials in Education Research*. Washington, DC: Brookings Institution Press.

Guess, H.A., Kleinman, A., Kusek, J.W. and Engel, L.W. (2002) *The Science of the Placebo: Toward an Interdisciplinary Research Agenda*. London: BMJ Publishing.

Guyatt, G.H., DiCenso, A., Farewell, V. *et al.* (2000) Randomized trials versus observational studies in adolescent pregnancy prevention, *Journal of Clinical Epidemiology*, 53: 167–74.

Harden, A., Oakley, A. and Oliver, S. (2001a) Peer-delivered health promotion by young people: a systematic review of different study designs, *Health Education Journal*, 60: 362–70.

Harden, A., Rees, R., Shepherd, J. *et al.* (2001b) *Young People and Mental Health: A Systematic Review of Research on Barriers and Facilitators*. London: EPPI-Centre Report, Social Science Research Unit, Institute of Education.

Hayes, R. (2003) Cluster randomised trials of sexual health interventions, in J. Stephenson, J. Imrie and C. Bonell (eds) *Effective Sexual Health Interventions: Issues in Experimental Evaluation*. Oxford: Oxford University Press.

Hodnett, E. and Roberts, I. (1966) Home-based social support for socially disadvantaged mothers (Cochrane Review), in *The Cochrane Library*, Issue 1. Oxford: Update Software.

Hunter, D. (1993) Let's hear it for R & D, *Health Service Journal*, 15 April: 17.

Jowell, R. (2003) *Trying it Out: The Role of 'Pilots' in Policy-Making*. London: Cabinet Office.

Kippax, S. (2003) Sexual health interventions are unsuitable for experimental evaluation, in J. Stephenson, J. Imrie and C. Bonell (eds) *Effective Sexual Health Interventions: Issues in Experimental Evaluation*. Oxford: Oxford University Press.

Kleijnen, J., Gøtzsche, P., Kunz, R.A. *et al.* (1997) So what's so special about randomisation?, in: A. Maynard and I. Chalmers (eds) *Non-random Reflections on Health Services Research*. London: BMJ Publishing.

Kunz, R., Vist, G. and Oxman, A.D. (2003) Randomisation to protect against selection bias in healthcare trials (Cochrane Methodological Review), in *The Cochrane Library*, Issue 1. Oxford: Update Software.

Lilford, R. and Jackson, J. (1995) Equipoise and the ethics of randomisation, *Journal of the Royal Society of Medicine*, 88: 552–9.

Morrison, K. (2001) Randomised controlled trials for evidence-based education: some problems in judging 'what works', *Evaluation and Research in Education*, 15: 69–83.

Mosteller, F. and Boruch, R. (eds) (2002) *Evidence Matters: Randomized Trials in Education Research*, Washington, DC: Brookings Institution Press.

MRC (Medical Research Council) (2000) *A Framework for Development and Evaluation of RCTs for Complex Interventions to Improve Health*. London: Medical Research Council.

MRC (Medical Research Council) (2002) *Cluster Randomised Trials: Methodological and Ethical Considerations*. London: Medical Research Council.

Oakley, A. (1992) *Social Support and Motherhood: The Natural History of a Research Project*. Oxford: Basil Blackwell.

Oakley, A. (1998a) Public policy experimentation: lessons from America, *Policy Studies*, 19(2): 93–114.

Oakley, A. (1998b) Living in two worlds, *British Medical Journal*, 316: 482–3.

Oakley, A. (1998c) Experimentation in social science: the case of health promotion, *Social Sciences in Health*, 4(2): 73–89.

Oakley, A. (2000a) *Experiments in Knowing: Gender and Method in the Social Sciences*. Cambridge: Polity Press.

Oakley, A. (2000b) Paradigm wars: some thoughts on a personal and public trajectory, *International Journal of Social Research Methodology*, 2(3): 247–54.

Oakley, A. (2001) Evaluating health promotion: methodological diversity, in S. Oliver and G. Peersman (eds) *Using Research for Effective Health Promotion*. Buckingham: Open University Press.

Oakley, A. and Fullerton, D. (1996) The lamp-post of research: support or illumination? in A. Oakley and H. Roberts (eds) *Evaluating Social Interventions*. Ilford: Barnardos.

Oakley, A., Fullerton, D., Holland, J. *et al.* (1995) Sexual health interventions for young people: a methodological review, *British Medical Journal*, 310: 158–62.

Oakley, A., Roberts, I., Turner, H. and Rajan, L. (2002) *A Feasibility Study for a Randomised Controlled Trial of Daycare for Preschool Children*. London: Social Science Research Unit Report, Institute of Education.

Oakley, A., Strange, V., Toroyan, T. *et al.* (2003) Using random allocation to evaluate social interventions: three recent UK examples, *Annals of the American Academy of Political and Social Science*, 589: 170–89.

Oakley, A., Strange, V., Stephenson, J. *et al.* and the RIPPLE study team (2004) Evaluating processes: a case study of a randomised controlled trial of sex education, *Evaluation*, 10(4): 440–462.

OECD (Organization for Economic Cooperation and Development) (2003) *Educational Research and Development in England*. New challenges for educational research, knowledge, management. Paris: OECD.

Pawson, R. and Tilley, N. (1997) *Realistic Evaluation*. London: Sage.

Pope, C. and Mays, N. (1995) Reaching the parts other methods cannot reach: an introduction to qualitative methods in health and health services research, *British Medical Journal*, 311: 42–5.

Ray, K.L. and Hodnett, E.D. (2001) Caregiver support for postpartum depression (Cochrane Review), in *The Cochrane Library*, Issue 2. Oxford: Update Software.

Rees, R., Harden, A., Shepherd, J., Brunton, G., Oliver, S. and Oakley, A. (2001) *Young People and Physical Activity: A Systematic Review of Research on Barriers and Facilitators.* London: EPPI-Centre Report, Social Science Research Unit, Institute of Education.

Ross, D.A. and Wight, D. (2003) The role of randomized controlled trials in assessing sexual health interventions, in J. Stephenson, J. Imrie and C. Bonell (eds) *Effective Sexual Health Interventions: Issues in Experimental Evaluation.* Oxford: Oxford University Press.

Rowland, D., DiGiuseppi, C., Roberts, I. *et al.* (2002) Prevalence of working smoke alarms in local authority inner-city housing: randomised controlled trial, *British Medical Journal,* 325: 998–1001.

Rychetnik, L., Frommer, M., Hawe, P and Shiell, A. (2002) Criteria for evaluating evidence on public health interventions, *Journal of Epidemiology and Community Health,* 56: 119–27.

Sheldon, T. and Oakley, A. (2002) Why we need randomised controlled trials, in L. Duley and B. Farrell (eds) *Clinical Trials.* London: BMJ Publishing.

Shepherd, J., Harden, A., Rees, R. *et al.* (2001) *Young People and Healthy Eating: A Systematic Review of Research on Barriers and Facilitators.* London: EPPI-Centre Report, Social Science Research Unit, Institute of Education.

Speller, V., Learmonth, A. and Harrison, D. (1997) The search for evidence of effective health promotion, *British Medical Journal,* 315: 361–3.

Stephenson, J. and Imrie, J. (1998) Why do we need randomised controlled trials to assess behavioural interventions? *British Medical Journal,* 316: 611–13.

Stephenson, J., Imrie, J. and Bonell, C. (eds) (2003a) *Effective Sexual Health Interventions: Issues in Experimental Evaluation.* Oxford: Oxford University Press.

Stephenson, J.M., Oakley, A., Charleston, S. *et al.* (1998) Behavioural intervention trials for HIV/STD prevention in schools: are they feasible? *Sexually Transmitted Infections,* 74: 405–8.

Stephenson, J.M., Oakley, A., Johnson, A.M. *et al.* (2003b) A school-based randomized controlled trial of peer-led sex education in England, *Controlled Clinical Trials,* 24(5): 643–57.

Strange, V., Forrest, S. Oakley, A. and the RIPPLE Study team (2001) A listening trial: 'qualitative' methods within experimental research, in S. Oliver and G. Peersman (eds) *Using Research for Effective Health Promotion.* Buckingham: Open University Press.

Strange, V., Forrest, S., Oakley, A. and the RIPPLE Study team (2002a) What influences peer-led sex education in the classroom? A view from the peer educators, *Health Education Research,* 17: 327–38.

Strange, V., Forrest, S., Oakley, A. and the RIPPLE Study team (2002b) Peer-led sex education: characteristics of peer educators and their perceptions of the impact on them of participation in a peer education programme, *Health Education Research,* 17: 339–50.

Strange, C., Allen, E., Oakley, A., Stephenson, J., Bouell, C., Johnson, A. and the RIPPLE Study team (in press), Integrating process with outcome data in a randomised controlled trial of sex education, *Evaluation.*

Thomas, J., Sutcliffe, K., Harden, A. *et al.* (2003) *Children and Healthy Eating: A Systematic Review of Barriers and Facilitators.* London: EPPI-Centre, Social Science Research Unit, Institute of Education, University of London.

Thomas, K.B. (1987) General practice consultations: is there any point in being positive? *British Medical Journal,* 294: 1200–2.

Thomson, H., Hoskins, R., Petticrew, M., Ogilvie, D., Craig, N., Quinn, T. and Lindsay, G. (2004) Evaluating the health effects of social interventions, *British Medical Journal,* 328: 282–5.

Toroyan, T., Roberts, I. and Oakley, A. (2000) Randomisation and resource allocation: a missed opportunity for evaluating health care and social interventions, *Journal of Medical Ethics,* 26: 319–22.

Toroyan, T., Roberts, I., Oakley, A. *et al.* (2003) Effectiveness of out-of-home day care for disadvantaged families: randomised controlled trial, *British Medical Journal,* 327: 906–9.

Tudor Hart, J. and Dieppe, P. (1996) Caring effects, *Lancet,* 347: 1606–8.

Wiggins, M., Oakley, A., Roberts, I. *et al.* (2004) The Social Support and Family Health study: a randomised controlled trial and economic evaluation of two alternative forms of postnatal support for mothers living in disadvantaged inner city areas, *Health Technology Assessment Monograph,* 8 (32).

Wight, D. and Obasi, A. (2003) Unpacking the 'black box': the importance of process data to explain outcomes, in J. Stephenson, J. Imrie and C. Bonell (eds) *Effective Sexual Health Interventions: Issues in Experimental Evaluation*. Oxford: Oxford University Press.

Zoritch, B., Roberts, I. and Oakley, A. (1998) The health and welfare effects of day-care: a systematic review of randomised controlled trials, *Social Science and Medicine*, 47: 317–27.

12 Area-based studies and the evaluation of multilevel influences on health outcomes

Graham Moon, S.V. Subramanian, Kelvyn Jones, Craig Duncan and Liz Twigg

Introduction

At root, much health research is concerned with individual people, events, interventions or programmes. For example, interest is frequently focused on the identification of regularities underpinning variations in the mortality or morbidity of individuals. Equally a comparison might be made between the therapeutic impact on individuals of a new drug and standard treatment regime using the traditional randomized controlled trial (RCT) (see Chapter 5). These 'individual-level' studies can be contrasted with those that have an explicit focus on geographical areas: what are often termed 'ecological' studies (see Box 12.1). This second type of study

> ### Box 12.1 Ecological studies
>
> Studies in which the unit of analysis is a geographical area or organizational entity. Ecological studies can be contrasted with individual studies, which, as the name suggests, have individuals as the basic unit of analysis.

manifests itself most simply through the production of choropleth maps comparing health outcomes between areas. Ecological studies are most common in health geography but are also typical of descriptive epidemiology and studies of health inequality. Good recent examples include Shaw *et al.* (1999) and Mitchell *et al.* (2000).

This chapter looks beyond the simplistic dichotomization of the individual and the ecological and offers an assessment of current directions in health research concerned with areas, places or geographies. This assessment focuses mainly on methodological issues regarding the analysis of area effects. An initial section briefly considers the nature of ecological analyses. This is used to introduce a more substantial assessment of the shortcomings of the ecological approach and the difficulties entailed in untangling area effects on health. From this assessment, and the concern to look beyond the dichotomization of the individual and the aggregate, it is concluded that an understanding of area effects must implicate both individual and ecological factors. To this end, the third substantive section of the chapter examines multilevel modelling, explaining what it does and outlining its scope in health research. A short conclusion summarizes the contentions of the chapter.

Ecological studies

Numerous health research studies have used an ecological design to examine variations or inequalities from a geographical perspective. Subject matter has ranged across mortality, morbidity, health-related behaviour and health service topics. Source data have generally been derived from routine officially-collected sources. The finding of area differences in the health status of populations has long been established. Research has consistently shown that people in different geographical areas apparently experience different degrees of ill health. Curtis and Jones (1998) provide a useful review of the field.

In the case of mortality the spatial scale of these ecological studies has been both national and more localized, with variations being considered between relatively large regions as well as between smaller spatial units. Curtis (1995) summarizes this work, while Illsley and Le Grand (1993) exemplify national-scale work. They examined ten-year age-specific death rates in England at seven points from 1930 to 1990 and found that, while a north-south gradient persisted in older age groups, it faded in younger age groups. Further work on this theme has corroborated the continued existence of a north-south divide in mortality at certain ages and indicated the lack of recent progress in narrowing this divide (Drever and Whitehead 1995). Subregional analyses document similar, often entrenched, patterns of inequality, as do more localized studies. Both are conventionally based on comparisons between local government units, though local studies may equally use census or postal geographies. An urban penalty is a frequent finding: urban and metropolitan areas tend to experience higher rates of mortality and morbidity than rural areas (Mullen 1992).

What factors underpin these observed geographical variations? Why does a map of mortality (or any other health issue) reveal geographical variation? Ecological studies examine this question by 'associative analyses', seeking correlations with other variables measured at the same geographical scale or building multiple regression models that seek to summarize the relationship between an areal outcome measure and a set of candidate predictors. Candidature in both these approaches is driven by theory and, nowadays, has increasingly implicated the social environment, particularly via measures of deprivation and structural perspectives on the causation of ill health (Townsend *et al.* 1988a; Acheson 1998; Shaw *et al.* 1999). To avoid problems arising from small numbers and to ensure statistical reliability, both approaches commonly work with extremely coarse geographies.

The majority of correlational associative analyses link deprivation to the calculation of simple areal rates that control for population composition by disaggregating or standardizing on the basis of personal characteristics, most typically to allow for the impact of age and sex on the health variable. Examples from research on health-related behaviour include Blaxter (1990), Dunbar and Morgan (1987) and Balarajan and Yuen (1986). Since this work only considers a very narrow range of characteristics at any one time, it provides only a limited insight into the nature of areal

variation. To this end, a smaller number of studies have adopted the more sophisticated regression modelling strategy, allowing for varying population compositions
by including age and sex as predictor variables alongside other variables (Braddon *et
al.* 1988; Whichelow *et al.* 1991). This latter approach has the advantage of making
clear the contribution of demography to health inequalities; Asthana *et al.* (2004)
show how the contribution of age and sex to health variations usually exceeds that
of deprivation.

The measures of deprivation employed in these analyses are many and varied,
capturing different aspects of deprivation such as those derived from educational
disadvantage, poor housing, tenure status or unemployment. Mostly these data are
obtained from national censuses though some may be aggregated from larger routine surveys, providing sample sizes are sufficient to permit generalization at the
desired spatial scale of analysis. In UK-based ecological analyses, much use is also
made of composite indicators of deprivation. These offer a single-figure summary
of several separate deprivation measures. Perhaps the best known of these composite
indicators is the Jarman 'under-privileged area index' (Jarman 1984). This uses
standard scores, weighting and linearization to summarize eight measures in a single
composite indicator designed to capture family doctor workload; over time it has
mutated into an indicator of deprivation though it is not without its critics (Senior
1991). Other similar indicators include the Townsend (Townsend *et al.* 1988b;
Ben-Shlomo *et al.* 1996) and Carstairs indices (Carstairs and Morris 1991). Both are
less controversial as indicators of deprivation. A rather different methodological
strategy underpins the construction of the UK Office of the Deputy Prime
Minister's Indices of Deprivation, but with similar results (see Box 12.2).

Box 12.2   The Indices of Multiple Deprivation

The Indices of Deprivation 2004 are measures of deprivation for every 2001 Census
Super Output Area and local authority area in England. They comprise seven
domains (income, employment, heath deprivation and disability, education, skills and
training deprivation, barriers to housing and services, living environment deprivation
and crime). These are combined into a single deprivation score and rank for each
area. There are also six summary measures for county councils, an Income Deprivation Affecting Children Index and an Income Deprivation Affecting Older People
Index.

Using data on mortality for 1989–93 in each of over 350 English local authorities, Drever and Whitehead (1995) exemplify the use of a composite deprivation
indicator as an aid to understanding health variations. They found a significant
relationship between mortality and the then Department of the Environment's
1991 deprivation index, equating high mortality with greater deprivation. This
relationship was strongest for males and was broadly consistent across age groups.
Another example, at a more localized spatial scale, is provided by Eames *et al.* (1993).
They relate several alternative social deprivation indices to premature mortality
using over 8000 English electoral wards as their ecological unit. They suggest that
the effects of deprivation are not limited to the poorest areas and also note that the
impact of deprivation on health varies across the country, being greatest in parts of
the North and in Central South-West London and least in East Anglia. There is a

consistent relationship between ill health and deprivation, with the highest mortality rates found in inner-city areas and suburban local authority housing estates.

As an alternative to single or composite measures of deprivation, some ecological studies use area typologies. Examples of UK area typologies include those derived by National Statistics from census data and commercial classifications such as ACORN classification, developed by CACI Limited (CACI 2003) or MOSAIC (Experian 2004). These typologies classify areas on the basis of a cluster analysis of area-based statistical measures. Clusters, or groups of areas, are internally homogeneous but different from other clusters. They are generally given names that reflect their key characteristics. Cluster identification depends on the variables selected and the clustering methodology as well as choice of areal unit, but the resulting area typologies highlight underlying ecological structuring within a population that is related to many aspects of human behaviour, including health. Meltzer *et al.* (2000) provide a recent example. They used ACORN to examine the proportion of children with a mental disorder in relation to area type. They found that areas characterized as 'striving' (low income, less prosperous) had rates of childhood mental disorder nearly 250 per cent above those found in 'thriving' (wealthy) areas. Other examples of the use of multivariate classifications include Shouls *et al.* (1996) and Wiggins *et al.* (1998). While this work has successfully linked a health differential to the social milieu of an area type, it is not clear what aspect of these classifications it is that brings about a health differential.

Traditionally in health and deprivation research, ecological studies have been used to help develop explanations of health inequalities. The areal basis to ecological analysis has however attracted little attention in its own right. 'Geography' has generally been used simply as a framework for identifying patterns or as a means of organizing data. Yet this usage is far from unproblematic. Mitchell (2001) notes the tendency to conflate small-area administrative divisions with more organic, functional and theoretically relevant notions of neighbourhood. Mitchell *et al.* (2000) have emphasized the advantages that come from working with areas of relatively equal population size or social homogeneity. Perhaps most importantly, the work of Openshaw (1983) on the modifiable areal unit problem (see Box 12.3)

Box 12.3   The modifiable area unit problem

'Since any study area over which data are collected is continuous, it follows that there will be a tremendous number of different ways by which it can be divided into non-overlapping areal units for the purpose of spatial analysis' (Openshaw 1983). The number of different zones for which *n* individuals can be aggregated is huge even for small values of *n*. The possibilities reduce but remain large if aggregation is constrained to ensure that neighbouring individuals are in the same zone. Crucially, each different aggregation can yield a different result.

---

serves as a reminder that the size and configuration of areal units can directly influence the results of associative analyses, to the extent of rendering statistically significant associations insignificant and, at the extreme, changing the direction of relationships.

Notwithstanding these difficulties, it is clear that ecological studies imply variations between places in terms of health outcomes. Places are (seemingly) different.

However, a key question is hidden in this innocuous statement. Is it place that makes the difference? At issue is the extent to which the spatial differences evident in ecological studies are simply a reflection of the differing social profiles of the resident populations within their areal units or whether there is something about an area which has an independent effect on health in its own right: a so-called 'area effect'. It is to area effects that attention now turns.

Area effects

If place makes a difference to health, health outcomes depend not only on individual characteristics (age, gender, class and so on) but also on place, the setting, 'ecology', or surrounding environment in which individuals live and work. A key interpretive question is the extent to which the observed place differences are 'area' or 'ecological' effects or merely a result of different types of people living in these places. To put it another way, do people of similar characteristics experience different health outcomes in different places?

Much ecological research is unable to answer such questions because it has conflated the genuinely ecological and the 'aggregate'. Hampson (1991) directly equates the two, claiming that the unique distinguishing feature of ecological studies is that they are empirical investigations involving a group of individuals as the unit of analysis. Real ecological effects would indisputably operate at the areal level, reflecting predictors and associated mechanisms operating at, and solely at, an areal level. The search for such measures and their assessment in properly designed studies is a current area of considerable research (Macintyre and Ellaway 2000; Ellen *et al.* 2001; Macintyre *et al.* 2002). Among the candidate measures for genuine ecological status might be those that capture the efficiency and effectiveness of area-based policy or the procedures of local service providers, the closure or out-migration of significant employers, measures of community stress, and indicators of community social capital. In a crude sense these ecological measures, particularly the last two, provide the empirical case for community development as a strategy for raising or maintaining the chances of good health.

Aggregate area effects, in contrast, equate the effect of an area with the sum of the many individual effects associated with the people living within the area. In this situation the key interpretive question posed above becomes particularly apposite. If common membership of an area by a set of individuals brings about an effect that is over and above that resulting from individual characteristics, then there may indeed be an area effect: the whole may be more than the sum of the parts. If this does not happen, it is individual factors that matter, not area effects. To assume an area effect on the basis of evidence derived from aggregate data is to commit the 'ecological fallacy' of transferring results from aggregates to individuals (see Box 12.4). As Figure 12.1 shows, the aggregate relation may even be of the opposite sign to the individual relations on which it is based. As Susser (1973) points out, the term

---

Box 12.4   Analytical fallacies

Ecological fallacies assume that the results of ecological studies apply to *individuals*, whereas **atomistic fallacies** assume that the results of individual studies apply *between areas*.

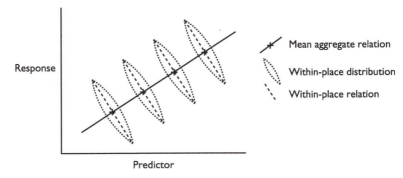

Figure 12.1   Reversing relationships and the ecological fallacy

Source: Jones and Duncan (1995)

'ecological fallacy' is really a misnomer; he prefers 'aggregative fallacy'. Shared residence in an area does not necessarily mean that individuals will draw the same influences from it; those who are spatial neighbours are not always social neighbours who vary in their interactions with those who live close to them.

Many, perhaps the majority, of ecological analyses are in fact analyses of aggregate data. Area effects are potentially of importance, but they cannot be assessed through aggregate analysis. They cannot distinguish the difference a place makes from what is in a place (Jones and Moon 1993). As the classic paper by Robinson showed, there is no reason to suggest that a relationship that occurs at the aggregate level can be held to exist at the individual level (Robinson 1950). Taking a hypothetical example, high levels of illness may be associated with high levels of unemployment at the regional level, but people who are ill in regions with high unemployment may be those in work.

One result of the widespread recognition of the ecological fallacy was a turn to survey methods and studies using the individual as a unit of analysis. Work at the individual level risks missing important area effects. If no attempt is made to incorporate measures relating to area characteristics then the 'atomistic fallacy' (Alker 1969) (see Box 12.4) is committed in which research completely ignores the situated nature of individual action and outcomes. This decontextualized research strategy not only denies area effects (and other collective impacts on health) but, in its individualistic approach, has had undoubted resonance with much neo-liberal health policy-making. Thus, Thomas (1993) declared that *The Health of the Nation* (Department of Health 1988), a policy developed by the British Conservative Party, viewed health-related behaviour as 'a matter of individual responsibility' and that 'behaviours are not placed in context' but rather are conceptualized in traditionally narrow epidemiological terms.

Composition and context

As a further basis for unpacking ideas about area effects, Macintyre (Macintyre *et al.* 1993; Macintyre 1995) has usefully distinguished between 'compositional', 'collective' and 'contextual effects' (see Box 12.5). The first refers to the idea that place differences are an artefact of differential socioeconomic composition. A purely compositional explanation for observed area variations in smoking would be that the sort of people whose personal and household characteristics are associated with

> **Box 12.5   Composition and context**
>
> **Composition** is the properties of individuals living *within* an area, also linked to the idea of *people deprivation*, whereas **context** is the properties of an area and may vary *between areas*. It is also linked to the idea of *place deprivation*.

high smoking rates tend to live in certain sorts of regions or localities, and this is why rates there are high; the people would smoke wherever they lived, and the place itself has no effect on their likelihood of smoking. A compositional effect has been invoked to explain differences in mortality between subjects in the Paisley/Renfrew study (in the West of Scotland) and in the Whitehall study (in London and the South East of England); it was argued that observed differences between the study populations were due to differences in the distribution of types of people in the two study populations, not to other differences between the West of Scotland and South East of England (Davey Smith *et al.* 1995).

Collective effects relate to the 'social miasma' by which individuals conform to the behaviour of the dominant group living in an area. The third term, contextual, represents the situation where place characteristics have a direct effect and can be equated with the 'genuine ecological effects' referred to above. Contextual effects may either impact on all residents equally, or more on some types of residents than others (for instance males as compared with females). Such influences might include climate, soil or water conditions, the built environment, publicly or privately provided amenities or facilities, sociocultural factors such as predominant religion or history, and the reputation of the area (Macintyre *et al.* 1993). Contextual explanations are perhaps most intuitively plausible when we compare countries: cultural differences in attitudes to smoking may in large part be the reason why middle-class professional men are far more likely to smoke in Paris than in San Francisco; and people in countries bordering the Mediterranean may be more likely to eat fresh fruit and salads all the year round than are those in Russia or Scotland, because of greater availability. The question is whether such explanations also apply to variations *within* countries, whether by regions, districts or neighbourhoods.

Work in social theory provides a start point. Anthony Giddens' structuration theory (Giddens 1984) draws attention to the way in which knowledgeable individuals draw upon social structures in their day-to-day living. Human agents operate within particular sociocultural milieux that contain a number of specific structural factors (conceptualized as rules and resources by Giddens) that stimulate and shape behaviour and constrain outcomes. By drawing on these, society and its constituent individuals produce patterns of behaviours and outcomes that also reproduce the structural factors that were involved. However, as these factors are as much a result of processes and a medium of those processes, there is always the possibility that they will be recreated differently as circumstances change. This recursive process is fundamentally context-specific and Giddens' theory emphasizes the way in which the interplay between individuals (agency) and social factors (structure/context) will be constituted differently at different times and in different settings. Giddens' work is complex and abstract but its (over) simplification here offers an important general reminder of the vitally important connections that exist between phenomena at a number of different levels. Processes operating at macro-levels need to be set alongside knowledgeable and capable human agents behaving at a micro-level.

Less conceptually, it is possible to discern four sets of mechanisms that may produce place differences: processes concerned with the physical environment, the cultural milieux, place deprivation and selective mobility. These are often highly interrelated. The first recognizes that people living in one part of a city or a region are likely to share common water supplies and experience similar levels of environmental pollution. The importance of such physical variables has, as noted earlier, long been recognized (Gardner 1973) but much of this literature has been based on aggregate data. Such ecological variables may then interact with household or individual characteristics such as lead plumbing or tobacco consumption to produce differential health outcomes.

Differences resulting from individual interaction with specific local cultures acknowledge that local specificity must be seen as integral to explanations of general social processes. Processes can never operate on the head of a pin in a geographically undifferentiated world; rather, social processes literally 'take place'. The juxtaposition of disparate forces in a place can create a qualitatively distinct setting which of itself can influence and modify the general processes. People and places exist in a recursive dialectic relationship: people create structures in the context of places; those structures then condition the making of people. People act individually and communally to create these local cultures through their everyday routines and institutional practices. This frames the local context which then provides the setting in which people learn to interpret and respond to general societal structures. As a 'general' process unfolds across space it interacts with places that have both a distinctive history and culture; as a result people change, places change and the uniqueness of place is maintained.

The basic distinction between composition and context is recalled in identifying area effects stemming from differences resulting from processes associated with place deprivation. Smith (1977) long ago summarized the distinction between people and place deprivation. In the former, people are deprived by virtue of their position in the socioeconomic system. In contrast, place-based deprivation refers to poor access to locationally specific goods and services. In the health literature, these arguments have been given a particular twist by Wilkinson (1996). He argues that material infrastructure and societal arrangements are geared through market forces to 'average' people. Thus, food retailing is increasingly arranged for those with a car. Consequently, those without cars have to shop at the more expensive remaining corner shops with their restricted range. Additional costs are incurred and additional effort is required to manage day-to-day tasks. Cummins and Macintyre (2002) and Wrigley (2002) provide empirical support for this argument in their work on the health effects of 'food deserts'. The basic conclusion is that, whatever one's personal characteristics, the opportunity structures in poorer areas are less conducive to health than those in better-off areas.

Differences resulting from the processes of selective mobility distinguish area effects stemming from the cumulative effects of individual mobility and the push and pull area effects of government policy and the market economy. As a result, certain groups of people are constrained while others are enabled; some places attract while others are regarded as 'sink estates' where few would choose to live. Different place-specific health outcomes may then occur as a result of the differential mobility of these different groups. These mechanisms for producing apparent differences between places have long been recognized as potentially important (Hill 1925) and research continues into such notions as the 'healthy migrant' hypothesis (Strachan *et al.* 1995; Brimblecombe *et al.* 1999, 2000; Dorling *et al.* 2000). Of course, contextual differences based purely on selective mechanisms may be seen as something of an artefact: studies of area effects on mortality are notoriously bedeviled by mobility in the years immediately prior to death. However, they also represent an important 'geographical sorting' of the population on which other processes of contextual differentiation may then operate.

These notions of contextuality have general relevance as they apply not only when the focus is on context as geographical setting but also when context is seen in terms of temporal (e.g. different time periods), administrative (e.g. health care administration areas), or institutional (e.g. hospital or clinic) settings. In terms of the last two cases, there are extremely important implications for health services research as they connect with the use of performance indicators. Variations in the performance of health service activities between different settings can be attributed to both the type of clients particular units serve (compositional effects) as well as the nature of the environment from and in which the service is provided (contextual or area effects) (Jones and Moon 1993; Leyland and Goldstein 2001).

Understanding area effects on health thus entails an acknowledgment of the existence of both compositional and contextual effects. The two are intricately connected (Macintyre and Ellaway 2000; Macintyre *et al.* 2002). Though there may be some genuine ecological effects, even these may be mediated or modified by composition. Much health-related data can therefore be expected to exhibit considerable non-stationarity (relationships between variables will not be consistent across all the geographic regions covered by the data); the parameters of association will vary spatially. While this differentiation can be due to model mis-specification or random sampling variation (Fotheringham 1997), it can also be reflective of area effects. To test for that eventuality requires an appropriate analytical strategy. Moreover, that strategy needs to recognize that area effects can be reactive or consensual. In the reactive case, individual and ecological effects operate in the 'opposite direction' while, in the consensual case, the effects are mutually reinforcing.

Some evidence for (real) area effects

Operationalizing ideas about composition and context and isolating the 'reality' of area effects has proved to be difficult and contentious. On the basis of a large-scale empirical study using the UK Health and Lifestyle Survey, Blaxter was convinced that contextual effects are important and that places matter in their own right. She wrote: 'while the health of manual men and women was almost always poorer than that of non-manual, it is clear that types of living area do make a difference' (1990). Fox *et al.* (1984) and Britton *et al.* (1990) replicated this conclusion using the UK Longitudinal Study and Webber and Craig's (1978) national typology of 36 different types of wards. In contrast, Sloggett and Joshi, also using the Longitudinal Study, have suggested that 'excess mortality associated with residence in areas designated as deprived . . . is wholly explained by the concentration in those areas of people with adverse personal or household socio–economic characteristics' (Sloggett and Joshi 1994). They found that a positive linear relationship between ward level deprivation and premature mortality largely disappeared when account was taken of individual socioeconomic characteristics. They support a compositional explanation for geographical variations in mortality although there remains a substantial and significant north-south difference in mortality in their analysis even after controlling for deprivation and individual social characteristics.

The evidence for contextual effects is therefore suggestive but equivocal. As a further example, regional differences in smoking and drinking in Britain have been observed for both men and women, standardized for age and socioeconomic group (Balarajan and Yuen 1986). However, these regional differences varied by sex and according to which measures of these behaviours were used. For example, the proportion that had never smoked did not differ by region for males, though it did for females. Both sexes showed significant variation by region in the proportions that had given up smoking. Standardized smoking ratios for heavy smoking showed a gradient from the North West to South East for both sexes. The suggestion from this and many other studies is that the effects of area or aspects of area on health vary according to individual characteristics, such as gender. This is also consistent with findings on socioeconomic and area variations in health as well as work on health-related behaviours. For example, studies have shown particularly marked health differences between rich and poor people in generally affluent places (Curtis 1995; Ecob 1996)

Thus the existing literature suggests that there may be some variation between areas not accounted for by compositional factors, and that the level of disadvantage or deprivation of the local area may have predictive power over and above individual factors. As Phillimore (1993) has argued: '[the] characteristics of places may be as important as the characteristics of people for an understanding of particular patterns of health'. He suggests that distinctive differences between places (in this case, Sunderland and Middlesborough) remain unexplained by standard accounts of the illness/deprivation nexus.

Moving forward

The arguments above represent the basic case for area effects on health. Just because health outcomes vary geographically, area effects are not necessarily present: compositional factors must be controlled but, once this is done, any remaining variation constitutes an area effect. Control must however be effective and comprehensive. Taken to an extreme, this position can be resolved to one in which area effects might be expected to 'disappear' once full and effective control for composition is made. To paraphrase the methodologist Gary King: 'if we really understood [health variations], we would not need to know much of contextual effects . . .' (1996). His argument finds an empirical parallel with the conclusion of Sloggett and Joshi (1994) that area effects reduce to the impact of composition.

King's is an important challenge to people interested in area effects. It can however be countered. It remains intuitively sensible to test for the possibility of area effects and intuitively plausible that the impact of the composition will vary by context. Unless contextual variables are considered, their direct effects and their indirect mediation by compositional variables cannot be identified. Moreover, composition itself has an areal dimension. Compositional estimates will be inefficient and biased if their inevitable spatial autocorrelation is not recognized in modelling strategies. Of course, controlling for individual factors can identify area effects, but the fact that individual (compositional) factors may 'explain' between-place variation serves as a reminder that real understanding of area effects is complex. Essentially, King's concentration on individuals as separate from their ecologies misses the important point that individuals' actions, choices and experiences are situated in the social-geographical places where they live their lives.

Undoubtedly, then, a key imperative in health research should be the declared aim of articulating the connections between the actions of individuals and the socioecological context in which these actions are performed. This argument suggests an approach that is multilevel, examining the circumstances of individuals at one level, and the contexts or ecologies in which they are located at another level and, crucially, doing so simultaneously. To gain a better understanding of area effects, all the relevant levels of analysis need to be considered at the same time.

Macintyre *et al.* (1993) posed the question: 'Should we be focusing on places or people?' They went on to argue that much health research has overplayed the distinction, given too much emphasis to the compositional and underplayed context. It should not be a case of one or the other, or too much of one and not enough of the other. Simultaneous consideration is essential for a proper understanding of the mechanisms by which places can affect people (Duncan *et al.* 1993).

Multilevel modelling

In the past 15 years multilevel modelling has emerged as the approach of choice within health research for the effective *simultaneous* consideration of composition and context and thus the definitive assessment of area effects on health-related outcomes (see Box 12.6). Its key advantage is that it is conceptually realistic as it

---

Box 12.6   Multilevel analysis

Also known as 'multilevel modelling', a form of statistical analysis akin to regression or generalized linear modelling but modified to work with data that has a hierarchical structure of, for example, people nested in areas. Crucially, it models the layers in the hierarchy simultaneously.

---

handles the micro-scale of composition and the macro-scale of contexts simultaneously within one model. By distinguishing the different 'levels' at which the determinants of health operate, multilevel models are able to treat the contexts identified in any one model as a random sample drawn from a larger underlying population. The procedures then make inferences about the variation among all contexts in the population using this random sample of contexts. Consequently, the variation between contexts is not treated as being fixed but, rather, as a random property that relates to a larger population (DiPrete and Forristal 1994; Hox and Kreft 1994; Blakely and Woodward 2000).

By the mid-1990s the value of the multilevel approach was beginning to be recognized within many different research areas associated with health and health care. Duncan *et al.* (1998), Rice and Leyland (1996) and Von Korff *et al.* 1992 provided reviews. Early health applications focused on institutional performance (Jones and Moon 1990, 1991; Jones *et al.* 1991; Leyland 1995; Leyland and Boddy 1997) and the geography of health-related behaviour (Duncan *et al.* 1993, 1996, 1998, 1999). More recently, the growth in output has been exponential and multilevel analysis has become a standard part of the quantitative health research armoury (Diez Roux 1998, 2000 2002) and the research emphasis has shifted to the complexity of area effects and elucidation of the impacts of social capital and income inequality on health (Subramanian *et al.* 2003c; Subramanian and Kawachi 2004). To this end the approach is now established across a range of disciplines concerned with social epidemology and software options are widely available (see Box 12.7).

> **Box 12.7 Multilevel software**
>
> Two bespoke packages offer a wide range of multilevel analysis capabilities: MLwiN and HLM. MLwiN from Harvey Goldstein's group (http://multilevel.ioe.ac.uk) has tended to be the choice in health research and now incorporates extensive Bayesian routines to improve estimation. HLM (Hierarchical Linear Modelling) is linked to Raudenbush and Bryk 2002. Multilevel analysis is also widely practised using SAS. Other possibilities exist, including a capability within Stata. A relatively up-to-date review is provided by de Leeuw and Kreft (2001).

Multilevel basics

Multilevel analysis requires data that contains measures of both composition and context. At the least, observations within a dataset need to have identifiers that distinguish the contextual setting(s) in which each observation is to be found. Such data are fairly widely available. Surveys, multicentre trials and the products of record linkage exercises typically possess the necessary properties. In Britain, examples include the longitudinal study (LS), the 1991 census Sample of Anonymized Records (SAR), the Health Survey for England (HSE) and the General Household Survey (GHS). British researchers have mainly used data from the routine large-scale surveys deposited in the national data archive. These surveys offer large sample sizes, generally in excess of 15,000 observations each year, and good designs with standardized question formats. Importantly, these designs incorporate hierarchical sampling with respondents drawn at random from randomly selected areas; this multilevel structure should be recognized in any analysis, notwithstanding its additional ability to enable the isolation of area effects.

Data for multilevel analysis are therefore relatively widely available. There are however two general problems that need to be noted and which apply in different ways to most sources. First, there is the matter of confidentiality restrictions. These may limit the availability of individual data, restricting release to a small number of cross-tabulations with limited dimensionality. For example, the dangers of identifying individuals in the census mean that only a few three-way cross tabulations are produced for small areas. Confidentiality may also mean that the identifiers of higher-level sampling units (areas) are not released. The fact that observations come from different areas may be known, but the actual identity of the areas may be confidential. In this situation the scope for linking-in further data to describe an area is lost. The characteristics of an area can only be estimated by aggregating the characteristics of the observations that lie within.

The second data problem that is frequently encountered in multilevel analysis concerns the definition of the higher-level areal units. As noted briefly above in the discussion of the shortcomings of ecological studies, the areas employed in such work rarely have much sociological meaning, though they often have administrative relevance. The same criticism can be applied to multilevel data sources. Area identifiers linked to sampling, such as postcode sectors, enable an insight into local area effects, but they work with areas that mean little to the public. Where such information is not available, perhaps for confidentiality reasons, the researcher can be left with very high-level administrative geographies. In an extreme case, the available areal indicators in the SAR are a relatively coarse, arbitrary sub-regional geography (Gould and Jones 1996).

Four graphical typologies can be used to outline the multilevel approach and show how it provides a framework for contextual analysis in health research that is technically robust. Consider a simple regression model in which it is hypothesized that cigarette consumption (the response variable) is a function of a person's age (the predictor variable). A traditional single-level ordinary least squares (OLS) regression analysis might generate the relationship shown in Figure 12.2a. Here the cigarette consumption/age relationship is shown as a straight line with a positive slope: older people consume more cigarettes. In this model the context in which the behaviour occurs is completely ignored: one single relationship is held to exist everywhere. In effect the model has explained everything in general and nothing in particular.

This can be rectified by recognizing the communities in which individuals live and using a two-level model with individuals at Level 1 nested within communities at Level 2. One possible result is shown in Figure 12.2b, a two-level 'random-intercepts' model. Here each of six different communities has its own cigarette consumption/age relation represented by a separate line. The single, thicker line represents the general relationship across all six communities. The parallel lines imply that, while cigarette consumption increases with age at the same rate in each place, some places have uniformly higher consumption rates than others. With the multilevel approach, therefore, we can see both the general relationship across all places and the particular relationship in specific places. In Figure 12.2c and d the situation is more complicated as the steepness of the lines varies from place to place. In Figure 12.2c the pattern is such that place makes very little difference for the elderly but there is a high degree of between-community variation in the cigarette consumption of the young. In Figure 12.2d there is a complex interaction between age and place. In some communities it is the young who have relatively high rates; in others it is the old.

The differing patterns of Figures 12.2b–d are simply achieved by varying the slopes and intercepts of the lines. If the vertical axis is centred at the mean age of individuals, the intercept represents the number of cigarettes consumed by a person of average age. The slope represents the increase in cigarette consumption associated with a unit increase in age. The key feature of multilevel models is that the communities are treated as a sample drawn from a population and their potentially different intercepts and slopes are treated as coming from two distributions at a higher level. A multilevel analysis summarizes these higher-level distributions in terms of two parts: a 'fixed' part that is unchanging across contexts, and a 'random' part that is allowed to vary. The fixed part gives the mean value of each distribution: the average slope and intercept across all communities (shown by the thick lines in Figure 12.2). The random part consists of variances that summarize the degree to which the community-specific slopes and intercepts differ from these average values.

By adopting a multilevel approach researchers are no longer restricted to working at a single level and this provides a number of substantive advantages. First, by combining individual and aggregate levels together in one analysis both the ecological fallacy (Robinson 1950) and the atomistic fallacy (Alker 1969) can be avoided. Working solely at an individual level means the context of local cultures is ignored, while working just at the aggregate level fails to capture individual variation fully. Second, by working at more than one level, the approach can start to separate compositional from contextual differences. Taking the example of smoking consumption, there may, nationally, be a tendency for older males to be heavy smokers. Consequently, high smoking places may simply result from the concentration of older males in certain locations. Alternatively, they could be a result of regional cultures that encourage smoking in all types of people. The former is a

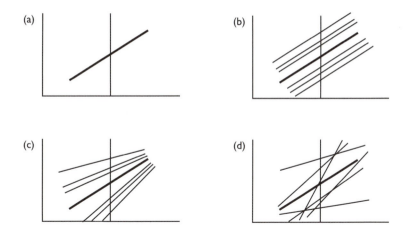

Figure 12.2 Varying slopes and intercepts: a graphical depiction of the multilevel model

Source: Duncan *et al.* (1996)

compositional difference related to the type of people contained within particular contexts. The latter is a contextual effect and refers to the difference arising irrespective of composition. A multilevel approach is able to separate these two effects and therefore has an important role to play in the examination of regional behavioral stereotypes.

By working at several levels simultaneously it becomes possible to allow for contextual variation in the predictor variables. Similar types of people (on the basis of individual characteristics) may not necessarily be behaving in the same way everywhere or experiencing the same health outcomes. The example above talks of the behaviour of people on average across all places and their specific behaviour in particular places. It is possible to model any variation found between places by including fixed variables at higher levels that reflect contextual characteristics. For example, a measure of community deprivation might be included to see whether it was a significant predictor of the variation between places in cigarette consumption by a person of average age. Additionally, cross-level interaction variables can be included as fixed effects. These capture situations where the characteristics of people and the characteristics of contexts interact to produce substantively different expressions of behaviour. For example, people of low social status may consume varying amounts of cigarettes depending upon the social composition of the area in which they live.

In terms of the potential for multilevel models to identify area effects, it is evident, thus far, that the basic methodological gain concerns the ability to 'control for' the impact on some health-related outcome of both the mean level of individual characteristics and the variability of those individual characteristics. The impact on area effects of this control can be evidenced in five fundamental ways. First, fixed part measures of the slopes associated with variables measuring higher-level characteristics indicate the independent effect of such measures having allowed for composition. Thus, to follow through the example above, the inclusion of an area measure of community deprivation in a model would enable the identification of the average effect of area deprivation on cigarette consumption, given the age of people living in an area.

Second, fixed part interactions between compositional and contextual variables (cross-level interactions) can be used to show how, on average, people with particular characteristics experience differential outcomes in the sorts of places indicated by the higher-level variable. Consider a two-level model (individuals in areas) with the response being the probability of an individual reporting limiting long-term illness and an individual predictor variable identifying low social class as opposed to high social class, and an area-level predictor, the percentage of high social class in an area. Cross-level interaction between the individual and the areal-level predictor can reveal a number of possibilities. There may be marked differences between low and high social class individuals in terms of their relationship to the area effect: it might even be negative for low social class but positive for high social class.

The three remaining parameters of interest when identifying area effects concern the random part of the model. It is important to stress that area effects are not only evidenced through fixed part terms; well-designed studies need to consider area effects in terms of the structure of variation. The random part of any model summarizes the variability of slopes, intercepts and their covariance – the degree to which slopes and intercepts are related. Returning to Figure 12.2, the cases shown would each have the same Level 1 random part: a variance term summarizing residual individual variation in cigarette consumption. However, they would differ in terms of their Level 2 random parts. Figure 12.2a is the result of a single non-zero intercept and slope. This is a single-level model and so there are no higher-level distributions: there is no variability between areas as the possibility has not been entertained in the model. Figure 12.2b has a set of intercepts but a single slope common to all areas. This simple third type of area effect would be captured by the random-part measure of intercept variation. The central empirical question concerning area effects is whether this higher-level variation remains significant when a range of appropriate and relevant individual variables (e.g. age, gender, income, class, employment status, housing tenure, educational background etc.) are included in an overall model to allow for the population composition of particular areas.

Figures 12.2c and d show variation in both intercepts and slopes. Measures capturing that variation would indicate area effects that imply both that areas differ and that they differ in relation to age. The fourth type of area effect thus concerns the extent to which slopes differ between areas: in Figure 12.2c age impacts on cigarette consumption much more in some areas than others. The degree of variation between areas changes according to age and does so in an increasing fashion.

The final type of area effect concerns the covariation of slope and intercept variation at the area level. In Figure 12.2c, the cigarette consumption/age relation is strongest in areas where consumption is higher on average; a steep slope is associated with a high intercept. The complex criss-crossing of Figure 12.2d is the result of a lack of pattern in the relationship between the variations in the slopes and intercepts. Overall therefore, the variation in area effects can be summarized by only three terms in the random part of the model. Importantly, this situation prevails whether there are 20 contexts or 200.

As well as looking at complexity in terms of between-area variation, it is also possible to look at variation between individuals. This is beyond the scope of this chapter but, besides being of substantive interest in its own right, complex between-individual heterogeneity can have important implications for estimates of between-area heterogeneity as there may be confounding across levels. What may appear to be higher-level area variability may in fact be between-individual, within-area heterogeneity (Bullen *et al.* 1997).

Just a little algebra

Thus far a graphical approach has been used to introduce the capabilities of multi-level models as a means of identifying area effects on health-related outcomes. Re-expressing these contentions as algebra is relatively straightforward, at least as far as they have been taken above. The fully-random models of Figures 12.2c and d in which both slopes and intercepts vary can be summarized in the equation:

$$Y_{ij} = \beta_0 + \beta_1 X_{ij} + e_{0ij} + u_{0j} + u_{1j}$$

There is a single outcome, cigarette consumption (Y) and a single individual-level predictor variable: age (X) centred about its mean. Y_{ij} represents the cigarette consumption of individual i in place j, X_{ij} is the centred age of individual i in place j. The terms β_0 and β_1 comprise the fixed part of the model and identify, respectively, the intercept (β_0) and the age-related slope (β_1). The β parameters can be interpreted as follows: β_0 is the consumption for individuals of average age. β_1 is the linear increase of consumption with age.

The random part of the model is identified by e_{0ij}, u_{0j} and u_{1j}. These are the 'random' departures from β_0 and β_1. The e_{0ij} captures the variations in *individual* cigarette consumption that are not accounted for by age: the individual 'random' term. They can be summarized by a single variance term, σ^2_{e0}. The u_{0j} identifies the variation in consumption at the *area* level, taking into account individual age and the 'residual' variation at the individual level; it can also be summarized by a single variance term, σ^2_{u0}. Finally, u_{1j} distinguishes the variation in the strength of the relationship between consumption and age across areas: the area-specific variability of the age-related slope (β_1). Its variance is σ^2_{u1}. Without this term, the graph of the equation would be that shown in Figure 12.2b. Not shown in the above equation, but implicitly present, is the covariation of the area-level slopes and intercepts: σ^2_{u10}.

This basic notation builds on the notions of a standard regression model and indicates all that is needed to interpret a simple multilevel model. It can readily be extended by adding additional fixed effects, β terms, measured on either a continuous scale or as a dummy variable, such as sex or the presence/absence of some areal attribute. It should also be noted that a range of different types of response variable can be handled (Rasbash *et al.* 2003). As well as the standard Gaussian model for continuous responses that has been introduced here, logit, log-log and probit models can be specified to model proportions and binary outcomes. Poisson and negative binomial distribution models are available to model counts, and multinomial and ordered multinomial models to model multiple categories.

A multitude of multilevel models

Figure 12.3 reveals the further generalizability of a multilevel approach by showing how the basic two-level structure can be extended to reflect a number of other more complex, yet frequently occurring and substantively interesting, data structures. The two-level structure of Figure 12.3a can be readily extended to the three-level structure of Figure 12.3b with individuals at Level 1 nested within local neighbourhoods at Level 2 and regions at Level 3. Variables can be included at each of the three levels making it possible, for example, to examine the cigarette consumption/age relation in the context of both local economic prosperity and regional economic prosperity. This extension of the framework to many levels is important as it ensures that any area effects are apportioned to the relevant level.

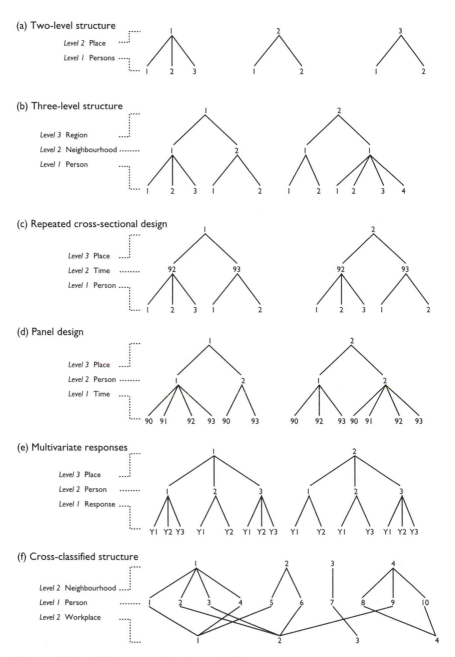

Figure 12.3   Different multilevel possibilities

Source: Duncan *et al.* (1998)

Rice *et al.* (1998) and Weich *et al.* (2004a, 2004b) have focused attention on household membership as a level between individuals and neighbourhoods.

There are many examples of these 'spatial' models in which people nest within areas. Recent examples include Subramanian and Kawachi (2003), Subramanian *et al.* (2003a) and Subramanian *et al.* (2004); Twigg *et al.* (2000a) demonstrate the utility of the approach in synthetic estimation. Moon and Barnett (2003) used a generalized binomial proportional–response model to compare Maori and Pakeha (European) smoking in New Zealand. They were able to work with a four-level model of individuals nested in census tracts, nested in larger census area units, nested in local government districts. The work concluded that, while Maori tend to smoke more than Pakeha, they actually smoke less than might be expected in districts where they form a large fraction of the population. This intriguing finding was linked to notions of relative inequality and prompted an ongoing project on the impact of segregation on smoking behaviour. An earlier example of the basic spatial multilevel model was Duncan *et al.* (1993). This work sparked a number of increasingly complex inquiries into area effects on smoking and drinking through its controversial conclusion that area was of negligible influence on either behaviour. This conclusion was derived from an analysis of the Healthy Lifestyle Survey (HALS) at three levels; individual, ward (local electoral districts, average population size around 5000) and region (22 in UK, average population around 2.5 million). Controlling for a number of individual characteristics reduced regional differences in smoking prevalence to 3 per cent either side of the national average, and average alcohol consumption to 10 per cent either side of the national average.

In passing, at this stage, it should be noted that the key issue in multilevel analysis is hierarchy. So far the focus has been on spatial hierarchies that build from people to local areas to larger regions. Each level in the hierarchy nests within a higher level. There is no reason however why this nesting need be spatial in an areal sense. The classic development of multilevel modelling was in educational research and saw pupils nested within classes within schools (Aitken and Longford 1986; Goldstein 1995). The obvious analogy is patients in wards in hospitals, or people in family doctor lists. These nestings are spatial in a 'point' sense: they link people to point locations rather than areas. Jones and Moon (1991) undertook such an analysis in their study of vaccination uptake and its variation between UK general practices after controlling for the individual characteristics of list members.

A further point to note is that hierarchies need not build from the individual. Area-based outcomes can be considered within higher-level regional contexts. In the absence of individual data, this approach can provide a sound way to control for both 'local' circumstances and the possibility of higher-level regional variations. Langford (1995) used this approach in a study of district-level variation in childhood leukaemia mortality. He worked with 1469 districts nested within 62 higher-level 'counties' and found little variation at the higher level once district variation had been accounted for. The small amount of higher-level variation was greatest for rural areas. The outcome measure was also associated with a high level of people in the armed forces. Langford used these findings to draw tentative conclusions about the relationship of leukaemia to population mixing in small communities.

Health researchers are also obviously interested in how outcome measures change over time (Goldstein *et al.* 1994). Moon *et al.* (2002) provide an exploratory example but the multilevel framework itself can be modified to understand context in terms of temporal settings. Figure 12.3c shows how a repeated cross-sectional design can be represented as a multilevel structure. Here, Level 3 in the hierarchy identifies areas, Level 2 is years and Level 1 is individuals. Thus, Level 2 represents repeated measurements of places. Such a structure can be used to examine outcome trends within higher-level units, taking account of their changing compositional make-up. A recent example of this design is provided by Jones and Jen (2004) who used data from the World Values Survey with self-rated health as the response variable and individuals at Level 1, survey years at Level 2 and the countries of the World Values Survey at Level 3. One of the bonuses in this design is that it is relatively robust to imbalance; countries do not have to report for every survey year.

Figure 12.3d shows another way in which time as context can be built into a multilevel analysis. In a repeated individual measures or 'panel design', Level 1 is the measurement occasion indexed by its time, Level 2 is the individual and Level 3 refers to areas. Thus, Level 1 represents repeated measurements of a group of individuals at particular times, while the characteristics of the individuals are recorded at Level 2. Such a structure allows the assessment of individual change within a contextual setting. Unlike conventional repeated measures methods which require a fixed set of repeated observations for all persons, both the number of observations per person and the temporal spacing among the observations may vary in a multilevel approach. Recent examples of the repeated individual measures design are provided by Neuendorfer *et al.* (2001) in a study of the effects, over time, of depressive symptoms in persons with Alzheimer's disease on depression in their family caregivers. They found that the rate of increase in caregiver depression was predicted by the rate of increase in patient depressive symptoms and by increases in patient dependency in activities of daily living. Other examples are provided by Hardy *et al.* (2003) and Sithole and Jones (2002); an extensive discussion is available in Singer and Willett (2003) whose fourth chapter gives explicit consideration to a muiltilevel panel model of alcohol consumption.

A further example of bringing in time as context in a multilevel framework concerns survival models where attention is focused on the time to an event. In these cases, the concern is with the survival of individuals (with particular characteristics) in particular contexts. An example would be the time a respondent stays alive after the beginning of a trial; this could be related to both individual and contextual characteristics. Such an approach requires special methods as the complete survival time is often unknown for many respondents. Jones *et al.* (2004) discuss this research direction.

Bringing in greater complexity

Conceptually, the same response measured at different times is no different from many responses measured at one time. Consequently, the multilevel framework can also be used to represent several different, though related, response variables. In the case of health research, this enables researchers to examine several different measures/dimensions of health status simultaneously. These different measures form a set of response variables at Level 1, which nest within individuals at Level 2, who nest within communities at Level 3. This form of multilevel structure is shown in Figure 12.3e. It is not necessary for measurements to be made on all individuals for all responses and the model can accommodate sets of responses that are a mixture of both categorical and continuous variables as well as situations where the responses are measured in the same way.

The multivariate multilevel model has great potential as researchers are often interested in two (or more) different, though related, dimensions of health. Duncan *et al.* (1996) and Twigg *et al.* (2000b) both provide case studies of the approach. The former examined the interrelation of the decision to smoke and the amount smoked, finding that areas with many smokers also tend to have people who smoke more. The latter investigated the simultaneous effect of individual demographic characteristics and sociostructural factors on self-reported problem drinking as revealed by CAGE scores and 'unsafe' levels of alcohol consumption. While the influence of key sociostructural variables was broadly similar for both unsafe alcohol consumption and high CAGE scores, there were notable exceptions when results were examined by tenure group: those in the rented sector were more likely to be problem drinkers as revealed by CAGE, but less likely to consume (unsafe) amounts of alcohol. Both dimensions of drinking behaviour were influenced by the consumption patterns of others in the household, with both likelihoods increasing as the average consumption of others in the household rose. The authors also found that the proportion of the population whose drinking behaviour might be classed as (potentially) problematic via the CAGE responses was substantially less than the proportion consuming above recommended 'safe' levels.

All the models considered so far have been strictly hierarchical, and contextual effects have nested within each other. Such a conception is frequently unrealistic and does not exhaust the possibilities of the multilevel formulation. Contextual sources of variation overlap and more than one may exist at each level. The resulting structure may be hierarchical, but the hierarchy is complex. Each lower-level unit may belong to more than one unit at the next higher level. In the case of health outcomes, an individual's health status may be influenced both by where they live and where they work. This can be modelled using a cross-classified structure with individuals at Level 1 and both neighbourhood and workplace at Level 2. This structure is shown in Figure 12.3f. Explanatory variables can be included for individual-level characteristics and for both Level 2 units. Substantively, this allows different contexts to be simultaneously modelled, making it possible to identify contextual settings that are having a confounding influence (Rasbash and Browne 2001). What appears as between-workplace variation may in fact really be between-neighbourhood variation.

Langford and Bentham (1996) provide an example of a multilevel cross-classified analysis. Their Level 1 was a geographical area, English health authorities, and their outcome measure was the standardized mortality ratio for males and females for each district. At Level 2 they had crossed measures for the region and for an area typology, the ACORN family. The main point of interest was that a district in any one region might be in any of the several ACORN families, and vice versa. From their study, they were able to conclude region accounts for approximately four times more variation in standardized mortality ratios (SMRs) than is explained by the ACORN classification and a clear north-south divide in excess mortality remains when both region and socioeconomic classification are modeled simultaneously.

Recently, attention has focused on the additional complexity that can result when higher-level units are defined by a membership made of lower-level units and that membership changes over time (Goldstein 2003). In the simple example of people nested within areas, an individual might move several times and any individual-level outcome might reflect area effects drawn from several contexts. Subramanian (2004) elaborates this model and Figure 12.4 provides a visual summary. Time measurements (Level 1) are nested within individuals (Level 2) who are in turn nested in neighbourhoods (Level 3). Importantly, individuals are assigned different weights for the time spent in each neighbourhood. For example, individual 25 moved from Neighbourhood 1 to Neighbourhood 25 during time period t1–t2, spending 20 per cent of her time in Neighbourhood 1 and 80 per cent in her new neighbourhood. This multiple-membership design should allow control of changing context as well as changing composition. It can also be extended to enable consideration of weighted effects of proximate contexts (Langford et al. 1999). So, for example, the geographical distribution of disease can be seen not only as a

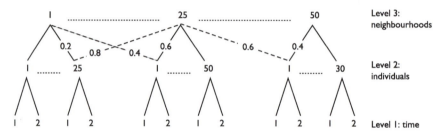

Figure 12.4   A repeated measures spatial multilevel model with multiple membership

Source: Subramanian (2004)

matter of composition and the immediate context in which an outcome occurs, but also a consequence of the impact of nearby contexts with nearer areas being more influential than more distant ones. As perhaps the ultimate extension of this idea, Goldstein (2003) talks of the modelling of area-level outcomes in which the area is conceptualized as having a multiple membership of individuals.

If multilevel models are constructed that are 'realistically complex' (Best *et al.* 1996) a better understanding of area effects and the ecology of health may result. Reaching this goal is likely to require a combination of different structures in any analysis. Incorporating both time and area in an analysis is central to this task. Few people stay forever in the same single context; most move from one to other. Meeting this challenge underlines the need for high-quality geo-referenced data.

Cautionary notes

Despite the considerable research attention that has focused on multilevel analysis, the approach is not without its problems. Nor is it without its critics and outstanding challenges. Three issues can be isolated. The first relates to sample sizes. To obtain reliable estimates of both within- and between-area variation, we require *many* individuals from *many* areas. The former allows a precise assessment of within-area relationships, the latter a precise assessment of between-area relationships, and the two together allow one to be distinguished from the other. Of course, there can be some compromise between the number of higher- and lower-level units, but the net result is that data requirements are substantial. Many studies will not be able to satisfy these criteria, particularly with regard to the number of contexts (sampled and distinguishable areas). It is important moreover to note that there are substantial technical implications if multilevel analyses are carried out when the number of higher-level units is small, including downwardly-biased variance estimates. Recent developments in Monte Carlo Markov Chain approaches to multilevel modelling (Goldstein 2003; Rasbash *et al.* 2003) can alleviate this problem somewhat but with a concomitant computational overhead.

The second issue relates to operationalizing context in terms of the hierarchical structure of particular datasets (Sampson and Morenoff 2002). This problem is most formidable in terms of analyses focusing on indeterminate spatial structures rather than more clearly defined institutional ones. Massey (1991) makes the central point: 'localities are not simple areas you can easily draw a line around'. Yet many health-based multilevel studies pay little attention to this warning and use the structure of the dataset to define higher-level units. These structures often derive from administrative boundaries and, while they may capture some notion of context, they often have no explicit theoretical justification in terms of the outcomes being studied.

Third, multilevel studies face a set of challenges in terms of their operationalization. The need for realistic complexity has already been noted. So too has the need to recognize that area effects are seldom caputured in a simple hierarchy but are themselves subject to autocorrelation with adjoining and overlapping areas. More straightforwardly, however, there is a need to counter a tendency to focus on the fixed effects in models by an enhanced consideration of the random part (Subramanian *et al.* 2003b). Complex variance-covariance structures are often necessary in order to understand fully the nature of area effects. An inevitable counterpoint of this tendency to complexity, necessary or not, must also be the development of robust procedures for model testing and diagnostic analysis (Langford and Lewis 1998; Leyland and Goldstein 2001).

Conclusions

This chapter has moved from an assessment of ecological studies, through a consideration of methodological issues associated with the notion of area effects, to an outline of the utility of multilevel models as a coherent framework for framing and testing ideas about contextuality and variability. A key strength of the multilevel framework is its considerable generality. It can be used to tackle a number of different and important questions of interest to health researchers. It is now increasingly recognized that area effects are complex. As Jones and Duncan (1996) note, there has been too much stress in health research on the stereotypical and the average and not enough on variability. There is seldom a single area effect; reality is heterogeneous: there are multiple area effects.

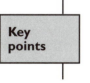

Key points

- Area-based studies run the risk of the ecological fallacy. There is no certainty that an observed difference between areas applies to all individuals within each area.

- Individual studies risk the atomistic fallacy. They are decontextualized and imply that everything is the same everywhere.

- Research into area effects (also known as contextual effects) needs to control for composition (the characteristics of the individuals within an area).

- Multilevel models provide a means of achieving such control and can be applied in a range of different designs that capture spatial, temporal and multiple settings.

- Realistically complex modelling is required to gain a better understanding of area effects.

Further reading

The statistical basis of multilevel modelling is set out in Goldstein (1995), Raudenbush and Bryk (2002), Snijders and Bosker (1999), Hox (2002), and Kreft and de Leeuw (1998). This latter is perhaps the simplest entry-level text. The websites of Goldstein's multilevel models project (http://multilevel.ioe.ac.uk) and Bryk and Raudenbush's 'hierarchical linear modelling' project (http://www.ssicentral.com/hlm/hlm.htm) are both helpful, particularly the former. Goldstein has collaborated with Leyland on a recent text setting out health applications in some detail (Leyland and Goldstein 2001). Throughout the chapter reference has been made to the authors' work applying multilevel models; a set of papers from the mid and late 1990s outline this work in the area of health-related behaviour (Duncan *et al.* 1993, 1996, 1998, 1999). Useful recent reviews of health-related multilevel modelling include Diez Roux (2000, 2001), Pickett and Pearl (2001) and Subramanian *et al.* (2003b). On area effects more generally, see Macintyre *et al.* (1993). For an alternative perspective on ecological analysis and a relief from health research, read King (1996).

References

Acheson, D. (Chair) (1998) *Independent Inquiry into Inequalities in Health: Report.* London: The Stationery Office.

Aitken, M. and Longford, N. (1986) Statistical modelling in school effectiveness studies, *Journal of the Royal Statistical Society A*, 149: 1–43.

Alker, H. (1969) A typology of ecological fallacies, in M. Dogan and S. Rokkan (eds) *Quantitative Ecological Analysis.* Cambridge, MA: MIT Press.

Asthana, S., Gibson, A. and Moon, G. *et al.* (2004) The demographic and social class basis of inequality in self-reported morbidity: an exploration using the Health Survey for England, *Journal of Epidemiology and Community Health*, 58: 303–7.

Balarajan, R. and Yuen, P. (1986) British smoking and drinking habits: regional variations, *Community Medicine*, 8: 131–7.

Ben-Shlomo, Y., White, I.R. and Marmot, M. (1996) Does the variation in the socio-economic characteristics of an area affect mortality? *British Medical Journal*, 312: 1013–14.

Best, N., Spiegelhalter, D., Thomas, A. and Brayne, C. (1996) Bayesian analysis of realistically complex models, *Journal of the Royal Statistical Society A*, 159: 232–342.

Blakeley, T. and Woodward, A. (2000) Ecological effects in multi-level studies, *Journal of Epidemiology and Community Health*, 54: 367–74.

Blaxter, M. (1990) *Health and Lifestyles.* London: Tavistock.

Braddon, F., Wadsworth, M., Davies, J. and Cripps, H. (1988) Social and regional differences in food and alcohol consumption and their measurement in a national birth cohort, *Journal of Epidemiology and Community Health*, 42: 341–9.

Brimblecombe, N., Dorling, D. and Shaw, M. (1999) Mortality and migration in Britain – first results from the British Household Panel Survey, *Social Science and Medicine*, 49: 981–8.

Brimblecombe, N., Dorling, D. and Shaw, M. (2000) Migration and geographical inequalities in health in Britain, *Social Science and Medicine*, 50: 861–78.

Britton, M., Fox, A., Goldblatt, P. *et al.* (1990) The influence of socio-economic and environmental factors on geographic variation in mortality, in M. Britton (ed.) *Mortality and Geography: A Review in the Mid-1980s.* London: HMSO.

Bullen, N., Jones, K. and Duncan, C. (1997) Modelling complexity: analysing between-individual and between-place variation – a multilevel tutorial, *Environment and Planning A*, 29: 585–609.

CACI (2003) Welcome to the new ACORN, www.caci.co.uk/acorn/default.asp (accessed 20 April 2004).

Carstairs, V. and Morris, V. (1991) *Deprivation and Health in Scotland.* Aberdeen: Aberdeen University Press.

Cummins, S. and Macintyre, S. (2002) Food deserts: evidence and assumption in health policy making, *British Medical Journal*, 325: 436–8

Curtis, S. (1995) Geographical perspectives on poverty, health and health policy in different parts of the UK, in C. Philo (ed.) *Off The Map: The Social Geography of Poverty in The UK.* London: Child Poverty Action Group.

Curtis, S. and Jones, I. (1998) Is there a place for geography in the analysis of health inequality? *Sociology of Health and Illness*, 20: 645–72.

Davey Smith, G., Shipley, M., Hole, D. *et al.* (1995) Explaining male mortality differentials between the West of Scotland and the South of England, *Journal of Epidemiology and Community Health*, 49: 541.

De Leeuw, J. and Kreft, I. (2001) Software for multilevel modelling, in A. Leyland and H. Goldstein (eds) (2001) *Multilevel Modelling of Health Statistics*. Chichester: Wiley.

Department of Health (1988) *The Health of the Nation*. London: HMSO.

Diez Roux, A. (1998) Bringing context back into epidemiology: variables and fallacies in multilevel analysis, *American Journal of Public Health*, 88: 216–22.

Diez Roux, A. (2000) Multilevel analysis in public health research, *Annual Review of Public Health*, 21: 171–92.

Diez Roux, A. (2001) Investigating neighbourhood and area effects on health, *American Journal of Public Health*, 91: 1783–9.

Diez Roux, A. (2002) A glossary for multilevel analysis, *Journal of Epidemiology and Community Health*, 56: 588–94.

DiPrete, T. and Forristal, J. (1994) Multilevel models: methods and substance, *Annual Review of Sociology*, 20: 331–57.

Dorling, D., Shaw, M. and Brimblecombe, N. (2000) Housing wealth and community health: exploring the role of migration, in H. Graham (ed.) *Understanding Health Inequalities*. Buckingham: Open University Press.

Drever, F. and Whitehead, M. (1995) Mortality in regions and local authority districts in the 1990s: exploring the relationship with deprivation, *Population Trends*, winter: 19–26.

Dunbar, G. and Morgan, D. (1987) The changing pattern of alcohol consumption in England and Wales 1978–1985, *British Medical Journal*, 295: 807–10.

Duncan, C., Jones, K. and Moon, G. (1993) Do places matter? A multilevel analysis of regional variations in health-related behaviour in Britain, *Social Science and Medicine*, 37: 725–33.

Duncan, C., Jones, K. and Moon, G. (1996) Health-related behaviour in context: a multilevel modeling approach, *Social Science and Medicine*, 42: 817–30.

Duncan, C., Jones, K. and Moon, G. (1998) Context, composition and heterogeneity: using multilevel models in health research, *Social Science and Medicine*, 46: 97–117.

Duncan, C., Jones, K. and Moon, G. (1999) Smoking and deprivation: are there neighbourhood effects? *Social Science and Medicine*, 48: 497–505.

Eames, M., Ben-Shlomo, Y. and Marmot, M. (1993) Social deprivation and premature mortality: regional comparison across England, *British Medical Journal*, 307: 1097–102.

Ecob, R. (1996) A multilevel modelling approach to examining the effects of area of residence on health and functioning, *Journal of the Royal Statistical Society A*, 159: 61–76.

Ellen, I., Mijanovich, T. and Dillman, K. (2001) Neighbourhood effects in health: exploring the links and assessing the evidence, *Journal of Urban Affairs*, 23: 391–408.

Experian (2004) *MOSAIC United Kingdom: The Consumer Classification for the UK*. London: Experian.

Fotheringham, A. (1997) Trends in quantitative methods 1: stressing the local, *Progress in Human Geography*, 21: 88–96.

Fox, A., Jones, D. and Goldblatt, P. (1984) Approaches to studying the effect of socio-economic circumstances on geographical differences in mortality in England and Wales, *British Medical Bulletin*, 40: 309–14.

Gardner, M. (1973) Using the environment to explain and predict mortality, *Journal of the Royal Statistical Society*, Series A, 136: 421–40.

Giddens, A. (1984) *The Constitution of Society*. Cambridge: Polity Press.

Goldstein, H. (1995) *Multilevel Statistical Models*. London: Edward Arnold.

Goldstein, H. (2003) Multilevel modelling of educational data, in D. Courgeau (ed.) *Methodology and Epistemology of Multilevel Analysis*. Amsterdam: Kluwer.

Goldstein, H., Healy, M. and Rasbash, J. (1994) Multilevel time-series models with applications to repeated-measures data, *Statistics In Medicine*, 13: 1643–55.

Gould, M. and Jones, K. (1996) Analysing perceived limiting long-term illness using UK census microdata, *Social Science and Medicine*, 42: 857–69.

Hampson, C. (1991) The utility of ecologic methodology in geographic studies of disease, *The Operational Geographer*, 9: 25–8.

Hardy, R., Kuh, D., Langenberg, C. and Wadsworth, M. (2003) Birthweight, childhood social class and change in adult blood pressure in the 1946 British birth cohort, *Lancet*, 362: 1178–83

Hill, A. (1925) Internal migration and its effect upon the death rates, *MRC Special Report Series*, 95: London: HMSO.

Hox J. (2002) *Multilevel Analysis: Techniques and Applications*. Hillsdale, NJ: Lawrence Erlbaum Associates

Hox, J. and Kreft, I. (1994) Multilevel analysis methods, *Sociological Methods and Research*, 22: 283–99.

Illsley, R. and Le Grand, J. (1993) Regional inequalities in mortality, *Journal of Epidemiology and Community Health*, 47: 444–9.

Jarman, B. (1984) Underprivileged areas: validation and distribution of scores, *British Medical Journal*, 289: 1587–92.

Jones, K. and Duncan, C. (1995) Individuals and their ecologies: analysing the geography of chronic illness within a multilevel modelling framework, *Health and Place*, 1: 27–40.

Jones, K. and Duncan, C. (1996) People and places: the multilevel model as a general framework for the quantitative analysis of geographical data, in P. Longley and M. Batty (eds) *Spatial Analysis: Modelling in a GIS Environment*. London: Pion.

Jones, K. and Jen, M-H. (2004) *Investigating the Absolute and Relative Income Hypothesis: Problems of Analysis and Measurement*. Bristol: School of Geographical Sciences, University of Bristol (mimeo).

Jones, K. and Moon, G. (1990) A multilevel model approach to immunisation uptake, *Area*, 22: 264–71.

Jones, K. and Moon, G. (1991) Re-assessing immunization uptake as a performance measure in general practice, *British Medical Journal*, 303: 28–31.

Jones, K. and Moon, G. (1993) Medical geography: taking space seriously, *Progress in Human Geography*, 17: 515–24.

Jones, K., Moon, G. and Clegg, A. (1991) Ecological and individual effects in childhood immunisation uptake: a multilevel approach, *Social Science and Medicine*, 33: 501–8.

Jones, K., Duncan, C. and Twigg, L. (2004) Evaluating the absolute and relative income, hypotheses: an exploratory analysis of deaths in the Health and Lifestyle Survey, in P. Boyle, (ed.) *The Geography of Health Inequalities in the Developed World*. Aldershot: Ashgate.

King, G. (1996) *A Solution to the Ecological Inference Problem: Reconstructing Individual Behavior from Aggregate Data*. Princeton, NJ: Princeton University Press.

Kreft, I. and de Leeuw, J. (1998) *Introducing Multilevel Modelling*, Thousand Oaks, CA: Sage.

Langford, I. (1995) A multilevel log-linear model of childhood leukaemia mortality, *Health and Place*, 1: 113–20.

Langford, I. and Bentham, G. (1996) Regional variations in mortality rates in England and Wales: an analysis using multilevel modelling, *Social Science and Medicine*, 42: 897–908.

Langford, I. and Lewis, T. (1998) Outliers in multilevel data, *Journal of the Royal Statistical Society A*, 161: 121–60.

Langford, I., Leyland, A., Rasbash, J. and Goldstein, H. (1999) Multilevel modelling of the geographical distribution of diseases, *Journal of the Royal Statistical Society*, C, 48: 253–68.

Leyland, A. (1995) Examining the relationship between length of stay and readmission rates for selected diagnoses in Scottish hospitals, *IMA Journal of Mathematics Applied in Medicine and Biology*, 12: 175–84.

Leyland, A. and Boddy, F. (1997) Measuring performance in hospital care: length of stay in gynaecology, *European Journal of Public Health*, 7: 136–43.

Leyland, A. and Goldstein, H. (eds) (2001) *Multilevel Modelling of Health Statistics*. Chichester: Wiley.

Macintyre, S. (1995). What are spatial effects and how can we measure them? in A. Dale (ed.) Exploiting national survey and census data: the role of locality and spatial effects, *CCSR Occasional Paper*, 12. Manchester: University of Manchester.

Macintyre, S. and Ellaway, A. (2000) Ecological approaches: rediscovering the role of physical and social environment in I. Kawachi, and L. Berkman (eds) *Neighbourhoods and Health*. New York: Oxford University Press.

Macintyre, S., MacIver, S. and Sooman, A. (1993) Area, class and health: should we be focusing on places or people? *Journal of Social Policy*, 22: 213–34.

Macintyre, S., Ellaway, A. and Cummins, S. (2002) Place effects on health: how can we conceptualise, operationalise and measure them? *Social Science and Medicine*, 55: 125–39.

Massey, D. (1991) The political place of locality studies, *Environment and Planning A*, 23: 267–81.

Meltzer, H., Gatward, R., Goodman, R. and Ford, T. (2000) *The Mental Health of Children and Adolescents in England*. London: The Stationery Office.

Mitchell, R. (2001) Multilevel modelling might not be the answer, *Environment and Planning A*, 33: 1357–60.

Mitchell, R., Dorling, D. and Shaw, M. (2000) *Inequalities in Life and Death: What if Britain Were More Equal?* Bristol: Policy Press.

Moon, G., Mohan, J., Twigg, L. *et al.* (2002) Catching waves: the historical geography of the general practice fundholding initiative in England and Wales, *Social Science and Medicine*, 55: 2201–13.

Moon, G. and Barnett, R. (2003) Spatial scale and the geography of tobacco smoking in New Zealand: a multilevel perspective, *New Zealand Geographer*, 59(2): 6–15.

Mullen, K. (1992) Area and health in cities: a review of the literature, *International Journal of Sociology and Social Policy*, 10: 1–24.

Neundorfer, M., McClendon, M., Smyth, K. *et al.* (2001) A longitudinal study of the relationship between levels of depression among persons with Alzheimer's disease and levels of depression among their family caregivers, *Journal Of Gerontology, Series B – Psychological Sciences And Social Sciences*, 56: 301–13.

Openshaw, S. (1983) The modifiable areal unit problem, *Concepts and Techniques in Modern Geography Series*, 38: Norwich: Geo Books.

Phillimore, P. (1993) How do places shape health? Rethinking locality and lifestyle in North-East England, in S. Platt (ed.) *Locating Health: Sociological and Historical Implications*. Aldershot: Avebury.

Pickett, K. and Pearl, M. (2001) Multilevel analyses of neighbourhood socioeconomic context and health outcomes: a critical review, *Journal of Epidemiology and Community Health*, 55: 111–22.

Rasbash, J. and Browne, W.J. (2001) Modelling non-hierarchical structures, in A.H. Leyland and H. Goldstein (eds) *Multilevel Modelling of Health Statistics*. Chichester: Wiley.

Rasbash, J., Steele, F., Browne, W. and Prosser, B. (2003) *A User's Guide to MLwiN, Version 2*. London: Institute of Education.

Raudenbush, S. and Bryk, A. (2002) *Hierarchical Linear Models: Applications and Data Analysis Methods*. London: Sage.

Rice, N. and Leyland, A. (1996) Multilevel models: applications to health data, *Journal of Health Services Research and Policy*, 1: 154–64.

Rice, N., Carr-Hill, R., Dixon, P. and Sutton, M. (1998) The influence of households on drinking behaviour: a multilevel analysis, *Social Science and Medicine*, 46: 971–9.

Robinson, W. (1950) Ecological correlations and the behaviour of individuals, *American Sociological Review*, 15: 351–7.

Sampson, R. and Morenoff, J. (2002) Assessing neighbourhood effects: social process and new directions in research, *Annual Review of Sociology*, 28: 443–78.

Senior, M. (1991) Deprivation payments to GPs: not what the doctor ordered, *Environment and Planning C*, 9: 79–94.

Shaw, M., Dorling, D., Gordon, D. and Davey Smith, G. (1999) *The Widening Gap: Health Inequalities and Policy in Britain*. Bristol: Policy Press.

Shouls S., Congdon, P. and Curtis, S. (1996) Geographic variations in illness and mortality: the development of a relevant area typology for SAR districts, *Health and Place*, 2: 139–56.

Singer, J. and Willett, J. (2003) *Applied Longitudinal Data Analysis: Modelling Change and Event Occurrence*. New York: Oxford University Press.

Sithole, J. and Jones, P. (2002) Repeated measures models for prescribing change, *Statistics in Medicine*, 21: 571–87.

Sloggett, A. and Joshi, H. (1994) Higher mortality in deprived areas: community or personal disadvantage? *British Medical Journal*, 309: 1470–4.

Smith, D. (1977) *Human Geography: A Welfare Approach*. London: Edward Arnold.

Snijders, T. and Bosker, R. (1999) *Multilevel Analysis: An Introduction to Basic and Advanced Multilevel Modeling*. London: Sage.

Strachan, D., Leon, D. and Dodgeon, B. (1995) Mortality from cardiovascular disease among interregional migrants in England and Wales, *British Medical Journal*, 310: 423–7.

Subramanian, S. (2004) The relevance of multilevel statistical methods for identifying causal neighbourhood effects, *Social Science and Medicine*, 58: 1961–7.

Subramanian, S. and Kawachi, I. (2003) The association between state income inequality and worse health is not confounded by race, *International Journal of Epidemiology*, 32: 1022–8.

Subramanian, S. and Kawachi, I. (2004) Income inequality and health: what have we learned so far? *Epidemiologic Reviews*, 26: 78–91.

Subramanian, S., Delgado, I., Jadue, L. *et al.* (2003a) Income inequality and health: multilevel analysis of Chilean communities, *Journal of Epidemiology and Community Health*, 57: 844–8.

Subramanian, S., Jones, K. and Duncan, C. (2003b) Multilevel methods for public health research, in I. Kawachi and L. Berkman (eds) *Neighbourhoods and Health*. New York: Oxford University Press.

Subramanian, S., Lochner, K. and Kawachi, I. (2003c) Neighbourhood differences in social capital: a compositional artefact or a contextual construct? *Health and Place*, 9: 33–44.

Subramanian, S., Nandy, S., Kelly, M. *et al.* (2004) Patterns and distribution of tobacco consumption in India: cross-sectional evidence from the 1998–9 national family health survey, *British Medical Journal*, 328: 801–6.

Susser, M. (1973) *Causal Thinking in the Health Sciences*. London: Oxford University Press.

Thomas, C. (1993) Public health strategies in Sheffield and England: a comparison of conceptual foundations, *Health Promotion International*, 8: 299.

Townsend, P., Davidson, N. and Whitehead, M. (1988a) *Inequalities in Health*. London: Penguin.

Townsend, P., Phillimore, P. and Beattie, A. (1988b) *Health and Deprivation: Inequality in the North*. London: Croom Helm.

Twigg, L., Moon, G. and Jones, K. (2000a) Predicting small-area health-related behaviour: a comparison of smoking and drinking indicators, *Social Science and Medicine*, 50: 1109–20

Twigg, L., Moon, G., Jones, K. and Duncan, C. (2000b) Consumed with worry: 'unsafe' alcohol consumption and self-reported problem drinking in England, *Health Education Research*, 15: 569–80.

Von Korff, M., Koepsell, T., Curry, S. and Diehr, P. (1992) Multilevel analysis in epidemiologic research on health behaviours and outcomes, *American Journal of Epidemiology*, 132: 1077–82.

Webber, R. and Craig, J. (1978) Socio-economic classification of local authorities, *Studies on Medical and Population Subjects*, 35.

Weich, S., Twigg, L., Holt, G. *et al.* (2004a) Contextual risk factors for the common mental disorders in Britain: a multilevel investigation of the effects of place, *Journal of Epidemiology and Community Health*, 57: 616–21.

Weich, S., Twigg, L., Holt, G. *et al.* (2004b) Geographic variation in the prevalence of common mental disorders in Britain: a multilevel investigation, *American Journal of Epidemiology*, 157: 730–7.

Whichelow, M., Erzinclioglu, S. and Cox, B. (1991) Some regional variations in dietary patterns in a random sample of British adults, *European Journal of Clinical Nutrition*, 45: 253–62.

Wiggins, R., Bartley, M., Gleave, S. *et al.* (1998) Limiting long-term illness: a question of where you live or who you are? A multilevel analysis of the 1971–1991 ONS longitudinal study, *Risk, Decision and Policy*, 3: 181–98.

Wilkinson, R. (1996) *Unhealthy Societies*. London: Routledge.

Wrigley, N. (2002) Food deserts in British cities: policy context and research priorities, *Urban Studies*, 39: 2029–40.

Mathematical models in health care

Jane P. Biddulph

Introduction

A model is a description of some system intended to predict what happens if certain actions are taken (Bratley *et al.* 1987). Model types include physical (sometimes called iconic), conceptual and mathematical.

Physical models

A typical example of a physical model is a wind tunnel to study the aerodynamics of an aeroplane wing. Bratley *et al.* (1987) suggest that engineers presumably use wind tunnels because they are sceptical as to whether differential equations (as a mathematical model of the system) adequately model the real system, or whether the differential equation solver available (computer software) is reliable.

Conceptual models

Conceptual models are often schematic. They describe general and major concepts and their interrelations, and therefore are useful to communicate ideas. These have been used to describe the organization and management of health care and health promotion. However, all research has an underlying conceptual framework/model. These form part of the research process, and provide a basis on which testable research can be formulated, even though the model itself is not testable.

Mathematical models

Edwards and Hamson (2001) describe a mathematical model as a model created using mathematical concepts such as functions and equations. However, due to the complexity of the mathematics involved, many mathematical models are not fully described mathematically in terms such as functions or equations. For this reason, the description that in a mathematical model the important aspect of the situation being modelled can be treated quantitatively (Hayden 2000) is potentially less confusing. Dean *et al.* (1997) distinguished mathematical models that are used to investigate problems and aid decision-making from statistical models: mathematical models are manipulated to explore potential solutions to a problem whereas statistical models are used for describing and simplifying data. Mathematical models that are used to investigate problems and aid decision-making are the focus of this chapter.

A model is almost always a simplification of the real system. This may be due to incomplete knowledge of the real system, difficulties in describing or collecting information on aspects of the system, or for economic reasons, in that it would just be too expensive to try and produce a model of any real system exactly. For a model to be useful it must adequately reflect the features of the system that are important to its application. A perfect model of the real system would produce exactly the same output measurements as the real system under the same inputs. The model in Figure 13.1, would not therefore be perfect as it has fewer inputs and different outputs.

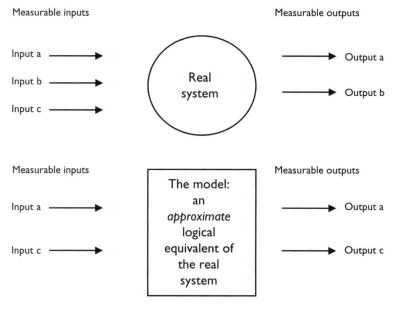

Figure 13.1   Real system and the model

Source: adapted from Bratley *et al.* (1987)

Uses of a mathematical model

With reference to mathematical models, a health care evaluation model has been defined by the ISPOR Task Force on Good Research Practices (Weinstein *et al.* 2003) as 'an analytic methodology that accounts for events over time and across populations, that is based on data drawn from primary and/or secondary sources, and whose purpose is to estimate the effects of an intervention on valued health consequences and costs'. The Task Force state that the purpose of the model is to reveal the relation between assumptions and outcomes, and that these assumptions include:

- structural assumptions about causal linkages between variables;
- quantitative parameters such as disease incidence, prevalence, treatment efficacy and effectiveness;

- survival rates;
- health state utilities;
- utilization rates;
- unit costs;
- value judgements that are valued by decision-makers.

The Task Force go on to say that 'a good study based on a model makes all of these assumptions explicit and transparent and states its conclusions conditionally upon them'.

Hethcote and Van Ark (1992) identified and described 15 purposes of epidemiological modelling and three limitations. These purposes and limitations are also applicable to many of the mathematical models used in health care, which would be described as epidemiological models by Hethcote and Van Ark. This is because epidemiology is the study of the distribution and determinants of disease prevalence in humans, and the functions of epidemiology include the building and testing of theories, and planning, implementing and evaluating detection, control and prevention programmes. Modelling plays an important role in these functions.

The 15 purposes of modelling, as identified by Hethcote and Van Ark (1992) are:

1 The model formulation process clarifies assumptions, variables and parameters.
2 The behaviour of precise mathematical models can be analysed using mathematical methods and computer simulations.
3 Modelling allows explorations of the effect of different assumptions and formulations.
4 Modelling provides concepts.
5 Modelling is an experimental tool for testing theories and assessing quantitative conjectures.
6 Models with appropriate complexity can be constructed to answer specific questions.
7 Modelling can be used to estimate key parameters by fitting data.
8 Models provide structures for organizing, coalescing and cross-checking diverse pieces of information.
9 Models can be used in comparing diseases of different types, or at different times, or in different populations.
10 Models can be used to theoretically evaluate, compare or optimize various detection, prevention, therapy and control programmes.
11 Models can be used to assess the sensitivity of results to changes in parameter values.
12 Modelling can suggest crucial data that needs to be collected.
13 Modelling can contribute to the design and analysis of epidemiological surveys.
14 Models can be used to identify trends, make general forecasts or estimate the uncertainity in forecasts.
15 The validity and robustness of modelling results can be assessed by using ranges of parameter values in many different models.

The three limitations identified by Hethcote and Van Ark (1992) are:

1 An epidemiological model is not reality; it is an extreme simplification of reality.
2 Deterministic models do not reflect the role of chance in disease spread and do not provide confidence intervals on results.
3 Stochastic models incorporate chance, but are usually harder to analyse than the corresponding deterministic model.

Some examples of mathematical models in health care

Mathematical models have been used to investigate a diverse range of aspects of the health care system. These include:

- A mathematical model of the anatomy, pathophysiology, tests, treatments and outcomes pertaining to diabetes, called 'Archimedes', that can be applied to a wide variety of clinical and administrative problems (Schlessinger and Eddy 2002; Eddy and Schlessinger 2003a). This health care model has undergone what must be one of the most comprehensive pieces of validation, in that a total of 74 validation exercises were conducted involving treatments and outcomes in 18 randomized controlled trials (RCTs). For 71 of the 74 exercises there were no statistically significant differences between the results calculated by the model and the results observed in the trial (Eddy and Schlessinger 2003b). This is an example of a model continuous in time, and represents biological variables continuously. The model is written in differential equations and the equations are programmed in Smalltalk (a programming language).

- A simulation model has been developed to assess the costs and effectiveness of a variety of screening strategies for colorectal cancer (Lejeune et al. 2003). The model, that intends to simulate biennial screening with the Hemoccult® test, is based on a decision tree analysis, using the Markov process. It estimates the annual medical and economic outcomes within a given cohort invited to participate in different screening strategies and within an non-screened cohort. Each cohort is followed from a given starting age, year by year until the age of 85 or until death. The model was validated with data from an independent RCT. For this trial, the observed mortality reduction was 18.0 per cent and the estimated mortality reduction was 18.4 per cent, indicating extremely close concordance.

- A discrete event simulation model of a hospital drug distribution system was constructed to explore the effects of different changes to the system on unavailability-related medication administration errors (Dean et al. 2001). The model was based on an 850-bed teaching hospital operating a ward pharmacy service typical of those in UK hospitals. The model was used to explore the effects of eight interventions on a 28-bed vascular surgery ward and a 16-bed renal medicine ward. An article by Dean et al. (1997) briefly discusses mathematical modelling and its potential applications in pharmacy.

- A study developed two models for HIV spread to investigate the impact of random screening and contact tracing. The researchers developed the models directly as differential equations, using approximations to estimate terms in their equations, rather than attempting to derive them from a stochastic or simulation model. The differential equations allowed them to quickly obtain insights into the dynamics of the two models. They found that the effectiveness of the intervention strategy varied strongly with the model and consequently the underlying aetiology of the disease transmission (Hyman et al. 2003). Various articles exist that discuss the use of mathematical models in exploring HIV, AIDS and sexually transmitted disease epidemiology (Aral and Roegner 2000; Stover 2000; Garnett 2002).

- The use of models to investigate drug resistance, such as antibiotic or antiviral drug resistance, is increasing as public health concern increases. Articles that discuss the roles of models in this type of investigation include Blower and Volberding (2002), who discuss what modelling can tell us about the threat of antiviral drug resistance.

Types of mathematical model

Dean *et al.* (1997) grouped mathematical models into six types (see Figure 13.2):

1 Deterministic, analytical
2 Stochastic, analytical
3 Deterministic, discrete-event, simulation
4 Stochastic, discrete-event, simulation
5 Deterministic, continuous-time, simulation
6 Stochastic, continuous-time, simulation

Although this grouping of model types is not universally used, it draws out some of the distinctive features of the various model types, and the terms for these features are often observed in the modelling literature.

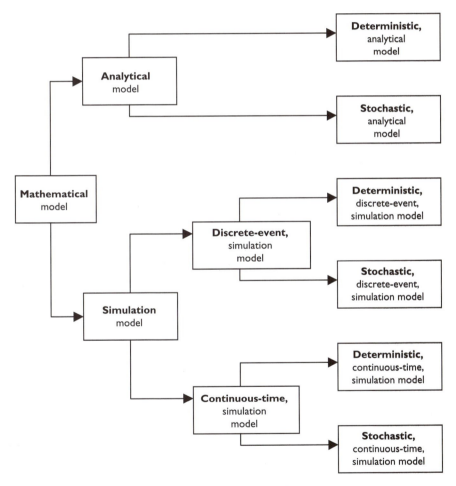

Figure 13.2   The six types of mathematical model

Source: adapted from Dean *et al.* (1997)

Analytical model versus simulation model

The analytical model has been described as a type of model that directly describes the relationships between inputs and outputs of a system and with which solutions are derived by using standard numerical methods, such as algebra and calculus (Dean *et al.* 1997). However, as the relationships become more complex, or more variables are involved, an analytical model may become too complicated to solve or possibly to describe with formulae, and with simplification, too unrealistic. These models generally need to be studied by means of simulation. In a simulation we use a computer to evaluate a model numerically (Law and Kelton 2000). However, if an analytical solution to a mathematical model is available and is computationally efficient, it is usually desirable to study the model in this way rather than via a simulation (Law and Kelton 2000). Many systems of interest are so complex that only through simulation can the system be represented in a valid way. Some models may contain components of each; analytical aspects within a simulation model.

Law and Kelton (2000) classified simulation models into those that are static or dynamic (in addition to those that are deterministic or stochastic, or continuous or discrete, as classified by Dean *et al.* 1997): 'A static simulation model is a representation of a system at a particular time, or one that may be used to represent a system in which time simply plays no role; examples of static simulations are Monte Carlo models . . . a dynamic simulation model represents a system as it evolves over time . . .' (Law and Kelton 2000). However, the authors noted that some writers define Monte Carlo simulation to be any simulation involving the use of random numbers.

Deterministic model versus stochastic model

In a deterministic model, once the inputs and relationships are described, the output is determined. Deterministic models do not reflect the role of chance. An example of this would be a deterministic computation of the number of people dying after five years in a cohort of 1000 people with an annual mortality rate of 10 per cent. Given that the annual mortality rate is assumed to be known, the proportion that have died over this time period can be calculated and is determined by the inputs. However, in a stochastic (probabilistic) model, random input components are incorporated (see Box 13.1). In the same example, this random incorporation might be by the computer generating a random number (1–100) from a uniform distribution for each simulated live individual in a given simulation year, and whether that person dies or not in the model is dependent on whether the random number generated is between 1–10 or 11–100, respectively. One of the advantages of this approach over deterministic computation is that 'fractional persons' will not have been computed. In this stochastic computation, the outcome for each of the 1000 people will be binary (dead or alive). As the concept of fractional person is absurd, a stochastic approach may often be preferred by health care modellers to remove the fractional person effect. Additionally, a stochastic approach may be preferred to

---

Box 13.1   Stochastic models

- Incorporate random input components.
- Many of the mathematical models in health care are stochastic, dynamic, discrete-event simulations.

represent the apparent randomness of, say, illness, response to treatment and death in populations.

Another way in which a random input variable maybe incorporated is when the parameter value itself is uncertain. In the example above, this would be the annual mortality rate, which might be the mean of a probability distribution with a range of values. Rather than use a single value, such as the mean, the probability of the occurrence of each of its possible values can be incorporated into the analytical or simulation model (Dean *et al.* 1997). The values that the parameter might take could be discrete (can take any value from a set of values) or continuous (can take any value within a range of values). However, as highlighted by Edwards and Hamson (2001), in practice the distinction between the two types is often blurred because a continuous variable will be measured to the nearest unit on some scale of measurement. Theoretical models for discrete random variables, such as the binomial distribution or Poisson distribution, are specified by a probability function. Theoretical models for continuous random variables, such as the normal distribution, are specified by a probability density function. However, rather than assume a theoretical model for the random input variable, actual data could be used in the form of a frequency table to calculate the probability of each of the values of the random variable occurring.

Discrete-event simulation versus continuous-time simulation

While state variables describe a system at a particular time, Law and Kelton (2000) describe discrete event simulation as the modelling of a system as it evolves over time by the representation in which the state variables change instantaneously at separate points in time. Consequently, the simulated system can only change through an event at specific points in simulated time, the event being an instantaneous occurrence. The same authors describe continuous simulation as the modelling over time of a system by a representation in which the state variables change continuously with respect to time. They suggest that typically continuous simulation models involve differential equations that give relationships for rates of change of the state variables with time.

Many of the mathematical models in health care use dynamic, stochastic, discrete-event simulation. (Some terms could be considered analogous with others.) An example of how representation in which the state variables change instantaneously at separate points in time works in practice in mathematical modelling in health care is through the common use of a Markov model to represent part of the system being modelled (see p. 300).

There are a variety of simulation software packages available. When selecting the appropriate simulation software, a software survey (e.g. via the online journal OR/MS Today) may be of use. Additionally, Law and Kelton (2000), discuss simulation software packages. Examples of simulation packages that have been cited in the medical literature include Extend v.3.2 by Dean *et al.* (1999) and @Risk v.3.5b by Eastman *et al.* (1997).

Law and Kelton (2000) categorized the features to consider when selecting simulation software into six groups, and discussed each:

- **General capabilities (including modelling flexibility and ease of use)**. The authors considered modelling flexibility, which is the ability to model a system whose operating procedures could have any amount of complexity, as the most important feature for a simulation software product to have.
- **Hardware and software considerations**. This includes the computer memory required, and compatibility with the machine.

- **Animation**. The authors suggested that the availability of built-in animation is one of the reasons for the increased use of simulation modelling.
- **Statistical features**. The authors stated that if a simulation product does not have good statistical analysis features then it is impossible to obtain correct results from a simulation study. Additionally, a must was a good random number generator.
- **Customer support and documentation**. This included the provision by the vendor of public training on the software on a regular basis, and the possibility of customized training. Good technical support, so that the purchaser could ask any questions on how to use the software, was also considered important, as was good documentation. However, the documentation, in the authors opinion, should be of a standard that makes it possible to learn a simulation package without taking a formal training course.
- **Output reports and plots**. This included the provision of a variety of graphics, and their exportability into other software packages. These other packages might be statistical, or those for producing reports.

Additional to these, cost may also be an important consideration.

Although there are a number of simulation packages, many modellers may opt to write the program in a computer language, such as Smalltalk (e.g. the Archimedes model for diabetes, see Schlessinger and Eddy 2002; Eddy and Schlessinger 2003a) or FORTRAN, rather than use a package.

Markov models in health care

Markov models (see Box 13.2) are state-transition models. They have often been used in mathematical models of health care to describe disease progression. Subjects in the mathematical model are allocated to one of the health states described, often according to other relevant characteristics, such as age and sex. The Markov model of disease progression is often schematically represented in the form shown in Figure 13.3. The arrows indicate the changes in health state that are possible. For example, a subject in the 'normal' disease-free state could transfer to the 'early stage of disease' state or the 'dead from other causes' state. (This is the probability of all cause mortality minus the probability of death from the disease being modelled.) The transitions that occur from one health state to another occur at defined time intervals, usually one year, according to transition probabilities (although continuous-time Markov models can be described). The state change is an instantaneous occurrence.

Markov models contain a finite number of mutually exclusive and exhaustive health states, having time periods of uniform length, and in which the probability of movement from one state to another depends on the current state and remains

---

Box 13.2   Markov models in health care

- Contain a finite number of mutually exclusive and exhaustive health states.
- The probability of movement from one state of another, which is dependent on the current state, is known as the transition probability or transition rate.
- In *Markov chain models*, the transition rates do not vary with simulated time.
- In *Markov process models*, the transition rates vary with simulated time.
- Markov models can be incorporated into decision trees.

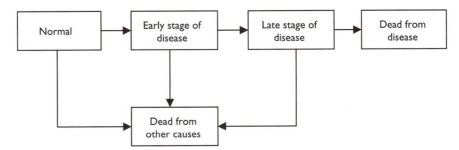

Figure 13.3   A hypothetical example of a Markov model used to describe disease progression

constant over time (Gold *et al.* 1996b). These are also called Markov *chain* models (Petitti 2000). However, in health care modelling we would often want the transition rate to vary with time as the subject's simulated age increases. We would probably want, at least, survival from the disease being modelled, and mortality from other causes, and maybe other state-to-state transitions, to vary with simulated age. Models that allow for systematic changes in transition probabilities as a function of simulated time rather than having constant transition probabilities are considered to be another type of Markov model and terms such as *semi-Markov models* (Gold *et al.* 1996b), *time-varying Markov models* (Gold *et al.* 1996b) and *Markov process models* (Petitti 2000) have been applied to these.

Differential and difference equations

Although not wishing to burden the reader with an undue number of mathematical terms, most reviews of the modelling literature will lead to some mention of differential and difference equations. Consequently, a very brief summary of their use is presented here. Fulford *et al.* (2001), usefully surmises that 'The difference between models leading to differential equations and those leading to difference equations is often expressed by saying that the former are continuous whereas the latter are discrete'. Consequently, in a continuous time model, the way in which a variable changes with time can be described by a differential equation. In a discrete event simulation, the way in which a variable changes with time can be described by a difference equation. For further detail on these areas, at a relatively novice level, Edwards and Hamson (2001) is recommended.

Decision analysis

Decision analysis is a systematic quantitative approach for assessing the relative value of one or more different decision options (Petitti 2000). In decision analysis, a decision tree is constructed, which schematically presents the sequence of decisions and chance events over time. Each chance event is assigned a probability. Alternative decision strategies are evaluated by calculating their average consequences. Historically, decision analysis was used by clinicians to make individual decisions about patients. However, this method is now widely used in the medical literature to evaluate both clinical and policy decisions (e.g. to screen or not to screen for a condition). It also often underpins cost-effectiveness analyses.

Figure 13.4 presents an example of a decision tree. This example is a simplified version of a decision tree that was presented in the medical literature (Shehata *et al.* 2004) to compare:

- not screening allogeneic blood donors for malaria (Strategy 1);
- using the standard questionnaire (Strategy 2);
- using the standard questionnaire followed by testing blood donors with risk factors for malaria with polymerase chain reaction (PCR) (Strategy 3); and
- screening all blood donors using PCR (Strategy 4).

The expected costs and the number of cases of malaria for each strategy were compared and incremental cost-effectiveness ratios were calculated as the cost per case of malaria averted. Figure 13.4, presents Strategies 1 and 4 only. It can be seen that the decision tree is built from left to right. In accordance with convention, the tree consists of decision nodes that are depicted by a square, and chance nodes that are depicted by circles. Outcomes are usually depicted as large rectangles but were absent from this tree. The branches from nodes are drawn at right angles. At a chance mode, the sum of the probabilities of each chance event must be equal to 1. The probabilities for each of the chance events are derived either from the literature, through study data, or via consensus expert opinion. Preferably the probabilities (0–1) for each of the chance events would be also displayed within the decision tree (e.g. Clark *et al.* 2000). The final analysis of the tree is relatively simple with the majority of the work involved often being in the formulation of the tree and the allocation of probabilities to each of the chance events. In our example, we want to calculate the probability of malaria transmission given each of the decision alternatives (no screening versus screening with PCR). To do this, we first need to calculate the probability of malaria transmission given each of the alternative routes in the tree. For the no screening decision option there is only one route leading to malaria transmission (or not) (and therefore one malaria transmission probability to

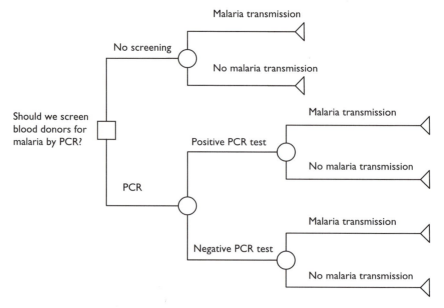

Figure 13.4   An example of a decision tree

Source: adapted from Shehata *et al.* (2004)

calculate), and for the screening with PCR decision option there are two routes (and therefore two malaria transmission probabilities to calculate). The probability is calculated by multiplying each of the chance probabilities along that route leading to the outcome of interest (e.g. malaria transmission). This is known as 'folding back' the decision tree. Then for each of the decision alternatives the probabilities of the same outcomes (in this example, malaria transmission) would be added to together. This is known as 'averaging'. Consequently, for the no screening option there is only one probability for malaria transmission, but for the screening option there are two, which are added together. From this the number of malaria cases expected with each option can be calculated.

In the original study on which this example is based the authors take this analysis further and perform a cost-effectiveness analysis to compare the outcome of the decision options in terms of cost per case of malaria averted. There are a number of very good sources that provide further examples of decision analysis in health care and practical guidance on applying decision analyses in health care: Sonnenberg (2003), Birmingham (2003), Petitti (2000), Detsky et al. (1997a, 1997b), Naglie et al. (1997) and Krahn et al. (1997). Additionally, for individuals new to decision analysis and therefore presenting work in this area, guidelines for verbal presentations of medical decision analyses are also available (Redelmeier et al. 1997).

There is a variety of software available to perform decision analysis including DATA 4.0 (2000), and TreeAge Pro (2004) from TreeAge Software, Inc., Williamstown, Massachusettes, Decision Maker 7.0 (Pratt Medical Group, Boston, Massachusetts), and SMLTREE 2.9 (Hollenberg JP. Roslyn, New York). Alternatively it may be possible to use a simple spreadsheet for the calculations depending on the complexity of the problem. When selecting the appropriate decision analysis software, software surveys may also be useful (e.g. via the online journal OR/MS Today).

The type of decision tree model in Figure 13.4 has several drawbacks that become apparent when we wish to model a system involving chronic diseases, such as cancer, or diabetes, where events such as a recurrence or stroke may occur more than one, or we wish to specify when events occur, or we need to change probabilities according to age or health status. To encompass each of these options would require separate branches of the decision tree, which would soon become very complicated and cumbersome. Rather than model each event as a separate branch of a very complicated tree, a more efficient mathematical representation is in the form of a Markov node. The incorporated Markov node leads to a Markov model. Guidance for incorporating Markov models in medical decision-making is provided by Sonnenberg and Beck (1993) and Naimark et al. (1997). Studies that have incorporated a Markov node in the decision tree model include the estimation of the long-term cost-effectiveness of a hypothetical screening programme for untreated amblyopia in 3-year-old children conducted by orthoptists in all German kindergartens in the year 2000 (König and Barry 2004), and a study to evaluate the health outcomes, costs and cost-effectiveness of vaccination with seven-valent pneumococcal conjugate vaccine, compared with no vaccination for children in Spain (Asensi et al. 2004).

Cost-effectiveness and cost-utility analysis

Many mathematical models used in health care incorporate an economic component, cost-effectiveness analysis (CEA) and cost-utility analysis (CUA) being the most frequently employed. The number of CEAs of health and medical interventions in the medical literature has grown considerably over the last ten years. The CEA

Registry (http://www.hsph.harvard.edu/cearegistry) identified 44 CUAs of life-saving interventions published between 1982 and 1991, and 490 published between 1992 and 2001.

CEA is an analytic tool in which costs and effects of a programme and at least one alternative are calculated and presented in a ratio of incremental cost to incremental effect (Gold *et al.* 1996b). Difference in costs between the alternative(s) (net costs) are divided by the difference in health outcomes (net effectiveness). In a CEA, health outcomes are expressed in units, such as number of cases of disease prevented, or number of life years gained. However, when we wish to compare health outcomes that are different, we need a universal unit. Quality-adjusted life years (QALYs) are used to overcome this problem in terms of health-related quality of life and survival for an individual. The term CUAs rather that CEA is often used to describe CEAs that use QALYs.

Box 13.3   Cost-utility analysis (CUA)

- Often used to describe cost-effectiveness analyses (CEAs) that use QALYs.
- The cost-utility ratio is an outcome of CUA. This ratio can be expressed as:

$$\frac{\text{Cost of intervention A} - \text{cost of intervention B}}{\text{No. of QALYs produced by strategy A} - \text{No. of QALYs produced by strategy B}}$$

What are QALYs?

QALYs are calculated from the product of a quality weight (a quantitative measure that reflects the desirability of living in the health state, typically where 0 = dead and 1 = full health) and the number of years the individual remains in that health state (Neumann *et al.* 2000). Consequently, one QALY is considered to be the equivalent to one year of perfect health. In a model of a system, QALYs that are obtained for each individual for each decision alternative are summed together. QALYs may also be discounted to adjust for time preference in that less weight is assigned to the quality weight, therefore reducing the number of QALYs as they occur further and further into the future. Each year in the future the quality weight will be devalued at a constant rate (the discount rate). Monetary costs in CEAs and CUAs can also be similarly discounted. See Lipscomb *et al.* (1996) and Petitti (2000) for discussions of discounting.

Various terms are frequently associated with quality weights such as utility, value and preference. Neumann *et al.* (2000) explain that preference is a general term used to describe the desirability of a set of outcomes. Values and utilities are different types of preference that depend on the elicitation method:

- **values** are measured under conditions of certainity (rating scale, time trade-off);
- **utilities** are measured under conditions of uncertainty that satisfy certain axioms of expected utility theory (standard gamble).

Neumann *et al.* (2000) go on to explain that the preference or quality weights that are produced from preferences developed with methods other than standard gamble are not technically utilities. In practice, the term *utility score* is frequently used instead of, say, quality weight, regardless of the method used.

The various ways that are used to determine preference or quality weights will not be comprehensively discussed in this chapter but include (Naglie *et al.* 1997):

Box 13.4   Formula for discounting quality weights

The net present value of a quality weight occurring $\times$ years in the future =

$$\frac{\text{Quality weight}}{(1 + D)^{\times}}$$

where D = discount rate (0–1) and the quality weight is also expressed between 0–1.

Example: If the quality weight is 1.0, and the discount rate is 5 per cent (0.05), what are the net present values of the quality weight for each of one to three years in the future?

Answer:

Year 1   0.95
Year 2   0.91
Year 3   0.86

- arbitrarily assigning a weight based on your judgement;
- having a group of experts reach a consensus on the estimates for the weights;
- searching for relevant published weights in the literature; or
- measuring directly, in appropriate subjects, using reliable and valid methods.

The CEA Registry (www.hsph.harvard.edu/cearegistry) contains a comprehensive catalogue of preference weights from published CUAs (Bell *et al.* 2001). It consists of 53 pages of preference weights for various health states, sorted by disease area and stating the measurement technique. The various methods used to measure preferences are described in Neumann *et al.* (2000), Pettiti (2000) and Gold *et al.* (1996a). However, it is acknowledged that the measurement of quality weight for health states may be affected by the technique used. In papers reporting utilities, it is often difficult to infer how the utility measurement was carried out (Stalmeier *et al.* 2001). Neumann *et al.* (1997) also highlighted the need for more rigour and consistency with respect to the methods used in estimating QALYs in CEAs, suggesting, at a minimum, that investigators should be more explicit about their methods so that readers can understand how the QALYs were constructed.

Finally, before we leave the QALY, it is worth noting that there are various problems associated with the concept of a QALY, which are comprehensively discussed by Nord (1999).

Mathematical models

Mathematical models (including decision analyses) are the basis of CEAs. In fact, for a novice in mathematical modelling, reading textbooks on CEAs in health and medicine will often lead to accessible explanations of mathematical modelling techniques, which may be preferable to reading textbooks on mathematical models as such.

Through a systematic search of the English-language medical literature that identified 522 original CUAs published from 1976 to 2001, the authors identified that the predominant modelling methods included simple decision tree analyses (36 per cent) and Markov models (47 per cent) (Olchanski *et al.* 2003). Through perusal of the CEA Registry reference list of CUAs from 1976 to 2001, many different examples of modelling techniques can be found.

The majority of appraisals made by the Appraisal Committee of the National Institute for Clinical Excellence (NICE) in England, which forms views on whether particular health technologies (drugs, surgical procedures, diagnostic techniques, devices, educational programmes etc.) are effective and cost-effective, and therefore whether they should be available free of charge, are informed by models. They have become an indispensable part of the analysis that the committee uses to reach many of its decisions (Akehurst 2003).

Steps in building a mathematical model

There is no set defined number of steps in building a mathematical model, but the processes involved in the development and use of a mathematical model can essentially be described in eight steps. These steps are not performed sequentially but iteratively, and therefore at various stages in the evolution of the mathematical model previous steps will be revisited as, say, refinements of the model occur. The eight steps, which will each be briefly discussed, are: formulation of the problem; model-building; data collection; refinement of the model; verification; validation; experimentation with the model; and use of the results. When building a mathematical model, it is recommended that this be done with regard to the report by Weinstein *et al.* (2003), and this feeds into the steps given below. However, one of the overriding messages is that of transparency, which can only occur through good, clear documentation of the model. If no one can understand how the model works, and the assumptions behind it, then this precludes valuable input and knowledge from others that can be utilized in the model. Garrison (2003) stated that 'It is important to recognize that the key principle of transparency can provide some measure of protection against the bad effects of bias and error, but it is clearly not a perfect solution'.

Formulation of the problem

This involves stating exactly what the purpose of the model is, exactly what you want the model to predict, and describing the important parts of the system. If the model involves a disease process, part of the formulation of the model will involve a scan of the medical literature to identify the relevant health states for the model, deducing the important relationships between the variables, establishing possible sources of parameter estimates, and identifying any important gaps in the knowledge and what you intend to do about them. However, the model should be as simple as possible. Garrison (2003) highlights the tendency of some modellers to begin by describing a detailed, exhaustive pathway of clinical consequences for which there are no data to make the estimates (and, more frequently in the past, to use expert panels to estimate everything), stating that these kinds of model are difficult to estimate and validate.

Model-building

This involves the selection of the type of model that will be used, which may be influenced by the problem defined above. As previously stated, software packages exist that can be used, although it is important not to underestimate the time that will be required to manipulate these appropriately. Additionally, the model can be written in a programming language. If the problem is complex and a simulation is being considered, then the time required to either write the program or utilise and build the model through a software package can be considerable. This will also involve some preliminary work on the presentation of output data from the model.

Data collection

Data collection involves the estimation of parameters and confidence intervals. It requires the setting up and collection of any data from the literature or studies that have either been specifically set up to, or are being used to, inform the study. It will also involve the explicit statement of assumptions of the model, and comprehensive documentation.

Refinement of the model

Given initial trial runs, changes in the model may be suggested, say to increase the complexity of the model, to modify how the data is input, or to modify the output. It may become apparent that some rethinking about the system is required if the output looks very different to what is expected given the input, suggesting that the system is not well represented by the model (validation, p. 307).

Verification

Verification is the checking that the program/formulae of the model is doing what the modeller thinks it is doing. This is also known as internal validity (Weinstein *et al.* 2003). Verification can be extremely difficult because if a model is extremely complex (and therefore so is the programme), it is difficult to say with absolute certainty, after numerous checks, that the programme is behaving completely as it should be.

Some tips to help with verification include:

- Does the output, given the input, look reasonable/likely?
- Vary one parameter at a time, and check to see if the model output looks reasonable/likely.
- If the model involves a random number generator, set this to a repeatable sequence of random numbers. This will reduce the variability of output between simulation runs so that changes in the output due to any model changes that have been incorporated when looking for bugs in the system are easier to detect.
- Putting the model under stress. This involves changing parameters to unlikely figures, which may cause any errors to become apparent (e.g. if a parameter value is 50 per cent, if this was set to, say, 0 per cent, what happens?).
- Write for output at various points in the programme to see if it makes sense.
- Have a programming partner. Sometimes you can stare at the programme for hours and you will not find where a bug is, or even if there is a bug, but talking through the problem with or perusal by someone who is also familiar with the programme may lead to a quicker resolution.

Validation

Validation involves checking that the model, correctly implemented, is a sufficiently close approximation to reality for the intended application (Bratley *et al.* 1987). Weinstein *et al.* (2003) allocate over a page of A4 to this subject, indicating the importance and perhaps confusion that can surround the validation of models. The task force behind this research grouped validation into three categories: internal validation; between-model validation; and external and predictive validation, and some of the main points are summarized below.

Internal validation

Included in this is the aforementioned verification, and when available, the use of independent data (input and output data) to investigate whether the model produces outputs consistent with those data.

Many models in health care don't have independent validation, and it is important to recognize that if a model is using all the input data from one source, then while it could reasonably produce the output expected, it may not be valid. Some models are constructed in such a way to preclude independent validation. A model of a national screening strategy might be an example of this. The model may use national data, being a simplification of the system, the former leading to a self-fulfilling prophecy of output and the latter precluding comparable outputs. However, recently, one of the most comprehensive pieces of validation on a health care model occurred (Eddy and Schlessinger 2003b). To validate the Archimedes model of diabetes and its complications for a variety of populations, organ systems, treatments and outcomes the authors simulated a variety of RCTs by repeating in the model the steps taken for the real trials and comparing the results calculated by the model with the results of the trial. Eighteen trials were chosen by an independent advisory committee. Half the trials had been used to help build the model; the other half had not. The latter trials comprise independent validations.

Between-model validation

The models should be produced independently of each other to permit tests of between-model corroboration. Discrepancies between model outputs should be explained and modellers should cooperate with others in comparing results and identifying and explaining discrepancies.

External and predictive validation

Models should be based on the best evidence available at the time they are built, and be able to predict intermediate and long-term outcomes from clinical trials or epidemiological studies. The ability of models to adapt to new evidence and scientific understanding should be regarded as a strength, not as a weakness of the modelling approach.

Additionally, Law and Kelton (2000) highlighted that a model that is valid for one purpose may not be for another, after all it is a simplification of a system given the purpose of the model. Finally, as previously stated, transparency may also help to validate the model by allowing others to contribute and form an informed opinion of the model.

Experimentation with the model

Once the model is verified and validated, experimentation with it would involve using it for its intended purpose to make predictions and investigate alternative strategies. Additionally, parameters should be varied, one at a time, to investigate the effects on predictions, in terms of robustness, and sensitivity analyses should be performed (see below).

Use of the results

The results may be used in practice to inform decisions.

Sensitivity analysis and robustness

Sensitivity analysis evaluates the stability of the conclusions of an analysis in relation to assumptions made during the analysis (Petitti 2000). It is used to look at sources of uncertainty in the model. Any results obtained that vary greatly with relative changes in a parameter might not be considered robust.

Weinstein *et al.* (2003) suggests that:

- All modelling studies should include extensive sensitivity analysis.
- When possible, sensitivity analyses within models that use Monte Carlo simulations should set the random number generator to a repeatable sequence of random numbers for each sensitivity analysis to minimize random simulation error.
- If cohort simulation is used, sensitivity analysis may be done using probabilistic (Monte Carlo, second-order) simulation, using the specified probability distributions of parameter inputs.

Uncertainty can be categorized as first-order or second-order, and these are terms frequently used in the literature on sensitivity analysis. One of the most useful explanations of these terms is provided by Stinnett and Paltiel (1997), who state:

First-order uncertainty reflects the inherent stochastic nature of a trial; even if the probability of an event is known with certainty, the outcome of any particular trial is unknown a priori. First-order uncertainty ('Will the toss of a fair coin result in a head or a tail?') persists even when the probability distribution of outcomes is known with certainty ('Heads and tails are equally likely, the probability of each being 50%'). Second-order uncertainty corresponds to uncertainty in the parameters of the probability distribution of outcomes. For example, one may be unsure whether a coin being tossed is fair; in such an instance, there is uncertainty not only surrounding the outcome of the toss but also with regard to the likelihood of each possible outcome.

Two types of sensitivity analyses that are frequently observed are:

- **One-way (univariate) sensitivity analysis** – the assumed value of variables in the model are varied, one at a time, while the values of the other variables remain fixed.
- **Two-way (bivariate) sensitivity analysis** – the model outputs for every combination of values of two variables are calculated, while the values of the other variables remain fixed. Graphs are often used to present the results.

Probabilistic methods, such as the Monte Carlo method, may be used. In these, for the uncertain parameters under investigation, a random draw from the distribution of possible parameter values would occur. Consequently, a second-order Monte Carlo simulation would involve the generation of a random number to determine the parameter value, such as the annual mortality rate from a distribution of possible rates, and the generation of a random number to determine whether that event occurs, such as whether the simulated person dies or lives, determined by the value of the random number relative to the value of mortality rate. For further discussions on sensitivity analysis, Petitti (2000) and Manning *et al.* (1996) are of use.

Conclusions

This chapter has described the types and uses of mathematical modelling in health care. A model has been defined as a description of some system intended to predict what happens if certain actions are taken. A mathematical health care evaluation model has been defined by Weinstein *et al.* (2003) as 'an analytic methodology that accounts for events over time and across populations, that is based on data drawn from primary and/or secondary sources, and whose purpose is to estimate the effects of an intervention on valued health consequences and costs'. There are several distinctive types of mathematical model. Many of those used in health care use dynamic, stochastic or discrete-event simulation and several simulation software packages are available.

Key points

- A *model* has been defined as a description of some system intended to predict what happens if certain actions are taken.

- Many of the mathematical models in health care use dynamic, stochastic and discrete event simulation. A *dynamic* model represents a system as it evolves over time. A *stochastic* model incorporates random input components. In a *discrete-event* model, the system state variables change instantaneously at separate points in time.

- A *simulation* model is used when the system relationships become more complex, or more variables are involved, and an *analytical* model may become too complicated to solve or possibly to describe with formulae, and with simplification, too unrealistic. In a simulation, we use a computer to evaluate a model numerically.

- *Decision analysis* has been defined as a systematic quantitative approach for assessing the relative value of one or more different decision options. A *decision tree* schematically presents the sequence of decisions and chance events over time, and conventions exist on the presentation of these trees.

- Simulation and decision analysis *software* exists but is not a prerequisite. The alternative is programming in a computer language.

- *Markov models* contain a finite number of mutually exclusive and exhaustive health states with movement from one state to another, which is dependent on the current state. In Markov *chain* models, the transition rates do not vary with simulated time. In Markov *process* models, the transition rates vary with simulated time. Markov models can be incorporated into decision trees to reduce the complexity.

- *Mathematical models* (including decision analyses) are the basis of cost-effectiveness analyses.

- *Verification* is the checking that the programme/formulae of the model is doing what the modeller thinks it is doing.

- *Validation* is checking that the model, correctly implemented, is a sufficiently close approximation to reality for the intended application.

- All modelling studies should include *sensitivity analyses*, which are the evaluation of the stability of the conclusions of an analysis to assumptions made in the analysis.

Further reading

Edwards, D. and Hamson, M. (2001) *Guide to Mathematical Modelling*. Basingstoke: Palgrave. This book is aimed at the first or second year level in an undergraduate degree course in mathematical sciences, and suggests that the amount of prerequisite mathematics and statistics is quite modest. It attempts to demystify and make accessible many modelling techniques through the numerous examples contained within. Although some novices to mathematics might find some sections difficult to completely understand, and the book is not focused on modelling in medicine and health, it will provide a useful explanation of techniques that at least will help in the interpretation of some modelling studies.

Gold, M.R., Seigel, J.E., Russell, L.B. and Weinstein, W.C. (eds) *Cost-Effectiveness in Health and Medicine*. Oxford: Oxford University Press. The editors claim that this book provides a detailed discussion of the theoretical background underlying areas of controversy, and uses theory to guide explicit recommendations for study conduct. Also, that it will be an important resource for cost-effectiveness analysts in medicine and public health who wish to improve the quality and comparability of their studies. It does this in a very accessible way, which novices could follow. Although many of the principles apply to modelling in general, in medicine and health, this generalist approach is not the focus of the book.

Petitti, D.B. (2000) *Meta-analysis, Decision Analysis and Cost-effectiveness analysis: Methods for Quantitative Synthesis in Medicine*, 2nd edn. Oxford: Oxford University Press. This book claims to be a lucid introduction and will serve the needs of students taking introductory courses that cover these subjects. It completely fulfils these aims. It is a very well written, easy to read book, with the use of many examples throughout to explain concepts. It will be especially useful for those interested in decision analysis and CEA, although many of the principles apply to modelling, in general, in medicine and health.

Weinstein, M.C., O'Brien, B., Hornberger, J. *et al.* (2003) Principles of good practice for decision analytic modelling in health-care evaluation: report of the ISPOR task force on good research practices – modelling studies, *Value in Health*, 6(1): 9–17. This is an excellent, easy to read article for anyone planning to undertake modelling work in health care, including novices. It provides useful tips, and guidelines for conducting and reporting modelling studies.

References

Akehurst, R.L. (2003) Making decisions on technology availability in the British National Health Service – why we need reliable models, *Value in Health*, 6: 3–5.

Aral, S.O. and Roegner, R. (2000) Mathematical modelling as a tool in STD prevention and control: a decade of progress, a millennium of opportunities, *Sexually Transmitted Diseases*, 27: 556–7.

Asensi, F., De Jose, M., Lorente, M. *et al.* (2004) A pharmacoeconomic evaluation of seven-valent pneumococcal conjugate vaccine in Spain, *Value in Health*, 7: 36–51.

Bell, C.M., Chapman, R.H., Stone, P.W. *et al.* (2001) An off-the-shelf help list: a comprehensive catalog of preference scores from published cost-utility analyses, *Medical Decision Making*, 21: 288–94.

Birmingham, C.L. (2003) Clinical decision analysis and anorexia nervosa, *International Journal of Law and Psychiatry*, 26: 719–23.

Blower, S. and Volberding, P. (2002) What can modelling tell us about the threat of antiviral drug resistance? *Current Opinion in Infectious Diseases*, 15: 609–14.

Bratley, P., Fox, B.L and Schrage, L.E. (1987) *A Guide to Simulation*, 2nd edn. New York: Springer-Verlag.

Clark, W.F., Churchill, D.N., Forwell, L. *et al.* (2000) To pay or not to pay? A decision and cost-utility analysis of angiotensin-converting-enzyme inhibitor therapy for diabetic nephropathy, *Canadian Medical Association Journal*, 162: 195–8.

Dean, B., Barber, N., van Ackere, A. and Gallivan, S. (2001) Can simulation be used to reduce errors in health care delivery? The hospital drug distribution system, *Journal of Health Services Research and Policy*, 6: 32–7.

Dean, B.S., Gallivan, S., Barber, N.D. and van Ackere, A. (1997) Mathematical modelling of pharmacy systems, *American Journal of Health-System Pharmacy*, 54: 2491–9.

Dean, B.S., van Ackere, A., Gallivan, S. and Barber, N.D. (1999) When should pharmacists visit their wards? An application of simulation to planning hospital pharmacy services, *Health Care Management Science*, 2: 35–42.

Detsky, A.S., Naglie, G., Krahn, M.D. *et al.* (1997a) Primer on medical decision analysis: part 1, getting started, *Medical Decision Making*, 17: 123–5.

Detsky, A.S., Naglie, G., Krahn, M.D. *et al.* (1997b) Primer on medical decision analysis: part 2, building a tree, *Medical Decision Making*, 17: 126–35.

Eastman, R.C., Garfield, S.A., Javitt, J.C. *et al.* (1997) Model of complications of NIDDM. I: model construction and assumptions, *Diabetes Care*, 20: 725–34.

Eddy, D.M. and Schlessinger, L. (2003a) Archimedes: a trial-validated model of diabetes, *Diabetes Care*, 26: 3093–101.

Eddy, D.M. and Schlessinger, L. (2003b) Validation of the Archimedes diabetes model, *Diabetes Care*, 26: 3102–10.

Edwards, D. and Hamson, M. (2001) *Guide to Mathematical Modelling*. Basingstoke: Palgrave.

Fulford, G., Forrester, P. and Jones, A. (2001) *Modelling with Differential and Difference Equations*. Cambridge: Cambridge University Press.

Garnett, G.P. (2002) An introduction to mathematical models in sexually transmitted disease epidemiology, *Sexually Transmitted Information*, 78: 7–12.

Garrison, L.P. (2003) The ISPOR good practice modelling principles – a sensible approach: be transparent, be reasonable, *Value in Health*, 6: 6–8.

Gold, M.R., Patrick, D.L., Torrance, G.W. *et al.* (1996a) Identifying and valuing outcomes, in M.R. Gold, J.E. Seigel, L.B. Russell and M.C. Weinstein (eds) *Cost-effectiveness in Health and Medicine*. Oxford: Oxford University Press.

Gold, M.R., Seigel, J.E., Russell, L.B. and Weinstein, M.C. (1996b) Glossary, in M.R. Gold, J.E. Seigel, L.B. Russell and M.C. Weinstein (eds) *Cost-effectiveness in Health and Medicine*. Oxford: Oxford University Press.

Hayden, B.W. (2000) Mathematical models, in B.W. Hayden, *Discrete Mathematics: Its Nature and Uses*. Plymouth State College: web version of fall 2000, www.mathpc04.Plymouth.edu/ch1.pdf. (Accessed 19 April 2004.)

Hethcote, H.W. and Van Ark, J.W. (1992) *Modeling HIV Transmission and AIDS in the United States*. (Originally published in 1992 by Springer-Verlag as *Lecture Notes in Biomathematics*. The publisher has now returned the copright to the authors and they have placed it in the public domain at www.math.uiowa.edu/~hethcote/) (accessed 19 April 2004).

Hyman, J.M., Li, J. and Stanley, E.A. (2003) Modeling the impact of random screening and contact tracing in reducing the spread of HIV, *Mathematical Biosciences*, 181: 17–54.

König, H-H. and Barry, J-C. (2004) Cost-utility analysis of orthoptic screening in kindergarten: a Markov model based on data from Germany, *Pediatrics*, 113: e95–108.

Krahn, M.D., Naglie, G., Naimark, D. *et al.* (1997) Primer on medical decision analysis: part 4: analyzing the model and interpreting the results, *Medical Decision Making*, 17: 142–51.

Law, A.M. and Kelton, W.D. (2000) *Simulation Modeling and Analysis*, 3rd edn. New York: McGraw-Hill.

Lejeune, C., Arveux, P., Dancourt, V. *et al.* (2003) A simulation model for evaluating the medical and economic outcomes of screening strategies for colorectal cancer. *European Journal of Cancer Prevention*, 12: 77–84.

Lipscomb, J., Weinstein, M.C. and Torrance, G.W. (1996) Identifying and valuing outcomes, in M.R. Gold, J.E. Seigel, L.B. Russell and M.C. Weinstein (eds) *Cost-effectiveness in Health and Medicine*. Oxford: Oxford University Press.

Manning, W.G., Fryback, D.G. and Weinstein, M.C. (1996) *Reflecting uncertainity in cost-effectiveness analysis*, in M.R. Gold, J.E. Seigel, L.B. Russell and M.C. Weinstein (eds) *Cost-effectiveness in Health and Medicine*. Oxford: Oxford University Press.

Naglie, G., Krahn, M.D., Naimark, D. *et al.* (1997) Primer on medical decision analysis: part 3: estimating probabilities and utilities, *Medical Decision Making*, 17: 136–41.

Naimark, D., Krahn, M.D., Naglie, G. *et al.* (1997) Primer on medical decision analysis: part 5: working with markov processes, *Medical Decision Making*, 17: 152–9.

Neumann, P.J., Zinner D.E. and Wright, J.C. (1997) Are methods for estimating QALYs in cost-effectiveness analyses improving? *Medical Decision Making*, 17: 402–8.

Neumann, P.J., Goldie, S.J. and Weinstein, M.C. (2000) Preference-based measures in economic evaluation in health care, *Annual Review of Public Health*, 21: 587–611.

Nord, E. (1999) *Cost-value Analysis in Health Care: Making Sense Out of QALYs*. Cambridge: Cambridge University Press.

Olchanski, N.V., Rosen, A.B., Chapman, R. *et al.* (2003) *25 Years of Cost-utility Analyses: State of the Field* (http://www.hsph.harvard.edu/cearegistry/abstracts/sgim2003-overview.pdf) (accessed 19 April 2004).

Petitti, D.B. (2000) *Meta-analysis, Decision Analysis and Cost-effectiveness Analysis: Methods for Quantitative Synthesis in Medicine*, 2nd edn. Oxford: Oxford University Press.

Redelmeier, D.A., Detsky, A.S., Krahn, M.D. *et al.* (1997) Guidelines for verbal presentations of medical decision analyses, *Medical Decision Making*, 17: 228–30.

Schlessinger, L. and Eddy, D.M. (2002) Archimedes: a new model for simulating health care systems: the mathematical formulation, *Journal of Biomedical Informatics*, 35: 37–50.

Shehata, N., Kohli, M. and Detsky, A. (2004) The cost-effectiveness of screening blood donors for malaria by PCR, *Transfusion*, 44: 217–28.

Sonnenberg, A. (2003) Decision analysis in clinical gastroenterology, *American Journal of Gastroenterology*, 99: 163–9.

Sonnenberg, F.A. and Beck, R. (1993) Markov models in medical decision-making: a practical guide, *Medical Decision Making*, 13: 322–39.

Stalmeier, P.F.M., Goldstein, M.K., Holmes A.M. *et al.* (2001) What should be reported in a methods section on utility assessment? *Medical Decision Making*, 21: 200–7.

Stinnett, A.A. and Paltiel, A.D. (1997) Estimating CE ratios under second-order uncertainty: the mean ratio versus the ratio of means, *Medical Decision Making*, 17: 483–9.

Stover, J. (2000) Influence of mathematical modelling of HIV and AIDS on policies and programs in the developing world, *Sexually Transmitted Diseases*, 27: 572–8.

Weinstein, M.C., O'Brien, B., Hornberger, J. *et al.* (2003) Principles of good practice for decision analytic modelling in health-care evaluation: report of the ISPOR task force on good research practices – modelling studies, *Value in Health*, 6: 9–17.

14 Economic evaluation of health care

Jackie Brown

Introduction

New or modified health care interventions can often offer significant gains to patients but the resources required to provide such interventions are limited. The use of scarce resources, whether these are people's time, equipment or buildings, has an opportunity cost in terms of the benefits forgone as a result of denying the use of these resources for competing health care interventions. A *health care intervention* is taken here to mean a form of service delivery as well as a specific treatment. As patients and the public cannot be offered all that is technically feasible or potentially beneficial, choices have to be made in the provision of health care (Buxton 1993; Drummond *et al.* 1998).

Efficiency is concerned with making choices so as to derive the maximum total benefit from the limited resources available. It is not about cost-cutting. Like evidence-based medicine, which emphasizes the need to make use of the best available formal evidence on effectiveness, health economics stresses the need to formally assess the implications of choices over the deployment of resources rather than relying on educated guesses or 'gut feelings'. A number of economic evaluation techniques are available to aid this formal assessment and help identify the most efficient allocation of resources (Torrance *et al.* 1996; Drummond *et al.* 1998). Moreover, economic evaluations are increasingly being used to augment clinical evaluation (Elixhauser *et al.* 1993; Pritchard 1998). In many counties, such as the UK, Australia and Canada for example, the pharmaceutical industry is forced to present economic arguments to regulatory and reimbursement concerns (Weinstein 1995). Agencies funding research, such as the UK Medical Research Council (MRC), also expect an economic evaluation to have been considered explicitly in proposed clinical trials.

This chapter discusses the principles underlying economic evaluation, the alternative types of economic evaluations and their appropriate use, methods of outcome measurement and valuation, as well as costing health care. In discussing how the results might be interpreted, the 'decision rules' for efficiency are explained. Finally, the chapter discusses some research design and implementation issues.

Principles of economic evaluation

Two features characterize an economic evaluation. The first is its consideration of both the costs (resource use consequences) as well as the health outcomes (non-resource use consequences). The second is its concern with alternative options in the delivery of health care. These might be in terms of the method of treatment – for example, surgery versus medical treatment or alternative drug treatments. Other options, depending on the intervention being evaluated, might relate to the type of personnel delivering the treatment, such as a nurse or a doctor, and/or the location of treatment, for example, outpatient or inpatient. Economic evaluation is the systematic comparison of both the costs (the resource use consequences) and the health outcomes (non-resource use consequences) of the feasible alternative options.

Health services generally have some kind of existing practice with regard to treatment. Hence it is the change in costs and outcomes of the alternatives, including current practice, which is relevant. Economic evaluation thus takes an incremental approach such that the results are presented as the difference in costs compared to the difference in outcomes of the options under appraisal.

A number of textbooks set out the broad principles which govern the way in which costs and outcomes should be handled within an economic evaluation (e.g. Sloane 1995; Gold *et al.* 1996b; Drummond *et al.* 1998; Drummond and McGuire 2001). The precise methods used to identify, measure and value the costs and outcomes will depend on the type of economic evaluation used, which in turn depends on the question being posed and the framework of analysis used to answer that question.

Type of economic evaluation and the rules of efficiency

As highlighted above, economic evaluation is not just about costs, but the relationship between costs and outcomes. A number of different types of economic evaluation methods exist. Each values resource use in monetary terms, but, as shown in Table 14.1, differs in how the outcomes of the alternative options are measured or valued (Torrance *et al.* 1996; Drummond *et al.* 1998).

Table 14.1 Types of economic evaluation

Type of economic evaluation	*Measurement/valuation of outcomes*
Cost-minimization analysis	Evidence from other sources, such as clinical trials, that the outcomes of the alternative interventions being evaluated are similar in all important aspects
Cost-consequence analysis	Various relevant clinically based and/or patient-based outcomes
Cost-benefit analysis	Monetary units
Cost-effectiveness analysis	Natural units (e.g. life years gained, cased detected)
Cost-utility analysis	Utility, usually QALYs gained

Cost-minimization analysis

The simplest type of analysis is cost-minimization analysis. This is used where it can be shown, for example from trial data, that there is good evidence that the outcomes of interest are similar for the alternative options under appraisal. Where this is the case it is only necessary to show differences in the resource costs between the alternatives, the least costly option being the most efficient one. For example, Coast *et al.* (1998) conducted a cost-minimization analysis of 'hospital at home' versus acute hospital care for medically stable elderly patients. The study was carried out alongside a pragmatic randomized clinical trial (RCT) which found the effectiveness, measured in terms of mortality, functioning, quality of life and satisfaction of care, to be similar between the two approaches to care (Richards *et al.* 1998).

Cost-consequence analysis

Cost-consequence analysis uses a mixture of relevant clinically-based measures, such as survival and symptom-free days, as well as patient-based measures relating to symptoms and or quality of life. An efficient option is thus one that is either less costly and 'overall' at least as effective as its alternative; or costs the same and is 'overall' more effective that its alternative; or is 'overall' more effective and more costly, but the additional benefit is thought worth the additional cost. An alternative is 'overall' more effective if it fairs better on at least one outcome measure and no worse on another. Where an intervention fairs better on one outcome and worse on another, decision-makers will have to make value judgements about the trade-offs in outcome to assess the overall value of effectiveness. Whether decision-makers' values are appropriate and whether they can cope with the cognitive burden, however, is a source of concern. Some means of combining the various outcomes is thus required (Drummond *et al.* 1998).

Cost-benefit analysis

In principle, cost-benefit analysis is the most comprehensive economic evaluation technique available. It requires both the resource use and non-resource use consequences of an intervention to be valued in monetary terms. A health care intervention that has a positive net value, in monetary terms, is thus an efficient one. Where many alternatives are being compared, the implication is that priority should be given to the intervention with the greatest net value. The results of a cost-benefit analysis are sometimes presented as cost-benefit ratios such that a ratio of less than 1 is efficient. Neither cost-benefit ratios nor benefit-cost ratios are generally recommended, however, because of inconsistencies in what is classified as a cost and what is classified as a benefit. Presenting the net value instead avoids this problem (Garber *et al.* 1996; Drummond *et al.* 1998).

In theory, because cost-benefit analysis values all the outcomes in monetary terms, it allows for efficiency comparisons across health and other sectors of society. The theoretical advantages, however, tend to be outweighed by the practical disadvantages of valuing the outcomes in monetary terms.

The most common means of assigning a monetary value to health consequences are the *willingness to pay* and *human capital* approaches. Willingness to pay (contingent valuation) uses survey methods to present respondents with hypothetical scenarios about the health care interventions under evaluation. The respondents are asked to think about the benefits associated with the intervention and reveal the maximum about they would be willing to pay for it. Although the number of published willingness to pay studies is growing, most are experimental, exploring conceptual issues regarding how willingness to pay should be measured – for example, to avoid bias and take account of uncertainty in health outcomes (Gafni 1991; Neumann and Johannesson 1994; O'Brien and Viramontes 1994; O'Brien and Gafni 1996; Drummond et al. 1998).

The human capital approach essentially values health resulting from the intervention in terms of the affected individuals' productive value. This is the present value of their future earnings (Weisbrod et al. 1980; Drummond et al. 1998). There are, however, practical and theoretical problems associated with the approach. For example, imperfections exist in the labour market causing inequalities in pay and hence inequalities in the value of health between individuals. In addition it is argued that the human capital approach, which restricts the impact of an intervention to productivity in the labour market, is not consistent with the principles of welfare economics, which has a wider view of the utility consequences beyond productivity. Hence the willingness to pay approach is generally preferred although, as highlighted above, still has conceptual problems (Mishan 1971; Drummond et al. 1998). Hence, despite the common use of the term cost-benefit analysis, in practice because of the practical difficulties and social dislike of putting a monetary value on life and suffering, cost-benefit studies are rarely undertaken.

Cost-effectiveness analysis

Cost-effectiveness analysis is appropriate where the health consequences of alternative interventions being appraised are expected to differ but can be measured in a uni-dimensional natural unit reflecting the health gains, such as life years gained or cases detected. No attempt is made to value the outcomes.

The incremental costs and effects of a health care intervention compared to some relevant alternative can be depicted graphically in a cost-effectiveness plane as shown in Figure 14.1 (Black 1990). Quadrants II and IV depict situations of dominance. In Quadrant II, the new intervention dominates, meaning it is either less costly and at least as effective as the alternative(s) or more effective and costs no more than the alternative(s). Similarly, in Quadrant IV the existing health care intervention dominates. These situations of dominance are, however, relatively rare. On the other hand, it is more common for a new intervention to be more (or less) effective but also cost more (or less) than the alternative(s) under appraisal, as depicted in Quadrants I and III. Here, where dominance does not exist, the results are presented as an incremental cost-effectiveness ratio (ICER). This can be expressed mathematically as:

$$ICER = \frac{C_A - C_B}{E_A - E_B}$$

Where C_A is the cost associated with the new intervention and C_B the cost associated with current treatment. Similarly, E_A is the effectiveness associated with the new intervention and E_B is the effectiveness associated with current treatment. Such a cost-effectiveness ratio may be, for example, the additional cost per additional case detected (Bryan et al. 1995; Drummond et al. 1998; Johnston and Brown 1999).

This then raises the issue as to what is an acceptable incremental cost-effectiveness ratio. An indication of what has been acceptable historically is useful but, essentially, a value judgement has to be made as to what society is willing to pay for an additional unit of effect (Laupacis et al. 1992). Graphically, in Figure 14.1, those interventions with incremental cost effectiveness ratios below the maximum acceptable cost-effectiveness ratio in Quadrants I or II will be deemed efficient. This area changes, of course, as the maximum acceptable cost-effectiveness ratio changes.

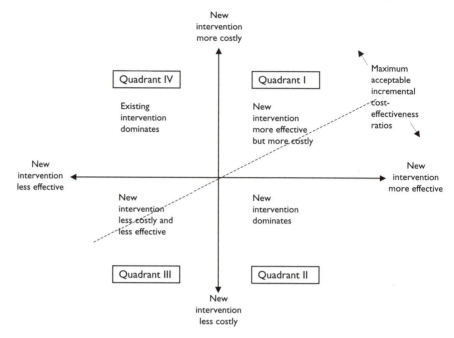

Figure 14.1   The cost–effectiveness plane

Source: adapted from Black (1990)

Cost-effectiveness analysis is appropriate for addressing technical efficiency – i.e. the most efficient intervention for treating a particular condition, for example, treating breast cancer. It can also be used for making comparisons across conditions whose effects are measured in the same units. Theoretically, however, it is more limited than cost-benefit analysis, as comparisons cannot be made across conditions where different outcome measures are used. Moreover, it is unlikely that a uni-dimensional measure of effectiveness will capture all the important effects.

Cost-utility analysis

Cost-utility analysis, by measuring the health effects in a generic unit, allows a broader comparison across different conditions. Essentially, cost-utility analysis can be considered a special case of cost-effectiveness analysis whereby the effects of the intervention are measured in terms of utility.

Utility reflects the preference of individuals or society. In the context of health care evaluation it refers to the value placed on a specific health status or an improvement in health status. The quality adjusted life year (QALY) is the most common measure of utility. It incorporates an interventions impact on survival as well as health-related quality of life. The quality of life associated with a health state is valued on a scale of 0 to 1, where death is assigned a value of 0 and full health a value of 1. The duration of each health state is then multiplied by its utility value. Where an intervention leads patients to experience a number of consecutive health states, the weighted durations are summed to give the total number of QALYs or QALY profile. This can be presented mathematically as:

$$\text{Total QALYs} = \Sigma^n_t \, v_1 d_1 + v_2 d_2 + v_3 d_3 \ldots v_n d_n$$

Where $v_{1 \ldots n}$ is the utility value for health states $1 \ldots n$, respectively, and $d_{1 \ldots n}$ is the duration of the respective health states.

The QALYs gained with a new intervention compared with existing treatment is thus estimated as the difference in respective QALY profiles. This is depicted graphically in Figure 14.2, which provides an example of a QALY profile for a new intervention and one for the current treatment. With the new intervention patients live longer and die on average at time t_1, compared to time t_0 with the current treatment. In this example, patients experience some decrease in quality of life with the new intervention. The area Q between the QALY profiles depicts this. After this decrease in quality of life patients then experience an improvement with the new intervention, as depicted by the area P between the QALY profiles. The total QALYs gained attributable to the new intervention is thus the area P minus area Q (Williams 1985).

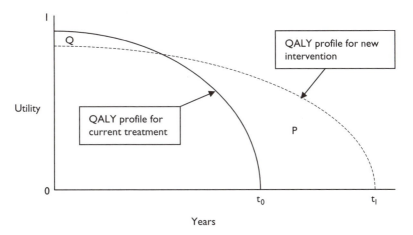

Figure 14.2   Example of a QALY profile for a new and current treatment

Eliciting utility values

A number of techniques exist to elicit values for specific health states; the three most widely used being the *standard gamble*, the *time trade-off* and the *visual analogue* or *rating scale*. The standard gamble is the classical method based on the axioms of expected utility theory (von Neumann and Morgenstern 1947; Torrance 1986). If a chronic health state is being valued, it asks respondents to consider a hypothetical choice between certainty in the chronic health state for life and a gamble. The gamble has two possible outcomes: full health (valued as 1) for life, or death (valued as 0). The probability of full health p is varied systematically, with the use of visual aids such as a probability wheel, until the respondent is indifferent between the certainty in the chronic health state for life and the gamble. At the point of indifference the chronic health state is valued as p. In the extreme case, for example, if the respondent values the chronic health state equivalent to good health, he would only accept the gamble if there were no probability of dying and the probability of full health were 1, equivalent to the value assigned to full health. The standard gamble approach can be adapted to take account of temporary health states, i.e. those followed by good health, and health states valued worse than death (Gold *et al.* 1996a; Drummond *et al.* 1998).

The time trade-off method requires the respondent to make choices between two certain outcomes. When a chronic health state is valued, the respondent is asked to choose between spending the rest of his or her life in the chronic health state or a shorter amount of time in full health. The amount of time in full health is varied systematically, again using visual aids, until the respondent is indifferent between the longer time in the chronic health state and less time in good health. The chronic health state is then valued as the shorter life expectancy in full health at the point of indifference divided by the life expectancy in the chronic health state. In the extreme case, for example, if the chronic health state is valued equivalent to good health, the respondent would be unwilling to give up any time in the chronic health state, hence the value of the chronic health state would be 1, the same as the value assigned to full health. The time trade-off approach can also be adapted to take account of temporary health states and for health states valued worse than death (Gold *et al.* 1996a; Drummond *et al.* 1998).

The visual analogue, or rating scale, requires the respondent to assign a number on a scale to the health state. The scale is often represented on a line on a page with clearly defined end-points represented by 0 and 100, which are then rescaled on a 0 to 1 scale. The approach can accommodate temporary health states and health states worse than death. Although simpler in its administration than either the standard gamble or time trade-off methods, it is often argued to be inferior as it does not employ the notion of choice and lacks theoretical foundation (Dolan 2001).

Generic classification instruments

Valuing health states using the methods described above is time-consuming, however. Rather than develop study-specific descriptions of health states, which then have to be valued, pre-scored multi attribute health status classification systems, such as the EuroQol EQ-5D (Brooks 1996), Quality of Well-Being (Kaplan and Anderson 2004) or Health Utilities Index (Gold *et al.* 1996a; Drummond *et al.* 1998) are often used. The EQ-5D, for example, is essentially a short questionnaire in which a patients classifies his or her current health status according to five domains: mobility, self-care, usual activities, pain/discomfort and anxiety/depression. Each domain consists of three levels and the patient indicates the level corresponding to their health state for each of the domains. The patient's health state is then valued according to a tariff originally obtained, using the time trade-off method, from a sample of the UK adult population (Brooks 1996; Drummond *et al.* 1998).

There is debate over *whose* values are appropriate. While it is increasingly being accepted that the values of the general public should be used for decision-making, since the public bears the costs associated with health care provision, others argue that it is only those experiencing the health state who actually know what it is like. In reality the distinction is not clear-cut as members of the general population experience and have experienced varying degrees of ill health in their lives (Dolan 1999, 2001).

As with cost-effectiveness analysis, an efficient intervention is one that is less costly and is *at least* as effective than the alternative(s), or *more* effective and costs no more than the alternative(s). Where this is not the case, the additional costs and QALYs gained with an intervention are presented in terms of an incremental cost-utility ratio. Again this raises the question as to what is an acceptable incremental cost per QALY gained. It is generally recognized, for example, that the UK National Institute for Clinical Excellence (NICE) has recently revised its threshold of acceptance to around £20,000 per QALY gained (see www.nice.org.uk).

Costing health care interventions

Costing involves identifying, measuring and valuing the resources incurred and avoided as a result of undertaking a particular health care intervention, the purpose being to value, in monetary terms, all the resource changes needed to produce a certain health outcome as a result of the intervention. Thus the sacrifices can be weighed against the gains of the intervention to determine the relative desirability of the intervention (Brouwer *et al.* 2001).

Identifying resource use

Resource costs include those incurred by the health service as a result of the intervention, for example, the cost of health care personnel, medical facilities and any diagnostic tests, drugs and supplies. Other sectors of society, such as social services, may also incur similar types of cost. In addition, patients are likely to incur out of pocket expenses related to receiving their treatment, such as the cost of travelling to and from their place of treatment or for childcare or dietary changes. The time a patient spends seeking care or receiving treatment is also a resource cost as is an informal carer's time and their out of pocket expenses incurred as result of their caring activities.

More controversial is the inclusion of productivity costs, that is, the costs associated with the lost, or decreased, ability to undertake paid and/or unpaid work or take part in leisure activities as a result of illness (Luce *et al.* 1996; Sculpher 2001). For a comprehensive review of the issues see Sculpher (2001). He distinguishes the following components of productivity costs: those incurred by the individual suffering from the illness as a result of lost work and leisure time, the external tax effects (the value of gross minus net income), the cost to the employer of the recruitment and training of a replacement worker and the effect on the previously unemployed replacing the ill individual. Most of the literature leads to the conclusion that an element of productivity cost should be included in economic evaluations, but differs on what should be included. The frictional cost method, for example, which was developed by some Dutch health economists, focuses mainly on the valuation of lost time from paid work. With the existence of involuntary employment in the labour market, it assumes that a previously unemployed individual can replace the lost productivity of an ill individual. Although there will be a cost incurred by the employer as a result of recruiting and training the previously unemployed individual, productivity loss will only occur during this 'friction' period of replacement (Koopmanschap and van Inveld 1992; Koopmanschap *et al.* 1995; Koopmanschap and Rutten 1996). The approach does not go uncriticized, however, with others arguing that the concept of a replacement worker may not be so simple in practice (Weinstein *et al.* 1997; Sculpher 2001). Nonetheless, the literature does tend to agree that when a generic outcome measure such as the QALY is used then the effect of lost leisure time to the individual is captured in theory, at least, by the outcome measure (Sculpher 2001).

Resource costs have also been classified in terms of direct and indirect costs, but this has led to confusion. Direct costs are those changes in resource use directly attributable to the intervention or treatment regimen. Although what is understood as direct hospital costs tends to be consistent, the inclusion of patients' and others' time costs is inconsistently classified as a direct cost, sometimes being termed as an indirect cost. Productivity gains or losses related to illness or death are generally referred to as indirect costs, but the term indirect cost is still open to many interpretations. Accountants for example refer to overheads and fixed costs as indirect costs (Luce *et al.* 1996; Drummond *et al.* 1998; Brouwer *et al.* 2001).

The range of resource costs included in the analysis will depend on the viewpoint, or perspective, of the study (Luce *et al.* 1996; Drummond *et al.* 1998; Brouwer *et al.* 2001). Generally, health economists argue that a societal perspective should be taken, such that all the important costs are included in the analysis, regardless of which sectors of society incur the costs. Often, however, studies adopt a narrower health service perspective, thus ignoring the costs incurred by patients, social and voluntary services, for example. If such excluded costs are substantial, however, then what appears to be an efficient use of resources from the narrower perspective of the health service may in fact be inefficient from a wider societal perspective.

The resource costs included in the analysis will also depend on the time horizon of the study. Ideally, the time horizon chosen should capture all the major resource use changes of the intervention under study (Luce *et al.* 1996; Brouwer *et al.* 2001). The inclusion of future resource use for diseases unrelated to the intervention under study, but which occur during an extended survival period as a result of the intervention, remains controversial (Luce *et al.* 1996; Johnston 2002). A theoretical case can be made for the inclusion of such costs as the intervention affects the way resources are used in the future. In practice, however, this would imply opposing a prevention programme, such as smoking cessation, because those spared a premature death from smoking-related causes would consume health care resources, unrelated to smoking, in the future. It might be argued, however, that future therapeutic decisions should be considered on their own merits. Also on a practical level, data may not be adequate to capture such future resource use. It is also worth noting that, if future health service resources are included then the future non-health service resources should also be considered (Luce *et al.* 1996; Drummond *et al.* 1998).

Measuring resource use

After identifying the costs to be included in an analysis, the next step is to measure the volume of resource use. The level of detail will depend on the approach taken. With a gross or macro-costing approach, resource use is broken down into larger components, such as inpatient days. With micro-costing the separate resource items are detailed. In general, this will include consideration of the staff time, consumable items, capital equipment and buildings plus the overheads and is referred by some as the 'bottom up' approach. Special surveys may be needed to collect such data if it is not readily available from other sources such as budget statements.

Gross-costing obviously has the advantage that it is requires less of the researcher's time, however, it provides less insight into the relationship between the scale of activity and unit costs. The choice of approach depends on the level of precision required. Both micro- and gross-costing methods are often used within one study for different resource use events. Macro-costing can provide an overall impression of the total costs, but micro-costing will be more important where costs between the alternatives under appraisal are likely to diverge or occur in the present. Future costs are likely to be less certain even with micro-costing (Luce *et al.* 1996; Brouwer *et al.* 2001).

Valuing resource use

In theory, to reflect a societal valuation of the sacrifice of the resources used to provide a health care intervention, the resources used should be valued at their opportunity cost – that is, the value in their best alternative use. In a competitive market this would be equivalent to the market price. Where market prices are not available, tariffs are frequently used, especially where a gross-costing approach is taken. They should only be used, however, where there is a clear indication that they reasonably approximate to actual costs and they contribute to a small amount of the total cost of the intervention being evaluated. In practice, tariffs are often used as means of allocating resources to health care providers without any real relationship to the costs of providing the service (Luce *et al.* 1996; Brouwer *et al.* 2001).

If published data on costs are not available, or are not thought to be generalizable, micro-costing of the opportunity cost of the separate resource use items, such as staff time and capital equipment, will be necessary. Market prices are often used to value such items, but where market prices do not exist, as in the case of a voluntary carer's time, an imputed market price such as the cost of a professional alternative can be used to reflect the opportunity cost of a carer's time. All costs should be presented at prices consistent with a specified year (Luce *et al.* 1996; Brouwer *et al.* 2001).

Just as not all costs require money outlays so not all money outlays imply a cost. Transfer payments, such as social benefits, are simply transfers from one sector of society to another. They do not reflect the use of resources and are therefore not real economic costs and should thus be excluded from the economic analysis. The issue is less clear where prices are used to estimate the opportunity cost of resources. It may be argue here that social transfers such as income tax or VAT are important to the decision-maker as they make up the full cost to the health service (Brouwer *et al.* 2001). The importance will depend on the perspective of the study.

A further consideration in the valuation of resource use is average versus marginal costs. Average costs include fixed costs, such as the cost of the building and over-heads, which do not vary with increased output. In the short run, therefore, the marginal costs of producing one additional unit of outcome would exclude the fixed costs. In the long run, however, average costs may be more appropriate as there will come a point where increased output requires expansion of the fixed costs. The fixed costs will then become variable. The analyst needs to consider the time horizon of the study and whether fixed costs are likely to become variable in the future (Luce *et al.* 1996; Brouwer *et al.* 2001).

It can be seen from the above discussion that the process of costing is complex. The analyst must ultimately decide on the appropriate method in the light of available data and the importance of the cost component in the context of the total cost of the intervention. It is therefore important that the analyst states clearly how the resources were identified, measured and valued.

Research design and implementation issues

Framework of analysis

Economic evaluations rely on good evidence on outcomes. Since RCTs are the clinical gold standard, health economists often turn to trials as an initial source of data. Clinical trials offer a relatively easy means of collecting economic data. The EuroQol EQ-5D (Brooks 1996), for example, can be added to other quality of life questionnaires used in a trial.

Clinical trials also offer a means of collecting data on resource use. The data collection forms will need to be well thought out in advance of the study and are best incorporated into the case record forms routinely collected throughout the trial. Care will be needed, however, to exclude the costing of events that are proto-col driven, such as outpatient visits scheduled specifically to monitor patients in the trial. Resource use should reflect the resources incurred in the service situation. A further issue arises from the fact that centres participating in trials are self-selective with an interested in research. Resource use data taken from a clinical trial may, therefore, have limited generalizablility if participating centres are not representative of centres in the wider population or other countries (Wilke *et al.* 1998; Raikou *et al.* 2000).

A further limitation of data collected in trials, generally, is the length of the clinical trial. Costs and health outcomes may occur beyond the trial time period. They can be taken into account through modelling the longer-term consequences. In any case, where trial data are not available or feasible, modelling the clinical pathways and the resource-generating events will be a necessary alternative. The modelling may be informed, for example, by the published literature, registry data and specially-designed surveys, or by adding follow-up measurement to the initial clinical trial. In some cases it will be necessary to resort to expert opinion. A tension nonetheless often exists between the pressure to use only evidence obtained directly from clinical trials and the need of the economist to model the broader consequences of the interventions (Gold *et al.* 1996a; Brouwer *et al.* 2001).

Dealing with uncertainty

In practice, uncertainty is widespread in economic evaluations. Methodological uncertainties were highlighted above, for example, concerning whose utility values are appropriate, the inclusion of productivity costs, future costs and the discount rate used. Other uncertainties highlighted were the generalizablility, or transferability, of findings to other settings. Also, given the complex process of cost and health outcome estimation, their values are invariably imprecise.

The standard way to deal with these uncertainties is to conduct sensitivity analyses, whereby the component of interest is varied by a meaningful amount. If the main results are insensitive to such variation then the analyst can conclude that their findings are robust. Sensitivity analyses are often used to determine those parameters where further data collection is required to give more precise estimates. One parameter is often varied at a time, but it may be meaningful to vary more than one parameter at a time or to conduct an extreme scenario analysis (Briggs *et al.* 1994; Briggs and Sculpher 1995; Manning *et al.* 1996; Briggs 2001).

Where utility and resource use data are collected at the patient level, for example, from patients within a clinical trial, uncertainty can be handled with statistical analysis. The alternative approaches have been much debated in the literature (Briggs and Sculpher 1995). Although resource use data are stochastic, thus allowing such analyses, it should be noted that unit costs are generally deterministic requiring sensitivity analysis to address their uncertainties.

Where data are synthesized using decision analytic models, uncertainty in the parameter estimates can be addressed through probabilistic sensitivity analysis. Each parameter in the model is assigned a distribution chosen to represent uncertainty in the parameter. The model is run many times. During each run the model simultaneously selects at random a value for each parameter from its assigned distribution using Monte Carlo simulation. The proportion of Monte Carlo simulations or runs favouring each treatment option can then be estimated for differing values assigned to the health outcome (Briggs 2001).

Dealing with time preference

As individuals and, collectively, as a society we are not indifferent as to when costs and benefits arise. A degree of positive time preference is exhibited. Individuals and society prefer to experience benefits now rather than later and would prefer to postpone costs. Time preference is evidenced, for example, by the existence of real interest rates (after allowing for inflation) paid on money saved. Economic evaluations take account of time preference by discounting future costs and benefits to their present value. For example:

$$PV = C_0 + \frac{C_1}{(1+r)^1} + \frac{C_2}{(1+r)^2} + \ldots + \frac{Cn}{(1+r)^n}$$

Where PV is the present value, C is the cost (or benefit) incurred each time period for time $t = 0$ to $t = n$ and r is the discount rate (Drummond *et al.* 1998).

Discounting is not without its concerns, however, and there is ongoing discussion, among other things, over what discount rate should be used and whether health benefits should be discounted at the same rate as monetary costs (Cairns 2001). Nonetheless, current practice and recommended guidelines generally suggest that future costs and health benefits should be discounted at the same rate and most guidelines suggest a discount rate of between 3 and 5 per cent. For example, the UK Treasury currently recommends a rate of 3.5 per cent per annum for discounting costs and benefits of public sector projects (http://greenbook.treasury.gov.uk).

Conclusions

A number of economic evaluation techniques are available to aid efficient decision-making. Each is concerned with evaluating two or more options and systematically compares both the costs and health outcomes. They differ, however, in terms of how the health outcomes are measured or valued. Only cost-utility analysis and cost-benefit analysis, by the nature of how the health outcomes are valued, allow comparisons across treatment areas.

When conducting an economic evaluation, it is important to consider the perspective of the study and the time horizon of analysis, as these will influence the costs included. Methodological uncertainties exist, for example, concerning whose utility values are appropriate, whether productivity costs and future costs should be excluded, the appropriate discount rate for costs and benefits, and the generalizablility of findings from trial data to other settings. Modelling may be needed as an alternative or adjunct to data collected in clinical trials. Given the methodological uncertainties and complex process of cost and health outcome estimation it is important that the analyst states clearly how the resources used and how health outcomes were identified, measured and valued and that uncertainty is addressed through sensitivity and/or statistical analyses as appropriate.

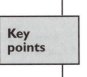

Key points

- A number of economic evaluation techniques are available to aid efficient decision-making.

- Each is concerned with evaluating two or more health care options and systematically compares both the costs and health outcomes.

- The techniques differ in terms of how the health outcomes are measured or valued.

- Only cost-utility analysis and cost-benefit analysis, by the nature of how health outcomes are valued, allow comparisons across treatment areas.

- The perspective of the study and the time horizon of analysis will influence the costs included.

- The analyst needs to state clearly how the resources used and health outcomes were identified, measured and valued.

- Modelling may be needed as an alternative or adjunct to data collected in clinical trials.

- Uncertainty needs to be addressed through sensitivity and/or statistical analyses, as appropriate.

References

Black, W.C. (1990) The CE plane: a graphic representation of cost-effectiveness, *Medical Decision Making*, 10: 212–14.

Briggs, A. (2001) Handling uncertainty in economic evaluation and presenting results, in M. Drummond and A. McGuire (eds) *Economic Evaluation in Health Care: Merging Theory with Practice*, pp. 172–235. Oxford: Oxford University Press.

Briggs, A. and Sculpher, M. (1995) Sensitivity analysis in economic evaluation: a review of published studies, *Health Economics*, 4: 355–71.

Briggs, A., Sculpher, M. and Buxton, M. (1994) Uncertainty in the economic evaluation of health care technologies: the role of sensitivity analysis, *Health Economics*, 3: 95–104.

Brooks, R. (1996) EuroQol: the current state of play, *Health Policy*, 37: 53–72.

Brouwer, W., Rutten, F. and Koopmanschap, M. (2001) Costing in economic evaluations, in M. Drummond and A. McGuire (eds) *Economic Evaluation in Health Care: Merging Theory with Practice*, pp. 68–93. Oxford: Oxford University Press.

Bryan, S., Brown, J. and Warren, R. (1995) Mammography screening: an incremental cost effectiveness analysis of two-view versus on-view procedures in London, *Journal of Epidemiology and Community Health*, 49: 70–8.

Buxton, M. (1993) Scarce resources and informed choices, in D. Ashton (ed.) *Future Trends in Medicine*, pp. 36–9. London: Royal Society of Medicine Press Ltd.

Cairns, J. (2001) Discounting in economic evaluation, in M. Drummond and A. McGuire (eds) *Economic Evaluation in Health Care: Merging Theory with Practice*, pp. 236–55. Oxford: Oxford University Press.

Coast, J., Richards, S.H., Peters, T.J. *et al.* (1998) Hospital at home or acute hospital care? A cost minimisation analysis, *British Medical Journal*, 316: 1802–6.

Dolan, P. (1999) Whose preferences count? *Medical Decision Making*, 19: 482–6.

Dolan, P. (2001) Output measures and valuation in health, in M. Drummond and A. McGuire (eds) *Economic Evaluation in Health Care: Merging Theory with Practice*, pp. 46–67. Oxford: Oxford University Press.

Drummond, M. and McGuire, A. (2001) *Economic Evaluation in Health Care: Merging Theory with Practice*. Oxford: Oxford University Press.

Drummond, M.F., O'Brien, B., Stoddart, G.L. and Torrance, G.W. (1998) *Methods for the Economic Evaluation of Health Care Programmes*. Oxford: Oxford University Press.

Elixhauser, A., Luce, B.R., Taylor, W.R. *et al.* (1993) Health care CBA/CEA: an update in the growth and composition of the literature, *Medical Care*, 31, Suppl: js1–js11.

Gafni, A. (1991) Using willingness-to-pay as a measure of benefit: what is the relevant question to ask in the context of public decision-making? *Medical Care*, 29: 1246–52.

Garber, A.M., Weinstein M.C., Torrance, G.W. and Kamlet, M.S. (1996) Theoretical foundations of cost-effectiveness analysis, in M.R. Gold, J.E. Siegel, L.B. Russell and M.C. Weinstein (eds) *Cost-effectiveness in Health and Medicine*, pp. 25–53. Oxford: Oxford University Press.

Gold, M.R., Patrick, G.W., Torrance, G.W. *et al.* (1996a) Identifying and valuing outcomes, in M.R. Gold, J.E. Siegel, L.B. Russell and M.C. Weinstein (eds) *Cost-effectiveness in Health and Medicine*, pp. 82–134. Oxford: Oxford University Press.

Gold, M.R., Siegel, J.E., Russel, L.B. and Weinstein, M.C. (1996b) *Cost-effectiveness in Health and Medicine*. Oxford: Oxford University Press.

Johnston, K. (2002) Modelling the future costs of breast screening, *European Journal of Cancer*, 37: 1752–8.

Johnston, K. and Brown, J. (1999) Two-view mammography at incident screens: cost effectiveness analysis of policy options, *British Medical Journal*, 319: 1097–102.

Kaplan, R.M. and Anderson, J.P. (2004) The general health policy model: an integrated approach, in B. Spilker (ed.) *Quality of life and Pharmacoeconomics in Clinical Trials*, pp. 309–22. Philadelphia, PA: Lippincott-Raven.

Koopmanschap, M.A. and van Ineveld, B.M. (1992) Towards a new approach for estimating indirect costs of disease, *Social Science and Medicine*, 34: 1005–10.

Koopmanschap, M.A., Rutten, F.F.H., van Inveld, B.M. and van Roijen, L. (1995) The friction cost method for measuring indirect costs of disease, *Journal of Health Economics*, 14: 171–89.

Koopmanschap, M.A. and Rutten, F.F.H. (1996) Indirect costs: the consequence of production loss or increased costs of production, *Medical Care*, 34: DS59–68.

Laupacis, P., Feeny, D., Detsky, A.S. *et al.* (1992) How attractive does a new technology have to be to warrant adoption and utilisation? Tentative guidelines for using clinical and economic evaluations, *Canadian Medical Association Journal*, 146: 473–81.

Luce, B.R., Manning, W.G., Siegel, J.E. and Lipscomb, J. (1996) Estimating costs in cost-effectiveness analysis, in M.R. Gold, J.E. Siegel, L.B. Russell and M.C. Weinstein (eds) *Cost-effectiveness in Health and Medicine*, pp. 176–213. Oxford: Oxford University Press.

Manning, W.G., Fryback, D.G., and Weinstein, M.C. (1996) Reflecting uncertainty in cost-effectiveness analysis, in M.R. Gold, J.E. Siegel, L.B. Russell and M.C. Weinstein (eds) *Cost-effectiveness in Health and Medicine*, pp. 247–75. Oxford: Oxford University Press.

Mishan, E.J. (1971) Evaluation of life and limb: a theoretical approach, *Journal of Political Economy*, 79: 687–706.

Neumann, P. and Johannesson, M. (1994) The willingness-to-pay for in-vitro fertilization: a pilot study using contingent valuation, *Medical Care* 32: 686–9.

O'Brien, B. and Gafni, M. (1996) When do the 'dollars' make sense? Toward a conceptual framework for contingent valuation studies in health care, *Medical Decision Making*, 16: 288–99.

O'Brien, B. and Viramontes, J.L. (1994) Willingness-to-pay: a valid and reliable measure of health state preference? *Medical Decision Making*, 14: 289–97.

Pritchard, C. (1998) *Trends in Economic Evaluation*, OHE Briefing no. 36. London: Office of Health Economics.

Raikou, M., Briggs, A., Gray, A. and McGuire, A. (2000) Costing methodology: centre-specific or average unit costs in multi-centre studies? Some theory and simulation, *Health Economics*, 9: 191–8.

Richards, S.H., Coast, J., Gunnell, D.J. *et al.* (1998) Randomised controlled trial comparing the effectiveness and acceptability of an early discharge hospital at home scheme with acute hospital care, *British Medical Journal*, 316: 1796–1801.

Sculpher, M. (2001) The role of estimating productivity costs in economic evaluation, in M. Drummond and A. McGuire (eds) *Economic Evaluation in Health Care: Merging Theory with Practice*, pp. 94–112. Oxford: Oxford University Press.

Sloane, F.A. (1995) *Valuing Health Care: Costs, Benefits and Effectiveness of Pharmaceuticals and Other Medical Technologies*. Cambridge: Cambridge University Press.

Torrance, G.W. (1986) Measurement of health state utilities for economic appraisal, *Journal of Health Economics*, 5: 1–30.

Torrance, G.W., Siegel, J.E. and O'Brien, B. (1996) Framing and designing the cost-effectiveness analysis, in M.R. Gold, J.E. Siegel, L.B. Russell and M.C. Weinstein (eds) *Cost-effectiveness in Health and Medicine*, pp. 54–81. Oxford: Oxford University Press.

Von Neumann, J. and Morgenstern, O. (1947) *Theories of Games of Economic Behaviour*. Princeton, NJ: Princeton University Press.

Weinstein, M.C. (1995) From cost-effectiveness ratios to resource allocation: where to draw the line? in F.A. Sloane (ed.) *Valuing Health Care: Costs, Benefits, and Effectiveness of Pharmaceuticals and Other Medical Technologies*, pp. 77–97. Cambridge: Cambridge University Press.

Weinstein, M.C., Siegel, J.E. and Garber, A.M. (1997) Productivity costs, time costs and health-related quality of life: a response to the Erasmus group, *Health Economics*, 6: 505–10.

Weisbrod, B.A., Test, M.A. and Stein, L.I. (1980) Alternatives to mental hospital treatment: economic cost-benefit analysis, *Archives of General Psychiatry*, 37: 400–5.

Wilke, R., Glick, H., Polsky, D. and Schulman, K. (1998) Estimating country-specific costs-effectiveness from multi-national trials, *Health Economics*, 7: 481–94.

Williams, A. (1985) Economics of coronary artery bypass grafting, *British Medical Journal*, 291: 326–9.

Part 3
Multidisciplinary research measurement

15 Psychological approaches to measuring and modelling clinical decision-making

Clare Harries and Olga Kostopoulou

Introduction

The aim of this chapter is to introduce the reader to a range of methods used to describe and evaluate clinical decision-making. We describe five different approaches, the information that is gleaned from them and the theoretical models and assumptions that underlie them.

Why study clinicians' decision-making?

Researchers, clinicians, educationalists and health policy workers may be interested in measuring and modelling clinical decision-making for a variety of different reasons. They may wish to identify cognitive, emotional and situational factors that influence clinical judgement and decision-making and information-processing style. They may be interested in identifying aspects of clinicians' judgement and decision-making that might be improved (Poses *et al.* 1986), discovering differences in practice between different health regions (Tape *et al.* 1991), identifying sources of disagreement between individuals (Kirwan *et al.* 1983c, 1986) or discovering the role that clinicians play in inequalities in health care (Schulman *et al.* 1999) and the influence of non-clinical information on decision-making (McKinlay *et al.* 1996; Schulman *et al.* 1999). They may wish to identify changes in cognition as expertise develops (Elstein *et al.* 1978; Boshuizen *et al.* 1991; Schmidt and Boshuizen 1993), or they may wish to capture the steps in expert judgement and decision-making with a view to feeding that behaviour into a computerized expert system (e.g. De Dombal 1984; Shortliffe 1991), setting a gold standard (e.g. Kirwan *et al.* 1983a), or teaching others (e.g. Boreham 1989; Harries and Gilhooly 2003).

Clinicians as experts

It is a caricature within the domain of the psychology of medical decision-making that clinicians (and humans in general) are buffoons, limited by their information-processing capacity, psychophysical perception of probability and utility, and by the inappropriate associations that they rely on and the strategies that they choose to use. Reports on physicians' cognition focus on systematic errors and problems with the perception of probability – and therefore diagnosis, understanding of information, choice and judgement (Dawson and Arkes 1987; Dawson *et al.* 1988; Hamm and Zubialde 1995; Chapman and Elstein 2000). This emphasis on the potential pitfalls of intuitive judgement and the use of rules of thumb may justify wariness where lives, health and reputations are at stake. But it is not the only take on the psychology of judgement and decision-making. For example, researchers operating within a Brunswikian tradition emphasize judges' achievement, and accuracy, measuring performance in context – i.e. taking into account the nature of the environment and task (Bursztajn and Hamm 1979; Hamm 1988); though see Dhami *et al.* (2004). In keeping with this, experts' ability to pick up important underlying patterns using intuitive processes is emphasized in work on scripts and pattern recognition (Abernathy and Hamm 1995; Hamm *et al.* 2000; Hamm 2003). Simple heuristics (rules of thumb) have been identified that perform as well as more complicated models in a natural environment (Gigerenzer *et al.* 1999; Gigerenzer and Selten 2002): even with limited working memory we may use optimal strategies. Other research has non-judgementally described clinicians' judgement and decision-making (e.g. process approaches and those focusing on reasoning); or studies the expert clinician as the gold standard (e.g. naturalistic decision-making).

Several criteria have been used to identify 'experts' (Shanteau *et al.* 2003). For example, they are accredited, identified as experts by their peers or by society, have factual knowledge, and may well have several years of experience. Many clinicians meet all of these criteria, and nearly all clinicians meet at least one. However, these criteria are less than ideal: clinicians may not keep up to date with new developments after accreditation, or their performance may deteriorate post-qualification for other reasons. A clinician may be known by peers and patients as an expert because they are charismatic and confident rather than because of their successful treatment rates. Experience has been found to increase a person's confidence in their own performance, but does not necessarily lead to an improvement in that performance (Goldberg 1968; Harvey *et al.* 1987). Several researchers have argued that experts should at least show consistency in their judgements (test-retest reliability), should show agreement with other experts, and should be able to discriminate between different cases (Shanteau *et al.* 2003). Many studies report wide variation in clinicians' judgements and in the policies they use. This, and consistency, appears to be related to the nature of the expert's task: domains associated with unaided judgements on humans in dynamic situations, with poor or no outcome feedback and with little agreement on gold standards, are associated with poor test-retest reliability (Shanteau 1992; see Ashton 2000 for a recent review on test-retest reliability in experts). Experts and sub-expert clinicians may have the same factual knowledge but apply it to cases in different ways – with different associated degrees of success (Patel *et al.* 1990).

Several researchers have investigated the automaticity that develops with experience (e.g. Schneider and Shiffrin 1985). Such automatization implies that experienced judgement and decision-making is fast and unlikely to be controlled by conscious thought or accessible to verbalization. This mode of decision-making is more intuitive than analytical, more like perception than reasoning (Kahneman 2003) and more likely to be disrupted by introspective thinking aloud (McMackin and Slovic 2000). In problem-solving in chess and physics, experts' highly structured knowledge leads to better problem representation than that of novices, better memory for cases and forward reasoning, whereby the information provided in a case leads directly to the correct solution or judgement (see Green and Gilhooly 1992 for a summary of this research).

Such a characterization of expertise would lead to investigations of expert judgement and decision-making that do not rely on verbalization, that focus on the mental representations in long- and short-term memory and that minimize interruption of the natural process. In the field of health care however, the characterization of expert judgement and decision-making is less straightforward. In the complex area of medicine, decision-makers may face high objective uncertainty, often lacking both probability information and gold standards. They may bring in colleagues' or others' opinions, are required to record formally the reasoning behind their decisions or explain it to colleagues and patients, and may rely on decision aids. Again, they process information differently depending on its presentation and the task conditions (Hamm 1988). Such a continuum of modes of information processing is captured in Hammond's cognitive continuum shown in Figure 15.1.

In medicine, arguably, frequently encountered and straightforward cases will lead to the type of automatized 'recognition-primed decision-making' seen in many domains of expertise (Lipshitz *et al.* 2001) and similar to perceptual processes (Kahneman 2003). With experience, people acquire a large repertoire of patterns or schemata which enable them to recognize and immediately categorize new situations as familiar or not (Schmidt *et al.* 1990; Charlin *et al.* 2000). Experts reason forward from case information to a judgement or decision (Patel and Groen 1986), or base their recognition of a pattern on a few forceful features (Grant and Marsden 1987), when all the information is presented. However, where information about a case arrives in parts (as it does when a patient enters a clinic or doctor's surgery with a presenting complaint), and does not immediately fit a classic pattern, their

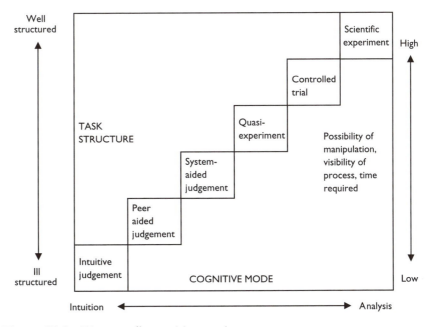

Figure 15.1   Hammond's cognitive continuum

Source: Hamm (1988). Reproduced with permission

reasoning, like that of novices, is better characterized as 'hypothetico-deductive': a few hypotheses are generated early on and evidence for (and, ideally, against) these is sought (Elstein *et al.* 1978). Pattern recognition or script activation (Charlin *et al.* 2000) may be seen as the first (hypothesis-generating) step of a hypothetico-deductive process, while partial pattern matching, or failure to match at all, leads to generation of multiple possible hypotheses. If time and opportunity allows, atypical cases, or cases in which stakes are high, are likely to encourage more analytic and systematic information processing (Chaiken *et al.* 1989).

In addition, clinicians of intermediate levels of experience have been found to recall case information better than less or more experienced clinicians (Claessen and Boshuizen 1985; Patel and Groen 1986; Boshuizen and Schmidt 1992). This has been explained by hypothesizing that because they lack a sufficiently broad repertoire of patterns, they use a deeper, more effortful level of processing, trying to apply their pathophysiological knowledge. Contact with patients leads to functional changes in knowledge: causal knowledge about disease consequences is accumulated, pathophysiological knowledge gets encoded into 'illness scripts' and episodic memories of actual cases are stored (Schmidt and Boshuizen 1993). This suggests that the information used to match patterns, or to generate and distinguish between hypotheses, will be functionally different with different degrees of experience. The variety and difficulty of cases seen in a health care setting leads to a variety of information-processing approaches. This in turn necessitates a variety of research methods, including those that investigate the organization of information or knowledge structures in memory (Charlin *et al.* 2000). In the following sections we discuss the situations in which each approach to modelling and measuring clinicians' decision-making might be more, or less, successful.

Interviews and focus groups

The results of interviews with clinicians differ depending upon the specificity of the questions asked, and this differs depending upon the purpose of the study. Studies asking general questions about information processing reveal both general and specific accounts. For example, using semi-structured interviews, DiCaccavo and Reid (1995) asked 36 GPs how they made decisions. Five of them indicated that they were not aware of how they used information, stating for example, '. . . it all goes into a dark box and makes a decision – which sometimes mystifies me . . .'. Eleven indicated the same, but more subtly: they explained how they negotiated management decisions with their patients, once they themselves had already decided on courses of action. Twelve gave general explanations talking in terms of tailoring the decision to the patients' needs and expectations or using their medical training and experience. Eight of the doctors gave scientific theories about their decision-making, including references to pattern recognition, algorithms, decision trees and personal protocols.

In another study, Andre *et al.* (2002) asked GPs in focus groups to discuss their use of 'rules of thumb' ('heuristics'). Classic heuristics are characterized as intuitive processes similar to perception (Kahneman 2003).[1] GPs concurred with the notion that many heuristics are implemented 'unconsciously', but, despite this, GPs in every group were able to recount specific examples. The explicit simple rules that they mentioned included patterns of symptoms suggestive of a particular disease or rules of thumb within which the steps to make a diagnosis had been abbreviated. Such open questioning reveals what clinicians believe and how they reason about their reasoning. Accounts may use the same terms as researchers themselves use (to hypothesize about clinicians' behaviour) but cannot be assumed to concur in the meaning of those terms.

Analyses to test the veracity of clinicians' descriptions of their own behaviour are rare but research on self-reports suggests that they are necessary (see Box 15.1). Accounts are often insufficiently specified to know when they are false (e.g. Andersson *et al.* 2002). When descriptions are specific to *types* of decision or case, group comparisons can be made, or predictions can be tested for individuals. For example, research assessing GPs' views on asthma treatment found that both those who believed that they were applying the guidelines and those who stated unfamiliarity with the guidelines described similar departures from them when asked about specific practices (Veninga *et al.* 1998). Quantitative information elicited in interviews is often worse than other sources at predicting actual behaviour. But such mismatches may lie in the assumptions as to how information is combined (Harries and Harvey 2000; Harries *et al.* 2000). Process rules elicited from interviews may also be used to predict judgements. From an interview with an expert consultant physician, following a think-aloud procedure with three 'paper patients' with migraine attacks (see p. 338), Boreham (1989) formed a set of 'production rules' ('if . . . then' rules). These were applied to seven new computer-simulated cases. The derived rules were reported to be effective at bringing seizures down in hypothetical patients, but comparisons with the original physician's behaviour were not reported.

Interviews that focus on specific instances (specific patient cases) increase specificity and avoid generalizations over what may be different decision-making procedures (see Box 15.1) but again tests of veracity are rare. While Boreham's interviews were based on paper-presented cases that had been seen relatively recently, van Thiel *et al.* (1997) investigated physicians' retrospective accounts of a specific real-life decision they had made to terminate a patient's life. Here interviews complemented the use of questionnaires. Discussion went beyond patient characteristics leading to an end-of-life decision and explored with whom the decision was discussed, and the reasoning behind it. This is a *critical incident approach* (one of the techniques used in naturalistic decision-making studies, see p. 348): it uses interviews to investigate the factors, reasoning and processes involved in recent memorable (effective or ineffective) decision-making situations. The resulting accounts are not always specific or predictive as they are subject to memory biases, but may illuminate some aspects of the decision situation. In another example, Dempsey and Bekker (2002) used an interview alongside GPs' proforma reporting of decisions to refer for emergency admission over four weeks, and their notes on a handful of specifically memorable prior incidents. They used qualitative analysis to identify themes influencing decision-making across GPs. These revealed the perceived constraints on the GPs' referral behaviour (see Box 15.2).

Interviews are useful, in that they allow an in-depth exploration and pursuit of the reasoning behind particular decisions. They can be used to complement other methods, either at the start of a programme in order to, for example, identify what information is relevant to the decision, the decision-making goals, the influence of underlying knowledge or other extraneous and constraining factors (that could feed into a task analysis – see Box 15.2), or to answer questions that other methods generate, for example by revealing interpretations of information. Arguably, they cannot be relied upon to be valid explanations, nor descriptions of underlying processes. Clinicians may have forgotten the specifics of the situation, the nature of the information processing, they may never have had access to it or they may be trying to generalize on the basis of one or more memorable situations. But even speculative hypotheses from someone who was there at the time of decision-making may yield useful insights into decision-making processes and the decision-making situation.

Box 15.1   Self-insight: what can we tell from what clinicians tell us about how they make judgements and decisions?

The debate about the usefulness of clinicians' (and others) verbalizations will run and run. Thirty years ago, Nisbett and Wilson (1977) demonstrated both that people *don't* report the influence of factors that seem to influence their choice, and that they *do* report the influence of factors that *don't* appear to influence their choice. People's accounts of their own behaviour were thought to represent *a priori* and socially-held theories. Ericsson and Simon (1984) agreed that retrospective reports were subject to forgetting and self-hypothesizing[2] (and idealizing). By this measure, descriptions of judgement and decision-making policies and behaviour gleaned in interviews are unlikely to be veridical – they are unlikely to match participants' actual behaviour. In keeping with this, a large number of judgement analysis studies that have asked participants to retrospectively report how their judgements were influenced by the available information suggested that self-insight is poor (Slovic and Lichtenstein 1971; Brehmer and Brehmer 1988). While clinicians and others' stated weights predict their actual decisions to some degree they are inferior to objective models calculated by researchers (though both depend upon the difficulty of the judgement task).

In fact, ratings of cue influence tend to have a systematic relationship to objective measures of cue influence: people list being influenced by many more cues than appear to be statistically influential and cues that are influential are a sub-set of those that are stated to be influential. Work in judgement analysis suggests that the apparently poor self-insight is less a matter of forgetting and more a problem of translating what you know into a verbalized policy. People seem to be able to pick the model of their own behaviour out when it is presented alongside those of others (Reilly and Doherty 1989, 1992; Reilly 1996; Harries *et al.* 2000). In particular, part of the problem of a retrospective account is the need to generalize one model that fits what may have been subtly different ways of using information on different cases (Harries and Harvey 2000; Lagnado *et al.* 2004).

But Ericsson and Simon (1980) argued that concurrent reports (those elicited from people while decision-making, judgement-making or problem-solving) could be more useful, as long as the information processing was not automatic, one-step, or a matter of recognition. One of the rationalizations for the clinical judgement analysis is precisely that people's behaviour is likely to be well-practised and automatized (a characterization also found in naturalistic decision making); but many clinical judgement situations are not so simple and require more than intuitive behaviour. In these circumstances, people's concurrent verbalizations, gleaned during a task, may give more accurate descriptions. Crucially, a distinction is made between asking participants to simply think aloud during their judgement- and decision-making – a process that slows, but does not change, behaviour (Denig and Haaijer-Ruskamp 1994), and asking them to reflect (analytically) on it. This latter approach has been found to change behaviour, though not necessarily for the better (Wilson and Schooler 1991; McMackin and Slovic 2000). For a review of different types of on- and off-line verbal reports, see Cooke (1994).

Box 15.2   What can we conclude from judgements on hypothetical cases?

The use of hypothetical cases to examine clinical judgement and decision-making is common but provokes many researchers and practitioners to question the generalizability of study results to real life behaviour (e.g. Morrell and Roland 1990). In fact, hypothetical cases are a heterogeneous category – they come presented on paper or computer (often generically referred to as 'paper patients'), as a robotic system or in the flesh and have the form of vignettes, scenarios, dynamic simulations or standardized patients (in which an actor presents as a patient). Issues of face validity (physical fidelity) may be confused with those of construct validity (psychological fidelity). The use of standardized patients is laudable, and their high fidelity means that, unflagged, they pass unnoticed within a clinician's case load (Rethans et al. 1991a, 1991b). Understandably, given their high fidelity, tests of the validity of standardized patients are hard to find. Moreover, they are limited in the range of conditions that they can simulate and they suffer from the 'first visit' bias. For example, a study of walk-in centres found that a small number of conditions could be managed equally effectively (if not more) by nurses and GPs but did not attempt to simulate chronic conditions such as diabetes, asthma and heart disease which account for a large part of a GP or nurse workload in primary care (Grant et al. 2002).

Unless a clinician is used to making judgements on the basis of summarized information (e.g. giving a second opinion or deciding on a referral (Harries and Gilhooly 2003) or information presented verbally by a colleague, the use of vignettes or 'paper patients' is certainly superficially unlike an interaction with the real thing (low fidelity). Although some degree of interpretation will have been involved, cases may be *plausible* ones, on which a reasonable judgment or decision can be made. Comparisons of performances on paper and real cases give a mixed message that cannot be generalized. Studies that apparently show low usefulness of paper cases tend to focus on differences in information search patterns. Studies that report high validity of paper cases do so on the basis of a good match between judgements on paper and real versions of a case. Certainly, results showing that in *one* study the paper cases developed were valid do not mean they will be so for *all* cases.

The onus is on the researcher to test the validity of their hypothetical cases. But such measurements are not easy. Where the same real cases are later presented on paper, consistency of response may be artificially high due to recognition. Correspondence between behaviour on paper and real cases needs to be measured in the context of correspondence between two judgments on any second presentation of a case (test-retest reliability). (See Kirwan et al. 1983b, 1983c). One possibility is to analyse the psychological demands of the task. Task analysis (analysing activity as a hierarchy of goals and sub-goals with their associated operations and plans) can indicate how similar behaviour in the study and behaviour in real life are (Shepherd 1998). As goals are identified, the constraints associated with their attainment emerge. Constraints can take the form of (lack of) skills, knowledge, information available, inappropriate design, time limits etc. In clinical environments, management priorities, staff shortages, computer delays/availability/usability, access to diagnostic tests, drug/treatment costs, bed availability and national targets are constraints often encountered. Constraints affect performance as they influence the strategies that people employ to attain their goals. They may also pose limitations on the solutions that are proposed to improve performance. While some constraints can be built into the task, or occur naturally, others may be incorporated tacitly by suggesting that participants assume that situations are similar to their usual setting. However, whether they do assume this or not is again hard to assess.

As a minimum indication of the validity of the approach, clinicians' willingness to engage in solving a case, their qualitative assessments of the plausibility of a case and their assessments as to how similar their behaviour was on the cases and in real life, can be collated retrospectively.

Process approaches

Unofficially, or officially, many investigators of clinical decision-making will begin by observing it. Analysis of video-recorded consultations, or notes made by an observer *in situ*, reveal what information was explicitly sought, what was communicated, the physical environment, the artefacts used and the non-verbal interactions that accompany the process of clinical reasoning, its timing, process and nature. Although such observations feed into the development of clinician checklists, interviews, structural analysis and experimental designs, they may also be used as the basis of process tracing studies in their own right.

Process tracing is a general term that characterizes a variety of methods that were developed to track the reasoning process as it unfolds over time, leading to a decision (see Box 15.3). Process tracing attempts to answer questions such as what information is searched for, how long it is attended to and how it is interpreted, and

---

Box 15.3   Process tracing refers to a multiplicity of methods

- **Asking participants to think aloud** while they are solving a problem and trying to infer their reasoning processes from the transcripts of their verbalizations.
- **Asking participants to cooperate with each other** in order to solve a problem and studying the protocols of these verbal exchanges (e.g. Suchman 1987).
- **Withholding information until it is specifically requested** and trying to infer people's knowledge and whether they apply previously taught rules from the information that they request (e.g. Duncan and Shepherd 1975; Marshall *et al.* 1981; Duncan and Praetorius 1987). This is also known as active information search (AIS) (Huber *et al.* 1997), and conversational analysis (Williamson *et al.* 2000).
- **Recording the participants' observable activity and its consequences on the system** in terms of responses of the dynamic variables – for example, pressure, temperature – under control. These are known as 'behavioural protocols' (Woods 1993) and have mainly been used to study supervisory

control. They can however be used in similar clinical situations, such as managing the anaesthetized patient during surgery (Lighthall *et al.* 2003). Inferences regarding intentions, knowledge and reasoning are difficult on the basis of behavioural protocols, therefore domain experts can be asked to observe episodes of behaviour or review behavioural protocols and help interpret the behaviour of the participants

- **Recording participant's behaviour on complex case simulations** ('microworlds') (Brehmer and Dörner 1993).
- **Recording the pattern of participants' information search or selection** on computer or paper presented information boards (Westenberg and Koele 1994).
- **Recording participants' eye gaze.** For example, Carmody *et al.* (1984) cited in Cooke (1994) used eye movement protocols to investigate the X-ray scanning patterns of radiologists. Unsworth (2001) used head-mounted recording equipment to record the information attended to by occupational therapists.

can therefore support inferences about information use and its impact on decisions. Importantly, by externalizing covert aspects of the decision-making process, it can capture the step-by-step, configural nature of information use often missed by methods based on statistical analysis of the outcome (see p. 341) and interviews.

Process tracing techniques may be *verbal* or *non-verbal* or may involve a combination (e.g. behavioural protocols). They have been employed in different forms in the study of clinical reasoning: as *stimulated recall* (Elstein *et al.* 1978), where participating physicians view and comment on their videotaped clinical encounters, as *think aloud* (Elstein *et al.* 1978; Kassirer *et al.* 1982; Moskowitz *et al.* 1988; Hassebrock and Prietula 1992; Denig *et al.* 2002; Backlund *et al.* 2003), and as *explanation protocols* (Patel and Groen 1986; Norman *et al.* 1989), where participants are asked to explain the pathophysiology of a case. Non-verbal process tracing techniques include *tracking eye movement* and gaze direction which can reveal information search patterns (Carmody *et al.* 1984 cited in Cooke 1994; Unsworth 2001). Figure 15.2 gives an example of the process tracing data gathered as a consultant in respiratory medicine encounters a hypothetical patient with chronic obstructive pulmonary disease (COPD).

Two issues are important in investigations of decision-making. We have already raised the issue of the truthfulness (veracity or match to the actual decision-making) of the description of a person's decision-making behaviour. In addition however, process tracing studies need to address the fact that in investigating behaviour, with hypothetical cases or manipulations introduced to externalize internal processes, we may change its nature (reactivity) (Russo *et al.* 1989) and limit generalizations to the target behavioural situation (see Box 15.2). Validity of verbalizations can be checked against a simultaneous log of the observable behaviour, verbal and non-verbal (Bainbridge 1999). Just because something is not mentioned, it does not mean that it has not happened or is not known. When Carmody *et al.* (1984) cited in Cooke (1994) recorded eye movements to investigate how radiologists scanned X-rays, a significant discrepancy was found between experts' verbal reports of their scanning behaviour and their eye movements. In a non-clinical example, Biggs *et al.* (1993) found that analysis based on information search suggested that less information was searched (e.g. 7 rather than 13 pieces of information) and greater intradimensional search occurred than was suggested by financial analysts' verbalizations.

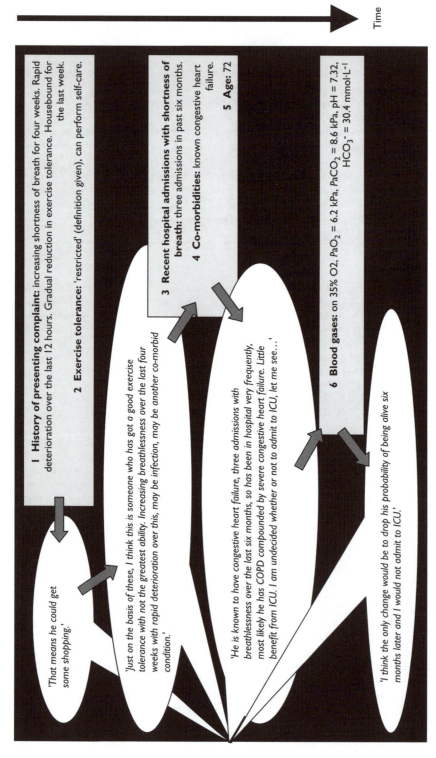

Figure 15.2 Process tracing of a clinical decision about whether to admit a patient with COPD in acute respiratory failure to the intensive care unit (ICU). The boxes present the information that the clinician requested sequentially to make his decision.

Source: adapted from Kostopoulou and Wildman (2004)

Reactivity can be guarded against by comparing the performance of silent versus verbalizing participants (or information selecting versus usual mode of processing). Simple reports of the content of working memory (thinking aloud) are unlikely to change behaviour and may yield useful descriptions. However, certain tasks are not conducive to concurrent verbalization, for example, if they involve verbal communication, high cognitive load, automatized or highly compiled performance or time pressures. Non-verbal process tracing techniques can be used to study some of these situations (see Box 15.3). These also need tests of reactivity. Similarly, the nature of clinical work usually precludes the use of process tracing during real-life decisions, but retrospective reports on recorded patient encounters can be obtained. For confidentiality and standardization purposes, actors are likely to be used rather than real patients (Elstein *et al.* 1978).

Process tracing studies have revealed a number of findings (Ford *et al.* 1989) Firstly, people commonly use non-compensatory information processing strategies – making decisions on the basis of key information. These may precede compensatory information use whereby different items of information are integrated together and each has an impact on the judgement. In fact, participants' information use has been classified into many different specific strategies for combining information. Secondly, as task complexity increases, the proportion of information searched decreases, and the mean search time decreases also. But variability in search patterns across cases tends to increase: participants search for very little information on some cases and much more on others. As time pressure increases (the time for the task is less), less information is searched for and it is processed faster. As the range of options and attributes available increases, information search decreases. Results of process tracing studies also differ depending upon the response mode. Rating judgements (such as assessing how bad a patient's arthritis is, or how likely a certain patient is to commit suicide) leads to greater information search than choice judgements (such as choosing which of two patients has worse arthritis, or which is more likely to commit suicide). In addition, choice judgements lead to greater intradimensional (attribute-wise) search. For example, past history of suicide attempts would be compared across patients, rather than examining all information about one patient at a time. Where process tracing is based on information search on an information board matrix of options and attributes there are also display format effects.

Process tracing is immensely useful in that it elicits a step-by-step breakdown of information processing that is easy to put into action (see p. 338). Information combination strategies do not need to be assumed, but emerge. Process tracing is invaluable for building decision models for prediction and it can also be used to confirm predictions (e.g. whether people will change their decision strategy under time pressures, or whether attributes of options are searched for and evaluated sequentially when choices are made). There are pros and cons of analyses that are based on just one or a few cases. There is less effort on the part of the participant in that they have fewer cases to decide upon but generalizations are limited to similar cases. The task effects listed above emphasize the importance of realism of task and judgement, and tests of reactivity.

Structural approaches

Structural approaches are those that statistically analyse the relationship between judgements or decisions made, and information about the clinician, client or setting. Because of this 'outcome-oriented' approach they are also known as 'black-box' approaches (Elstein *et al.* 1978). Some of these analyses are useful for pulling out general patterns across settings. For example, statistical analyses of decisions (prescription, treatment etc.) by clinician or region show how as clinician characteristics or regional characteristics vary, different proportions of decisions are made with resulting changes in patient satisfaction ratings (Lundkvist *et al.* 2002). Other structural analyses are based on more case-specific information.

Judgement analysis[3] has been used in a clinical context for 50 years. (See Hammond 1955 for an early publication; see e.g. Wigton 1988, 1996; Engel *et al.* 1990 for overviews of the approach and Harries 2002 for a more recent update.) Like process tracing and conjoint analysis (see Chapter 16), judgement analysis models the influence of case information on judgement or decision-making. Endemic in judgement analysis is the concept of the clinician as an intuitive expert, whose behaviour must be observed without interrupting the flow, and whose verbalizations may be a far cry from the automatic information processing underlying their skilled behaviour. Like conjoint analysis, the focus is on statistically measuring how, as case information varies, the judgement or decision varies. To understand the essence of judgement analysis, see the changes in information across the hypothetical cases shown in Figure 15.3, and the resulting changes in clinical judgements. Changes suggest that the judgements are strongly influenced by the patients' age and by their gender, separately.

Although the use of information is relatively clear in the example shown in Figure 15.3, in practice, covariation of information on a case, and the number of pieces of information that vary from case to case, call for more formal analysis, and collection of data over a large number of cases. Experts recommend five to ten cases per item of information[4] if cue use is analysed with multiple linear regression or other regression techniques (Howell 1992; Cooksey 1996).

Judgement analysis emphasizes the importance of analysing each individual's judgement-making separately ('idiographic analysis'). Brunswik advocated the use of a meaningful sample size of data from any one participant in their natural environment (rather than one piece of data from large numbers of participants in order to be able to draw general conclusions about that individual's behaviour) (Hammond and Stewart 2001). There is an emphasis on an individual's ability to exploit the natural relationships between pieces of information in the environment, for example by using a small number of cues with high predictive value, or substituting hard to access cues with others that approximate them.

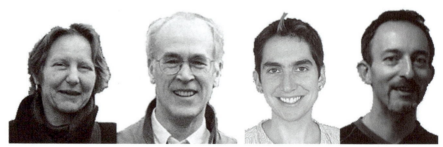

Four people present to a doctor with identical symptoms (chronic cough with green phlegm of one week's duration). She judges her likelihood of prescribing an antibiotic as follows:

80%	40%	40%	20%

Figure 15.3   Judgement analysis: judgements vary as information on a case varies

However, in practice, there is often a trade-off between naturally sampled behaviour (collected on real cases), and modelling each person's behaviour separately: researchers tend to either emphasize natural sampling, but combine results across individuals (Tape *et al.* 1991), or model each individual's behaviour, but using hypothetical or paper-based cases (e.g. Chaput de Saintonge and Hathaway 1981) (see Box 15.2 and Dhami *et al.* 2004, for a discussion of representativeness in studies of cognition).

The importance of the structure of the environment (that is, the relationship between cues) for understanding clinicians' judgement and decision-making was formalized in the development of the lens model and the lens model equation (Hursch *et al.* 1964; Tucker 1964). Figure 15.4 depicts how well a physician is able to judge pneumonia by the correlation between their judgements and some criterion measure or gold standard (pneumonia as indicated in a radiograph). Both the judgement and the gold standard are modelled in terms of the information available, using the same statistical techniques. The two models capture the essence of the physician's judgement strategy and what's predictable in the environment, respectively. By examining the relationship between the models, the fits of the models and the relationship between the parts of the judgement and environment that are not captured in the models, we can see how much of a person's performance can be explained by the difficulty of the judgement situation (the predictability of the environment), by their inconsistency or by their use of a sub-optimal strategy. Tape *et al.* (1991) demonstrated that physicians in three different states differed in their ability to predict pneumonia in their patients ($r_A = 0.41, 0.66$ and 0.55 in Illinois, Nebraska and Virginia respectively) but also found that pneumonia was harder to predict in some states than in others ($R_E = 0.39, 0.64, 0.59$ in Illinois, Nebraska and Virginia respectively). Comparison of the regression models of pneumonia and judgements of pneumonia showed that physicians used different but locally appropriate information in diagnosing pneumonia in the three states.

Seventeen years ago, in a review of 30 years of research using judgement analysis,

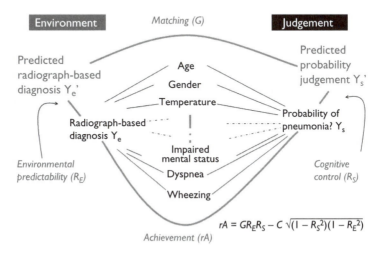

$$rA = GR_ER_S - C\sqrt{(1 - R_S{}^2)(1 - R_E{}^2)}$$

Figure 15.4 The lens model and lens model equation are used in judgement analysis to understand a clinician's judgements in the context of the predictability of the environment and covariation between cues.

Source: based on Tape *et al.* (1991)

Brehmer and Brehmer (1988) concluded that linear models are good fits of the data, that judges tend to show moderate test-retest reliability, poor to moderate self-insight, poor to moderate agreement with each other and that most judges (most clinicians in particular) appear to use only a handful of cues (see also Slovic and Lichtenstein 1971). Since then, other non-linear models have been explored, and the degree of self-insight shown has been found to be good in some studies. Only wide variation in professionals' judgements and their limited consistency is a remaining conclusion.

The use of repeated hypothetical cases facilitates measurement of *consistency* (in this case, test-retest reliability) of judgement.[5] Consistency of judgement (commonly r = 0.6) is not so much a product of the judge, but of the interaction between the judge and the task. For example, GPs showed different degrees of test-retest reliability on different tasks (mean r_{tt} = 0.35, 0.71 and 0.30 when they were judging the probability of prescribing lipid lowering drugs, migraine drug prescription or HRT for different hypothetical computer-presented cases) (Harries *et al.* 1996). Consistency and differences in information use and decision thresholds will affect *agreement*. Agreement on judgements over the same hypothetical cases varies depending on the task. For example, concordance W = 0.25, 0.56 and 0.37 when GPs judged the probability of prescribing lipid-lowering drugs, migraine drugs or HRT on common sets of cases (Harries *et al.* 1996). Variation in consistency also influences how well any model will be able to *fit* an individual's behaviour (their cognitive control). Again this varies between tasks. For example, mean R_S = 0.23, 0.55 and 0.31 on the three prescription tasks mentioned above.

The use of regression techniques to model individuals' behaviour (and that of the environment) has caused controversy over the years (Hammond 1996). Linear models have been found to be extremely good fits to the data, matching judgements on original sets of data, and predicting them on hold out cases better than other models. Even simple linear models are extremely useful for predicting judges' behaviour and capturing other data (Dawes and Corrigan 1974; Dawes 1979).[6] Linear models of experts' judgements usually indicate that only a handful of cues (three to five) within the capacity of our working memory are significant.[7] Rather than suggesting that all the information is weighted and added, linear models suggest that clinicians base their judgements on a few forceful features (see also Gale and Marsden 1985; Grant and Marsden 1987).

However, despite these advantages, and their compatibility with memory constraints, linear models are objected to because, in many people's eyes they are psychologically implausible. Linear models assume that, on every case, information will be used linearly, and will be weighted and added in the same way – as if a clinician just applied a scoresheet to make a judgement for each client she or he sees. This model contrasts with the non-linear patterns and configural cue use found in judges' verbal descriptions of their own information use, and also in process tracing studies. For example, whereas a linear model of a clinicians' behaviour might include influence of cholesterol level and attitude to treatment separately (those with high cholesterol and an explicit request both contribute to the likelihood of getting lipid lowering treatment), a clinician's verbal report might suggest (somewhat obviously) that a patient's attitude to treatment only has an effect if they have a high enough cholesterol level to be considered for treatment. The explicit policy is configural in that the use of one piece of information depends upon the value of another piece of information. It is non-compensatory in that low cholesterol levels will determine the decision, no matter what the levels of the other pieces of information.

Researchers have tested a variety of models within judgement analysis (Cooksey 1996). While linearity is partly a matter of coding in a statistical model, and configural cue use can be captured by using dummy variables, the inclusion of these usually adds little if anything to the fit of regression models, and it is not always clear which non-linear and configural patterns should be included in a model. Einhorn (1970) found that non-compensatory models were better fits than standard linear additive models for his three physician participants. Inclusion of the interactions specified by an individual about their own behaviour adds no more to the fit of their model than it does to others' models who do not mention the configural pattern of cue use (Harries 1995; Harries *et al.* 2000). Where fit is improved, researchers have argued that this is likely to be overfitting.[8] (However, see the section on choosing methods on p. 350.)

Dhami and Harries (2001) used *fast and frugal models* to describe GP's judgements (see also Gigerenzer *et al.* 1999; Kee *et al.* 2003). Like regression models, these are structural models in that they are based on the statistical structure of the relationship between the information available and judgements, without requiring verbalization or monitoring of information acquisition patterns, but the analysis results in a simple step-by-step description (see Figure 15.5).[9] These models performed comparatively to linear regression models in predicting professionals' behaviour, but are more psychologically plausible in suggesting that different information might come into play in different cases (see also Harries and Harvey 2000).

Conjoint analysis also does not assume a linear model. The use of conjoint analysis to examine clinical judgement and decision-making is relatively uncommon,

GP-1's matching heuristic

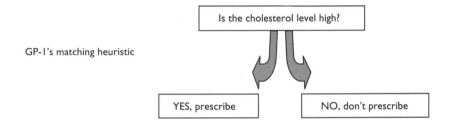

GP-1's logistic regression model

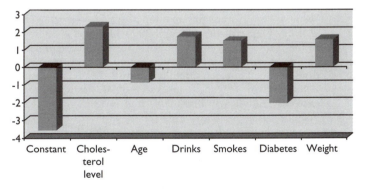

Figure 15.5 The simple heuristic of this expert clinician is easy to understand and apply to new cases. It performs as well as the logistic regression model in predicting clinician's judgements.

Source: adapted from Dhami and Harries (2001)

although it is increasingly popular as a basis for examination of patients' preferences and valuation of options in decision-making (see Chapter 16). It is also occasionally used to examine clinicians' non-clinical judgements, such as choice of speciality (Thornton 2000; Scott 2001). Conjoint analysis is based on judgements on a carefully constructed set of hypothetical cases that allow for capture of the 'partworths' of each cue – utility at each of its levels. So linearity of cue use is not assumed, but simplification of cues into different levels is necessary. For example, Wigton et al. (1986) used a fractional factorial design of conjoint analysis within a lens model framework to examine physicians' diagnosis of pulmonary embolism. Physicians appeared to have a threshold whereby low and medium levels of a cue differed little, but high levels had an impact on decision-making. This non-linear cue use would show up in a functional plot of each cue against the judgement. While Wigton used conjoint analysis within a lens model framework, Chinburapa et al. (1993) used it in conjunction with an experimental between-subjects manipulation of accountability and task complexity. As task complexity increased, the use of non-compensatory strategies for choosing drugs increased, suggesting that regression-based additive models would be less appropriate.

Studies by Wigton and Chinburapa presented physicians with cases one at a time, as patients would be seen during diagnosis and drug prescription decision-making. More recently, Hill et al. (2004) have used a *discrete choice* analysis (see Chapter 16) to examine surgeons' prioritization of patients for carotid endarectomy. A model was formed across all physicians, though each physician made a choice for 21 pairs of patients. The information processing during decision-making is reported by the authors as showing physicians' underlying knowledge patterns.

Issues of veridicality and reactivity also arise in analysis based on structural models. While models paramorphically predict the data well, the usefulness of their description can be questioned (Birnbaum 1973). Task effects, descriptive and procedural effects demonstrated in process tracing studies and in experimental studies question the generalizability of models of behaviour based on cases appearing in different combinations or on which different judgements are made to the clinician's usual experience (Shafir et al. 1993; Redelmeier and Shafir 1995).

Experimental approaches

While systemic problems are often blamed for errors in clinical practice (Donchin et al. 1995; Department of Health 2000; Dovey et al. 2002), experimental approaches to the study of judgement and decision-making emphasize the potential pitfalls of clinical reasoning. Many, though not all, demonstrations of errors and biases derive from between-subject, carefully controlled experiments.

Studies on diagnosis suggest that if participants consider more diagnoses explicitly, rather than implicitly, their judgements of the likelihood of each of the diagnoses changes. Unpacking the 'all other' category reduces the perceived likelihood of the focal diagnosis (Tversky and Koehler 1994). Even experienced physicians, asked to assess the likelihood that a 22-year-old woman with stomach pain had gastroenteritis, ectopic pregnancy, or none of the above, rated gastroenteritis as significantly more likely than expert physicians who assessed the likelihood that she had gastroenteritis, ectopic pregnancy, appendicitis, pyelonephritis, pelvic inflammatory disease, or none of the above (mean probability rating = 31 per cent versus 16 per cent) (Redelmeier et al. 1995). Experimental studies also demonstrate that participants have a tendency to base their diagnoses on information that is typical of a disease (pseudodiagnostic), rather than diagnostic of it. For example, Klayman and

Table 15.1 Pseudodiagnostic reasoning: by considering the symptoms that are *typical* of a disease, participants are misled into thinking that a patient with a harsh cough is likely to have proxititis

Percentage of patients with each disease, showing each symptom

		Proxititis	Zymosis
Cough	Dry	60%	90%
	Harsh	40%	10%

Brown (1993) asked people to estimate the probability that a patient with a harsh cough has proxititis (one of two equally likely hypothetical diseases), given that although a dry cough is more common than a harsh cough in those with proxititis, a harsh cough is much more common in those with than without proxititis (see Table 15.1); that is, a harsh cough is a diagnostic but not typical symptom of proxititis. A similar bias was shown in physicians by Wolf *et al.* (1985). Experiments have also demonstrated that those seeking rather than being given information are more likely to use it in their diagnostic judgements (Redelmeier *et al.* 2001). In sum, clinicians like other humans tend to show confirmation bias: using rules of thumb that may often be useful, they search for and accept information that will confirm their focal diagnosis, tend to discount information that disconfirms the focal diagnosis or confirms an alternative, and do not revise probabilities of preferred diagnoses sufficiently in the light of new evidence ('conservatism'). Physicians in experiments also show hindsight bias: those who are told what the correct diagnosis was judge that it was more likely on the basis of the presenting symptoms than those who are not told the correct diagnosis before they judge likelihood (Dawson *et al.* 1988).

Clinicians have also been shown to be prone to framing bias when making decisions on hypothetical cases. McNeil *et al.* (1988) found that the proportion of physicians opting for surgery over radiation therapy for a hypothetical lung cancer scenario was significantly higher when information was presented in terms of survival than in terms of mortality rates. In surgery, but not radiation therapy, only 90 out of 100 people would survive treatment (10 would die). This phenomenon illuminates the nature of the value function underlying our preferences. Like perception of the light coming from a match in a dark or a well-lit room, our perception of the value of options shows diminishing sensitivity to change. Gains or losses are perceived relative to a reference point, rather than outright, and there is a kink in the value function at the point of this reference point so that losses drop away quickly, their effect looming as a significant change (Kahneman and Tversky 1979; Tversky and Kahneman 1992). This relationship is shown in Figure 15.6.

Controlled experiments also demonstrate some of the problems with clinicians' risk perception. Participants responses to scenarios show the use of simple heuristics and a categorical perception of risk (see Chapter 16 and Kahneman *et al.* 1982). Their judgements of likelihood reveal the influence of context and of risk format on understanding of risk. For example, 60 per cent of physicians judged the 'rare' side-effects of beta-blockers to be 1/1000, but 20 per cent of physicians judged 'rare' side-effects of antihistamines to be 1/1000 (Timmermans 1994).

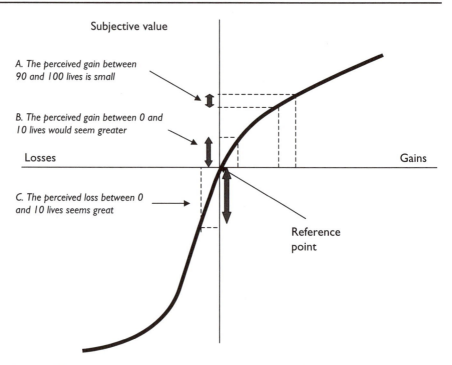

Figure 15.6   Prospect theory value function suggests that we value outcomes as gains or losses relative to a reference point; we show diminishing sensitivity to changes in gains (A versus B) or losses, but losses loom larger than gains (C versus B)

Naturalistic decision-making

Naturalistic decision-making (NDM) emerged as a separate research paradigm in the late 1980s and enjoyed considerable popularity in the 1990s. Even though it borrows heavily from other research traditions, it was born out of a reaction to the limited ability of experimental methodologies to study complex, real-life tasks. Tasks typically studied by NDM researchers are dynamic (involve changes in time), continuous (involve cycles of action–monitoring–feedback activity rather than single decisions), potentially stressful (involve time constraints, risk and uncertainty) and are usually carried out by cooperating teams. Examples of domains studied include fire chiefs, a host of different types of military personnel (Klein 1998) and offshore oil installation managers (Flin *et al.* 1996).[10] In the clinical domain, anaesthetic decision-making has been the subject of numerous NDM studies that have looked at how domain knowledge and information about the patient are acquired and used (e.g. Norros and Klemola 1999; Anceaux and Beuscart-Zephir 2002; Smith *et al.* 2004). Investigators in the USA and Belgium have used full-scale anaesthetic simulators both for research and educational purposes (Nyssen and De Keyser 1998; Lighthall *et al.* 2003). Neonatal intensive care has been studied using NDM approaches, for example the insightful early detection of neonatal abnormalities by nurses (Crandall and Gretchel-Reiter 1993) and the potential for error created by the fragmentation of tasks between shifts and between staff (Kostopoulou and Shepherd 2000). Surgical teams in action have been observed to identify threats to patient safety and features of successful performance (Helmreich and Schaefer 1994; Carthey 2003). The decision-making of critical care nurses has been investigated to identify influential contextual factors (Bucknall 2003; Currey and Botti 2003). Finally, less 'dramatic' decision-making situations have been studied to aid selection of drug infusion pumps in hospitals (Keselman *et al.* 2003).

NDM is largely descriptive in its approach and has mainly (but not exclusively) used qualitative methodologies to study phenomena of interest. It employs a host of methodologies, also used in ethnography, human factors and non-traditional cognitive science approaches (e.g. situated action, activity theory, distributed cognition – Nardi 1996), observations, interviews, questionnaires, recordings of performance (video or audio), analyses of critical incidents, think-aloud reports, task analyses, walk-throughs and talk-throughs.[11] The aim of these and other more or less formalized methods is to enable researchers to understand the environment where task performance unfolds, the goals of the individual and the organization, the artefacts, the organization of work and allocation of tasks, communications and interactions between people, and the demands and constraints on performance that all these factors impose, as well as the skills and knowledge required and the difficulties experienced. Performance and error cannot be understood outside the environment where they naturally occur. NDM also uses simulation and laboratory-based techniques, whereby participants interact with computer-presented dynamic systems to study specific aspects of cognitive task performance (e.g. Randel *et al.* 1996).

The over-reliance of the NDM approach on verbal data has been criticized, given the inadequacy of verbal data to uncover underlying cognitive processes (e.g. Bainbridge 1999). Other methodological concerns have been the numerous uncontrolled variables under study, and subjectivity in interpretation. As NDM researchers themselves acknowledge (Lipshitz *et al.* 2001), there is a need to develop theory and models and more rigorous methodologies, without losing sight of the real world. This is not an easy endeavour.

The most well-known model of NDM research is the recognition-primed decision making (RPDM) model (Klein *et al.* 1993, Klein 1998). According to this, when experienced decision-makers are faced with a situation requiring a decision, they recognize the situation as familiar or not. RPDM is not especially concerned with the cognitive mechanism of this recognition process; it could be pattern matching, prototype matching, partial matching or analogical reasoning. It can also be conceptualized as 'forward reasoning' (e.g. Elstein *et al.* 1978; Patel and Groen 1986). Recognition quickly leads to decision and action. Again, the model is not very specific about how this happens. It could be in the form of 'if-then rules' or as part of the pattern that has been recognized (in the sense of patterns having direct links to actions). RPDM suggests that experienced decision-makers do not evaluate concurrently the relative advantages and disadvantages of several courses of action. Instead, they adopt the first workable solution that comes to mind. This has been explained on the basis of Simon's (1990) concept of 'satisficing'. The way decision-makers check that this solution is workable is by playing it through a mental simulation to ensure that it works without any 'side-effects'. If it doesn't seem to work, it is either adjusted or rejected and an alternative solution is brought to mind for evaluation. Therefore, RPDM assumes that when evaluation of alternatives takes place it is sequential, a 'singular evaluation approach' (Klein 1998) rather than concurrent.

However, if there is no immediate recognition of the situation at hand, even experienced decision-makers have to gather more information, evaluate different options (Klein 1998) and even perform comparative evaluation (compare and contrast between options). It is suggested that this is done when people have to justify their decisions. So, having to explain a decision to a patient may make the clinician follow a more analytical mode of reasoning. Or it may make them simply promote their version of events, adding weight to their mental simulation (see Schwartz *et al.* 2004 for a recent demonstration of the negative effects of accountability).

Expert decision-making tends to be viewed as 'the gold standard' within the NDM paradigm, even though it is acknowledged that experts make mistakes. It is not however explained well what the gold standard is when experts disagree, as seems to be the case in uncertain situations (Shanteau *et al.* 2003), or how expertise is acquired.

In its consideration of non-cognitive factors that may lead to erroneous performance, NDM speaks with a human factors language (e.g. workload, inexperience, inappropriate design). Elstein (2001) suggests that the value of NDM is in focusing attention on the organizational factors affecting performance. In addition, NDM seems to have brought ethnographic/qualitative methodologies to the attention of behavioural and classical decision researchers and promoted a discussion about the value of these as opposed to or in combination with structured laboratory experimentation (see the whole of the *Journal of Behavioral Decision Making*, special issue 2001).

Choosing methods

The approaches described above are diverse. From a pragmatic perspective, method choice might be guided by ease of implementation, reactivity, veracity and generalizability. *Ease of implementation* boils down to personal preferences, situational constraints and participant preferences. All methods require effort: while analysis of process tracing data is time-consuming, the construction of vignettes and simulated cases needs careful analysis before any data is collected. Experimental methods and interviews need careful development of theoretical foci as well as materials. The situation of interest itself may pose limitations on the range of methods that can be employed. Naturalistic decision-making, including recordings of activity and observations, can be employed in settings such as the consulting room, the operating theatre or accident and emergency departments. In such settings of high activity, decision-making situations arise with high frequency. We may however be interested in specific types of decisions that arise less frequently, such as how GPs assess suicide risk in depressed patients, how doctors assess suitability of certain types of patients for surgery or intensive care treatment, or how neonatal nurses respond to a neonate in respiratory distress in intensive care. These decisions may not occur frequently and their occurrence cannot be predicted. They do not therefore lend themselves to observation and may need to be simulated in order to be studied. Patient confidentiality is another reason for employing simulations of decision situations. Finally, if we aim at manipulating features of the decision situation or the decision-maker, using simulation avoids harm to patients.

Issues of *reactivity* also arise with every method: Any approach that alters the circumstances under which a decision is made *may* also alter the way the decision is made. The onus is on the researcher to demonstrate that explicitly observed behaviour, behaviour while thinking aloud, or performance on hypothetical cases differs little from that occurring naturally on similar or identical cases (see Box 15.2). Failure to take into account the usual task constraints may limit generalization, but even encouraging participants to make a judgement rather than a decision, to consider options one at a time rather than side by side, or to consider more than the usual number of options, has been shown to lead to different information use (see Chapter 16).

The onus is also on the researcher to demonstrate the *veracity* of the resulting model, but this will interact with the model *generalizability* and the usefulness of the model. A model's fit to the original judgements and its ability to predict judgements on new cases is limited as a measure of veracity and as a basis for model choice (Dhami and Harries 2001). For example, when structural models are compared with think-aloud protocols, they are better predictors of the judgement or decision they are modelling, but do not inform us about other behavioural steps in the process, nor about how information is interpreted (e.g. Einhorn *et al.* 1979). Fit may be a useful yardstick if the purpose of the research is to capture the non-random aspects of the judgement for assessment in judgement analysis, or for feeding into an automated system, or setting a gold standard.

A model's match to the process of judgement and decision-making, and its capture of the influences on judgement and decision-making is harder to identify, but is more relevant in considering the educational, comparative or evaluative purposes of examining clinical judgement. Often (though not always), influences and processes are implicit – their only elucidation being in the formation of the model. One solution to this problem is to compare the descriptions derived from multiple approaches or models.

At a global level such cohesion of findings can be seen in the similar characterization of changes in information processing as a result of changes in task demands. For example, both process tracing studies and structural analysis suggest that under time pressure, and stress, when information load is increased, and when cases are judged side by side, rather than one at a time, information is less likely to be weighed up comparatively – non-compensatory information processing is encouraged (Billings and Marcus 1983; Maule and Svenson 1993; Reiskamp and Hoffrage 1999).

At a more specific level, the use of different complementary tasks may not always be feasible. For example, it makes little sense to trace the processes underlying quick judgements made under time pressure, or made often. Similarly, it makes little sense to try to statistically model information use during difficult or rare decisions without the aid of simulated cases. There is unlikely to be sufficient variation along common lines to draw firm conclusions. But when analyses are carried out on different measurements from the same judgements (e.g. think-aloud protocols versus structural analysis or information collection), differences in characterizations may reflect a focus on different aspects or different levels of the process (Einhorn *et al.* 1979; Biggs *et al.* 1993). Or they may reflect different tasks being carried out – different judgements being made – on the same case. When Harries (1996) interviewed occupational therapists about their behaviour during an earlier think-aloud study, she found that some of the information considered at the time of reviewing cases for referral prioritization was actually being considered in relation to a treatment decision. Information search may relate to multiple judgements on a case, or to multiple goals. The differences between these judgement processes may be missed if only a process tracing study is carried out, and the existence of multiple goals may be missed in the focus on single judgements rife in structural analyses. Naturalistic decision-making and task analysis can help to build up a contextual framework and these can be used to complement results emerging from other techniques. In an investigation of the role of doctors' decision-making in age-related inequalities, Bowling *et al.* (2004; Harries *et al.* 2004) used idiographic judgement analyses, process tracing and interviews to ascertain the multiple steps and decisions in treating patients presenting with chest pain and how patient characteristics influence each of these steps.

The significance of different characterizations of clinical judgement and decision-making (as information integration, script following, pattern recognition, hypothesis-testing, storytelling), as a function of task, experience, level of description or rhetoric is a matter of debate (see Witteman *et al.* 2004). Those modelling with the aim of using the resulting descriptions for education, to distinguish between clinicians or to examine other aspects of the process may also want to take into account psychological plausibility, and the ease with which models are understood (their transparency) (Dhami and Harries 2001; Harvey 2001). While transparency[12] is partly in the eye of the beholder, psychological plausibility is measured against what else we know about human behaviour given situational constraints. Troublingly, part of what we know is the result of models of (and experiments on) behaviour. When the results of different approaches concur they are easier to accept into a coherent picture of expert clinical reasoning.

Conclusions

We have introduced various different approaches to modelling and measuring clinician judgement and decision-making. These approaches complement each other, being more or less suited to different situations and focusing on different aspects of the judgement and decision-making task and situation. Together, they help to build up a larger picture of how clinical reasoning may change with situation, with experience and with information about the client.

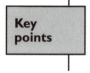

Key points

- Clinical decision-making may be measured in order to identify cognitive, emotional and situational factors that influence clinical judgement and decision-making, and information processing style.

- There are many diverse approaches to collecting information on, and analysing, decision-making.

- The results of interviews with clinicians on their decision-making differ depending on the specificity of the questions asked.

- Analyses to test the veracity of clinicians' descriptions of their own behaviour are necessary (e.g. a log of observable behaviour, recorded eye movements).

- Process tracing encompasses methods to track and break down the process of decision-related reasoning, step by step, as it unfolds over time. Process tracing techniques may be verbal or non-verbal or a combination of these.

- Structured approaches statistically analyse the relationship between the decisions made and information about the clinician, the client and the setting; judgement analysis is used to model the influence of case information on judgements made, or decision-making.

- Issues of veridicality and reactivity arise in analysis based on structural models.

- While systemic problems are often blamed for errors in clinical practice, carefully controlled experiments have emphasized the potential pitfalls of clinical reasoning.

- Naturalistic decision-making methods are largely descriptive and have mainly incorporated qualitative methods of investigation; simulation and laboratory-based computer exercises are also used.

- Choice of method can be guided by ease of implementation, reactivity, veracity and generalizability.

Notes

1 Examples of heuristics include the judgement of frequency by ease of retrieval of exemplars in implementation of the availability heuristic (Kahneman *et al.* 1982), and the use of simple name recognition to judge which of two cities is largest, in the absence of factual knowledge (Gigerenzer *et al.* 1999).
2 Flanagan (1991) argues that any *causal* account of behaviour is inevitably a hypothesis.
3 Studies using this technique also refer to it as social judgement theory, lens model analysis, policy capturing, and may also refer to the commonly used statistics–regression analysis. Policy capturing is arguably a misleading term in that a model (by necessity) paramorphically simulates the judge's behaviour rather than capturing it, and the judge's use of information is not necessarily explicit or idealized, as the term 'policy' might suggest.
4 We use the terms *item of information*, *cue* and *variable* interchangeably in this section.
5 Where real rather than hypothetical cases are used, some measure of consistency can be gained by modelling each half of the data, comparing the models and observing the fit of the resulting models on the other half of the data. Similarly, agreement between clinicians can be compared by comparing the predicted judgements of models of their behaviour on new or unmodelled data.
6 In fact, the predictions from models of clinicians and other experts consistently turn out to be better (more accurate) than the original judgements of the clinician (Meehl 1954, 1965). This phenomenon, known as 'bootstrapping' (since the judge is being pulled up by their bootstraps) can be explained in terms of the small amount of inconsistency or random error in a person's judgement-making.
7 Researchers often use the full linear model with non-zero but statistically insignificant weights to predict judgements. This would result in overfitting of original data, but reduce performance on hold-out sets (see Dhami and Harries 2001 for a critique of this practice).
8 Overfitting is when a model of a set of data captures some of its random elements. When predictions are made from the model on a hold-out sample of cases (those not included in the original set), the fit of the model is significantly reduced. To measure this effect many studies either use holdout sets of data, or use cross-validation whereby models are formed on two halves of a dataset and their ability to predict the other half of the data is measured.
9 Fast and frugal models are simple in that the description of information use is easy to understand, and few cues (often just one) are involved. Forty years ago, researchers argued that the good fit of regression models reflected humans' tendency to simplify the world around them and base judgements on main effects rather than interactions (regression models are after all good models of the environment, as well as of the judge). However, mathematical complexity and cognitive complexity are not necessarily the same thing (Einhorn 1971), and neurologically information may be processed easily in a manner that is paramorphic to mathematically complex weighting and adding.
10 For applications of such methodologies in various domains see Greenbaum and Kyng (1991), Kirwan and Ainsworth (1992), Klein *et al.* (1993), Lipshitz *et al.* (2001). Note that authors may not necessarily use the term 'naturalistic decision-making' but the methods described have been extensively used by NDM researchers.
11 Staff literally walk around a realistic setting to demonstrate how they perform their tasks (walk-throughs), or talk through what they do, using some kind of memory aid (e.g., a diagram of their workspace) without being at the normal work setting.
12 Transparency in this case is ease of comprehension and applicability of a model.

Acknowledgements

The work of Olga Kostopoulou is supported by a National Primary Care Post-doctoral Award from the Department of Health, Research and Development and the Healthcare Foundation.

Further reading

General

Goldstein, W.M. and Hogarth, R.M. (1997) *Research on Judgment and Decision Making: Currents, Connections and Controversies*. Cambridge: Cambridge University Press.

Harvey, N. (ed.) (2001) Studying judgement: models and methods, *Thinking and Reasoning*, 7 (special issue).

Thompson, C. and Dowding, D. (eds) (2002) *Clinical Decision Making and Judgement in Nursing*. Edinburgh: Churchill Livingstone.

Process-tracing techniques

Elstein, A.S., Shulman, L.S. and Sprafka, S.A. (1978) *Medical Problem Solving: An Analysis of Clinical Reasoning*. Cambridge, MA: Harvard University Press.

Juslin, P. and Montgomery, H. (eds) (1999) *Judgment and Decision Making: Neo-Brunswikian and Process-Tracing Approaches*. Mawah, NJ: Lawrence Erlbaum.

Structural approaches

Cooksey, R. (1996) *Judgment Analysis: Theory, Methods, and Applications*. London: Academic Press.

Experimental approaches

Chapman, G.B. and Elstein, A.S. (2000) Cognitive processes and biases in medical decision-making, in G.B. Chapman and F.A. Sonnenberg (eds) *Decision Making in Health Care: Theory, Psychology, and Applications*. Cambridge: Cambridge University Press.

Naturalistic decision-making

Journal of Behavioral Decision Making (2001) Special issue on naturalistic decision-making.

Klein, G. (1998) *Sources of Power: How People Make Decisions*. Cambridge, MA: MIT Press.

Resources

www.sjdm.org: Society for Judgement and Decision Making – follow links to teaching websites and other related links.

www.brunswik.org: judgment analysis–related website.

References

Abernathy, C. and Hamm, R.M. (1995) *Surgical Intuition: What it is and How to Get It*. Philadelphia, PA: Hanley and Belfus.

Anceaux, F. and Beuscart-Zephir, M.C. (2002) Anesthetic preoperative consultation: information gathering management and role of the data selected on anesthesia process planning, *Travail Humain*, 65: 59–88.

Andersson, S.J., Lindberg, G. and Troein, M. (2002) What shapes GPs' work with depressed patients? A qualitative interview study, *Family Practice*, 19: 623–31.

Andre, M., Borgquist, L., Foldevi, M. and Molstad, S. (2002) Asking for 'rules of thumb': a way to discover tacit knowledge in general practice, *Family Practice*, 19: 617–22.

Ashton, R.H. (2000) A review and analysis of research on the test-retest reliability of professional judgment, *Journal of Behavioral Decision Making*, 13: 277–94.

Backlund, L., Skånér, Y., Montgomery, H. *et al.* (2003) Doctors' decision processes in a drug-prescription task: The validity of rating scales and think-aloud reports, *Organizational Behavior and Human Decision Processes*, 91: 108–17.

Bainbridge, L. (1999) Verbal reports as evidence of the process operator's knowledge, *International Journal of Human-Computer Studies*, 51: 213–38.

Biggs, S.F., Rosman, A.J. and Sergenian, G.K. (1993) Methodological issues in judgment and decision-making research: concurrent verbal protocol validity and simultaneous traces of process, *Journal of Behavioral Decision Making*, 6: 187–206.

Billings, R.S. and Marcus, S.A. (1983) Measures of compensatory and noncompensatory models of decision behavior: process tracing versus policy capturing, *Organizational Behavior and Human Performance*, 31: 331–52.

Birnbaum, M.H. (1973) The devil rides again: correlation as an index of fit, *Psychological Bulletin*, 79: 239–42.

Boreham, N.C. (1989) Modelling medical decision-making under uncertainty, *British Journal of Educational Psychology*, 59: 187–99.

Boshuizen, H.P.A. and Schmidt, H.G. (1992) On the role of biomedical knowledge in clinical reasoning by experts, intermediates and novices, *Cognitive Science*, 16: 153–84.

Boshuizen, H.P.A., Hobus, P.P.M., Custers, E.J.F.M. and Schmidt, H.G. (1991) Cognitive effects of practical experience?, in A.E. Evans and V.L. Patel (eds) *Advanced Models of Cognition for Medical Training and Practice*. New York: Springer.

Bowling, A., Harries, C. and Harvey, N. *et al.* (2004) *The Extent of Inequalities in Treatment Between Age Groups Within the NHS*. End of award report for ESRC funded project R000238247.

Brehmer, A. and Brehmer, B. (1988) What have we learned about human judgment from thirty years of policy capturing?, in B. Brehmer and C.R.B. Joyce (eds) *Human Judgment: The SJT View*. Amsterdam: Elsevier.

Brehmer, B. and Dörner, D. (1993) Experiments with computer-simulated microworlds – escaping both the narrow straits of the laboratory and the deep blue sea of the field study, *Computers in Human Behavior*, 9: 171–84.

Bucknall, T. (2003) The clinical landscape of critical care: nurses' decision-making, *Journal of Advanced Nursing*, 43: 310–19.

Bursztajn, H. and Hamm, R.M. (1979) Medical maxims: two views of science, *The Yale Journal of Biology and Medicine*, 52: 483–6.

Carmody, D.P., Kundel, H.L. and Toto, L.C. (1984) Comparison scans while reading chest images – taught, but not practiced, *Investigative Radiology* 19: 462–6.

Carthey, J. (2003) The role of structured observational research in health care, *Quality and Safety in Health Care*, 12: 13ii–16.

Chaiken, S., Liberman, A. and Eagly, A.H. (1989) Heuristic and systematic information processing within and beyond the persuasion context, in J.S. Uleman and J.A. Bargh (eds) *Unintended Thought*. New York: Guilford Press.

Chapman, G.B. and Elstein, A.S. (2000) Cognitive processes and biases in medical decision making, in G.B. Chapman and F.A. Sonnenberg (eds) *Decision Making in Health Care: Theory, Psychology, and Applications*. Cambridge: Cambridge University Press.

Chaput de Saintonge, D.M. and Hathaway, N.R. (1981) Antibiotic use in otitis media: patient simulations as an aid to audit, *British Medical Journal*, 283: 883–4.

Charlin, B., Tardif, J. and Boshuizen, H.P.A. (2000) Scripts and medical diagnostic knowledge: theory and applications for clinical reasoning instruction and research, *Academic Medicine*, 75: 182–90.

Chinburapa, V., Larson, L.N., Brucks, M. *et al.* (1993) Physician prescribing decisions: the effects of situational involvement and task complexity on information acquisition and decision making, *Social Science and Medicine*, 36: 1473–82.

Claessen, H.F.A. and Boshuizen, H.P. (1985) Recall of medical information by students and doctors, *Medical Education*, 19: 61–7.

Cooke, N.J. (1994) Varieties of knowledge elicitation techniques, *International Journal of Human–Computer Studies*, 41: 801–49.

Cooksey, R. (1996) *Judgement Analysis: Theory, Methods, and Applications.* London: Academic Press.

Crandall, B. and Gretchel-Reiter, K. (1993) Critical decision method: a technique for eliciting concrete assessment indicators from the intuition of NICU nurses, *Advances in Nursing Science,* 16(1): 42–51.

Currey, J. and Botti, M. (2003) Naturalistic decision making: a model to overcome methodological challenges in the study of critical care nurses' decision making about patients' hemodynamic status, *American Journal of Critical Care,* 12: 206–11.

Dawes, R.M. (1979) The robust beauty of improper linear models in decision making, *American Psychologist,* 34: 571–82.

Dawes, R.M. and Corrigan, B. (1974) Linear models in decision making, *Psychological Bulletin,* 81: 95–106.

Dawson, N.V. and Arkes, H.R. (1987) Systematic errors in medical decision making: judgment limitations, *Journal of General Internal Medicine,* 2: 183–7.

Dawson, N.V., Arkes, H.R., Siciliano, C. et al. (1988) Hindsight bias: an impediment to accurate probability estimation in clinicopathologic conferences, *Medical Decision Making,* 8: 259–64.

De Dombal, F. (1984) Computer-aided diagnosis of acute abdominal pain: the British experience, *Revue d'Epidemiologie et de Sante Publique,* 32: 50–6.

Dempsey, O.P. and Bekker, H.L. (2002) Heads you win, tails I lose: a critical incident study of GPs' decisions about emergency admission referrals, *Family Practice,* 19: 611–16.

Denig, P. and Haaijer-Ruskamp, F.M. (1994) 'Thinking aloud' as a method of analysing the treatment decisions of physicians, *European Journal of Public Health,* 4: 55–9.

Denig, P., Witteman, C.L.M. and Schouten, H.W. (2002) Scope and nature of prescribing decisions made by general practitoners, *Quality and Safety in Health Care,* 11: 137–43.

Department of Health (2000) *An Organisation with a Memory.* London: The Stationery Office.

Dhami, M.K. and Harries, C. (2001) Fast and frugal versus regression models of human judgement, *Thinking and Reasoning,* 7: 5–23.

Dhami, M.K., Hertwig, R. and Hoffrage, U. (2004) The role of representative design in an ecologial approach to cognition, *Psychological Bulletin,* 130(6): 959–88.

DiCaccavo, A. and Reid, F. (1995) Decisional conflict in general practice: strategies of patient management, *Social Science and Medicine,* 41: 347–53.

Donchin, Y., Gopher, D. and Olin, M. et al. (1995) A look into the nature and causes of human errors in the intensive care unit, *Critical Care Medicine:* 294–300.

Dovey, S.M., Meyers, D.S., Phillips, R.L. Jr et al. (2002) A preliminary taxonomy of medical errors in family practice, *Quality & Safety in Healthcare,* 11: 233–8.

Duncan, K.D. and Praetorius, N. (1987) Knowledge capture for fault-diagnosis training, *Advances in Man–Machine Systems Research,* 3: 165–78.

Duncan, K.D. and Shepherd, A. (1975) A simulator and training technique for diagnosing plant failures from control panels, *Ergonomics,* 18: 627–42.

Einhorn, H.J. (1970) The use of nonlinear, noncompensatory models in decision making, *Psychological Bulletin,* 73: 221–30.

Einhorn, H.J. (1971) Use of nonlinear, noncompensatory models as a function of task and amount of information, *Organizational Behavior and Human Performance,* 6: 1–27.

Einhorn, H.J., Kleinmuntz, D.N. and Kleinmuntz, B. (1979) Linear regression and process-tracing models of judgment, *Psychological Review,* 86: 465–85.

Elstein, A.S. (2001) Naturalistic decision-making and clinical judgment, *Journal of Behavioral Decision Making,* 14: 363–5.

Elstein, A.S., Shulman, L.S. and Sprafka, S.A. (1978) *Medical Problem Solving: An Analysis of Clinical Reasoning.* Cambridge, MA: Harvard University Press.

Engel, J.D., Wigton, R., LaDuca, A. and Blacklow, R. (1990) A social judgment theory perspective on clinical problem solving, *Evaluation and the Health Professions,* 13: 63–78.

Ericsson, K.A. and Simon, H.A. (1980) Verbal reports as data, *Psychological Review,* 87: 215–51.

Ericsson, K.A. and Simon, H.A. (1984) *Protocol Analysis: Verbal Reports as Data.* Cambridge, MA: MIT Press.

Flanagan, O.J. (1991) Cognitive science and artificial intelligence: philosophical assumptions and implications, in O.J. Flanagan (ed.) *The Science of the Mind,* 2nd edn. Cambridge, MA: MIT Press.

Flin, R., Slaven, G. and Stewart, K. (1996) Emergency decision-making in the offshore oil industry, *Human Factors*, 88(2): 262–77.

Ford, J.K., Schmitt, N., Schechtman, S.L. *et al.* (1989) Process tracing methods: contributions, problems, and neglected research questions, *Organizational Behavior and Human Decision Processes*, 43: 75–117.

Gale, J. and Marsden, P. (1985) Diagnosis: process not product, in M. Sheldon, J. Brooke and A. Rector (eds) *Decision-Making in General Practice*. Basingstoke: Macmillan.

Gigerenzer, G. and Selten, R. (2002), *Bounded Rationality: The Adaptive Toolbox*. Cambridge, MA: MIT Press.

Gigerenzer, G., Todd, P.M., and The ABC Research Group (1999) *Simple Heuristics That Make Us Smart*. Oxford: Oxford University Press.

Goldberg, L.R. (1968) Simple models of simple processes? Some research on clinical judgments, *American Psychologist*, 23: 483–96.

Grant, C., Nicholas, R., Moore, L. and Salisbury, C. (2002) An observational study comparing quality of care in walk-in centres with general practice and NHS Direct using standardised patients, *British Medical Journal*, 324: 1556.

Grant, J. and Marsden, P. (1987) The structure of memorized knowledge in students and clinicians: an explanation for diagnostic expertise, *Medical Education*, 21: 92–8.

Green, A.J.K. and Gilhooly, K.J. (1992) Empirical advances in expertise research, in M.T. Keane and K.J. Gilhooly (eds) *Advances in the Psychology of Thinking*, vol. 1. London: Harvester Wheatsheaf.

Greenbaum, J. and Kyng, M. (1991) *Design at Work: Cooperative Design of Computer Systems*. Hillsdale, NJ: Laurence Erlbaum Associates.

Hamm, R.M. (1988) Clinical intuition and clinical analysis: expertise and the cognitive continuum, in J. Dowie and A. Elstein (eds) *Professional Judgment: A Reader in Clinical Decision Making*. Cambridge: Cambridge University Press.

Hamm, R.M. (2003) Medical decision scripts: combining cognitive scripts and judgment strategies to account fully for medical decision making, in D. Hardman and L. Macchi (eds) *Thinking: Psychological Perspectives on Reasoning, Judgment and Decision Making*. Chichester: Wiley.

Hamm, R.M. and Zubialde, J. (1995) Physician's expert cognition and the problem of cognitive biases, *Primary Care*, 22: 181–212.

Hamm, R.M., Scheid, D.C., Smith, W.R. and Tape, T.G. (2000) Opportunities for applying psychological theory to improve medical decision making: two case histories, in G.B. Chapman and F.A. Sonnenberg (eds) *Decision Making in Health Care: Theory, Psychology and Applications*. Cambridge: Cambridge University Press.

Hammond, K.R. (1955) Probabilistic functioning and the clinical method, *Psychological Review*, 62: 255–62.

Hammond, K.R. (1996) Upon reflection, *Thinking and Reasoning*, 2: 239–48.

Hammond, K.R. and Stewart, T.R. (2001) *The Essential Brunswik*. New York: Oxford University Press.

Harries, C. (1995) Judgement analysis of patient management: general practitoners' policies and their self-insight, Ph.D. thesis, University of Plymouth.

Harries, C. (2002) Clinical judgement analysis: a one day international meeting, *Newsletter of the European Association for Decision Making*: 4–10.

Harries, C. and Harvey, N. (2000) Taking advice, using information and knowing what you are doing, *Acta Psychologica*, 104: 399–416.

Harries, C., Evans, J. St. B.T., Dennis, I. and Dean, J. (1996) A clinical judgement analysis of prescribing decisions in general practice, *Le Travail Humain*, 59: 87–111.

Harries, C., Evans, J. St. B.T. and Dennis, I. (2000) Measuring doctors' self-insight into their treatment decisions, *Applied Cognitive Psychology*, 14: 455–77.

Harries, C., Bowling, A., Forrest, D. and Harvey, N. (2004) *How Does a Patient's Age Affect Physician Decision Making?* Unpublished report. London: Department of Psychology, University College London.

Harries, P.A. (1996) A study to identify, in the field of community mental health, the factors influencing occupational therapists' decision making as to whether or not to accept a referral, M.Sc. thesis, University of Exeter.

Harries, P.A. and Gilhooly, K. (2003) Improving clinical judgments using captured policy, paper presented at 19th Annual Meeting of Brunswick Society, Vancouver, Canada, November.

Harvey, N. (ed.) (2001) Studying judgement: models and methods, *Thinking and Reasoning*, 7 (special issue).

Harvey, N., Garwood, J. and Palencia, M. (1987) Vocal matching of pitch intervals: learning and transfer effects, *Psychology of Music*, 15: 90–106.

Hassebrock, F. and Prietula, M.J. (1992) A protocol-based coding scheme for the analysis of medical reasoning, *International Journal of Man–Machine Studies*, 37: 613–52.

Helmreich, R.L. and Schaefer, H. (1994) Team performance in the operating room, in M.S. Bogner (ed.) *Human Error in Medicine*, 1st edn. Hillsdale, NJ: Lawrence Erlbaum Associates.

Hill, M.D., Foss, M.M., Tu, J.V. and Feasby, T.E. (2004) Factors influencing the decision to perform carotid endarectomy, *Neurology*, 62: 803–5.

Howell, D.C. (1992) *Statistical Methods for Psychology*, 3rd edn. Belmont, CA: Duxbury Press.

Huber, O., Wider, R. and Huber, O.W. (1997) Active information search and complete information presentation in naturalistic risky decision tasks, *Acta Psychologica*, 95: 15–29.

Hursch, C.J., Hammond, K.R. and Hursch, J.L. (1964) Some methodological considerations in multiple-cue probability studies, *Psychological Review*, 71: 42–60.

Kahneman, D. (2003) A perspective on judgment and choice: mapping bounded rationality, *American Psychologist*, 58: 697–720.

Kahneman, D. and Tversky, A. (1979) Prospect theory: An analysis of decision under risk, *Econometrica*, 47: 263–91.

Kahneman, D., Slovic, P. and Tversky, A. (1982) *Judgment Under Uncertainty: Heuristics and Biases*. Cambridge: Cambridge University Press.

Kassirer, J.P., Kuipers, B.J. and Gorry, G.A. (1982) Toward a theory of clinical expertise, *American Journal of Medicine*, 73: 251–9.

Kee, F., Jenkins, J., Patterson, C. *et al.* (2003). Fast and frugal models of clinical judgment in novice and expert physicians, *Medical Decision Making*, 23: 293-300 .

Keselman, A., Patel, V.L., Johnson, T.R. and Zhang, JJ. (2003) Institutional decision-making to select patient care devices: identifying venues to promote patient safety, *Journal of Biomedical Information*, 36: 31–44.

Kirwan, B. and Ainsworth, L.K. (1992) *A Guide to Task Analysis*. London: Taylor & Francis.

Kirwan, J.R., Chaput de Saintonge, D.M., Joyce, C.R.B. and Currey, H.L.F. (1983a) Clinical judgment analysis: practical application in rheumatoid arthritis, *British Journal of Rheumatology*, 22(supplement): 18–23.

Kirwan, J.R., Chaput de Saintonge, D.M., Joyce, C.R.B. and Currey, H.L.F. (1983b) Clinical judgment in rheumatoid arthritis: I. Rheumatologists' opinions and the development of 'paper patients', *Annals of the Rheumatic Diseases*, 42: 644–7.

Kirwan, J.R., Chaput de Saintonge, D.M., Joyce, C.R.B. and Currey, H.L.F. (1983c) Clinical judgment in rheumatoid arthritis: II. Judging 'current disease activity' in clinical practice, *Annals of the Rheumatic Diseases*, 42: 648–51.

Kirwan, J.R., Chaput de Saintonge, D.M., Joyce, C.R.B. *et al.* (1986) Inability of rheumatologists to describe their true policies for assessing rheumatoid arthritis, *Annals of the Rheumatic Diseases*, 45: 156–61.

Klayman, J. and Brown, K. (1993) Debias the environment instead of the judge: an alternative approach to reducing error in diagnostic (and other) judgment, *Cognition*, 49: 97–122.

Klein, G. (1998) *Sources of Power: How People Make Decisions*. Cambridge, MA: MIT Press.

Klein, G.A., Orasanu, J., Calderwood, R. and Zsambok, C.E. (1993) *Decision Making in Action: Models and Methods*. Norwood, NJ: Ablex.

Kostopoulou, O. and Shepherd, A. (2000) Fragmentation of care and the potential for human error in neonatal intensive care, *Topics in Health Information Management* (special edition of *Human Error in Clinical Information Systems*), 20: 78–92.

Kostopoulou, O. and Wildman, M. (2004) Sources of variability in uncertain medical decisions in the ICU: a process tracing study, *Quality and Safety in Health Care*, 13: 272–80.

Lagnado, D., Newell, B.R., Shanks, D.R. and Kahan, S. (2004) Insight in multiple cue probability learning. Poster presented at the Experimental Psychology meeting, University of Oxford, 31 March.

Lighthall, G.K., Barr, J., Howard, S.K. *et al.* (2003) Use of a fully simulated intensive care unit environment for critical event management training for internal medicine residents, *Critical Care Medicine*, 31: 2437–43.

Lipshitz, R., Klein, G., Orasanu, J. and Salas, E. (2001) Focus article: taking stock of naturalistic decision making. *Journal of Behavioral Decision Making*, 14(5): 331–52.

Lundkvist, J., Akerlind, I., Borgquist, L. and Molstad, S. (2002) The more time spent on listening, the less time spent on prescribing antibiotics in general practice, *Family Practice*, 19: 638–40.

Marshall, E., Scanlon, K.E., Shepherd, A. and Duncan, K.D. (1981) Panel diagnosis training for major-hazard continuous-process installations, *The Chemical Engineer*, 365: 66–9.

Maule, A.J. and Svenson, O. (1993) *Time Pressure and Stress in Human Judgment and Decision Making*. New York: Plenum Press.

McKinlay, J.B., Potter, D.A. and Feldman, H.A. (1996) Non-medical influences on medical decision making, *Social Science and Medicine*, 42(5): 769–76.

McMackin, J. and Slovic, P. (2000) When does explicit justification impair decision making? *Applied Cognitive Psychology*, 14: 527–41.

McNeil, B., Pauker, S.G. and Tversky, A. (1988) On the framing of medical decisions, in D.E. Bell, H. Raiffa and A. Tversky (eds) *Decision Making: Descriptive, Normative and Prescriptive Interactions*. Cambridge: Cambridge University Press.

Meehl, P.E. (1954) *Clinical Versus Statistical Prediction*. Minneapolis, MN: University of Minnesota Press.

Meehl, P.E. (1965) Seer over sign: the first good example, *Journal of Experimental Research in Personality*, 1: 27–32.

Morrell, D.C. and Roland, M.O. (1990) Analysis of referral behaviour: responses to simulated case histories may not reflect real clinical behaviour, *British Journal of General Practice*, 40: 182–5.

Moskowitz, A.J., Kuipers, B.J. and Kassirer, J.P. (1988) Dealing with uncertainty, risks, and tradeoffs in clinical decisions, *Annals of Internal Medicine*, 108: 435–49.

Nardi, B.A. (1996) Studying context: a comparison of activity theory, situated action models, and distributed cognition, in B.A. Nardi (ed.) *Context and Consciousness: Activity Theory and Human–Computer Interaction*, Cambridge, MA: MIT Press.

Nisbett, R.E. and Wilson, T.D. (1977) Telling more than we can know: verbal reports on mental processes, *Psychological Review*, 84(3): 231–59.

Norman, G.R., Rosenthal, D., Brooks, L.R. *et al.* (1989) The development of expertise in dermatology, *Archives of Dermatology*, 125: 1063–8.

Norros, L. and Klemola, U.M. (1999) Methodological considerations in analysing anaesthetists' habits of action in clinical situations, *Ergonomics*, 42: 1521–30.

Nyssen, A.S. and De Keyser, V. (1998) Improving training in problem solving skills: analysis of anesthetists' performance in simulated problem situations, *Le Travail Humain*, 61: 387–401.

Patel, V.L. and Groen, G.J. (1986) Knowledge based solution strategies in medical reasoning, *Cognitive Science*, 10: 91–116.

Patel, V.L., Groen, G.J. and Arocha, J.F. (1990) Medical expertise as a function of task difficulty, *Memory and Cognition*, 18: 394–406.

Poses, R.M., Cebul, R.D. and Wigton, R.S. (1986) Feedback on simulated cases improves doctors' probability estimates, abstract, *Clinical Research*, 34: 832A.

Randel, J.M., Pugh, H.L. and Reed, S.K. (1996) Differences in expert and novice situation awareness in naturalistic decision making, *International Journal of Human–Computer Studies*, 45: 579–97.

Redelmeier, D.A. and Shafir, E. (1995) Medical decision making in situations that offer multiple alternatives, *Journal of the American Medical Association*, 273: 302–5.

Redelmeier, D.A., Koehler, D.J., Liberman, V. and Tversky, A. (1995) Probability judgment in medicine: discounting unspecified possibilities, *Medical Decision Making*, 15: 227–30.

Redelmeier, D.A., Shafir, E. and Aujla, P.S. (2001) The beguiling pursuit of more information, *Medical Decision Making*, 21: 376–81.

Reilly, B.A. (1996) Self-insight, other-insight, and their relation to interpersonal conflict, *Thinking and Reasoning*, 2: 213–24.

Reilly, B.A. and Doherty, M.E. (1989) A note on the assessment of self-insight in judgment research, *Organizational Behavior and Human Decision Processes*, 44: 123–31.

Reilly, B.A. and Doherty, M.E. (1992) The assessment of self-insight in judgment policies, *Organizational Behavior and Human Decision Processes*, 53: 285–309.

Reiskamp, J. and Hoffrage, U. (1999) When do people use heuristics and how can we tell?, in

G. Gigerenzer, P. Todd and The ABC Research Group (eds) *Simple Heuristics that Make Us Smart*. New York: Oxford University Press.

Rethans, J.-J., Drop, R., Sturmans, F. and Van der Vleuten, C. (1991a) A method for introducing standardized (simulated) patients into general practice consultations, *British Journal of General Practice*, 41: 94–6.

Rethans, J.-J., Sturmans, F., Drop, R. and Van der Vleuten, C. (1991b) Assessment of the performance of general practitioners by the use of standardized (simulated) patients, *British Journal of General Practice*, 41: 97–9.

Russo, J.E., Johnson, E.J. and Stephens, D.L. (1989) The validity of verbal protocols, *Memory and Cognition*, 17: 759–69.

Schmidt, H.G. and Boshuizen, H. (1993) On aquiring expertise in medicine, *Educational Psychology Review*, 5: 205–21.

Schmidt, H.G., Norman, G.R. and Boshuizen, H.P. (1990) A cognitive perspective on medical expertise: theory and implication, *Academic Medicine*, 65: 611–21.

Schneider, W. and Shiffrin, R. (1985) Categorization (restructuring) and automatization: two separable factors, *Psychological Review*, 92: 424–8.

Schulman, K.A., Berlin, J., Harless, W. *et al.* (1999) The effect of race and sex on physicians' recommendations for cardiac catheterization, *The New England Journal of Medicine*, 340: 618–26.

Schwartz, J., Chapman, G.B., Brewer, N. and Bergus, G.R. (2004) The effects of accountability on bias in physician decision making: going from bad to worse, *Psychonomic Bulletin and Review*, 11: 173–8.

Scott, A. (2001) Eliciting GPs' preferences for pecuniary and non-pecuniary job characteristics, *Journal of Health Economics*, 20: 329–47.

Shafir, E., Simonson, I. and Tversky, A. (1993) Reason-based choice, *Cognition*, 49: 11–36.

Shanteau, J. (1992) Competence in experts: the role of task characteristics, *Organizational Behavior and Human Decision Processes*, 53: 252–66.

Shanteau, J., Weiss, D.J., Thomas, R.P. and Pounds, J. (2003) How can you tell if someone is an expert? Performance-based assessment of expertise, in J. Shanteau and S. Schneider (eds) *Emerging Perspectives on Judgment and Decision Research*. Cambridge: Cambridge University Press.

Shepherd, A. (1998) HTA as a framework for task analysis, *Ergonomics*, 41: 1537–52.

Shortliffe, E.H. (1991) Medical informatics and clinical decision making: the science and the pragmatics, *Medical Decision Making*, 11: s2–14.

Simon, H.A. (1990) Invariants of human behavior, *Annals of Reviews in Psychology*, 41: 1–19.

Slovic, P. and Lichtenstein, S. (1971) Comparison of Bayesian and regression approaches to the study of information processing in judgment, *Organizational Behavior and Human Performance*, 6: 649–744.

Smith, A., Goodwin D. and Mort, M. (2004) Expertise in practice: an ethnographic study exploring acquisition and use of knowledge in anaesthesia, *British Journal of Anaesthesia*, 91: 319–28.

Suchman, L.A. (1987) *Plans and Situated Actions: The Problem of Human–Machine Communication*. Cambridge: Cambridge University Press.

Tape, T.G., Heckerling, P.S., Ornato, J.P. and Wigton, R.S. (1991) Use of clinical judgment analysis to explain regional variations in physicians' accuracies in diagnosing pneumonia, *Medical Decision Making*, 11: 189–97.

Thornton, J. (2000) Physician choice of medical speciality: do economic incentives matter? *Applied Economics*, 32: 1419–28.

Timmermans, D. (1994) The roles of experience and domain of expertise in using numerical and verbal probability terms in medical decisions, *Medical Decision Making*, 14: 146–56.

Tucker, L. (1964) A suggested alternative formulation in the developments by Hursch, Hammond, and Hursch, and by Hammond, Hursch, and Todd, *Psychological Review*, 71: 528–30.

Tversky, A. and Kahneman, D. (1992) Advances in prospect-theory – cumulative representation of uncertainty, *Journal of Risk and Uncertainty*, 5: 297–323.

Tversky, A. and Koehler, D.J. (1994) Support theory: a nonextensional representation of subjective probability, *Psychological Review*, 101: 547–67.

Unsworth, C.A. (2001) Using a head-mounted video camera to study clinical reasoning, *American Journal of Occupational Therapy*, 55: 582–8.

van Thiel, G.J.M.W., van Delden, J.J.M., de Haan, K. and Huibers, A.K. (1997) Retrospective study of doctors' 'end of life decisions' in caring for mentally handicapped people in institutions in the Netherlands, *British Medical Journal*, 315: 88–91.

Veninga, C.C.M., Denig, P., Heyink, J.W. and Haaijer-Ruskamp, F.M. (1998) General practitoners' views on the treatment of asthma, *Huisarts Wet*, 41: 236–40.

Westenberg, M.R.M. and Koele, P. (1994) Multi-attribute evaluation processes: methodological and conceptual issues, *Acta Psychologica*, 87: 65–84.

Wigton, R.S. (1988) Applications of judgment analysis and cognitive feedback to medicine, in B. Brehmer and C.R.B. Joyce (eds) *Human Judgment: The SJT View*. North Holland: Elsevier Science.

Wigton, R.S. (1996) Social judgement theory and medical judgement, *Thinking and Reasoning*, 2: 175–90.

Wigton, R.S., Hoellerich, V.L. and Patil, K.D. (1986) How physicians use clinical information in diagnosing pulmonary embolism: an application of conjoint analysis, *Medical Decision Making*, 6: 2–11.

Williamson, J., Ranyard, R. and Cuthbert, L. (2000) A conversation-based process tracing method for use with naturalistic decisions: an evaluation study, *British Journal of Psychology*, 91: 203–21.

Wilson, T.D. and Schooler, J.W. (1991) Thinking too much: introspection can reduce the quality of preferences and decisions, *Journal of Personality and Social Psychology*, 60: 181–92.

Witteman, C.L.M., Harries, C., Bekker, H.L. and Van Aarle, E.J.M. (2004) *Telling Tales About Psychodiagnostic Decision Making*. Unpublished.

Wolf, F.M., Gruppen, L.D. and Billi, J.E. (1985) Differential diagnosis and the competing hypotheses heuristic: a practical approach to judgment under uncertainty and Bayesian probability, *Journal of the American Medical Association*, 253: 2858–62.

Woods, D.D. (1993) Process-tracing methods for the study of cognition outside of the experimental psychology laboratory, in G.A. Klein, J. Orasanu, R. Calderwood and C.E. Zsambok (eds) *Decision Making in Action: Models and Methods*. Norwood, NJ: Ablex.

16 Approaches to measuring patients' decision-making

Clare Harries and Anne Stiggelbout

Introduction

With the increasing encouragement of patients' involvement in decision-making there has also been increasing interest in studying and facilitating such decision-making (Broadstock and Michie 2000; Pierce and Hicks 2001). The purpose of this chapter is to introduce a series of methods that can be used to help a patient and carer, policy-maker or researcher, understand an individual's or society's preferences for different treatments or states of health, in the context of health care decision-making.

Models of decision-making come from different disciplines. They are rooted in social psychology, cognitive psychology, psychophysics, economics and mathematics. This chapter describes four approaches to examining patient decision-making. We first describe *holistic methods* – those that elicit overall preferences for health states or treatments. Second we describe methods that elicit *values for aspects of health* or of treatments either in and of themselves or for the purpose of valuing overall health states or treatments. Establishing preferences is not a straightforward procedure, but requires an understanding of some of the psychological processes that underlie judgement and decision-making. In our third section, we describe those approaches that predict intentions from *attitudes and beliefs*. Finally, we turn to methods that seek to describe the process of patient decision-making. We present each method in brief, give recent examples of use of the method and papers in which the method is presented more fully. The measurement techniques are described in the context of a discussion of the psychological mechanisms involved in preferences for health states and treatments and with reference to the multiple reasons for studying patient decision-making.

Why study patient decision-making?

There are several reasons to study patient decision-making. One is to help individuals express how they feel both about potential outcomes and about available options to facilitate informed, shared or physician-as-agent decision-making (Gafni *et al.* 1998; Robinson and Thomson 2001; Dowie 2002). The preferences may feed into a decision analysis to identify the best option for the patient. Alternatively, the elicitation process itself may act as a decision aid, helping people evaluate the meaning of the options and to compare and contrast them. A second important reason for identifying patient preferences is to optimize decision-making at health policy level. Individuals' health state preferences, also called utilities, can feed into a decision analysis to identify which treatment options are most efficacious, and can be analysed to calculate which are most cost-effective. In this way, preferences can be fed into local policy guidelines tailored to certain patient groups or local populations, or they can be applied at a national level to inform national guidelines and balance out spending *within* a national health service, or *across* areas of national public expenditure (Stiggelbout 2000). Once quantified, it is easier to evaluate the relative merits of reducing unemployment, building new roads or screening men for prostate cancer. Finally, we wish to mention scientific purposes to assess preferences, determinants of preferences and cognitive, emotional and social processing of information in decision-making. Do preferences of the young differ from those of the elderly; do women who conceive through *in-vitro* fertilization have different preferences regarding prenatal testing than women who conceive spontaneously? Such analysis has useful implications for information presentation in and outside the clinic.

Arguably, the most crucial distinction in health care decision-making is between preferences used in decision-making at the level of an individual and those used for groups or for a society. These situations differ. Firstly, at the level of the individual patient, very strict criteria hold regarding the reliability of the measurement methods, if one wishes to base a decision purely on the result of the methods. At the individual level, methods are mostly used for process purposes, to help patients clarify their values. They function as decision *aids*, not as decision-*makers*. Ultimately, the decision is made using various sources of input, including the information from the aid. At the group level, less strict criteria hold, since one can compensate for lack of reliability by taking larger sample sizes to obtain precise estimates. Secondly, societal preferences and valuations tend to differ from those of individuals in particular health states.[1] Whose utilities should be used for making policy decisions about nationally-funded health treatments is a matter of debate (Dolan 1999).

In studying patient preferences, health professionals, researchers and policymakers may address what state patients would prefer to be in or what value they place on that state or treatment, and how they value each aspect of that health state, or each aspect of a treatment. We will consider methods relevant to this in the next two sections. Difficulties lie in addressing each of these questions. Fifty years of research on decision-making has revealed that preferences are generally not preexisting, waiting to be revealed, but that we tend to construct our preferences as we go along or during the elicitation (Payne *et al.* 1992; Slovic 1995). In the process of constructing preferences, individuals are very vulnerable to aspects of the elicitation process, and are thus influenced by the set of options on offer (e.g. Redelmeier and Shafir 1995; Hsee *et al.* 1999; Zikmund-Fisher *et al.* 2004), by how they are offered (e.g. McNeil *et al.* 1988; Welkenhuysen *et al.* 2001; Bergus *et al.* 2002) and by when they are offered and the state one is in at the time (Loewenstein *et al.* 2003). These effects are discussed in Boxes 16.1 to 16.4. We shall return to this and describe the process of decision-making later.

Valuing health states and treatments: holistic techniques

We can distinguish two different approaches to measuring global health state or treatment preferences. The holistic approach, which will be discussed in this section, requires the respondent to assign values to each possible health state or treatment, where a state or treatment represents a combination of many attributes. The decomposed approach enables the investigator to obtain values for all health states or

Box 16.1   The psychology of decision-making: probability

The perception of *probability* or risk has a prominent place in research on patients' judgement and decision-making. Health decision-making is decision-making under uncertainty; probability is an important component in expected utility theory, and people have a tendency to be risk averse. In fact, there are individual differences in risk attitude (Rosen *et al.* 2003) and changes in risk attitude that depend upon positive or negative framing (Kahneman and Tversky 1979).

Research suggests that we are insensitive to changes in risk (overestimating small risks and underestimating larger risks), and that we tend to perceive risk categorically rather than as a continuum (an outcome is understood as either risky or certain) (see Lloyd 2001 for a review of this literature). Subjective probability functions reflect these characteristics (see Tversky and Kahneman 1992; Ayton and Wright 1994; Fox and See 2003) but risk perception is dependent on how it is presented (Gigerenzer 2003). This has prompted a large body of research on risk communication in health care (e.g. Lloyd 2001; Julian-Reynier *et al.* 2003). Such information can be communicated numerically, verbally, and graphically. Numerical risk is often poorly understood, particularly if expressed as probabilities, relative frequencies, or ratios (Timmermans and Henneman 2002). Risks expressed with common denominators facilitate comparison of different outcomes (Grimes and Snively 1999), and frequentistic information facilitates understanding in comparison to percentages, or probabilities (Gigerenzer 2003; Gigerenzer and Edwards 2003). Risk perception and risk attitude also depend upon experience in the task domain (Harries and Harvey 2000a; Weber *et al.* 2004). While informative in terms of a direction or quality of information (Teigen and Brun 1999), verbal probability terms are notoriously vague – each term translating to a whole range of numerical probabilities (Timmermans 1994; Berry *et al.* 2003). The use of graphics is popular but systematic research on their effects is limited (Timmermans *et al.* 2004).

treatments without requiring the judge to assign values to every one. It expresses the overall value as a decomposed function of the attributes. We discuss this approach in the next section. The main focus of this section will be on methods for health *state* valuation, but in some instances these are used for the valuation of *treatments* as well.

Holistic valuations of health states encompass a valuation of the quality of life of those states, and the valuations are therefore sometimes called preference-based measures of quality of life (see Chapter 14), as distinct from descriptive measures of quality of life, such as the Short Form-36 (SF-36) (see Chapter 18). The methods can either be used to have respondents value hypothetical health states, or to have patients rate their own current health (or more commonly their health over the past week).

Several methods exist to assess preference-based measures of quality of life. The first two that we will discuss measure the *utility* of a health state, that is, a cardinal measure of the strength of an individual's preference for particular outcomes when faced with uncertainty (Torrance and Feeny 1989). A distinction is usually made in the decision-making literature between utilities, or strengths of preferences under uncertainty, and values or strengths of preferences under certainty (Keeny and Raiffa 1976). This concept of utilities dates from the 1940s when a normative model for decision-making under uncertainty, expected utility theory, was developed (Von Neumann and Morgenstern 1944).[2] This model calculates the utility that can be expected from each option in terms of the utility of its outcomes, and the probability with which they will occur. In most decisions in health care, outcomes may occur with a certain probability, and the decision problem is thus a problem of choice under uncertainty. Decision analysis is indeed firmly grounded in expected utility theory, and the most common use of utilities is in decision analyses. In such analyses the strategy of preference is calculated by combining the utilities of the outcomes with the probabilities that the outcome will occur (for more information see Hunink *et al.* 2001 and Chapter 13). An important application of utilities is the QALY, or quality adjusted life year, in which each year spent in a health state is multiplied by its utility, and the adjusted life years are summed (see also Chapter 14). Not all preference-based methods adhere to the axioms of expected utility theory, but the ones with less theoretical underpinnings have been developed to provide a more feasible approach.

The *standard gamble* (SG) (see Figure 16.1) has long been seen as the gold standard, since it adheres to the axioms of expected utility theory. It is based on the principle that a person will be willing to accept a risk in order to obtain good health, if he or she feels that the health state under evaluation is undesirable. The respondent is offered the hypothetical choice between the sure outcome (the health state to be valued, for one's remaining life expectancy) and the gamble, with probability p of obtaining the best possible outcome (optimal health, for one's remaining life expectancy, defined as 1) and a probability $(1 - p)$ of the worst possible outcome (usually immediate death, defined as 0). By varying p, the value is obtained at which

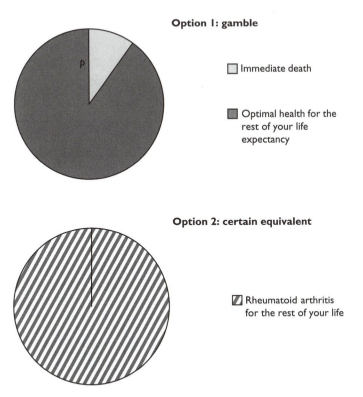

Figure 16.1 Which would you choose? Standard gamble methods adjust p until you feel indifferent between these two choices, but participants' risk aversion leads to over-valuing of health states

the research participant feels the sure outcome and the gamble to be equivalent (in expected utility terms, 'indifferent'). The utility for the sure outcome, the health state to be valued, is equal to the value of p at the point of indifference ($U = p \times 1 + (1 - p) \times 0 = p$). Thus, for example, a woman is asked to rate the state 'rheumatoid arthritis' (which may or may not be her present health state). If she is indifferent to the choice between her remaining life in that state and a gamble with a probability of 0.90 that her remaining life will be in optimal health and a probability of 0.10 of immediate death, her utility for that health state is 0.90 ($0.90 \times 1 + 0.10 \times 0$). When research participants are not rating their own health, the health state needs to be described in a scenario, which is generally framed in terms of physical, emotional, and social functioning.

Through the use of probability the concept of risk, or uncertainty, is introduced in the method. The utility measured with a SG therefore reflects not only the respondents' preference for life in the health state, but also their attitude towards risk. The use of probabilities has proven to be a major drawback of the method, since respondents have difficulties relating to probabilities (see Box 16.1). Moreover, respondents have been shown to transform probabilities: they tend to overweight small probabilities and underweight large ones.[3] In most examples in health, small probabilities of bad outcomes (such as death) occur, which thus tend to be over-weighted, leading to extremely risk-averse answers. Respondents are generally unwilling to accept a small probability $1 - p$ of death, and thus assign too high a utility. Ceiling effects subsequently limit the ability of the SG to discriminate between health states. The extreme risk aversion seen in the SG has led researchers to use an alternative method, the time trade-off.

Box 16.2   The psychology of decision-making: time

Time has a fundamental role to play in health care because health is experienced in time and because changes in health occur at particular time points (and delay of outcomes leads to discounting of their value) (Chapman 2003). Research on inter-temporal choice suggests that we have a limited ability to predict our future preferences and utilities. For example, attendees for an AIDS test overestimated the impact of a positive or negative test on how they'd feel five weeks following the result (Sieff et al. 1999 cited in Loewenstein and Angner 2003). Part of this phenomenon reflects lack of appreciation of our ability to adapt. In a notorious study Brickman et al. (1978) found that those who had won the Lottery rated their happiness as little different from those in a control group and little above those who had become paraplegic. Generally, people tend to overestimate how good a good experience will be, and how bad a bad experience will be. To explain these errors in utility forecasting researchers have suggested that we tend to anchor our judgement to our current emotional state (a type of visceral emotional anchoring associated with projection bias). We lack awareness of our ability to adapt to new circumstances, focus on particular aspects of our new circumstances and the value of health states or other outcomes is reduced as the time before they occur increases (Loewenstein et al. 2003; Wilson and Gilbert 2003).

Anchoring to our current state means that we cannot properly conceive of what it is to be in pain, not in pain, hungry, not hungry etc. if we are not currently in that state (an intrapersonal empathy gap: Read 2001). For example, Christensen-Szalanski (1984) found that the majority of women who one month before labour expressed a preference to avoid anaesthesia during labour actually opted for it, but one month later expressed the same preference for its avoidance as before labour (see Chapman and Elstein 2001). Asking patients post-treatment for retrospective evaluations of earlier poor health states will change their anchor point. But controlling for this reference point, and attempting to broaden the attributes focused on does not seem to aid intra- or interpersonal utility assessment (Baron *et al.* 2003).

Different discount rates have a particular impact when good and bad outcomes are likely to occur at different points in time, as in when choosing between virtues (long-term benefits but short-term unpleasantness, typical of good health practices) and vices (short-term pleasantness and long-term costs typical of practices that are bad for our health) (Read *et al.* 1999; Read 2001). When deciding well in advance we can clearly distinguish the relative merits of outcomes occurring at different points in time. But as the point of choice nears in time, immediately rewarding outcomes seem relatively good.

Importantly for health state valuation, our retrospective assessments of a series of experiences also seem to be *duration independent* – i.e. not influenced by the amount of *time we spent in the series of health states*. For example, Redelmeier and Kahneman (1996) collected retrospective and real-time evaluations of pain by patients undergoing colonoscopy or lithotripsy. Retrospective evaluations depended upon peak pain and pain during the final few minutes of the procedure, not duration of pain. In a more recent randomized controlled trial, half of 682 patients had the tip of their colonoscopy tube left resting uncomfortably, but not painfully, in their rectum for a few minutes at the end of the procedure. The whole procedure lasted longer but was rated as less unpleasant and less aversive. These patients were significantly more likely to attend for repeat colonoscopy (Redelmeier *et al.* 2003). Preferences for a happy ending seem to contradict preferences for better outcomes earlier. When thinking about sequences of outcomes in abstract, participants seem to prefer to have the same migraine pain fading off over an hour rather than increasing over an hour. The preference for a happy ending seems to coincide both with what participants expect to happen and what they consider appropriate. Preferences for sequences of health over a lifetime do not show preferences for getting fitter and more healthy as old age creeps on (Chapman 2000; Read and Powell 2002).

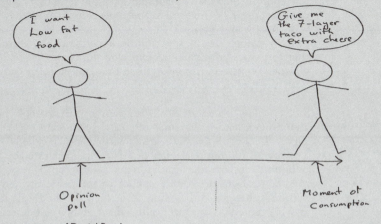

Figure courtesy of Daniel Read

**Option 1: X years in optimal   Option 2: 15 years with
health, then death   rheumatoid arthritis, then death**

Figure 16.2   Which would you choose? Time trade-off methods adjust X until you feel indifferent between these two choices. Arguably, time-related biases in participants' responses tend to cancel each other out

In the *time trade-off* (TTO) method (see Figure 16.2) a research participant is asked to choose between their remaining life expectancy in the health state to be valued and a shorter life span in optimal health. In other words, they are asked whether they would be willing to trade years of their remaining life expectancy for improved health. As an example, let's say a 65-year-old woman has a remaining life expectancy (according to national life tables) of 15 years. She is asked how many years X in a state of optimal health she considers equivalent to a period of 15 years (her remaining life expectancy) in the state 'rheumatoid arthritis'. By varying the duration of X the point is found where she is indifferent to the choice between the two options. The simplest and most common way to transform this optimal health equivalent X into a utility (ranging from 0 to 1) is to divide X by 15.

This method often better reflects the clinical situation at hand than the SG. Patients' willingness to trade life years is generally larger than their willingness to accept risk, resulting in TTO scores generally being lower than SG scores for the same states.

Both for the SG and for the TTO, elicitation becomes more complex when temporary states are to be valued. The regular (chronic) procedure assumes that the health state to be valued is followed by death. Temporary states are generally followed by either good health or another disease state. Therefore, a two-step procedure is needed to assess the utility. In the first step the state is valued relative to an anchor state, and in the second step the anchor state is valued relative to perfect health and death (see Drummond *et al.* 1997 or Jansen *et al.* 1998 for details on the procedure). Since many treatment states are temporary, and this procedure is quite complex, the TTO method has been developed specifically to value treatments, and is further discussed on p. 372.

Even though strictly speaking no uncertainty is involved in the method, and it therefore does not adhere to expected utility theory, in practice TTO scores are generally considered utilities, since they are preference-based. This is in contrast with scores of the next method, the visual analogue scale.

The *visual analogue scale* (VAS) is a rating scale, a simple method that can be self-administered and is therefore often used to obtain evaluations of health states in surveys (see Figure 16.3). Research participants are asked to rate the state by placing a mark on a 100mm horizontal or vertical line, anchored by death (usually on the left or bottom) and optimal health (on the right or top). The preference is the number of millimetres from the 'death' anchor to the mark, divided by 100. An alternative version is that of a verbal rating scale, such as 'On a scale where 0 represents death and 100 represents optimal health, what number best describes your health over the past week?' The preference score is then the number divided by 100.

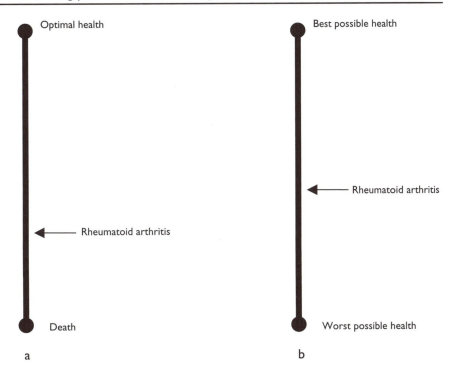

Optimal health

Best possible health

Rheumatoid arthritis

Rheumatoid arthritis

Death

Worst possible health

a

b

Figure 16.3   How would you rate your rheumatoid arthritis? Visual analog scales with anchors at death (a), or the worst possible health state (b), are simple tools for people to express how they value particular health states but results require statistical transformation to be used as decision utilities

Sometimes best possible health and worst possible health are used as anchors, especially in surveys where researchers think it may be threatening to patients – such as those with metastasized cancer – to 'mark themselves' on a death–well scale, or when health states are thought to be worse than death. See Box 16.4 for a discussion of the implication of these response changes.

The VAS does not reflect any trade-off that a research participant may be willing to make in order to obtain better health, neither in terms of risk nor in years of life. It can therefore not be considered a preference-based method. Transformations of VAS scores have been proposed to approximate true SG or TTO utilities. A power model has been proposed by Torrance (1976) to transform aggregate VAS scores into aggregate TTO scores: $TTO = 1 - (1 - VAS)^{1.61}$. In a later study a similar function was proposed for a transformation from VAS into SG scores: $SG = 1 - (1 - VAS)^{2.27}$ (Torrance *et al.* 1996). Most studies have found similar functions, but the coefficients seem to be context-dependent (see Torrance *et al.* 2001 for an editorial on the usefulness of the VAS).

Magnitude estimation is a scaling method that was developed by psychophysicists to overcome the limitations of the rating scales, i.e. the lack of ratio–level measurement and the tendency of respondents to use categories equally often (verbal scale), or not to use the upper and lower ends of the scale (VAS). The respondent is given a standard health state and asked to provide a number or ratio indicating how much better or worse each of various other states is compared with the standard. For example, the research participants are instructed to assign the number 10 to the first case, the standard. Then a case that is half as desirable receives the number 5 and a case that is regarded as twice as desirable is given the number 20. Magnitude estimation is seldom used, since it is not based on any theory of measurement and since the scores have no obvious meaning in the context of decision-making. They do not reflect utility, and as such cannot be used in decision analyses.

Box 16.3   The psychology of decision-making: option and information presentation effects

Infamous in the psychology of judgement and decision-making are examples of violations of the principle of description invariance: when the same information is presented differently, participants show different preferences. Most notoriously, how options are *framed* (e.g. positively or negatively) affects their evaluation. For example, focusing respondents' attention on probability of survival, rather than the complimentary probability of death, can lead to different preferences (McNeil *et al.* 1988). Losses have a greater influence than gains. In addition, participants tend to show risk aversion when dealing with gains (they prefer a sure gain to an equivalent risky gain), but are risk-seeking when dealing with losses (they prefer a risky loss to a sure loss of equivalent value) (Kahneman and Tversky 1979; Tversky and Kahneman 1992). Crucially, losses and gains are seen relative to a reference point. Thus it is that healthy women have been shown to be risk-seeking when considering a short number of years of life (*Loss* relative to life expectancy) but risk-averse when considering a larger number of years of life (*Gain* relative to life expectancy) (Verhoef *et al.* 1994).

In addition to presentation effects, the *range of options* on offer to respondents affects preferences such that generalizations cannot be made beyond the set of options studied. For example, evaluating options singly can result in opposite preference patterns to when they are judged side by side, and adding an extra option can change the order of preference of the current set of options seen. These two phenomena have at their root an explanation in terms of reason-based choice (Shafir *et al.* 1993). Patients, physicians and all of us seek reasons for judging one option as superior to another. Thus, a middle-aged woman may be a priority for surgery when there is just her and an older man, but the man may be prioritized if there is another middle-aged woman also awaiting surgery (Redelmeier and Shafir 1995). Attributes that are hard to evaluate when options are viewed on their own become more meaningful sources of discrimination when two options are judged side by side. For example, Zikmund-Fisher *et al.* (2004) gave a series of hypothetical patient decision-making situations to participants who either judged the option alone or judged two options together. When evaluated side by side the number of operations a physician had performed became salient, was evaluated differently and was more influential on participants' rating of potential eye surgeons. Such problems of poor attribute evaluation due to unfamiliarity can be attenuated by providing participants with suitable references such as the average score on a particular attribute (Hsee *et al.* 1999).

Combined together the results above suggest that the 'losses' highlighted in distinguishing between options will have greater impact than comparative 'gains'. This is compatible with the wide body of research that addresses the role of anticipated regret and anticipated disappointment on our decision-making (see Connolly and Reb 2003 for some examples).

Box 16.4   The psychology of decision-making: procedural effects

How people are asked to respond to options inevitably affects their preferences. This is a violation of the principle of procedural invariance. Asking a person which of two options they least prefer or would reject (framing of the response mode) leads to greater influence of negative attributes; asking which option they would prefer, or which to keep, leads to greater influence of positive attributes on judgement-making (Shafir *et al.* 1993). Explained in terms of reason-based choice, this also shows a *compatibility* effect whereby attributes are relatively over-influential if they are compatible with the judgement being made. Labels attached to the ends of response scales can create similar compatibility effects, are associated with anchoring (whereby responses are artificially near to an anchor point) and can lead to apparent discrepancies because of our tendency to spread multiple responses evenly over the scale offered (Parducci's range-frequency effect: Parducci 1965, 1990).

Compatibility has been used to account for differences in preferences underlying *judgements versus choice*. The task of matching (whereby participants alter an attribute until two alternatives are equivalent) seems to emphasize the influence of the attribute being altered, whereas choice shows greater influence from the most prominent attribute. Sumner and Nease (2001) found that most participants preferred 30 years with migraine for six days per month to living for 20 years with migraine for four days per month if they were asked to choose between the two experiences. But they preferred the latter if they were asked to alter the number of days with migraine for 30 years to make it equivalent to the 20-year experience. Making a judgement in terms of days of migraine increases the influence of this information on decision-making. Similarly, costs become salient in judgements of willingness to pay, and duration information salient in time trade-off judgements.

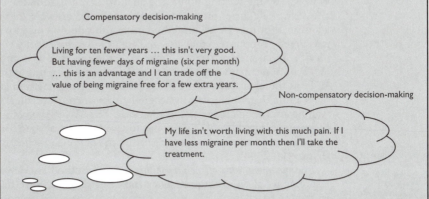

Change in response mode from judgement to choice also changes how information is combined (*strategy compatibility*). When judging options, participants exhibit compensatory strategies – combining several relevant pieces of information to come to an overall judgement (illustrated). But in choosing between options, comparative judgements encourage lexicographic information processing whereby the choice is made on the basis of the first most important and informative piece of information. If this is not a decisive factor then the next most important piece of information is examined. This is non-compensatory: different attributes cannot trade-off against each other. The use of such simple decision rules, revealed both in process tracing based on information search and via experimental paradigms has been associated particularly with participants' intuitive judgements (Maule and Svenson 1993; Chaiken *et al.* 1989; Kahneman 2003). Although preferences may satisfy, rather than optimize (Simon 1986), there is also a suggestion that such simple strategies can exploit the natural structure in the decision environment to produce optimal decisions (Gigerenzer *et al.* 1999).

A different variant, called the *person trade-off* has gained popularity among health economists and policy-makers (Nord 1995). It was formerly known as the equivalence method, and the task is to determine how many people in health state X are equivalent to a specified number of people in health state Y. From a policy perspective, the person trade-off seeks information similar to that required by policy-makers. It has been used in the elicitation of disability weights for disabililty-adjusted life years (DALYs), a measure used by the World Health Organization as a summary measure of population health (Murray and Acharya 1997).

The *willingness to pay* (WTP) is a method used primarily by health economists. To value health states, it asks the respondents what amount, or what percentage of, their household income they would be willing to pay to move from a less desirable state to a state of optimal health. More frequently WTP is used to assess respondents' willingness to pay for treatments and services. It is most commonly used in cost-benefit analyses, in which all outcomes are expressed in monetary terms, in contrast to cost-effectiveness analyses, in which health outcomes are expressed in QALYs. As is the case for magnitude estimation and the person trade-off method, this method does not result in a utility.

The results of the WTP are strongly influenced by the income of the respondent as well as by the starting point (the anchor) that is used in the elicitation (or by the answering categories provided if multiple choice answers are given in a survey). In addition, they may be of limited use in health care systems in which patients do not pay directly for services they use, and are not used for considering the value of these services in monetary terms. These validity problems have limited the use of the WTP until now, however, despite these limitations, an important application of the WTP is the elicitation of the value of *time*. In many decision analyses, patient time plays a role (e.g. time spent in hospital either during a medical procedure, or in the waiting room, or during a consultation). The WTP elicits the amount of money that patients would be willing to pay to save the time needed for these purposes, and can be incorporated in the numerator (costs) of the cost-effectiveness ratio (van den Brink *et al.* 2004).

The *treatment trade-off* or *probability trade-off* method assesses, in a holistic manner, respondents' strength of preference for a treatment (relative to another treatment). In this approach, preferences for combined process and outcome paths are elicited in the following way. The patient is presented with two clinical options, for example treatments A and B, which are described with respect to the chances of benefits and side-effects, and is asked to state a preference for a treatment. If treatment A is preferred, the interviewer systematically either increases the probability of benefit from treatment B, or reduces the probability of benefit from treatment A (and vice versa if treatment B is preferred). The particular aspects of the treatments that are altered in this way, and the direction in which they are changed, are decided upon beforehand, according to the clinical characteristics of the problem and the nature of the research question (Llewellyn-Thomas 1997). For example, these may include the probability of side-effects of treatment, risk of recurrence or chance of survival. The relative strength of preference for a treatment is assessed by determining the patient's willingness to accept side-effects of that treatment or forego benefits of the alternative treatment. This general approach has been adapted specifically to a variety of treatment decisions. Examples are decisions about adjuvant chemotherapy in breast cancer (Levine *et al.* 1992), benign prostatic hypertrophy (Llewellyn-Thomas *et al.* 1996), treatment of lupus nephritis (Fraenkel *et al.* 2002) and radiotherapy for breast cancer (Whelan *et al.* 1995).

The resulting preference scores are idiosyncratic to the original decision problem, and only the strength of preference for treatment A relative to treatment B is obtained, not a utility. For formal decision analysis this approach is therefore not suitable. However, for decision support it seems appropriate as it is tailored to the clinical problem at hand, and will reflect the real life situation more than a utility assessment. This method has indeed been used 'at the bedside' using decision boards as visual aids. It seems a promising way to help patients who wish to engage in decision-making to clarify and communicate their values.

Valuing health states and treatments: decomposition techniques

Decomposed methods to value health states or treatments express the overall value of these as a decomposed function of the health state or treatment attributes. For example, an eye surgery option can be classified in terms of how qualified a surgeon is, how long the waiting list is, what the average complication is and the time till recovery (Ross *et al.* 2003). The relative value patients place on each of these attributes will determine, for example, whether they are prepared to wait for a long time for a highly qualified surgeon, or would rather be seen immediately but by a junior doctor.

Decomposed models that reveal how a patient values different attributes can be based on statistical inference or on explicit decomposition, and have several purposes.[4] Firstly, as in the case of *multi-attribute utility theory* (MAUT), discussed below, relative importance ratings for attributes can be used to identify global preferences for health states or treatments. Secondly, where there are individual differences in preferences, or the health care worker's and patient's preferences differ, the values underlying those preferences can be identified. Such an analysis can highlight the key issues that carers should raise when discussing treatments with patients (e.g. Ross *et al.* 2003). For example, conjoint analysis revealed that lack of energy or 'pep' is the most important determinant of preferences for management of non-metastatic prostate cancer (Sculpher *et al.* 2004). With this in mind, patient treatment could focus on increasing energy levels. Such analysis may thus identify new treatment packages that, for minimum cost or effort, create a much preferred alternative. Thirdly, knowledge of other patients' preference patterns may aid individuals making choices about their own treatment (Sculpher *et al.* 2004).

The best-known application of a decomposed method is that based on MAUT, which uses explicit decomposition (see Figure 16.4). Decision analysts developed MAUT in the early 1960s when they felt the need to expand methods of decision analysis to situations where multiple competing objectives were seen, rather than a single well-defined objective such as survival. Each attribute of a health state (or similarly of a treatment) is given an importance weight. Next, respondents score how well each health state (or treatment) does on each attribute. These scores are weighted by the importance of the attributes and then summed over the attributes to give an overall multi-attribute score for each state or treatment. For this

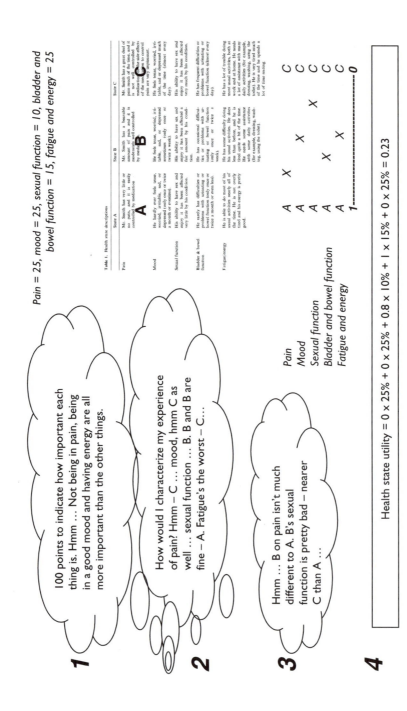

Figure 16.4 Illustration of the elicitation of utilities for prostate cancer patients' health states by Chapman et al. 1999. Two patients may describe their experience in similar terms (steps 2 and 3) but because of different relative importance ratings, their utilities will differ. Table reproduced with permission.

summation, the theory specifies utility functions and the independence conditions under which they would be appropriate.

Chapman *et al.* (1999) give an example of a MAUT model for prostate cancer. Calculation of the utility of different patients' health states is illustrated in Figure 16.4. The patient with prostate cancer first divides 100 points to illustrate the relative importance of each of five attributes, then rates his own health on each of those attributes by identifying which of three descriptions is most like his own experience. Finally, he rates the middle option on each attribute to show how good or bad it is in comparison with the other two health states. MAU scores were computed by multiplying, for each attribute, the level by importance weight, and summing across attributes. MAU scores did not correlate with TTO scores for the patients' current health on a 0–1 death-optimal health scale, but they did correlate with TTO scores that had been standardized relative to the utilities for the best and worst states. TTO values on an absolute scale may incorporate additional factors beside the value for current health, such as the willingness to trade longevity for health, a factor that is not usually included in the MAUT model.

Several decomposed methods use statistical inference to identify the way information is combined to form a global assessment of a health state or treatment. For example, *functional measurement* (related to *conjoint analysis* – Kreiger *et al.* 2001 – see p. 376), based on Anderson's information integration theory, in theory allows one to test the underlying subjective processes by which respondents process information. For example, information may be combined by adding (as in MAUT), or by averaging (Anderson 1971). The measurement process provides a validation of the derived scale values, which is an advantage of this method that other decomposed methods do not have. Due to logistical difficulty of functional measurement, researchers often assume an additive process, rather than carrying out an analysis of the mode of information processing. See Froberg and Kane (1989) and Veit *et al.* (1982).

Most methods of statistical inference assess preferences for health states or treatments and use regression models to infer the parameters of the model, assuming an additive linear process. Usually, judges are asked to evaluate a set of multi–attribute health states, then the subjective weights and scale values of a simple utility model are estimated using regression procedures. Next, the model thus estimated can be used to infer health state preferences from attributes.

The *analytical hierarchy process* (AHP) decomposes options into a hierarchy of criteria that include a person's ultimate goal for the decision. Firstly, participants identify their ultimate goal (e.g. maximum possible health and well-being), and their sub–goals (criteria) that contribute to that (e.g. avoiding side-effects, decreasing risk of cancer). Participants compare options in a pairwise fashion in terms of these criteria: they give them a rating to indicate which is better, or whether they are similar. These pairwise ratings can be combined to give each option a score in terms of each criteria, and to work out how the attributes describing an option contribute to achieving the criteria. They then prioritize those critera, giving them a weight to indicate how much they contribute to achieving the ultimate goal (Dolan and Bordley 1991; Dolan 1995; Carter *et al.* 1999). These can be combined to give each option a score in terms of the ultimate goal.

Both MAUT and statistically inferred regression methods have found well-known applications in health state classification systems (Feeny *et al.* 1995). The two most frequently used systems are the Health Utilities Index (Torrance *et al.* 1996) and the EuroQoL EQ-5D (Dolan 1997; Busschbach *et al.* 1999). *Health indexes* are customarily composed of two components: a descriptive system and a formula for assigning a utility to any unique set of responses to the descriptive system. The descriptive system consists of a set of attributes, and a health state is described by indicating the appropriate level of functioning on each attribute. For instance, in the EuroQoL EQ-5D the attributes, or domains, are mobility, self-care, usual activities, pain/discomfort and anxiety/depression. Each domain is divided into three levels of severity, corresponding to no problem, some problem and extreme problem. By combining one level from each of the five domains, a total of 3 to the power 5 (i.e. 243), health states are defined.

The formula is generally based on utilities that have been obtained in part from direct measurement and in part from application of multi–attribute utility theory (as in the Health Utilities Index) or statistical inference (as in the EQ-5D), to fill in values not measured directly. In both instances, only a limited number of valuations have been obtained from the surveyed population, usually the general public.

Health state classification systems or health indexes have been developed for use in cost-effectiveness analysis from a societal perspective. For these analyses, utilities are required from a representative sample of the general public, since the purpose generally is to inform the allocation of public resources (Gold *et al.* 1996). Pre-measured utilities from samples of the general public have been obtained for these systems, as described above, and the formula can be found in the literature (Russell *et al.* 1996). It suffices to map the treatment outcomes (the health states) onto the descriptive system using information from patients, and to use the scoring formula, with the pre-measured values from the general public, to obtain utilities from the general public as required in the cost-effectiveness equation. In this way, standardization over studies is obtained. All researchers use the same utility set, and cost-effectiveness ratios are comparable.

Of more recent date is a scoring formula based on the Short Form-36 (SF-36) descriptive health status instrument. Researchers in the UK have created from the SF-36 a six-dimensional health classification system called the SF-6D (Brazier *et al.* 2002). A representative sample of the general population valued a sample of the 18,000 health states, and statistical inference was used to obtain the utility scoring formula. Since the SF-36 is the most widely used health status instrument, the preference-based measure created from it has the potential to considerably extend the scope for undertaking economic evaluation in health care using existing and future SF-36 datasets. Utilities for use in cost-effectiveness analyses have become available for many conditions in this way.

Valuing aspects of health states and treatments

Whereas the ultimate aim of techniques such as MAUT is to assess preferences for health states or treatments via decomposition, other techniques aim to measure how treatment or health state attributes are valued. Judgement analysis, conjoint analysis, discrete choice experiments and the repertory grid method, as well as the process tracing techniques described on p. 381 each examine how aspects of a treatment or health state influence preferences.

Conjoint Analysis has been widely used to examine consumer preferences, particularly in marketing (Green and Srinivasan 1978) and its use in examining patient preferences is increasing with the availability of both generic and specialist software.[5] The principle of conjoint analysis is that evaluations of options are compared to reveal the importance of differences between them.[6] Similar to the statistically-based decomposition techniques described above, participants judge hypothetical cases (health states or treatments) that are described in terms of combinations of attributes at particular levels (see Figure 16.5). Statistical analysis reveals the relative importance weights of attributes and identifies sets of attribute level utilities.

TREATMENT A	TREATMENT B
One-off payment of £400	One-off payment of £300
No problems maintaining an erection	No problems maintaining an erection
No problems with physical energy	No problems with physical energy
No loss of libido	No loss of libido
Two months greater life expectancy than B	Two months less life expectancy than A
Mild diarrhoea	No diarrhoea
Mild hot flushes	Mild hot flushes
Breast swelling and tenderness	Breast swelling and tenderness

Figure 16.5 In statistical decomposition techniques respondents choose or rate health states or treatment options. Septuagenarian men with non-metastatic prostate cancer chose between examples similar to the ones above to reveal what they value in a treatment

Source: adapted from examples in Sculpher *et al.* (2004)

In a full factorial design, all possible options, involving every combination of attribute levels, would be created[7] and judged. But this creates a large number of options (over a thousand in the prostate cancer example in Figure 16.5). In a fractional factorial design each attribute is varied across options independently of changes in the other attributes (an orthogonal design) and a more reasonable number of cases are created. Interactions between attributes cannot be measured but there is evidence that these add little, if anything, to the fit of the model (Ryan and Farrar 2000). Most researchers simplify the set of options by choosing few attributes, few levels of the attributes, and by using a fractional factorial rather than a full factorial design.

Conjoint analysis studies elicit one of three types of respondent judgement. Most commonly, options are seen one pair at a time and a choice is made between them (hence the name 'conjoint analysis'). Options are paired according to the original full or fractional factorial design, or, in adaptive conjoint analysis – with the use of special software – they are paired according to a set of stated attribute weights and responses to previous options (Fraenkel *et al.* 2001, 2004). Fewer judgements are required if each option is be paired with the same alternative, such as the status quo. For example, Ryan and Farrar (2000) present an example in which orthodontic patients made 15 choices between their current treatment option and alternatives defined in terms of waiting time, and local or hospital location of first and second appointments. Instead of choices between pairs of options a participant might rank many options in order of preference. Or they might rate each option individually according to how attractive it is. See Boxes 16.3 and 16.4 for a discussion of the implications of these changes in option presentation and response.

Discrete choice experiments are variations on forced-choice conjoint analysis with their roots in economics (Ryan *et al.* 2001). Analysis of the data is based on random utility theory. *Judgement analysis* is technically similar to conjoint analysis but has its roots in a Brunswikian tradition of psychology, seeking to describe participants' natural judgement processes, as they happen, rather than what they would prefer if they had a range of options (see Chapter 15).

The type of analysis carried out depends upon the judgements made about the options, but most are regression based. Where discrete choices are made, log probit models are used to analyse the relationship between propensity to choose one option over another and the difference between options on each dimension.

Random effects probit models can be used to analyse the results from all individuals in one model, taking repeated measures into account (Ratcliffe *et al.* 2004). Alternatively, preliminary analysis can be based on each individual's judgements or choices separately (idiographic analysis) and then calculating group average weights or average attribute level utilities. Ranked options and judgemental ratings of options can be regressed onto the raw dimension values of each option using multiple linear regression.

It is common practice to exclude judgements from participants who show poor test-retest reliability, inconsistency of preferences, or 'irrationality' by making judgements contrary to basic assumptions (e.g. participants who favour more pain over less pain, all other things being equal) (see San Miguel *et al.* 2005 for a recent exploration of the reasons behind this). Some randomness in responses is to be expected, and is taken into account in analysis. With carefully explained materials administered by interview, 2 per cent of data may show such errors, though 5–10 per cent is more usual with survey-based materials.

More controversial is the treatment of data from respondents who do not trade attributes against each other. Many respondents make such lexicographic or non-compensatory choices whereby for example the decision is based on one factor (see Box 16.4). This may reflect the range of cases participants have seen – they may be willing to trade, but not with these levels of these attributes (Viney *et al.* 2002) – but may also be part of a natural mode of choice behaviour found within models of bounded rationality (Lloyd 2003). Interestingly, forcing participants to make choices allows measurement of the marginal differences in utility caused by changes in different attributes, but may discourage trading, in comparison to elicitation of participants' matching or evaluation judgements (see Box 16.4).

In an article in a special supplement of *Quality in Health Care*, Frewer *et al.* (2001) proposed the use of *repertory grid techniques* as a 'bottom-up' approach to analysing what is of more or less importance to patients choosing between treatments. While conjoint analysis and other statistical inference techniques have their roots in psychophysics, perception and cognition, repertory grid techniques emerged from Kelly's construct theory in social psychology (Kelly 1955).[8] Repertory grids have been used to assess patients' quality of life measures in relation to their previous and desired states of health (see Patel *et al.* 2003 for a critical literature review). In the statistical inference techniques discussed above, option attributes are defined or identified by the researcher prior to analysing their relative importance. In the case of *analytical hierarchy process* this may happen after discussion with respondents. In repertory grid analysis the defining attributes, and their hierarchical combinations, emerge from participants' contrasts between options.

Repertory grid analysis involves four steps. Firstly, in a series of judgements a participant indicates which of three options (such as treatments) differs from the other two, and in what way. This is repeated for all possible triplets of options. Secondly, each option is rated to indicate to what degree it has this characteristic. Thirdly, characteristics are rated to indicate how important they are. Fourthly, a grid of options by characteristics (termed 'constructs') is analysed, using simple frequency counts (the number of times a particular construct appears in the option set or the number of overlapping constructs that options have), or using some sort of computer-based cluster analysis. Principal components analysis identifies the correlations between patterns of constructs for each option to reveal which are similar to each other and which constructs tend to co-occur and form a principal component. *Generalized procrustes analysis* (GPA) is similar to principal components analysis but can summarize results across participants even if they have not produced an identical set of constructs.

For example, Rowe *et al.* (2005) used repertory grid analysis to identify how patients perceived seven angina treatment options. Each of 21 patients was shown triplets of possible options[9] and stated reasons that one differed from the other two. For example, keyhole surgery might be categorized as 'risky' in contrast to drugs to prevent symptoms and reduce risks of heart attack and drugs to treat symptoms only. Each patient only judged three possible sets of triplets, but then rated each option in terms of the constructs that had emerged from these initial contrasts. GPA analysis placed options on a two-dimensional graph, distinguishing doing nothing from doing something, and clustering drug treatments distinct from surgical treatments. When constructs were mapped onto these components some were clearly defined and participants showed agreement: having treatment was linked with maintaining lifestyle and was not worthless whereas no treatment was linked with being a burden. Having surgery was invasive, experimental and involved anaesthesia, but having drugs was easy, convenient and reversible. Plots of other constructs revealed individual differences. For example, risky, frightening, positive experiences and preference fell in different positions on the map depending on the participant.

As it is, repertory grid analysis focuses on how a patient perceives the set of available options. Arguably, it could be used with both patients and expert physicians to highlight differences in the relevant option components, difficult decision points (Baker 1996), and with a view to correcting any misunderstandings (on either part). Health care professionals may have misunderstood why a patient has particular preferences or inclinations. Patients may have misunderstood exactly which treatments are more or less safe, dangerous or long-lasting.

Predicting patient decisions from attitudes, beliefs and judgements

The methods described above emerge generally from either an expected utility theory framework of decision-making in which each option is decomposed into its outcomes and their respective probabilities of occurrence and utilities or from an information integration framework of decision-making in which options are decomposed into objective or subjective attributes. People's choices, or their decisions about their behaviour (their intended actions), can also be understood in terms of their attitudes, beliefs and judgements about treatments or outcomes. Frameworks such as in the *health belief model, protection motivation theory*, the *theory of reasoned action* and the *theory of planned behaviour* are seen as useful bases for changing health-related behaviour. These models differ subtly from each other: each includes an attitude or cost-benefit component as an important determinant of people's behaviour but the models vary according to the other determinants included in each (Armitage and Conner 2000).

The theory of reasoned action (TRA) (Fishbein and Ajzen 1975) is similar to expected utility theory in that two main elements are assessed: (a) belief or probability that particular outcomes will occur, and (b) the evaluation of these outcomes. Sutherland *et al.* (1998) applied TRA to cancer patients' preferences for participating in a hypothetical chemotherapy trial. They observed two sets of beliefs for participating: (a) pro-social beliefs (e.g. benefit future patients, help research) and (b) pro-self beliefs (e.g. prolong life, side-effects). They also stress the importance of assessing idiosyncratic beliefs, that is, beliefs that are unique for each patient. TRA provides a framework to analyse the cognitive cost-benefit structure for patients' preferences for adjuvant chemotherapy. But in particular, TRA considers the importance of the role of the subjective norm. This encapsulates the influence of important other people on a patient's preferences: their views on the behaviour or outcome, and the patient's desire to comply with their views are measured. In the context of participating in a chemotherapy trial, Sutherland *et al.* (1998) observed that ten different other persons could have an impact on the decision to participate (e.g. family doctor, surgeon, partner, family members). Siminoff and Fetting (1991) also found that patients relied heavily on their physicians to make treatment decisions. TRA's extension – the theory of planned behavior (TPB) (Ajzen 1991) additionally emphasizes the importance of behavioural control or self-efficacy (perceived ability to carry out the behaviour) as an influential factor in decision-making.

Protection motivation theory (PMT) consists of an appraisal of the threat (susceptibility and severity) of a health state and the ability to cope. This latter component, similar, but not identical to perceived barriers and benefits in the health belief model (see below), consists of response-efficacy (the usefulness of the behaviour) as well as self-efficacy (perceived ability to carry out the behaviour). Its usefulness in explaining or predicting behaviour, and in the design of interventions is significant, but limited (Armitage and Conner 2000) and there is some suggestion that the threat appraisal component is less useful than the coping appraisal component for predicting behaviour (Milne *et al.* 2000). PMT's conceptualization of the threat of a health state includes susceptibility (equivalent to the perceived probability that the state will occur) and severity. For example, the probability and severity of a recurrence or metastasis may influence preferences for adjuvant chemotherapy. In this context the risk attitude of patients may also be relevant: some people are more willing than others to take risks in the short term in order to gain in the long term.

Finally, the Health Belief Model (HBM) suggests that decisions about behaviour are determined by a number of specific components. Perceived susceptibility to the health state (again equivalent to a perception of probability of it occurring) and perceived severity of that state together make up perceived threat of the health state. Perceived benefits of a behaviour or intervention and perceived barriers to the behaviour or intervention together make up an evaluation of the behaviour. Finally health motivation and cues to action are also predictive of whether or not a health-related behaviour will be carried out. The theoretical framework of the HBM has been useful for designing interventions (e.g. Oliveria *et al.* 2004), and for understanding specific reasons for lack of compliance with current treatments (e.g. Sage *et al.* 2001).

The psychological models and theories in this section are useful frameworks for thinking about health decision-making and health interventions, but their predictive and descriptive ability as theories or models has been questioned. They have been tested via the administration of questionnaires that seek to measure the relevant attitudes, beliefs and cognitions in each individual. Although researchers with particular interests emphasize the positive, in a review of five years of published research on the models mentioned above, Ogden (2003) points out that none make specific predictions, and all papers report support for the relevant theory or model they are testing, even when some components of the theory or model are not found to be significant.

Describing the process of and influences on judgement and decision-making

We now turn to approaches that seek to describe the process of a patient's decision making. Many studies have used *focus groups* (Unson *et al.* 2003) and *in-depth retrospective interviews* to ascertain how a decision was or is made (e.g. Hudak *et al.* 2002; Harcourt and Rumsey 2004) or how the decision situation is or was perceived

(Walter and Britten 2002). Although a useful complement to other techniques, the problems of forgetting and *post hoc* rationalization, as well as the self-hypothesizing that is inevitable with considerations of underlying cause have been well debated in psychology and philosophy (Ericsson and Simon 1980, 1984; Flanagan 1991; see also Chapter 15). Analysis of interviews across patients can be used to yield thematic influences on decision-making. Others have advocated the analysis of *think-aloud protocols* or *information acquisition patterns* to ascertain how information is sought and interpreted, and how it influences decision-making. Such techniques are collectively known as *process tracing techniques*. While commonly used to examine health professionals' decision making (see Chapter 15), their use with patients raises ethical issues due to the potential disruption of the consultation and the cognitive burden at what may be a difficult time for patients. The result of process tracing may be a series of if-then statements (production rules), though verbal protocols from patients thinking aloud during decision-making might also be analysed qualitatively to ascertain the themes appearing in a person's narrative. It is important that process tracing techniques describe what the decision-maker actually does (it is veridical) and that it does not change their behaviour (reactivity). There is evidence that reflective, analytical thinking aloud may change behaviour – but this may be for the better, or for the worse (Wilson and Schooler 1991; McMackin and Slovic 2000).

Finally, some researchers have used more *naturalistic* and observational approaches to examine patients' cognitive and emotional strategies during decision-making. For example, in an examination of the information processing, emotions and cognitions associated with the use of a decision aid, Bekker *et al.* (2003) analysed transcripts of midwife-patient interaction during consultations about prenatal diagnostic testing. Similarly, Caspi *et al.* (2004) studied the themes emerging in the decision-making processes of patients seeking alternative therapies.

These methods are in some cases in the spirit of the naturalistic decision-making (NDM) approach usually used with experts (such as emergency-room surgeons, firefighters etc.) working under time pressure on significant problems. NDM encompasses a collection of tools, including interviews, observations and even computerized simulations, with the aim of studying decision processes in as naturalistic or realistic setting as possible. See Lipshitz *et al.* (2001) and, for a discussion of the potential use of NDM in examining patient decision-making, see Broadstock and Michie (2000).

As well as the practically oriented methods described above, researchers have also carried out epidemiological-style statistical analyses to identify correlates of particular decision-making preferences or practices (e.g. Staradub *et al.* 2002). They have carried out carefully designed experiments that reveal the information processing and potential biases in patients' decision-making (e.g. Zikmund-Fisher *et al.* 2004). And they have used questionnaires to elicit explicitly the perceived pros and cons, risks and benefits of different options, perceptions of probability and of harm, responsibility and anticipated regret (Wroe *et al.* 2004). The results of these feed into our understanding of the psychology of decision making (see Boxes 16.1–4).

Importantly, the use of process tracing and think-aloud techniques, focus groups, interviews and dialogue analysis may reveal key influences on decision-making that may not have appeared in choices between scenarios, rating, or questionnaires used in other approaches. For example, Unson *et al.* (2003) found that adherence is affected by differences in perceptions of the seriousness of non-adherence, doubts regarding the competence of the health care worker and respondents' own perceptions of their vulnerability. Hudak *et al.* (2002) reveal from interviews the perception of elderly people that their poor health state is a normal part of the ageing process, not bad enough for treatment, and that their physicians would have suggested that they had treatment if their condition merited it. Although such studies demonstrate the strong influence of physicians' advice (Gurmankin *et al.* 2002), advice-based decision-making is an important but relatively neglected topic in decision research (Yaniv 2004).

Choosing between methods

The descriptive methods above serve to *elucidate* a patient's preferences, and the reasoning behind those preferences. Research in the psychology of judgement and decision-making suggests that the methods will also *establish* a patient's preferences, since we tend to construct our preferences as we go along (Payne *et al.* 1992; Slovic 1995), seeking and evaluating reasons for different choices. We process information intuitively, using heuristics unless time and circumstances allow and potential gains or losses merit the effort of deliberate analysis (Hamm 1988; Chaiken *et al.* 1989; Kahneman 2003). Preferences are prone not only to the inconsistencies that are inherent in making judgements (and all subjective measures) but also show specific influences associated with probability (Box 16.1), time (Box 16.2), how information is presented (Box 16.3) and how judgements are made (Box 16.4). The implications of these findings for describing and measuring patient decision-making are import-ant and are increasingly being used to understand and explain patterns of responses and discrepancies in results between different methods (e.g. Chapman and Elstein 2001; Redelmeier *et al.* 2001a, 2001b; Bleichrodt 2002; Lloyd 2003).

The methods described in the approaches above have been developed for differ-ing aims. Here we shall discuss their use in relation to the reasons for studying patients' decision-making that we introduced at the beginning (see Figure 16.6).

Scientific interest and describing and predicting health decision-making

Most of the techniques mentioned above are relevant to (socio)scientific interest in that they advance our understanding of individuals' health-related behaviour and how this interacts with society's norms and the social and informational setting. It is easy to see how quantitative techniques feed into health policy decision-making formally and informally, but qualitative models and those describing and predicting decision-making also have a role to play. For example, researchers may analyse individual differences in health behaviours on the basis of individual differences in attitudes and cognitions with a view to changing behaviour by changing attitudes or cognitions, and may analyse the differences in information processing and other decision influences for the decision made and its outcome with a view to improving decision-making via process.

Policy decision-making and valuing health

Most of the holistic methods described in this chapter have been developed for use in decision analyses and cost-effectiveness analyses, to provide a measure of effectiveness in situations where more than two outcomes occur. In situations with two outcomes (such as alive and dead) it suffices to choose the option with the highest chance of the best outcome (e.g. that with the highest survival rate). In situations with more than two outcomes, outcomes need to be valued relative to one another. Utility provides such a valuation, on a scale from 0 to 1 (generally – but not necessarily – death to optimal health). Chapters 13 and 14 describe decision analysis and cost-effectiveness analysis in more detail.

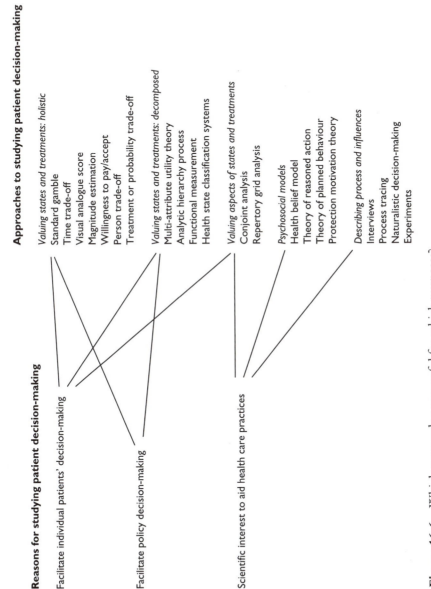

Figure 16.6 Which approaches are useful for which purposes?

To obtain decision utilities for policy decision-making, the researcher needs to choose from SG, TTO and VAS. The SG used to be considered the gold standard, but due to biases in the method, especially probability transformation, leading to utilities that are biased towards 1, the TTO seems to be most frequently used nowadays. Further, patients generally find it an easier and more acceptable method. Little is known about the biases that may operate in the TTO, but it has been argued that those occurring tend to cancel each other out. For example, time discounting makes it relatively easy to trade far-off life years in the TTO, and results in an underestimate of utility. But scale compatibility will overweight the response scale of duration in comparison to health state information, leading to unwillingness to trade life years, despite poor health. This results in a bias upwards. Bleichrodt (2002) presents a clear explanation of the possible biases operating in the SG and TTO.

As described above, a VAS score is not a decision utility, but nevertheless the VAS is frequently used, due to its ease of administration. SG and TTO are preferably administered in an interview, to minimize inconsistent and incoherent responses, whereas a VAS can be administered in a questionnaire. VAS is also potentially influenced by basic psychological phenomena (see Box 16.4). Values have been argued to be too low, since no trade-off is involved, and therefore transformations as described above need to be performed.

MAUT is used to infer utilities for health states (in the Health Utilities Index) and this is fed into decision analysis. Willingness to pay can be used in cost-benefit analysis and in cost-effectiveness analysis. In contrast, although applications of conjoint analysis may assess holistic values (for example on a 5–7 point scale), the focus of this method is on calculation of attribute utilities rather than assessment of utilities for particular health states or treatments. This, and the other valuation methods are not used in the context of decision analysis, since they do not result in a utility on a 0–1 scale. These methods have predominantly been used in health services research to assess correlates of preferences, such as sociodemographic characteristics of (potential) service users and to influence policy decision-making. Such information can feed into policy decision-making at a less mathematical level and is also of scientific interest.

Facilitating individual decision-making

It has been suggested that shared or informed decision-making (Bekker *et al.* 1999) is preferable to traditional physician-as-agent models in part because it's easier to transfer information about options to a patient than about a patient's values and preferences to the physician (Gafni *et al.* 1998).[10] Many of the methods described above can be used to facilitate individual patients' informed decision-making.

Although decision analysis on the basis of an individual patient's utilities derived from SGs may be questioned, the results of TTO-based assessments and MAUT assessments can and have been used in individuals' decision analysis and decision aids e.g. (Unic *et al.* 1998; Pell *et al.* 2002). Population-based utilities can be fed into decision rules to aid decision-making in specific decision situations (e.g. Robinson and Thomson 2000; Thomson *et al.* 2000).

An analytical approach may facilitate the trade-off of attributes, encourage consistency and reduce the impact of short-term emotional and social influences. However, some researchers have been wary of promoting an analytical decision approach that potentially impedes incorporation of relevant emotions (fear awaiting results, regret, anxiety), hard to quantify aspects of the treatment process (e.g. taking a pill every day for the rest of your life), and other intuitive and qualitative aspects of the decision-making process (Ubel and Loewenstein 1997; Ubel 2002). In support of this stance, there is evidence that explicit reasoning and consideration of the rationale behind decision-making may impede it (Wilson and Schooler 1991; Tetlock 1992; McMackin and Slovic 2000).

Although there is evidence that decision aids without an explicit utility assessment procedure facilitate decision-making (Bekker and Wong 2004), much of the intended merit of patient decision aids is to help reduce decision conflict and encourage decisions that are consistent with patients' values (in other words, to help patients work out how they value different attributes or goals and how to trade these off against each other). In keeping with this, evaluations of decision aids measure decision conflict (O'Connor 1995), regret (Feldman-Stewart *et al.* 1999) and satisfaction (Holmes-Rovner *et al.* 1996). Anxiety-based assessment measures appear to be less useful (Bekker *et al.* 2003), and satisfaction does not seem to increase with the use of decision aids (O'Connor *et al.* 1999). The focus of assessing decision facilitation then, is the experience of the decision-making process. This is not necessarily separate from the outcome of the decision in terms of rated well-being (Stalmeier *et al.* 2004).

Conclusions

This chapter has introduced several approaches to describing and measuring patients' judgement and decision-making. These approaches come from a number of different disciplines and have been applied with a number of different purposes. Research on patient decision-making aims to facilitate good decisions at a policy level, using systematic strategies to pin down underlying values. It also aims to facilitate a good decision-making experience at an individual level, helping patients to construct their preferences in the social, emotional and cognitive context.

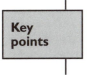

Key points

- Patient decision-making may be investigated in order to facilitate informed decision-making or to optimize decision-making at policy level.

- The process of preference elicitation may itself act as a decision aid, helping people evaluate the meaning of the options, and compare and contrast them.

- The holistic approach to measuring global health state or treatment preferences requires the respondent to assign values to each possible health state or treatment.

- The decomposed approach enables the investigator to obtain values for all health states or treatments without the assignation of values to every one. It expresses the overall value as a function of the health state or treatment attributes involved; the best known application of this method is MAUT.

- Several holistic methods exist to assess preference-based measures of quality of life: measures of the utility of a health state (a cardinal measure of the strength of an individual's preference for that health state when faced with uncertainty), such as the SG and TTO, and non-utility based measures such as visual analogue rating scales, magnitude estimation and willingness to pay.

- Other methods, including judgement analysis, conjoint analysis, discrete choice experiments, repertory grid methods and process tracing techniques each examine how aspects of a treatment or health state influence preferences.

- People's choices, decisions or actions can also be understood in terms of their attitudes and beliefs. Frameworks such as the HBM, PMT, TRA and the TPB are useful, theoretical bases for understanding people's choices or their decisions about their behaviour.

- Other approaches that aim to describe the process of patients' decision-making include focus groups, the analysis of think-aloud protocols or of information acquisition patterns (process tracing), as well as naturalistic and observational approaches.

- Preferences are prone to the inconsistencies inherent in judgement, and show influences associated with probability, time, how the information is presented and how judgements are made. Knowledge of these issues is increasingly used to explain response patterns and has important implications for describing and measuring patient decision-making.

Notes

1 Differences in health ratings of those in a health state and not in a health state parallel some of those shown in Box 16.1.
2 Centuries before this, Jeremy Bentham and other philosophers used the term 'utility' to refer to the pleasure or pain experienced at a particular moment in time. See Read (2004) for a discussion of the distinction between decision utilities and moment-by-moment experienced utilities.
3 Critical tests of expected utility in the decision theory literature have shown that it is not empirically valid. Based on these findings, a descriptive theory, prospect theory, has been developed by Kahneman and Tversky (1979) and Tversky and Kahneman (1992), among others, which provides an explanation for the commonly found overestimates in the SG (see Wakker and Stiggelbout 1995; Bleichrodt et al. 2001). Bleichrodt (2002) provides some reasonably accessible papers on this issue.
4 Psychologists have long been interested in the mismatch between people's explicit and statistically derived attribute weights. Judgement predictions based on statistical weights are more accurate than the judgements on which they are calculated, a phenomenon known as bootstrapping (Meehl 1954, 1965), and explicit weights seem to be an idealization compared with statistical weights (see Harries et al. 2000; Harries and Harvey 2000b). See also Chapter 15.
5 e.g. SPSS ORTHOPLAN procedure and Stated Preference Experiment Editor and Designer (SPEED; http://www.hpgholding.nl/software/speed.htm) for the design of the experiments and calculation of utilities; Sawtooth software (http://www.sawtoothsoftware.com/) for computer-based elicitation and calculation of utilities.
6 In adaptive conjoint analysis participants state which attributes are important, then judge options or states that vary along those important attributes.
7 Relevant attributes are identified on the basis of literature searches (Ryan et al. 2001a; Maddala et al. 2003), previous research (e.g. Fraenkel et al. 2001), interviews (Ross et al. 2003; Sculpher et al. 2004), focus groups, or discussions with experts (Ratcliffe et al. 2004).
8 Repertory grid has been used in social psychology to identify how individuals perceive themselves and others, and how they think others perceive them.
9 The seven treatment options were no treatment, three drug treatment options, balloon angioplasty, keyhole surgery and coronary artery bypass surgery.
10 Dowie (2002) argues for the assessment of patients' meta-preferences (their preferences for participation in the decision – as to how the decision should be made) in decision support systems.

Further reading

Chapman, G.B. and Elstein, A.S. (2000) Cognitive processes and biases in medical decision making, in G.B. Chapman and F.A. Sonnenberg (eds) *Decision Making in Health Care*. Cambridge: Cambridge University Press.

Hastie, R. and Dawes, R.M. (2001) *Rational Choice in an Uncertain World*. Thousand Oaks, CA: Sage.

Hunink, M., Glasziou, P., Siegel, J. *et al.* (2001) *Decision Making in Health and Medicine: Integrating Evidence and Values*. Cambridge: Cambridge University Press. See in particular Chapter 4.

Pierce, P.F. and Hicks, F.D. (2001) Patient decision-making behavior: an emerging paradigm in nursing science, *Nursing Research*, 50: 267–74.

Stiggelbout, A.M. (2000) Assessing patients' preferences, in G.B. Chapman and F.A. Sonnenberg (eds) *Decision Making in Health Care*. Cambridge: Cambridge University Press.

Resources

Medical Decision Making websites (patient decision making)

http://symptomresearch.nih.gov/chapter_4/chaauthorbio.htm. Chapter 4 of the *Interactive Textbook on Clinical Symptom Research on Patient Decision Making*, written by Hal Arkes.

http://www.smdm.org. Society for Medical Decision Making webpages.

http://www.nemc.org/medicine/cdm/. Division of Clinical Decision Making, Informatics and Telemedicine, Tufts–New England Medical Centre.

http://www.ohri.ca/centres/DecisionAids/default.asp. Ottawa Health Decision Centre.

References

Ajzen, I. (1991) The theory of planned behavior, *Organizational Behavior and Human Decision Processes*, 50: 179–211.

Anderson, N.H. (1971) Information integration and attitude change, *Psychological Review*, 78: 171–206.

Armitage, C.J. and Conner, M. (2000) Social cognition models and health behaviour: a structured review, *Psychology and Health*, 15: 173–89.

Ayton, P. and Wright, G. (1994) *Subjective Probability*. Chichester: Wiley.

Baker, D. (1996) Understanding the basis of treatment choices for varicose veins: a model of decision making with the repertory grid technique, *Quality in Health Care*, 5: 128–33.

Baron, J., Asch, D.A., Fagerlin, A. *et al.* (2003) Effect of assessment method on the discrepancy between judgments of health disorders people have and do not have: a web study, *Medical Decision Making*, 23: 422–34.

Bekker, H. and Wong, S.S. (2004) Evaluating the effectiveness of a leaflet to support women's decision making between termination methods, *Medical Decision Making*, 24(4): 430.

Bekker, H.L., Thornton, J.G., Airey, C.M. *et al.* (1999) Informed decision making: an annotated bibliography and systematic review, *Health Technology Assessment*, 3(1).

Bekker, H.L., Legare, F., Stacey, D. *et al.* (2003) Is anxiety a suitable measure of decision aid effectiveness? A systematic review, *Patient Education and Counselling*, 50: 255–62.

Bergus, G.R., Levin, I.P. and Elstein, A. (2002) Presenting risks and benefits to patients: the effect of information order on decision making, *Journal of General Internal Medicine*, 17: 612–17.

Berry, D.C., Raynor, D.K., Knapp, P. and Bersellini, E. (2003) Patients' understanding of risk associated with medication use, *Drug Safety*, 26: 1–11.

Bleichrodt, H. (2002) A new explanation for the difference between time trade-off utilities and standard gamble utilities, *Health Economics*, 11: 447–56.

Bleichrodt, H., Pinto, J.L. and Wakker, P. (2001) Making descritive use of prospect theory to improve the prescriptive use of expected utility, *Management Science*, 47: 1498–514.

Brazier, J., Roberts, J. and Deverill, M. (2002) The estimation of a preference-based measure of health from the SF-36, *Journal of Health Economics*, 21: 271–92.

Brickman, P., Coates, D. and Janoff-Bulman, R. (1978) Lottery winners and accident victims: is happiness relative? *Journal of Personality and Social Psychology*, 36: 917–27.

Broadstock, M. and Michie, S. (2000) Processes of patient decision making: theoretical and methodological issues, *Psychology and Health*, 15: 191–204.

Busschbach, J.J., McDonnell, J., Essink-Bot, M.L. and Van Hout, B.A. (1999) Estimating parametric relationships between health description and health valuation with an application to the EuroQol EQ-5D, *Journal of Health Economics*, 18: 551–71.

Carter, K.J., Ritchey, N.P., Castro, F. *et al.* (1999) Analysis of three decision-making methods: a breast cancer patient as a model, *Medical Decision Making*, 19: 49–57.

Caspi, O., Koithan, M. and Criddle, M.W. (2004) Alternative medicine or 'Alternative' patients: a qualitative study of patient-oriented decision-making processes with respect to complementary and alternative medicine, *Medical Decision Making*, 24: 64–79.

Chaiken, S., Liberman, A. and Eagly, A.H. (1989) Heuristic and systematic information processing within and beyond the persuasion context, in J.S. Uleman and J.A. Bargh (eds) *Unintended Thought*. New York: Guilford Press.

Chapman, G.B. (2000), Preferences for improving and declining sequences of health outcomes, *Journal of Behavioral Decision Making*, 13: 203–18.

Chapman, G.B. (2003) Time discounting of health outcomes, in G. Loewenstein, D. Read and D.F. Baumeister (eds) *Time and Decision: Economic and Psychological Perspectives on Intertemporal Choice*. New York: Sage.

Chapman, G.B. and Elstein, A.S. (2001) Cognitive processes and biases in medical decision making, in G.B. Chapman and F.A. Sonnenberg (eds) *Decision Making in Health Care: Theory, Psychology, and Applications*. Cambridge: Cambridge University Press.

Chapman, G.B., Elstein, A., Kuzel, T.M. *et al.* (1999) A multiattribute model of prostate cancer patients' preferences for health states, *Quality of Life Research*, 8: 171–80.

Christensen-Szalanski, J.J.J. (1984) Discount functions and the measurement of patients' values: womens' decisions during childbirth, *Medical Decision Making*, 4: 47–58.

Connolly, T. and Reb, J. (2003) Omission bias in vaccination decisions: where's the 'omission'? Where's the 'bias'?, *Organizational Behavior and Human Decision Processes*, 91: 186–202.

Dolan, J.G. (1995) Are patients capable of using the analytic hierarchy process and willing to use it to help make clinical decisions?, *Medical Decision Making*, 15: 76–80.

Dolan, J.G. and Bordley, D.R. (1991) Individualized patient decision-making using the analytic hierarchy process (AHP) – reliability, validity, and clinical usefulness, *Medical Decision Making*, 11: 322.

Dolan, P. (1997) Modeling valuations for EuroQol health states, *Medical Care*, 35: 1095–1108.

Dolan, P. (1999) Whose preferences count?, *Medical Decision Making*, 19: 4.

Dowie, J. (2002) The role of patients' meta-preferences in the design and evaluation of decision support systems, *Health Expectations*, 5: 16–27.

Drummond, M.F., O'Brien, B., Stoddart, G.L. and Torrance, G.W. (1997) *Methods for the Economic Evaluation of Health Care Programmes*, 2nd edn. Oxford: Oxford University Press.

Ericsson, K.A. and Simon, H.A. (1980) Verbal reports as data, *Psychological Review*, 87: 215–51.

Ericsson, K.A. and Simon, H.A. (1984) *Protocol Analysis: Verbal Reports as Data*. Cambridge, MA: MIT Press.

Feeny, D., Furlong, W., Boyle, M. and Torrance, G. (1995) Multi-attribute health status classification systems: Health Utilities Index, *Pharmacoeconomics*, 7: 490–502.

Feldman-Stewart, D., Brundage, M.D., McConnell, B.A. and Mackillop, W.J. (1999) Practical issues in assisting shared decision making, *Health Expectations*, 3: 46–54.

Fishbein, M. and Ajzen, I. (1975) *Belief, Attitude, Intention and Behavior: An Introduction to Theory and Research*. Reading, MA: Addison-Wesley.

Flanagan, O.J. (1991) Cognitive science and artificial intelligence: philosophical assumptions and implications, in O.J. Flanagan (ed.) *The Science of the Mind*, 2nd edn. Cambridge, MA: MIT Press.

Fox, C. and See, K.E. (2003) Belief and preference in decision under uncertainty, in D. Hardman and L. Macchi (eds) *Thinking: Psychological Perspectives on Reasoning, Judgement and Decision Making*. Chichester: Wiley.

Fraenkel, L., Bogardus, S. and Wittink, D.R. (2001) Understanding patient preferences for the treatment of lupus nephritis with adaptive conjoint analysis, *Medical Care*, 39: 1203–16.

Fraenkel, L., Bogardus, S. and Concato, J. (2002) Patient preferences for treatment of lupus nephritis, *Arthritis & Rheumatism*, 47: 421–8.

Fraenkel, L., Bogardus, S., Concato, J. *et al.* (2004) Patient preferences for treatment of rheumatoid arthritis, *Annals of the Rheumatic Diseases*, http://ard.bmjjournals.com

Frewer, L.J., Salter, B. and Lambert, N. (2001) Understanding patients' preferences for treatment: the need for innovative methodologies, *Quality in Health Care*, 10: 150–4.

Froberg, D.G. and Kane, R.L. (1989) Methodology for measuring health state preferences – I: Measurement strategies, *Journal of Clinical Epidemiology*, 42: 345–54.

Gafni, A., Charles, C. and Whelan, T. (1998) The patient–physician encounter: the physician as a perfect agent for the patient versus the informed treatment decision making model, *Social Science and Medicine*, 47: 347–54.

Gigerenzer, G. (2003) *Reckoning with Risk*. London: Penguin.

Gigerenzer, G. and Edwards, A. (2003) Simple tools for understanding risks: from innumeracy to insight, *British Medical Journal*, 327: 741–7.

Gigerenzer, G., Todd, P.M., and The ABC Research Group (1999) *Simple Heuristics That Make Us Smart*. Oxford: Oxford University Press.

Gold, M.R., Siegel, J.E., Russell, L.B. and Weinstein, M.C. (1996) *Cost-Effectiveness in Health and Medicine*. Oxford: Oxford University Press.

Green, P.E. and Srinivasan, V. (1978) Conjoint analysis in consumer research: issues and outlook, *Journal of Consumer Research*, 5: 103–23.

Grimes, D.A. and Snively, G.R. (1999) Patients' understanding of medical risks: implications for genetic counseling, *Obstetrics and Gynaecology*, 93: 910–14.

Gurmankin, A.D., Baron, J., Hershey, J.C. and Ubel, P.A. (2002) The role of physicians' recommendations in medical treatment decisions, *Medical Decision Making*, 22: 262–71.

Hamm, R.M. (1988) Clinical intuition and clinical analysis: expertise and the cognitive continuum, in J. Dowie and A. Elstein (eds) *Professional Judgement: A Reader in Clinical Decision Making*. Cambridge: Cambridge University Press.

Harcourt, D. and Rumsey, N. (2004) Mastectomy patients' decision-making for or against immediate breast reconstruction, *Psycho-Oncology*, 13: 106–15.

Harries, C. and Harvey, N. (2000a) Are absolute frequencies, relative frequencies or both effective in reducing cognitive biases? *Journal of Behavioral Decision Making*, 13: 431–44.

Harries, C. and Harvey, N. (2000b) Taking advice, using information and knowing what you are doing, *Acta Psychologica*, 104: 399–416.

Harries, C., Evans, J. St. B.T. and Dennis, I. (2000) Measuring doctors' self-insight into their treatment decisions, *Applied Cognitive Psychology*, 14: 455–77.

Holmes-Rovner, M., Kroll, J., Schmitt, N. *et al.* (1996) Patient satisfaction with health-care decisions: the satisfaction with decision scale, *Medical Decision Making*, 16: 56–64.

Hsee, C.K., Loewenstein, G.F., Blount, S. and Bazerman, M.H. (1999) Preference reversals between joint and separate evaluations of options: a review and theoretical analysis, *Psychological Bulletin*, 125: 576–90.

Hudak, P.L., Clark, J.P., Hawker, G.A. *et al.* (2002) You're perfect for the procedure! Why don't you want it? Elderly arthritis patients' unwillingness to consider total joint arthroplasty surgery: a qualitative study, *Medical Decision Making*, 22: 272–8.

Hunink, M., Glasziou, P., Siegel, J. *et al.* (2001) *Decision Making in Health and Medicine: Integrating Evidence and Values*. Cambridge: Cambridge University Press.

Jansen, S.J., Stiggelbout, A.M., Wakker, P. *et al.* (1998) Patients' utilities for cancer treatments: a study of the chained procedure for the standard gamble and time trade-off, *Medical Decision Making*, 18: 391–9.

Julian-Reynier, C., Welkenhuysen, M., Hagoel, L. *et al.* (2003) Risk communication strategies: state of the art and effectiveness in the context of cancer genetic services, *European Journal of Human Genetics*, 11: 725–36.

Kahneman, D. (2003) A perspective on judgment and choice: mapping bounded rationality, *American Psychologist*, 58: 697–720.

Kahneman, D. and Tversky, A. (1979) Prospect theory: an analysis of decision under risk, *Econometrica*, 47: 263–91.

Keeny, R.L. and Raiffa, H. (1976) *Decisions with Multiple Objectives: Preferences and Value Trade-offs.* New York: Wiley.

Kelly, G.A. (1955) *The Psychology of Personal Constructs.* New York: Norton.

Kreiger, A.M., Green, P.E. and Wind, Y. (2001) Thirty years of conjoint analysis: reflections and prospects, *Interfaces*, 31: s56–73.

Levine, M.N., Gafni, A., Markham, B. and MacFarlane, D. (1992) A bedside decision instrument to elicit a patient's preference concerning adjuvant chemotherapy for breast cancer, *Annals of Internal Medicine*, 117(1): 53–8.

Lipshitz, R., Klein, G., Orasanu, J. and Salas, E. (2001) Taking stock of naturalistic decision-making, *Journal of Behavioral Decision Making*, 14(5): 331–52.

Llewellyn-Thomas, H.A. (1997) Investigating patients' preferences for different treatment options, *Canadian Journal of Nursing Research*, 29: 45–64.

Llewellyn-Thomas, H.A., Williams, J.I., Levy, L. and Naylor, C.D. (1996) Using a trade-off technique to assess patients' treatment preferences for benign prostatic hyperplasia, *Medical Decision Making*, 16: 262–82.

Lloyd, A.J. (2001) The extent of patients' understanding of the risk of treatments, *Quality in Health Care*, 10: 114–18.

Lloyd, A.J. (2003) Threats to the estimation of benefit: are preference elicitation methods accurate? *Health Economics*, 12: 393–402.

Loewenstein, G. and Angner, E. (2003) Predicting and indulging changing preferences, in G. Loewenstein, D. Read and D.F. Baumeister (eds) *Time and Decision: Economic and Psychological Perspectives on Intertemporal Choice.* New York: Sage.

Loewenstein, G., Read, D., and Baumeister, D.F. (2003) *Time and Decision: Economic and Psychological Perspectives on Intertemporal Choice.* New York: Sage.

Maddala, T., Phillips, K. and Johnson, F. (2003) An experiment on simplifying conjoint analysis designs for measuring preferences, *Health Economics*, 12: 1035–47.

Maule, A.J. and Svenson, O. (1993) *Time Pressure and Stress in Human Judgement and Decision Making.* New York: Plenum Press.

McMackin, J. and Slovic, P. (2000) When does explicit justification impair decision making? *Applied Cognitive Psychology*, 14: 527–41.

McNeil, B., Pauker, S.G. and Tversky, A. (1988) On the framing of medical decisions, in D.E. Bell, H. Raiffa and A. Tversky (eds) *Decision Making: Descriptive, Normative and Prescriptive Interactions.* Cambridge: Cambridge University Press.

Meehl, P.E. (1954) *Clinical Versus Statistical Prediction.* Minneapolis, MN: University of Minnesota Press.

Meehl, P.E. (1965) Seer over sign: the first good example, *Journal of Experimental Research in Personality*, 1: 27–32.

Milne, S., Sheeran, P. and Orbell, S. (2000) Prediction and intervention in health-related behavior: a meta-analytic review of protection motivation theory, *Journal of Applied Social Psychology*, 30: 106–43.

Murray, C.J. and Acharya, A.K. (1997) Understanding DALYS (disability-adjusted life years), *Journal of Health Economics*, 16: 703–30.

Nord, E. (1995) The person-trade-off approach to valuing health care programs, *Medical Decision Making*, 15: 201–8.

O'Connor, A.M. (1995) Validation of a decision conflict scale, *Medical Decision Making*, 15: 25–30.

O'Connor, A.M., Rostrom, A., Fiset, V. *et al.* (1999) Decision aids for patients facing health treatment or screening decisions: systematic review, *British Medical Journal*, 319: 731–4.

Ogden, J. (2003) Some problems with social cognition models: a pragmatic and conceptual analysis, *Health Psychology*, 22: 424–8.

Oliveria, S.A., Dusza, S.W., Phelan, D.L. *et al.* (2004) Patient adherence to skin self-examination – effect of nurse intervention with photographs, *American Journal of Preventive Medicine*, 26: 152–5.

Parducci, A. (1965) Category judgment: a range-frequency model, *Psychological Review*, 72: 407–18.

Parducci, A. (1990) Response bias and contextual effects: when biased?, in J.-M.F. and M.G.J-P. Caverni (eds) *Cognitive Biases.* North Holland: Elsevier Science.

Patel, K.K., Veenstra, D.L. and Patrick, D.L. (2003) A review of selected patient-generated outcome measures and their application in clinical trials, *Value in Health*, 6: 595–603.

Payne, J.W., Bettman, J.R., Coupey, E. and Johnson, E.J. (1992) A constructive process view of decision making: multiple strategies in judgment and choice, *Acta Psychologica*, 80: 107–41.

Pell, I., Dowie, J., Clarke, A. *et al.* (2002) Development and preliminary evaluation of a clinical guidance programme for the decision about prophylactic oophorectomy in women undergoing a hysterectomy, *Quality and Safety in Health Care*, 11: 32–9.

Pierce, P.F. and Hicks, F.D. (2001) Patient decision-making behavior: an emerging paradigm for nursing science, *Nursing Research*, 50: 267–74.

Ratcliffe, J., Buxton, M., McGarry, T. *et al.* (2004) Patients' preferences for characteristics associated with treatments for osteoarthritis, *Rheumatology*, 43: 337–45.

Read, D. (2001) Intrapersonal dilemmas, *Human Relations*, 54: 1093–117.

Read, D. (2004) *Utility Theory from Jeremy Bentham to Daniel Kahneman*. London School of Economics working paper No. LSE OR 04–64. London: London School of Economics.

Read, D. and Powell, M. (2002) Reasons for sequence preferences, *Journal of Behavioral Decision Making*, 15: 433–60.

Read, D., Loewenstein, G. and Kalyanaraman, S. (1999) Mixing virtue and vice: combining the immediacy effect and the diversification heuristic, *Journal of Behavioral Decision Making*, 12: 257–73.

Redelmeier, D.A. and Kahneman, D. (1996) Patients' memories of painful medical treatments: real-time and retrospective evaluations of two minimally invasive procedures, *Pain*, 66: 3–8.

Redelmeier, D.A. and Shafir, E. (1995) Medical decision making in situations that offer multiple alternatives, *Journal of the American Medical Association*, 273: 302–5.

Redelmeier, D.A., Schull, M.J. and Hux, J.E. (2001a) Problems for clinical judgement 1: eliciting an insightful history of presenting illness, *Canadian Medical Association Journal*, 164: 647–51.

Redelmeier, D.A., Tu, J.V., Schull, M.J. *et al.* (2001b) Problems for clinical judgement 2: obtaining a reliable past medical history, *Canadian Medical Association Journal*, 164: 809–13.

Redelmeier, D.A., Katz, J. and Kahneman, D. (2003) *Pain*, 104: 187–94.

Robinson, A. and Thomson, R. (2000) The potential use of decision analysis to support shared decision making in the face of uncertainty: the example of atrial fibrillation and warfarin anticoagulation, *Quality in Health Care*, 9: 238–44.

Robinson, A. and Thomson, R. (2001) Variability in patient preferences for participating in medical decision making: implication for the use of decision support tools, *Quality in Health Care*, 10: 134–8.

Rosen, A.B., Tsai, J.S. and Downs, S.M. (2003) Variations in risk attitude across race, gender, and education, *Medical Decision Making*, 23: 511–17.

Ross, M.-A., Avery, A. and Foss, A. (2003) Views of older people on cataract surgery options: an assessment of preferences by conjoint analysis, *Quality and Safety in Health Care*, 12: 13–17.

Rowe, G., Lambert, N., Bowling, A. *et al.* (2005) Ascertaining patients' preferences for treatment for angina using a modified repertory grid method. *Social Science and Medicine*, 60: 2585–2595.

Russell, L.B., Gold, M.R., Siegel, J. *et al.* (1996) The role of cost-effectiveness analysis in health and medicine: Panel on Cost-Effectiveness in Health and Medicine, *Journal of the American Medical Association*, 276: 1172–7.

Ryan, M. and Farrar, S. (2000) Using conjoint analysis to elicit preferences for health care, *British Medical Journal*, 320: 1530–3.

Ryan, M., Bate, A., Eastmond, C. and Ludbrook, A. (2001) Use of discrete choice experiments to elicit preferences, *Quality in Health Care*, 10 (supplement): i55–60.

Sage, C.E., Southcott, A.M., and Brown, S.L. (2001) The health belief model and compliance with CPAP treatment for obstructive sleep apnoea, *Behaviour Change*, 18: 177–85.

San Miguel, F., Ryan, M. and Amaya-Amaya, M. (2005) Irrational stated preferences: a quantitative and qualitative investigation, *Health Economics*, 14, 307–322.

Sculpher, M.J., Bryan, S., Fry, P. *et al.* (2004) Patients' preferences for the management of non-metastatic prostrate cancer: discrete choice experiment, *British Medical Journal*, 328: 382–4.

Shafir, E., Simonson, I. and Tversky, A. (1993) Reason-based choice, *Cognition*, 49: 11–36.

Sieff, E.M., Dawes, R.M. and Loewenstein, G. (1999) Anticipated versus actual reaction to HIV test results, *American Journal of Psychology*, 112: 297–311.

Siminoff, L.A. and Fetting, J.H. (1991) Factors affecting treatment decisions for a life-threatening illness: the case of medical treatment of breast cancer, *Social Science and Medicine*, 32: 813–18.

Simon, H. (1986) Alternative visions of rationality, in H. Arkes and K.R. Hammond (eds) *Judgement and Decision Making: An Interdisciplinary Reader*. Cambridge: Cambridge University Press.

Slovic, P. (1995) The construction of preference, *American Psychologist*, 50: 364–71.

Staradub, V.L., Hseih, Y.-C. and Clauson, J. (2002) Factors that influence surgical choices in women with breast carcinoma, *Cancer*, 95: 1185–90.

Stalmeier, P.F.M. *et al.* (2004) On the evaluation of shared decision-making: the decision evaluation scales. Oral presentation at 9th biennial meeting of the European Society for Medical Decision Making, Rotterdam, June.

Stiggelbout, A.M. (2000) Assessing patients' preferences, in G.B. Chapman and F.A. Sonnenberg (eds) *Decision Making in Health Care*. Cambridge: Cambridge University Press.

Sumner, W. and Nease, R.F. (2001) Choice-matching preference reversals in health outcome assessments, *Medical Decision Making*, 21: 208–18.

Sutherland, H.J., Da Cunha, R., Lockwood, G.A. and Till, J.E. (1998) What attitudes and beliefs underlie patients' decisions about participating in chemotherapy trials? *Medical Decision Making*, 18: 61–9.

Teigen, K.H. and Brun, W. (1999) The directionality of verbal probability expressions: effects on decision, predictions, and probabilistic reasoning. *Organizational Behavior and Human Decision Processes*, 80: 155–90.

Tetlock, P.E. (1992) The impact of accountability on judgement and choice: toward a social contingency model, *Advances in Experimental Social Psychology*, 25: 331–76.

Thomson, R., Parkin, D., Eccles, M. *et al.* (2000) Decision analysis and guidelines for anticoagulant therapy to prevent stroke in patients with atrial fibrillation, *Lancet*, 355: 956–62.

Timmermans, D. (1994) The roles of experience and domain of expertise in using numerical and verbal probability terms in medical decisions, *Medical Decision Making*, 14: 146–56.

Timmermans, D.R.M. and Henneman L. (2002) The communication of genetic risks: What we know and what we need to learn. Essay for the programme "Sovietal Component of Genomics", NWO and Netherlands Genomic Initiative, The Hague.

Timmermans, D., Molewijk, B., Stiggelbout, A. and Kievet, J. (2004) Different formats for communicating surgical risks to patients and the effect on choice of treatment. *Patient Education and Counseling*, 54(3): 255–63.

Torrance, G.W. (1976) Preferences for health states: an empirical evaluation of three measurement techniques, *Socio-Economic Planning Science*, 10: 129–36.

Torrance, G.W. and Feeny, D. (1989) Utilities and quality-adjusted life years, *Journal of Technological Assessment in Health Care*, 5: 559–75.

Torrance, G.W., Feeny, D., Furlong, W.J. *et al.* (1996) Multiattribute utility function for a comprehensive health status classification system, Health Utilities Index Mark 2, *Medical Care*, 34: 702–22.

Torrance, G.W., Feeny, D. and Furlong, W. (2001) Visual analog scales: do they have a role in the measurement of preferences for health states? *Medical Decision Making*, 21: 329–34.

Tversky, A. and Kahneman, D. (1992) Advances in prospect-theory – cumulative representation of uncertainty, *Journal of Risk and Uncertainty*, 5: 297–323.

Ubel, P.A. (2002) Is information always a good thing? Helping patients make 'good' decisions, *Medical Care*, 40 (supplement): v39–44.

Ubel, P.A. and Loewenstein, G. (1997) The role of decision analysis in informed consent: choosing between intuition and systematicity, *Social Science and Medicine*, 44: 647–56.

Unic, I., Stalmeier, P.F.M., Verhoef, L.C.G. and Van Daal, W. (1998) Assessment of the time-tradeoff values for prophylactic mastectomy of women with a suspected genetic predisposition to breast cancer, *Medical Decision Making*, 18: 268–77.

Unson, C.G., Siccion, E., Gaztambide, J. *et al.* (2003) Nonadherence and osteoporosis treatment preferences of older women: a qualitative study, *Journal of Women's Health*, 12: 1037–43.

van den Brink, M., van den Hout, W.B., Stiggelbout, A.M. *et al.* (2004) Cost-utility analysis of preoperative radiotherapy in patients with rectal cancer undergoing total mesorectal excision: a study of the Dutch Colorectal Cancer Group, *Journal of Clinical Oncology*, 22: 244–53.

Veit, C.T., Rose, C.J. and Ware, J.E.J. (1982) Effects of physical and mental health on health-state preferences, *Medical Care*, 20: 386–401.

Verhoef, L., De Haan, A. and Van Daal, W. (1994) Risk attitude in gambles with years of life: empirical support for prospect theory, *Medical Decision Making*, 14: 194–200.

Viney, R., Lancsar, E. and Louviere, J. (2002) Discrete choice experiments to measure consumer preferences for health and healthcare, *Expert Review in Pharmacoeconomics Outcomes Research*, 2: 89–96.

Von Neumann, J. and Morgenstern, O. (1944) *Theory of Games and Economic Behavior.* Princeton, NJ: Princeton University Press.

Wakker, P. and Stiggelbout, A. (1995) Explaining distortions in utility elicitation through the rank–dependent model for risky choices, *Medical Decision Making*, 15: 180–6.

Walter, F.M. and Britten, N. (2002) Patients' understanding of risk: a qualitative study of decision-making about the menopause and hormone replacement therapy in general practice, *Family Practice*, 19: 579–86.

Weber, E., Shafir, S. and Blais, A.-R. (2004) Predicting risk sensitivity in humans and lower animals: risk as variance, or coefficient of variation, *Psychological Review*, 111: 430–45.

Welkenhuysen, M., Evers-Kiebooms, G. and d'Ydewalle, G. (2001) The language of uncertainty in genetic risk communication: framing and verbal versus numerical information, *Patient Education and Counseling*, 43: 179–87.

Whelan, T.J., Levine, M.N., Gafni, A. *et al.* (1995) Breast irradiation postlumpectomy: development and evaluation of a decision instrument, *Journal of Clinical Oncology*, 13: 847–53.

Wilson, T.D. and Gilbert, D.T. (2003) Affective forecasting, *Advances in Experimental Social Psychology*, 35: 345–411.

Wilson, T.D. and Schooler, J.W. (1991) Thinking too much: introspection can reduce the quality of preferences and decisions, *Journal of Personality and Social Psychology*, 60: 181–92.

Wroe, A.L., Turner, N. and Salkovskis, P.M. (2004) Understanding and predicting parental decisions about early childhood immunizations, *Health Psychology*, 23: 33–41.

Yaniv, I. (2004) Receiving other people's advice: influence and benefit, *Organizational Behavior and Human Decision Processes*, 93: 1–13.

Zikmund-Fisher, B.J., Fagerlin, A. and Ubel, P.A. (2004) Is 28% good or bad? Evaluability and preference reversals, *Medical Decision Making*, 24: 142–8.

17 Techniques of questionnaire design

Ann Bowling

Introduction

Questionnaires are printed or electronic documents used to collect information. They can be designed as structured or semi-structured (as opposed to the unstructured, in-depth interview formats used in qualitative research). Structured questionnaires involve the use of fixed questions, batteries of questions and/or measurement scales which are presented to respondents in the same way, with no variation in question wording, using closed questions (pre-coded response choices). It is assumed that each item means the same to each respondent. With structured, pre-coded formats, the information obtained from respondents is tailored by the questions asked and the response choices offered. Semi-structured questionnaires will also include a number of open-ended questions, to enable respondents to reply in their own words. This method enables respondents to raise other relevant issues not covered by the interview schedule. The strength of structured questionnaires is the ability to collect unambiguous and easy to count answers, leading to quantitative data for analysis. It is a relatively economical method, especially when used with large samples of people. The weakness of structured questionnaires is that pre-coded response choices may not be sufficiently comprehensive, and not all answers may be easily accommodated. Some respondents may therefore be 'forced' to choose inappropriate pre-coded answers.

Structured questionnaire design and scaling should be based on three well-established bodies of knowledge: the well-developed theories and methods of measurement from social science, which date back to the late eighteenth and early nineteenth century; the methods of scaling for the measurement of psychological attributes which were developed in the early twentieth century (e.g. Thurstone, Likert and Guttman techniques of scaling); and the scientific principles of measurement established by mathematical psychologists during the mid-twentieth century (see Crocker and Algina 1986; Nunnally and Bernstein 1994). These led to the establishment of rigorous methods of psychometric evaluation. The term *psychometric* is derived from the Greek *psyche* = mind and *metron* = measure. Psychometrics is the science of the measurement of mental functions. Psychometric theory dictates that when a concept cannot be measured directly (e.g. health status, quality of life – QoL – health-related quality of life – HRQoL), a series of questions which tap different aspects of the same concept need to be asked and then tested for their reliability (consistency) and validity (whether they measure what they purport to) –

their *psychometric properties*. The methods, as well as the techniques of, and common rules for, questionnaire design are described in this chapter.

Issues to consider

A questionnaire, any single question items and any full measurement scales contained within it, should have a clear relationship to the aims of the study. The measures used should be based on a clear conceptual model, and be reliable, valid and responsive to changes. Once testing has been completed and the scale judged to be satisfactory, the wording, items and layout should not be changed, otherwise the psychometric properties of the instrument may be affected and retesting will then be required. Preservation of the integrity of the instrument is also why interviewers using structured questionnaires must be trained to ask the questions in the same, standardized way, and not vary the wording or order.

The questions which the investigator needs to consider when designing and selecting measurement instruments are:

- What is it that the instrument measures?
- What type of population is it to be administered to? And what type of population was the measure developed for?
- How reliable and valid is the measure and how was it tested?
- Do population norms for the measure exist for comparative purposes?
- Is the measure sensitive to anticipated changes in the study population (e.g. in their health) if repeated over time?
- How acceptable is the measure to the study population? Are the questions easily completed? What is the likely rate of non-response to items? What time burden does it place on respondents, as well as on the research team?
- What level of data does the measure produce and do these fit with the required statistical analyses: nominal (numbers are used for classifications), ordinal (scale items stand in some kind of relation to each other), interval (the characteristics of an ordinal scale but the distances between any two numbers on the scale are of a known size) or ratio (the characteristics of an interval scale but the zero point is true and not arbitrary)?
- Is the measure available in alternate forms (self-completion and interviewer versions)?
- Has conceptual and linguistic equivalence been obtained in translated versions?

Translation of a research instrument into another language does not consist simply of translation and back translation before assessing its suitability for use. White and Elander (1992) have drawn attention to the most important principles of translation, which involve testing for cultural equivalence, congruent values and careful use of colloquialisms. They suggested the following practice: secure competent translators who are familiar with the topic; use two bilingual translators (one to translate and one to translate back to the original language, without having seen the original); assemble a review panel, composed of bilinguals, experts in the field of study and members from the population of interest, who should refine the translations and assess equivalence, congruence and any colloquialisms used. Apart from rigorous methods of translation and assessment for cultural equivalence, the psychometric properties of the instrument should be reassessed in each culture/country that the instrument is to be used in, including item-scale correlations, comparisons of missing responses, scale correlation with any existing gold standards or other similar instruments and analysis of the psychometric properties of the instrument in relation to sub-groups within the population of interest.

Given the complexity and expense of developing new measurement tools, most investigators prefer to use existing measures. Where additional items are required they should be included in the broader questionnaire to be administered and not embedded within an existing measurement scale, as the latter should have been carefully developed and tested for equivalence of meaning, acceptability, burden, question form, wording and order effects, reliability and validity, factor structure (dimensionality), as well as its scaling properties. Any changes to a tested instrument will necessitate it being retested.

Psychometric assessment for reliability and validity

It was pointed out earlier that psychometric theory dictates that when a concept cannot be measured directly, a scale comprising a series of questions that tap into different aspects of the concept should be developed and administered. The questions need to be derived from a larger pool of items (e.g. generated by the target population). In this process, the larger pool of items is reduced, using specific statistical methods, to form a scale of the domain of interest, and the resulting scale is tested to ensure that it measures the phenomenon of interest consistently (reliability), that it is measuring what it purports to measure (validity) and that it is responsive to relevant changes over time. The satisfaction of these conditions is most likely when the resulting instrument contains several items to measure the concept of interest in order to permit testing for internal consistency and to minimize random error.

Psychometric validation is the process by which an instrument is assessed for reliability and validity by mounting a series of defined tests on the population group for whom the instrument is intended. *Reliability* refers to the reproducibility and consistency of the instrument. It refers to the homogeneity of the instrument and the degree to which it is free from random error. There are certain parameters, such as test-retest, inter-rater reliability and internal consistency that need to be assessed before an instrument can be judged to be reliable. *Validity* is an assessment of whether an instrument measures what it aims to measure. It should have face, content, concurrent, criterion, construct (convergent and discriminant) and predictive validity. It should also be responsive to actual changes. Reliability affects validity. An unreliable scale inevitably has low validity. While small samples may be used for testing a measure for reliability, validity studies should use larger samples, and make comparisons with several other samples to assess stability. The concepts are described in detail by Streiner and Norman (2003). The types of reliability and validity are shown in Boxes 17.1 and 17.2.

In addition, measures should satisfy several other criteria: they should be responsive to change, and be precise. We also need to know how sensitive and specific measurement tools are. There is an unresolved debate about whether responsiveness is an aspect of validity (Hays and Hadhorn 1992). The concepts of *responsiveness*, *sensitivity* and *specificity* are interrelated and are defined in Box 17.3.

Factor structure

The *factor structure* of measurement tools needs to be assessed. Questions that deliberately tap different dimensions within a scale will not necessarily have high item-item or item-total reliability correlations. Therefore, given the importance placed on high internal reliability, factor analysis has traditionally been used to define a

Box 17.1   Reliability

- **Test-retest:** this is a test of the stability (reproducibility) of the measure over short periods of time in which it is not expected to change, by making repeated administrations of it. Cohen's (1968) kappa coefficient is used to test nominal data, weighted kappa for ordinal data and Pearson's correlations for interval level data. Kappa has a value of 0 if agreement is no better than chance, a negative value if worse than chance, and a value of unity (1) if there is perfect agreement. A low correlation can sometimes be difficult to interpret – it may reflect actual change rather than poor reliability of the measure. Confidence intervals should also be used to assess the size of the difference between the scores.
- **Inter-rater:** this is the extent to which the results obtained by two or more raters or interviewers agree for similar or the same populations. As above, the kappa test or Pearson's correlations, Spearman's rho and Kendall's tau may be used for the analysis. Fleiss (1981) suggested that a kappa result of less than 0.40 indicates poor agreement, 0.40–0.59 is fair agreement, 0.60–0.74 is good agreement and 0.75–1.00 is excellent agreement. An intra-class correlation coefficient (e.g. between raters, or subjects at different time periods) of, for example, 0.80 or more indicates that the scale is highly reliable.
- **Internal consistency:** this involves testing for homogeneity and is the extent to which the items (questions) relating to a particular dimension in a scale (e.g. physical ability) tap only this dimension and no other. The methods which should also be used are multiple form, split half, item-item and item-total correlations, and Cronbach's alpha (Cronbach 1951).
- **Multiple form:** the correlations for the (multiple) sub-domains of the scale, if they exist, are computed.
- **Split half:** if the instrument is divided into two parts, the correlations between the two are computed (not always possible if the items are not homogeneous and cannot be divided, or the scale's sub-domains measure different constructs).
- **Item-item and item-total:** these are the extent to which each of the items within a domain is correlated, and the extent to which each item within a domain correlates with the total score for that domain. Item-total correlations of below $r = 0.20$ are usually rejected in the development of measurement scales (Kline 1986).
- **Cronbach's alpha:** this produces an estimate of reliability based on all possible correlations between all the items within the scale. For dichotomous responses, the Kuder Richardson test can be used instead (Cronbach's alpha was derived from this). It is based on the average correlation among the items and the number of items in the instrument (values range from 0 to 1). It is an estimate of internal consistency. There is no agreement over the minimum acceptable standards for scale reliability. Some regard 0.70 as the minimally acceptable level for internal consistency reliability (Nunnally 1978), others accept > 0.50 as an indicator of good internal consistency (as well as of test-retest reliability) (Cronbach 1951; Helmstater 1964). A reliability coefficient of 0.70 implies that 70 per cent of the measured variance is reliable and 30 per cent is owing to random error. A low coefficient alpha indicates that the item(s) does not belong to the same conceptual domain.

> **Box 17.2 Validity**
>
> An instrument is assigned validity after it has been satisfactorily tested repeatedly in the populations for which it was designed. This type of validity is known as internal validity, as opposed to external validity, which refers to the generalizability of the research findings to the wider population of interest. The different forms of validity are described below; it should be noted that they are not all mutually exclusive (e.g. concurrent validity is part of criterion validity).
>
> - **Face:** this is often confused with content validity, but it is more superficial. It simply refers to investigators' subjective assessments of the presentation and relevance of the questionnaire: do the questions appear to be relevant, reasonable, unambiguous and clear?
> - **Content:** this is also a theoretical concept, but is more systematic than face validity. It refers to judgements (usually made by a panel) about the extent to which the content of the instrument appears logically to examine and comprehensively include, in a *balanced way*, the *full scope* of the characteristic or domain it is intended to measure.
> - **Criterion:** this covers correlations of the measure with another criterion measure, which is accepted as valid (referred to as the 'gold standard'). This is often not possible where there are no gold standards (e.g. of QoL), and proxy measures are used instead. Criterion validity is usually divided into two types: *concurrent* and *predictive validity*: Concurrent involves the independent corroboration that the instrument is measuring what it intends to measure (e.g. the corroboration of a physical functioning scale with observable criteria). Predictive means that the instrument should be able to predict(i) future changes in key variables in expected directions and (ii) hypothesized cross-sectional associations.
> - **Construct (convergent and discriminant):** this is the extent to which the instrument tests the hypothesis or theory it is measuring. There are two parts to construct validity: *convergent validity* requires that the scale should correlate with related variables; *discriminant validity* requires that the construct should not correlate with dissimilar variables.

small number of underlying dimensions, each of which contains items which group together in a consistent and coherent way (i.e. with sufficient consistency to each other).

Thus, factor analysis, like principal components analysis, is used in order to identify the separate factors (dimensions) that make up an instrument, and to describe how the items group together in order that they form a more manageable set of variables (factors or principal components) (e.g. a health status instrument would be made up of the dimensions of physical functioning, mental health, social role functioning and so on). These are assumed to reflect the underlying hypothetical constructs of the instrument (Streiner and Norman 2003). Orthogonal varimix rotation can then be used to choose the factors or principal components in such a way as to minimize their overlap (indicated by the amount of their shared variance) and thereby enhance interpretability of the instrument. The number of factors to extract is determined by their eigenvalues, statistical criteria of interpretability (Cattell 1966) and congruity with other studies. A factor is considered as important, and

Box 17.3 Other criteria that measures should fulfil

- **Responsiveness to change:** the instrument should be responsive to actual changes which occur in an individual or population over a period of time, particularly those of social and clinical importance. Responsiveness is a measure of the association between the change in the observed score and the change in the true value of the construct.
- **Precision:** the instrument should be capable of detecting *small changes* in an attribute.
- **Sensitivity:** this refers to the proportion of actual cases (such as people who actually have the target condition, e.g. clinical depression) who score correctly as positive cases on a measurement tool (e.g. who score as depressed on a scale purporting to measure depression); and the ability of the gradations in the scale's scores to adequately reflect actual changes.
- **Specificity:** this is a measure of the probability of correctly identifying a non-affected person with the measure, and refers to the *discriminative ability* of the measure. Thus, it refers to the proportion of people who are non-cases (e.g. do not actually suffer from clinical depression) and who are therefore correctly classified as negative with the measure (e.g. who are not actually depressed and who therefore do not score as depressed on the scale measuring depression). Again, the ability of the gradations in the scale's scores to reflect actual changes adequately is also important. When a measurement scale produces a continuous variable, the sensitivity and specificity of the scale can be altered by changing the cut-off point for detecting cases, although by raising the threshold for case detection the danger is that fewer genuine cases will be detected – and thus sensitivity is decreased. Bland (1995) has described the sample sizes required for reliable estimates of sensitivity and specificity, or positive predictive value (true positives) and negative predictive value (true negatives).
- **Sensitivity analysis:** this is a method of estimating the robustness of the conclusions of the study or its assumptions. Sensitivity analysis involves making plausible assumptions about the margins of error in the results in question and assessing whether they affect the implications of the results. The margins of error can be calculated using the confidence intervals of the results or they can be guessed.
- **Responsiveness and receiver operating characteristic (ROC) curves:** The *discriminant* ability of a scale possessing continuous data can be investigated using ROC curves. An ROC curve examines the degree of overlap of the distributions of the scale score for all cut-off points for defined groups, and the curve itself is a plot of the true positive rate against the false positive rate for each point on the scale (sensitivity plotted against one minus specificity). The degree of overlap between the defined groups is measured by calculating the area under the curve (AUC), and its associated standard error. The greater the total area under a plotted curve from all cut-off points, the greater the instrument's responsiveness. ROC curves can also be used to identify cut-off points for dichotomizing continuous scales, although it should be noted that all cut-offs are essentially arbitrary.

its items worthy of retention in the scale, if its eigenvalue (a measure of its power to explain variation between subjects) exceeds a certain value (1.5 is commonly taken).

In theory, exploratory factor analysis should be used in scale development in order to identify and discard items that are not correlated with the items of interest. Factor analysis is also used to confirm that the scale items principally load on to that factor and correlate weakly with other factors. However, it is important not to lose sight of the social and clinical significance of items. Where items are regarded as essential to the content validity of a measure, but they do not load on a cluster of interrelated variables, their retention as separate items in a questionnaire should be considered on theoretical grounds, or the instrument developed and tested further. Scale items should therefore be included in a measure according to the information they contribute.

Kessler and Mroczek (1995) showed that undue emphasis on internal consistency can also result in considerable overlap and redundancy of scale items. They suggested replacing factor analytic methods with regression techniques to identify the items that capture most of the variance of an underlying construct. For example, a measure of QoL is more valuable if it contains items that address the different components of QoL, rather than items with high internal consistency but which address just particular components of this concept. Factor analysis, then, can lead to solutions that operate against more socially and clinically important items of measurement. Coste *et al.* (1997), on the basis of a review of the literature, reported that, most commonly, factor analysis of the longer versions of measurement scales, and statistical correlations between the longer and shorter versions of a measure, are used to finalize the content of an instrument. Less often is there any apparent check on whether the information content has been retained (with the risk of reduced content validity).

An example of the development and testing of a measurement scale for patient-based outcomes in multiple sclerosis (MS) is given by Hobart *et al.* (2004). This is summarized in Box 17.4. Ideally, they would also have administered the instrument in a small-scale interview survey as well as a postal survey at Stage 2, and would have included non-MS Society members to increase the external validity of the measure (members may not be representative of all those with the condition). This would enable an interviewer to assess people's interpretations of the question wording (equivalence), their use of the response categories and whether they were comprehensive enough, and other relevant issues important to people which were not represented on the questionnaire.

Bias and error in measurement

There are many threats to the reliability and validity of a measure and its scaling, in addition to the many potential biases and errors in the conceptualization of the research idea, the design, sampling and process of the study, which can lead to systematic deviations from true population values (see Last 1988 for a description of the different types of bias). The types of bias and error which are common pitfalls in measurement are outlined next.

Acquiescence response set and response style bias refers to a person's manner of responding to questions, and is often known as 'yes-saying' to items regardless of their content. Respondents will more frequently endorse a statement than disagree with its opposite. Respondents can also get into a pattern of ticking the nearest response choice presented to them in a scale (e.g. the nearest left-hand column in the response scale which is often, for example, 'Strongly agree' – followed by 'agree, disagree, strongly disagree'), which can have the same effect as automatic

---

Box 17.4   Standard psychometric methods used to develop the Multiple Sclerosis Impact Scale

- **Stage 1 (item generation):** questionnaire items were generated from 30 patient interviews on the impact of MS on their lives, expert opinion and literature review.
- **Stage 2 (item reduction and scale generation):** the questionnaire developed in Stage 1 was administered by postal survey to 1530 randomly selected members of the MS Society. Standard item reduction techniques were used to develop a rating scale.
- **Stage 3 (psychometric evaluation):** the rating scale was evaluated for data quality, scaling assumptions, acceptability, reliability and validity in a separate postal survey of 1250 MS Society members. Responsiveness was evaluated in 55 people admitted to hospital for rehabilitation and intravenous steroid treatment of MS elapses.

The initial pool of 129 items was thus reduced to 29 questions in two domains (physical and psychological), and responses were tested for missing data, the percentage of respondents' scale scores that could successfully be generated for item test-retest reliability, item convergent and discriminant validity, distribution of responses (variability), any floor or ceiling effects and internal consistency (using Cronbach's alpha). Factor analysis was used to test the dimensions (two) and thus support the calculation of two summary scores.

'yes-saying'. The technique to overcome these problems is to prevent automatic 'yes-saying', regardless of item content, by making respondents think more about the question.

This can be done by balancing scale items with *both* negative and positive items (e.g. including both positive and negative attitude statements such as 'Choice of hospital for treatment is a patient's right' and 'Choosing a hospital for treatment is a waste of patients' time'), and by switching the response scale direction periodically in the measure itself, thereby alternating the wording of response choices so that the 'agree' or 'disagree' or the 'yes' or 'no' are not always in the same direction.

Interviewer bias. The interviewer can, subconsciously, or even consciously, bias respondents to answer in a certain way, for example, by appearing to hold certain values which can lead to a social desirability bias, or by asking leading questions. It is important to train interviewers carefully so that they retain a neutral approach, do not express their views, and conduct the interview in a standardized way, not altering the question wording or order in any way.

Observer or rater bias is due to the difference between the true situation and that recorded by the observer or rater owing to perceptual influences. This is a problem when measures are not self-completed by the target population (e.g. patients themselves) but are completed by proxies acting on their behalf. The method of using proxy raters is common in research on severe mental illness and palliative care.

Random measurement error simply means error due to chance. Measurement scales may contain a certain amount of random deviation, known as random measurement error, such as when respondents guess the answer rather than give a true 'don't know' reply, or give an unpredictably different response when interviewed on a different day or by a different interviewer. It is usually assumed that most measurement errors are in different directions and will cancel each other out in an overall scale score. It is important to use measurement scales which show a high level of reliability (repeatability), with minimal susceptibility to random error.

Reactive effects (awareness of being studied) refers to the effect of being studied upon those being studied. Their knowledge of the study may influence their behaviour (they may become more interested in the topic, pay more attention to it and become biased), or they may change their behaviour simply because someone (the investigator) is taking an interest in them. A 'guinea pig' effect occurs if, when people feel that they are being tested, they feel the need to create a good impression, or if the study stimulates interest not previously felt in the topic under investigation and the results are distorted. The term 'Hawthorne effect' derives from an early study where the people being investigated were believed to have changed in some way owing to the research process (Roethlisberger and Dickson 1939). It is often referred to as a 'reactive (Hawthorne) effect' (although it is now understood that the behaviour changes detected in this study were not due to observer error).

Recall (memory) bias relates to respondents' selective memories in recalling past events, experiences and behaviour, and *reporting bias* refers to respondents' failure to reveal the information requested (e.g. perhaps due to lack of motivation, embarrassment, feelings of threat or the sensitivity of the information).

Social desirability bias may exert a small but pervasive effect (people wish to present themselves at their best) and lead to a *response set* (the wish to give a preferred image and answer questions accordingly).

Systematic and total survey error

Finally, the various biases and errors inherent in a study are known as its *systematic error*. The errors in the study result in an estimate being more likely to be either above or below the true value, depending upon the nature of the (systematic) error in any particular case. The errors usually stem from selection bias in the sample, information bias (e.g. misclassification of subjects' responses owing to error or bias) or the presence of extraneous variables, which have not been taken into account in the study design and which intervene and confound the results. The *total survey error* equals the sum of all errors from the sampling method and data collection procedures. It should equal the difference between the sample survey estimate and the true or population value, and needs to be estimated. Estimation, however, is often difficult and generally only attempted in relation to large population surveys and censuses.

Piloting the questionnaire

Ideally, the items for inclusion in a questionnaire should have been generated at some stage from the population of interest, as well as from the relevant literature. The investigator should also hold meetings with 'experts' in the field and group discussions with members of the target group in order to ensure the validity of the coverage. The ideas and topics to be included in the questionnaire should be operationalized (developed into measures, e.g. questions, scales, and/or existing measures selected to tap them) and then the questionnaire should be more formally developed and piloted. Questions can first be tested on members of the research team or colleagues, in order to make initial assessments of comprehension, sense and so on, and then pre-piloted with a small group from the population of interest. Face-to-face piloting should continue with new sample members until the researchers are confident that the questionnaire requires no further changes. Piloting also acts as a check on potential interviewer errors (where face-to-face interviews is the method of choice). As well as analysis of the returned questionnaires, the interviewers, where used, should be consulted (in a focus group forum) about any aspects of the questionnaire that they feel need revising. Only when shared meaning, relevance, comprehension and comprehensiveness of response scales has been assessed in face-to-face interviews should questionnaires be tested in a mail or other self-administration method. The latter can be used as a check on whether certain items are missed by respondents (item non-response). Only by seeking feedback from them will the investigator know the cause of the missing responses (e.g. error due to poor questionnaire signposting of skips for items which are not relevant to certain groups) or respondents' perceptions that the items are not relevant to them, or they find them embarrassing, sensitive, threatening, or simply boring and not interesting.

If the questionnaire contains new, previously untested items, or has not been used before with the target population, then it will need to be fully tested face to face on a sample of people from the target population. Testing complete scales for reliability and validity involves a great deal of time, effort and expense; therefore, there is a strong argument in favour of using existing scales.

The covering letter

All researchers should give sample members a covering letter about the study to keep for reference, with reassurance that the organization and study are bona fide. The covering letter should be written on the organization's headed notepaper, include the name and address of the sample member and the identification (serial) number, and address the recipient by name. The letter should explain how the person's name was obtained, outline the study aims and benefits (concisely), guarantee confidentiality and be signed in blue ink (so it is not confused with a photocopy) in order to personalize it (which increases response).

Questionnaire layout

The use of electronic questionnaires is increasing. They can be viewed on laptop computers during interview studies; they can be programmed for client and/or staff self-completion within organizations (e.g. in hospital clinics); and they can be accessed via the internet. Internet and email-based questionnaires are common within organizations where people have access to computers. While internet surveys are increasing among market researchers in the USA, they are rare in Europe. This is due to the lack of complete sampling frames (lists of email addresses), low response rates and the large socioeconomic group and age biases among people with access to the internet and with email facilities (access is relatively low among people in lower socioeconomic groups and people aged over 65). Even in the USA only a small proportion of the population can be successfully contacted by electronic questionnaires outside their employment (Dillman 2000). The use of hard paper questionnaires is still common, and their most common use is within postal surveys. Whatever method is chosen, it is important that the layout and instructions on completion are clear.

Electronic questionnaires have the advantage that they can prevent the respondent moving on to the next question until previous questions have been completed, and they can prevent out of range answers being entered in error (e.g. if the electronic questionnaire instructs the respondent to enter '1' for positive and '2' for negative responses, and the respondent erroneously presses '3' instead of '2' to represent a 'no' response, the computer can bleep and display an error message). However, this method cannot prevent an error being made with in-range responses (e.g. if the responses are '1 = yes' and '2 = no', the respondent can still enter 1 for 'no' in error).

This section focuses on paper-based questionnaires, although the basic principles are applicable to all methods. If a paper questionnaire is to be used it is important that it has been printed clearly and professionally, and that it is visually easy to read and comprehend. The instructions for the respondent or interviewer should also be given clearly at the beginning – for example, whether answers are to be ticked, circled, written in or combinations. A thank-you statement should be given at the end of the questionnaire. It is also customary for the first few lines of a questionnaire to include the label 'Confidential', the respondent's unique identification number instead of their name and address (in order to preserve anonymity), the title of the study and a brief introduction. Any filter questions for items that do not apply to some respondents must be clearly labelled and all interviewers and respondents must understand which question to go to next.

Lower-case letters, rather than capitals, should be used for text (capitals can have a dazzling effect, and they can make it appear that the researcher is SHOUTING at respondents). There should be space for verbatim comments where appropriate (and all respondents can be asked to record any additional comments in a space provided). Coloured paper (e.g. yellow) may enliven a questionnaire, but the colour should not be dark (or the print will be more difficult to read), and dazzling colours should be avoided. A Cochrane Review on increasing response rates to postal questionnaires reported that the use of coloured paper increased response rates, as did the use of stamps and first-class postage, instead of franked envelopes for outward mailings, and follow-ups to non-respondents at three-week intervals with another copy of the questionnaire (i.e. and not just a reminder letter) (Edwards *et al.* 2001).

Questions must be numbered in order (1, 2 etc.), and sub-questions clearly labelled (e.g. as 1a, 1b, etc.). A question and its response categories should never be split over two pages, as this can lead to confusion. Each section of the questionnaire should form a module and be topic-based (e.g. questions should be grouped together by subject). The order of questions is important (see p. 417) and questions should not skip backwards and forwards between topics. This is more professional and less irritating for respondents. It is important to provide linking sentences when moving to new modules on the questionnaire: for example, 'The next questions ask about some personal details', 'These questions are about your health'.

Question form, order and wording

The form, order and wording of the questions can all affect the type of responses obtained from people (Schuman and Presser 1981). It is essential to be aware of this when designing questionnaires and selecting batteries of measurement scales. The skill of questionnaire design is to minimize these influences and the subsequent biases in the results.

Question form

Question form refers to the format of the question (e.g. closed with pre-coded scaled or dichotomous response choices which respondents select to represent their replies, or open-ended questions where respondents' own words are recorded), and the type of measuring instrument (e.g. single items, batteries of single items); more broadly it includes type of response scale and method of scaling.

The format of the questionnaire can affect the answer. While closed questions are simpler and quicker to administer and code than open-ended questions, the comprehensiveness of the response choices or scales selected for closed questions is important in order to prevent people's responses being forced into inappropriate categories. Closed questions, by giving respondents a range of possible answers from which to choose, can also give them clues (prompts) about the types of answers expected, which they might not have thought of themselves. If respondents are given structured, closed response choices from which to choose, then it is important to ensure that all reasonable alternative answers are included, as otherwise they will be unreported. Aided recall procedures (show cards displaying the pre-coded response choices which are handed to respondents) may be helpful if under-reporting is likely to be a problem, for example, where memories need prompting to recall past events or behaviour. Again the list of alternatives must be comprehensive to prevent under-reporting. This may not be realistic if a complex area is being investigated, and therefore open-ended questions may be more appropriate.

With questions asking about knowledge, open-ended questions are preferable to the provision of response choices in order to minimize successful guessing. (Similarly, postal questionnaires should also be avoided when asking questions about knowledge as they give respondents the opportunity to consult others, or to look up the answers.) Open-ended questions are also better than closed questions for obtaining information about the frequency of undesirable behaviour, or asking threatening questions (card sorting and responses in sealed envelopes may also be worth considering where the range of likely responses is known).

Types of structured response scales, followed by scaling, are described next.

Response scales

Researchers select response scales primarily on the basis of the ease of constructing, administering and analysing the scale. A response scale is simply the attachment of a number to response categories to collect, process and analyse responses. For example, responses could be on a continuum of 'Strongly agree = 1, Agree = 2, Neither agree nor disagree = 3, Disagree = 4, Strongly disagree = 5' against an 'attitude statement' (e.g. 'Surgery (for X condition) would improve my lifestyle'). Or respondents could be asked to tick one of a list of statements which best represents their opinion, as in the example:

> **Which _one_ of the following do you think should be the priority of health services?**
> *Better information for patients*
> *More choice of where to be treated*
> *Shorter waiting lists for treatment*
> *More comfortable waiting rooms*
> *Cleaner hospitals*
> *Shorter waits to see a doctor in clinics*

The first scale presents carefully ordered categories, while the second presents categories in no particular order. The first requires respondents to decide where they fit on a scale; the second requires respondents to compare each discrete category with the others before making a choice – a more difficult task.

The researcher needs to bear in mind the *burden of the exercise* when choosing response scales. The first example is a response scale in a *Likert format*. Likert scales have five- to seven-point ordered response categories placed against statements to which respondents indicate the extent of their agreement or disagreement ('Strongly agree' to 'Strongly disagree'). Another example of an ordered Likert format is 'None, Very mild, Mild, Moderate, Severe, Very severe' (e.g. to depict severity of pain). The responses may be numbered (e.g. None = 1 through to Very severe = 6), but this is simply a coding and the data collected remain ordinal – they have an inherent ordered sequence but the distance between different categories cannot be assumed to be the same (e.g. it cannot be assumed that that the difference in meaning between 'Strongly agree' and 'Agree' is the same as that between 'Strongly disagree' and 'Disagree').

The Likert scale response format is commonly used because it is easily understood and analysed (although constructing a full Likert attitude scale – as opposed to using the response format only – takes time). The Likert method is the most commonly used response choice format in health status and HRQoL scales, apart from dichotomous 'yes/no' formats. A scaled response format is always preferable to a dichotomous response format where there is a choice, because it will be more precise. For example, 'Are you able to walk? Yes/No?': people who have some difficulty walking but can still walk will reply 'Yes'. But if they could choose a response from a scale of difficulty (e.g. 'No, Slight, Moderate, Great difficulty, or Unable to walk at all') they could select either 'Slight', 'Moderate' or 'Great' difficulty, as appropriate. Thus the scaled response category is more sensitive and precise than a dichotomous category, and provides the investigator with more information.

Another popular method is the *visual analogue scale*, is which respondents are asked to place a mark on a line to indicate their response. The lines are usually horizontal and 10cm in length, and anchored at both ends with the extremes of the response used, either using categories (words) or numbers (see Box 17.5). Many measures of pain, symptoms and QoL use visual analogue scales, whereby the

---

Box 17.5   Visual analogue scale

Please mark the line with an **X** to indicate how you feel about your life as a whole:

So good, it could not be better _____ So bad, it could not be worse

Please place an **X** on the line to indicate your quality of life during the past week:

Lowest quality _____ Highest quality

Please mark the line with an **X** to indicate how you rate your health overall – 0 represents 'Poor health' and 10 represents 'Excellent health':

_____

Poor health 0 1 2 3 4 5 6 7 8 9 10 Excellent health

respondent makes a judgement of how much of the scale is equivalent to the intensity of their experience (e.g. severity of pain).

A variation on the simple visual analogue scale is the numeric scale in which the horizontal (or vertical) lines are bounded by numbers *and* adjectives at either end. The line may also have numerical values displayed at regular intervals along it (from 0 to 5, 0 to 10 or 0 to 100) in order to help respondents to intuitively understand the scale (this is known as a *numeric scale*). Numeric scales enable the use of more sophisticated and powerful statistics, although the achievement of a truly numeric scale on subjective topics is rare. Numerical scales should be used with caution as there is evidence that respondents are either drawn to them or see them as special in some way, and avoid them (Kubovy and Psotka 1976).

Categorical scales, using words as the descriptors as in Likert scales, show similar responsiveness as visual analogue scales. The evidence on whether respondents find categorical scales easier to understand than visual scales is contradictory, although categorical scales (e.g. in the form of five- or seven-point Likert scales) are generally preferred because of their ease of administration, analysis and interpretation (Jaeschke *et al.* 1990). As indicated earlier, a scaled response choice (e.g. 'Great difficulty' to 'No difficulty' with a task of daily living) is preferable to a dichotomous response choice (e.g. 'Yes, has difficulty/No, has no difficulty' with a task). The scaled response gives respondents more choice, it is generally more sensitive to changes (e.g. in difficulties with tasks before and after surgery), it has less ceiling or floor effects (e.g. over time, a respondent with difficulties could move from 'Some difficulty' to 'Great difficulty' in a scaled response, but can only reply 'Yes, have difficulty' in a dichotomous response), and more sophisticated statistical analyses is permitted.

A scaled response to a question (the response scale), which simply refers to the attachment of a number to a response category, is not the same as scaling, as in the development and analysis of a measurement scale (e.g. an attitude measurement scale). Scaling involves the *use of procedures* which enable the investigator to attach a numerical value to the response statements, and ultimately to the concepts being measured.

Scaling, then, is the assignation of numbers to responses (e.g. relating to attitudes, beliefs, perceptions) following a specified method and set of associated rules. Ideally the assignation would achieve an interval level of measurement. The reasons for scaling include the ability to test whether the measure of the target concept represents one or several dimensions, and for scoring, analysis and interpretation purposes, in order to be able to obtain a number that represents a person's attitude.

Levels of measurement

The statistical techniques that are permitted for use with a quantitative set of data are dependent on the *level of measurement* achieved by the instruments used in the study. The best instruments are those that yield quantitative values and make fine distinctions among respondents. Powerful statistical techniques can be used with data that have been collected using more sophisticated levels of measurement.

Following Stevens (1946, 1951), standard research procedures refer to nominal, ordinal, interval and ratio scales, defined by their numerical assignments. *Nominal* or *categorical* data do not have any underlying continuum, units or intervals with equal or ordinal (ranking) properties, and hence cannot be scaled. Instead, there are a number of discrete categories into which responses can be classified or 'coded', but as they cannot be placed in any ordering they have no numerical value or under-lying continuum (observations are simply grouped and not ranked). Examples of nominal scales are dichotomous and descriptive responses (e.g. binary yes/no; descriptors such as male, female; green, blue, red). *Ordinal* scales, in which observations are grouped and ranked, are commonly used levels of measurement. Technically, Likert scales are ordinal scales (e.g. 'Very happy, Fairly happy, Neither happy nor unhappy, Fairly unhappy, Very unhappy'). *Interval* data are achieved where observations are grouped and their ranks considered to be of equal intervals. *Guttman scales*, which are hierarchical or cumulative scales, claim to be interval scales (technically, this is questionable). Parametric statistical techniques that are applicable to interval scales are powerful. *Ratio data* are achieved where observations are grouped, and of equal intervals with a true zero point (e.g. weight). The most powerful statistical tests are applicable. The levels of measurement are summarized in Box 17.6.

Box 17.6   Levels of measurement

- **Nominal:** numbers are used for classifications such as male = 1 and female = 2.
- **Ordinal:** scale items stand in some kind of relation to each other, such as 'Very satisfied' through to 'Not very satisfied'.
- **Interval:** the characteristics of an ordinal scale but the distances between any two numbers on the scale are of a known size (e.g. temperature).
- **Ratio:** the characteristics of an interval scale but the zero point is true and not arbitrary (e.g. weight).

Scaling

Psychometric theory dictates that when a concept cannot be measured directly (e.g. attitudes or perceptions of health status, QoL), a series of questions which tap different aspects of the same concept need to be asked. An attitude is the tendency to evaluate something (psychologists call this the 'attitude object') in a particular way, usually positively or negatively. The 'attitude object' can be any aspect of life, including things (e.g. hospitals), people (e.g. doctors), behaviour (e.g. smoking cigarettes) or abstract ideas (e.g. perceived health status). This evaluative component is usually studied in relation to cognitive (beliefs), evaluative (feelings) and behavioural (action) components, which are not always consistent with each other.

Most measures of attitudes/perceptions/beliefs assess these by presenting respondents with sentences containing statements about the particular attitude being measured. As indicated earlier, the initial series of questions which have been developed to form a scale are tested and then reduced to remove redundant and inconsistent items, using specific statistical methods, to form a scale of the domain of interest. The resulting scale requires further testing to ensure that it measures the phenomenon of interest consistently (reliability), that it measures what it purports to measure (validity) and that it is responsive to relevant changes over time. The satisfaction of these conditions is most likely when the resulting instrument contains several items to measure the concept of interest in order to permit testing for internal consistency and to minimize random error.

Measurement scales involve a series of items about a specific domain that can be summed (sometimes weighted) to yield a score. If responses are averaged or summed across an appropriate set of questions, then a more valid measure than a single item question or battery of single items is obtained, because any individual item error or bias tends to be cancelled out across the items when averaged or summed. Therefore, items on the scale should measure different aspects of the same concept (i.e. they should all express a different belief about the area of interest, or a different aspect of the behaviour) so that they will not all be limited by the same types of error or question bias.

The statements for inclusion in attitude scales should assess favourable or unfavourable sentiments. Thus some items should be worded positively (e.g. 'Surgery is more likely to improve my quality of life than medication') and others negatively (e.g. 'Surgery is likely to have a bad effect on my lifestyle') (this may necessitate some reverse coding of items at the analysis stage in order for positive values/attitudes/perceptions to achieve scores at the customary high end of the scale). Similarly, forced choice questions should also be balanced and present alternative statements for respondents to choose from (e.g. 'I fear for the future of children today' and 'Children today will have a wonderful future'). It was pointed out earlier that this achieving of a balance of negative and positive 'attitude' statements in scales is standard procedure in research in order to lead people to think harder about the concept being measured and their attitudes – to minimize acquiescence bias (automatic endorsement of statements and 'yes-saying'), and a tendency to answer all the questions in a specific direction regardless of their content.

In relation to layout, the response categories should be balanced with extreme positive responses at one end of the scale and negative responses at the other end, representing the strength of the response (e.g. a rank order of 'Very satisfied' down to 'Not very satisfied') (see Box 17.7).

Box 17.7 Examples from the Life Orientation Test – R

	I agree a lot	I agree a little	I neither agree nor disagree	I disagree a little	I disagree a lot
In uncertain times, I usually expect the best	☐	☐	☐	☐	☐
If something can go wrong for me, it will	☐	☐	☐	☐	☐
I don't get upset too easily	☐	☐	☐	☐	☐
I'm always optimistic about my future	☐	☐	☐	☐	☐

Source: Scheier *et al.* (1994). Journal of Personality and Social Psychology 67: 1073.
© American Psychological Association. Reprinted with permission.

Again, it was pointed out earlier that sequences of questions asked with similar response formats are likely to produce stereotyped responses, such as a tendency to endorse the responses positioned on the far right-hand side or those on the far left-hand side of the questionnaire when they are displayed horizontally. Thus the direction of response scales should also be varied in order to minimize the likelihood of people going down the scale and ticking all the positive ('Agree') responses automatically. It is well established that respondents will more frequently endorse a statement than disagree with its opposite. This is not always straightforward to interpret. Cohen *et al.* (1996) reported that asking patients if they agreed with a negative description of their hospital experience produced a greater level of reported dissatisfaction than asking them if they agreed with a positive description. This explains why well-designed scales alternate the direction of the response codes to make people think about the question rather than automatically tick all the right-hand side response choices. Goldberg's General Health Questionnaire (GHQ) is a good example of the variation in the direction of the question wording and response categories (Goldberg and Williams 1988). There are several versions of this scale available (short to long) and the items in each version of the scale vary from positive to negative wording. The direction of the response categories also varies. The positive items have 'positive–negative' direction response choices and the negatively-worded items have reversed direction response choices for example, GHQ-30 asks 'Have you recently: Felt on the whole you were doing things well (Better than usual to Much less well); Felt that life isn't worth living (Not at all to Much more than usual)'.

The wording, format and direction of response categories used with different types of questions or scales *throughout* the questionnaire should also be varied, as the use of the same type of response scale throughout can again lead to *a response set*. The Short Form-36 questionnaire for measuring health status is a good example of this variation (see Ware *et al.* 1997). The response scales vary in type and in direction throughout, including, for example, 'Not at all/Slightly/Moderately/Quite a bit/ Extremely'; 'None/Very mild/Mild/Moderate/Severe/Very severe'; 'All of the time/Most of the time/Some of the time/A little of the time/None of the time'. Wagner *et al.* (1991) also varied response scale wording in their measure evaluating community health programmes ('Strongly agree to Strongly disagree' was changed to 'Agree strongly to Strongly disagree').

It is usual to provide between four and six response categories for each statement, and while the use of more enhances the discriminative ability of the measure, more than ten should be avoided to minimize respondent burden (leading to impaired ability to select an appropriate response). Respondents appear to be reluctant to use extreme categories or scale end-points. The effect is to moderate responses. For example, if people are asked to rate their health as 'Excellent, Very good, Good, Fair or Poor', many will avoid using the 'Excellent' and 'Poor' categories at the extremes and choose 'Very good' and 'Fair' instead.

Many investigators avoid a middle 'neutral' response category because some people (often up to 20–30 per cent) will 'sit on the fence' and choose the middle category in order to avoid making a statement on either side. Sometimes, however, the researcher will want to know genuine no opinion responses and include it (e.g. 'Neither agree nor disagree'). The placing of the neutral 'undecided' category is important. If an 'undecided' choice is placed in the middle of a scale, twice as many respondents are likely to chose it than if it is placed at the end (see Dillman 2000). There is some evidence that including a labelled middle category (e.g. 'Neither oppose nor favour') reduces positivity bias, by drawing responses from the positive end of the scale down to the middle point (see Tourangeau *et al.* 2000).

In the analysis, the responses to the statements are summed and in some cases weighted depending on whether research has established that the items have a relative importance to each other. For example, in the development phases of a health status scale, people might have rated pain as twice as important as sleeplessness in relation to their overall health; thus the researchers may wish to give pain twice the weight of sleeplessness in the scale scoring. The final score for the measurement scale should range from high to low for the same construct (e.g. the scores on a measure of perceived physical and mental functioning should be calculated separately for each of these dimensions as they are different constructs).

The most psychometrically sound measurement scales of perceived health status provide separate sub-scale scores for each dimension measured (e.g. the eight sub-domain scores of the SF-36: Ware *et al.* 1997). Some measures of health status (e.g. the Sickness Impact Profile: Bergner *et al.* 1981), sum all the dimensions together (e.g. to provide a single score for pain, physical functioning, mental functioning etc.)

in order to provide a global score. This practice leads to loss of internal consistency (because a person can score highly on the physical functioning items but low on the mental functioning items) and loss of information about the meaning of the score. Some scales also do this for the distinct purpose of providing a single score which is necessary for use in economic utility analyses (e.g. the EuroQol–EQ–5D, see EuroQol Group 1990).

Additive scores and weighting item scores

If the scale items lie on a single dimension, then it would be reasonable to suggest that they can be used to form a scale. The simplest, albeit crude, method of combining scale items is to add the item response scores to form a multi–item score. This is adequate for most purposes. For example, with knowledge questions, each correct answer can be given a value of 1 and each incorrect answer allocated 0, and the items added to form the score. With attitude scale responses, a numerical value can be attached to each class, such as 'Strongly agree = 4, Agree = 3, Disagree = 2, Strongly disagree = 1'. As indicated elsewhere, there is some debate about the appropriate value for middle scale values (e.g. 'Neither agree nor disagree' or 'Don't know' responses). If a value of 0 is assigned to these middle responses it is assumed that there is 'no opinion' or 'no knowledge', which might not be true: people often select these categories as an easy option. The problematic scoring of these responses is one reason why some investigators omit them and force respondents to make a decision one way or the other (a method which might encourage people to make a wrong decision). Many investigators allocate a middle scale value to 'No opinion' (e.g. 'Neither agree nor disagree') responses, as in Likert scales. In this case, the scale values would be: Strongly agree = 5, Agree = 4, Neither agree nor Disagree = 3, Disagree = 2, Strongly disagree = 1.

The crude addition of scores, which results in all items contributing equally to the multi–item scale score, makes the assumption that all items are of equal importance. This can be questioned in many existing scales, and it is often dubious to assume that there are equal intervals between each score, particularly if statistics appropriate for interval level data are then used. If some items are regarded as more important than others, they should be weighted accordingly (their scores are multiplied by X to enable them to count more). There is always the problem that with equal weightings it is unlikely that the domains have equal significance to different social groups and individuals within these, and if scales are weighted it is unlikely that the weightings will be equally applicable to different groups and individuals. While scoring and weighting should be tested for discriminative ability between groups of people, their validity will be at group, not individual, level. The issue of individualized measurement is increasingly topical and readers are referred to the volume by Joyce *et al.* (1999) for further discussion.

The statistical procedures that can be used to calculate appropriate weightings include factor analysis or principle components analysis, which identify the mathematical factors underlying the correlations between scale items, and can be used in the construction of appropriate sub–scales. However, there is increasing debate about the usefulness of weighting item scores, and there is evidence that complex weightings add little to the precision of the scoring (Jenkinson *et al.* 1991; Streiner and Norman 2003).

Methods of attitude scaling

The rules for scaling expressed attitudes depend on the method chosen. A scale can represent a concept on one or on several dimensions. A concept such as height can be measured along a single dimension (e.g. using numbers of inches or centimetres on a tape measure). The three major methods of unidimensional scaling are Thurstone (Thurstone and Chave 1929) (equal-appearing interval scaling), Likert (1932) (summative scaling) and Guttman (1950) (cumulative or hierarchical scaling) (see Procter 1993 for brief descriptions). A three-dimensional concept could be measured using a semantic-differential scale (Osgood *et al.* 1957). This method is based on a theory which states that objects can be rated along the dimensions of activity (e.g. active-passive), evaluation (e.g. favourable-unfavourable) and potency (e.g. powerful-powerless). For example, undergoing surgery might be rated by an individual as highly 'passive' *and* 'unfavourable', *and* as making them feel 'powerless'. With the finally developed scale, respondents are presented with pairs of diametrically opposed adjectives at either end of a (usually ten-point) scale and mark their position between the two extremes. These methods are all used in the development of scales measuring self-evaluations of health status, symptoms (e.g. pain) and HRQoL (see Bowling 2002, 2004 for fuller descriptions). Likert scales are the most popular, and are often known as rank order rating scales (e.g. 'Better-Same-Worse'; 'More-Same-Less'; 'Strongly agree-Agree-Neither agree nor disagree-Disagree-Strongly disagree'; 'Cannot do at all; Can do with great difficulty; Moderate difficulty; No difficulty'). The associated rules of scale measurement have been carefully developed by psychologists in relation to the measurement of attitudes, and these have been drawn on in the development and construction of scales measuring health beliefs and behaviours, and self-evaluations of health status and broader QoL.

The most commonly used attitude scales focus on the evaluative component (as described above), but psychologists are also interested in the cognitive component of attitudes. One technique of assessing these is 'thought listing' (Petty and Cacioppo 1981). For example, after listening to or seeing a message, people are asked to write down in a specified time all their thoughts which are relevant to it. These thoughts are then rated and categorized: for example, according to whether they agree or disagree with the issue. This leads to the development of understanding about the beliefs and knowledge underlying attitudes. Similar information can be obtained by carrying out content analyses of material or group discussions, and analyses of body reactions (language) as people listen to (and react to) the messages presented to them. Other variations of projective techniques include sentence completion exercises, uncaptioned cartoon completion and picture interpretation (see Oppenheim 1992).

Repertory grid techniques can be useful in providing information about people's individual constructs, interrelationships and changes in attitudes over time (Kelly 1955). With this technique, the investigator presents three stimuli (a triad), such as photographs, to the respondents and asks them to say which two are the most alike and in what ways, and how they differ from the third. The constructs which underlie the distinctions are dimensions of the opinion. Respondents then relate the constructs to each other to form a grid. The constructs are listed in a grid down the left-hand side. Across the top are the stimuli, to each of which the construct is to be applied. The investigator takes the respondent through the grid step by step, ticking underneath each object said to possess the construct. The value of this method is that the constructs come from the respondent – not from the investigator. If the procedure is repeated over time, then changes can be measured. This method is often used as pilot research for the development of semantic-differential scales. A modification of this method was used by Rowe *et al.* (2005) to assess patients' preferences for treatment. Angina patients were interviewed in order to elicit their personal reasons underlying preferences for various treatment options. Interviews followed a general repertory grid technique, in which seven treatment options were presented to patients in triads and patients were asked to state ways in which two were alike and different from the third. Treatments considered ranged from medication to invasive revascularization therapies, with a 'no treatment' option. Constructs were elicited which successfully distinguished between medical and surgical treatments included 'frightening', 'invasive', 'effective', 'quick', 'easy' and reversible'.

Another method of measuring attitudes and desired behaviour is by use of vignettes (which simply means illustration). Short descriptions of the topic of interest, or case histories of patients, are presented to people along with pertinent questions. For example, doctors may be presented with vignettes of patients and their presenting symptoms and asked what investigations and treatments they would request. Investigators usually structure the method by giving people a list of response choices, such as possible actions. One example of this method is the study of clinical judgements conducted by Harries *et al.* (2004) in which doctors were presented with hypothetical, electronic (computer-presented) patients with varying symptoms of cardiovascular disease and asked to make decisions about investigation and treatment. Patients' sociodemographic profiles were varied randomly across the vignettes, in order that their independent effects on clinical decision-making could be assessed.

Single-item questions

A single-item measure, by definition, is the use of a single question to measure the concept of interest. For example, the two most popular single-item, global health indicators in use are self-rated health status (see Box 17.8) and limited longstanding illness. Batteries of questions are a series of single items (rather than a specially constructed scale where responses can be summed), each relating to the same variable of interest. Each item is analysed and presented individually, not summed together.

Both multi- and single-item questionnaires have their advantages and disadvantages. Single-item measures are the simplest form of measurement and less

---

Box 17.8   Subjective health status

Over the last twelve months would you say your health has on the whole been:

Good . . . 1
Fairly good . . . 2
Not good . . . 3

(General Household Survey: Walker et al. 2001)

In general, would you describe your health as:

Excellent   ☐
Very good   ☐
Good   ☐
Fair   ☐
Poor   ☐

(Source: SF-36 Health Survey: Ware et al. 1993. Copyright © Medical Outcomes Trust. All rights reserved. Reproduced with permission of the Medical Outcomes Trust; www.qualitymetric.com)

burdensome for investigators and respondents. Their use can enhance high response and completion rates and speed data processing and analysis. On the other hand, a single item might not provide the detail which the investigator requires, and respondents might also find a single overall assessment of their situation (e.g. health or QoL) difficult: they are required to consider all aspects of the area being measured, while ignoring irrelevant features, and to differentially weigh them up to provide a single rating.

A frequently-asked question by clinical investigators is why instruments which aim to measure patients' perceptions of a phenomenon (e.g. of their health status, or HRQoL) contain multiple questions, when there is good evidence that a measure containing just a single, global question is likely to suffice. The issues are summarized by Bowling (2005), and are described below. Some researchers do not wish to use a lengthy instrument because their questionnaires are already fairly long, or the patient group of interest is severely ill or frail, and they wish to minimize the burden on the patients and on the research team. In such circumstances, single questions have the obvious advantage of brevity, of making less demands than multi-item measures on respondents, on interviewers (where used) and on data analysts.

Before the widespread use of lengthier measurement scales to tap health status and HRQoL, single-item, global questions were commonly used in population surveys. Over the past two decades a large industry worldwide has emerged to produce, bank and distribute increasing numbers of lengthy, psychometrically tested, multi-item and multi-domain measures of broader health status, QoL and HRQoL. But there is good evidence of acceptable levels of reliability and validity for single-item, global measures of these concepts, as well as of their ability to detect improvement or deterioration in specific medical conditions.

Self-rated health

At its most basic, the self-rated health item (see Box 17.8) consists of asking respondents to rate their health as 'Excellent, Good, Fair or Poor', although variations of this have been frequently used in surveys worldwide. In order to increase the question's ability to discriminate between groups, many researchers now insert a 'Very good' category in between the 'Excellent' and 'Good' response choices (given that many respondents are affected by social desirability bias and rate their health at the 'good' end of the scale spectrum). This question is also frequently used in social gerontology where the tradition is to ask respondents to rate their health in relation to their age. This prevents older respondents from assessing their health with reference to younger age groups, and inevitably rating it as sub-optimal, given research which shows that people spontaneously compare their health to reference groups (Kaplan and Baron-Epel 2003). However, in a comparison of two absolute questions, 'How do you regard your health?' and 'How would you rate your general health status?' with the comparative age question, 'How would you assess your general health status compared to that of others of the same age?', Eriksson et al. (2001) reported that people tended to overestimate their health in relation to others, and this effect *increased* with age. Thus the comparative question over-adjusts for age.

The self-rated health status single item has also been shown to be significantly and independently associated with specific health problems, use of health services, changes in functional status, mortality, age, socioeconomic status and recovery from episodes of ill health in all age groups (National Heart and Lung Institute 1976; Singer et al. 1976; Kaplan and Camacho 1983; Goldstein et al. 1984; Idler and Kasl 1995; Bierman et al. 1999; Greiner et al. 1999; Siegel et al. 2003). Investigators of the MacArthur field study of successful ageing in the USA, for example, reported that self-rated health (poor/bad ratings of health compared to excellent ratings) was a strong and significant predictor of mortality in the general sample, as well as in controlled analyses when the sample was divided into healthy and less healthy cohort samples (Schoenfeld *et al.* 1994). However, analysis of data from the Australian National Health Survey has shown that it does have some response instability when repeated in the same questionnaire (before and after other questions about health), although this might also reflect the biasing effect of question order (Crossley and Kennedy 2000).

Interpretation of the item at an individual level varies, depending on the referent being used by the respondent. Some people refer to specific health problems and others to general physical functioning when replying to the question (Meurer *et al.* 2001). Other research using anchoring vignettes (fixed descriptions of each response choice level, in order to increase consistency of respondents' interpretations of them), has found that their use provides a powerful tool for adjusting for the influence of varying expectations on self-ratings of health. This can enhance comparison of results (e.g. older and younger people with the same level of health might rank themselves differently on a health status scale due to varying expectations of health and ability by age) (Salomon *et al.* 2004).

Other single-item questions

The question, asking people if they have a 'longstanding illness, disability or infirmity', has been judged to be a valid measure for use in general health surveys, and shown to be associated with relevant health indicators, including specific health problems, serious health conditions and the single item on self-rated health (Manor *et al.* 2001). The question has, however, posed an enigma for researchers when comparing international data over time. A review of the use of the question in surveys by Bajekal *et al.* (2004) found that it produced estimates that were sensitive to factors related to the instrument (e.g. question wording and order effects), to the mode of data collection (e.g. interview or self-administered questionnaire), to the survey process (e.g. collection of data by proxy) and to the sponsorship and context of the survey. If single-item questions are to be relied upon, then attention to clear, simple and unambiguous wording at their design stage is obviously essential. For example, one of the most popular single-item measures of global well-being used by social scientists is a simple, single concept question on happiness (see Bradburn 1969; Blanchflower and Oswald 2001). This has been asked in the US General Social Survey to tap QoL since 1946: 'Taken all together, how would you say things are these days – would you say you are Very happy, Pretty happy, or Not too happy?' It shows stability over time and has fuelled intense international debate about happiness and relative deprivation across nations (Bowling 2005).

Visual analogue scales are also frequently used as single items. The visual analogue scale is commonly used in cancer, pain and QoL research as single items, batteries or scales (see Box 17.5). As pointed out earlier, the method uses lines, the length of which are taken to denote the continuum of some emotional or physical experience such as tiredness, pain, nausea or anxiety. The lines are usually horizontal and 10cm in length, with stops ('anchors') at right angles to the line at both extremes, representing the limits of the experience being measured (e.g. 'Severe pain' to 'No pain at all'). The respondent places a cross on the line to indicate their state, for example:

Severe pain ———— *X* ———— *No pain at all*

There are many references in the literature to the high levels of reliability, validity and sensitivity of this simple technique, including its ability to discriminate between healthy and sick people, its sensitivity to the stages of the disease progress and its ability to predict mortality. A QoL visual analogue scale has been reported to have good reliability, validity and responsiveness to change when used as a single item in studies of QoL and cancer, and correlated highly with longer multi-item scales of broader health status and symptoms (de Boer *et al.* 2004). For example, a QoL 'uniscale' is in widespread use, in which the respondent places a cross on a horizontal line to indicate their QoL during the past week (anchored at each end from 'Lowest quality' to 'Highest quality').

However, the majority of definitions and measures of health status, broader QoL and HRQoL have focused on their multidimensionality, and investigators prefer to use measures which contain several sub-domains and several items measuring each of the domains covered. It has been proposed by Fayers and Hand (2002) that QoL is more appropriately measured with a global single item. This is because multi-domain measures confound the dimensionality of these concepts with the multiplicity of their causal sources. Thus, in order that predictor and component variables can be separated, such concepts need to be considered as unidimensional, but with multiple causes. The unidimensional indicator is then logically the dependent variable in analyses, and the predictor variables include the range of pertinent multidimensional scale variables (e.g. social, psychological, functional ability etc).

Single items are, in any case, also useful as broad summary ratings of diverse aspects of respondents' health, QoL and HRQoL, especially where respondents might have improved on one domain (e.g. physical functioning) but not on another (e.g. mental functioning). Thus the additional use of a general, or global, summary question to capture overall attitudes or perceptions is recommended (e.g. after administering an attitude scale about patients' preferences for type of treatment, a general question should be used to directly ask them which they prefer overall). This can be used as a validity check on the scale (the two would be expected to provide high and significant correlations together), as well as providing a useful summary outcome measure. Single items are also generally accepted as useful in the assessment of health transitions (e.g. Since . . . would you say your health is 'Much better, Somewhat better, About the same, Somewhat worse, Much worse?').

Single or multi-item scales?

While single items have been shown to be sensitive to changes in condition, they may be insufficiently sensitive to detect subtle changes after treatment (e.g. if used in clinical trials) that a longer instrument could detect (Bernhard *et al.* 2001). Scales using multiple items are more stable and reliable (i.e. the items produce replies which are more consistent and less prone to distortion from sociopsychological biases) than single items, and more responsive to particular treatment effects (Fayers and Machin 2000). In particular, the use of multiple items enables random measurement error to be cancelled out, resulting in increased reliability and precision (Gardener *et al.* 1998). Responses can also be affected by other factors, including question wording, social desirability bias and interviewer bias, all of which can lead to measurement error. Social desirability bias exerts a small but pervasive influence in self-report measures. People may describe the variable (e.g. QoL) of interest in a way they think the investigator wants to hear, and people want to present themselves in the best possible way. Single items are also more difficult to test. For example, they cannot be tested for split half or multiple form reliability, but they can be tested for face and content validity and against other measures, and they can be subjected to test-retest and inter-rater reliability. Generally, where questionnaire length permits, scales are preferred to single items because their multiple items are suitable for statistical calculations using summed and weighted scores (e.g. pain might be given twice the weight of mobility in the scale score, if it is judged to be twice as important). On the other hand, there is a body of literature in psychology which demonstrates that there is little to be gained by complex weightings over simple summated scoring (see earlier).

The careful development work on health status batteries at Rand in the USA also demonstrated that a well-constructed multi-item scale (even with just five to ten items) is more sensitive to changes in patients' condition over time than any single-item measure (Manning *et al.* 1982; McHorney *et al.* 1992). In addition, multi-item measures can provide a complete profile of multidimensional phenomena, and can yield information on changes within the individual dimensions measured by the scale (e.g. physical functioning, psychological health), although at the cost of increased burden and the risk of asking irrelevant questions.

During the 1980s and 1990s, emerging patient-based health status and HRQoL measures were notable for their length, which was dictated by the rigours of the social science tradition of psychometric theory and testing. But from the mid-1990s onwards, scale developers increasingly acknowledged that the most popular measures were those which were brief and comprehensive, and that more practical measures were required, especially if they were to be administered in busy clinical settings or in the context of large trials and surveys. Hence there was a proliferation of increasingly short versions of existing measurement instruments, and more efficient summary measurement scales for use in the burgeoning health outcomes sphere. Probably the most well known example of this is the development of the Short Form-12 (i.e. 12 items) and the Short Form-8, both derived from the Short Form-36 health status questionnaire, as well as the development of summary measures of physical and mental health (see www.sf-36.org and www.rand.org). While the shorter versions of these short form scales are inevitably less sensitive than the full versions, their careful psychometric development and calibration, based on the most powerful items from the parent measures, has led to their retaining a high degree of accuracy, which has led in turn to their wide adoption in both research on clinical outcomes and population health.

Question order

Apart from the form of the questions and response type, the order and also the wording of questions can affect response and bias results. Detailed rules governing the design and ordering of questionnaires are found in texts by Sudman and Bradburn (1983) and Oppenheim (1992). One problem with self-administered questionnaires, however, is that respondents can read through them and negate the effects of deliberate ordering of questions.

Most questionnaires adopt a 'funnel' approach to question order. With this technique, the module starts with a broad question and progressively narrows down to specific issues; this process necessarily involves the use of filter questions to 'filter out' respondents to whom the specific questions do not apply and direct them or the interviewer to the next question which applies to them.

The main rules applying to the ordering of questions are: ask easy and basic (not sensitive or threatening) questions first; as answers can be influenced by previous answers, ask the most important questions first where no other rules apply; questions about behaviour should be asked before questions about attitudes (e.g. ask 'Have you ever smoked cigarettes?' before 'Do you think that smoking should be (a) permitted in restaurants or (b) banned in restaurants?'). In the case of undesirable behaviour, one technique is to ask whether the respondent has ever engaged in the behaviour before asking about current behaviour (e.g. 'Have you ever smoked cigarettes?' 'Do you smoke cigarettes now?'). This reduces under-reporting of current behaviour. Specific questions can also influence response to more general questions:

1 How satisfied are you with your health?
2 How satisfied are you with your life in general?

The above will produce different responses from:

1 How satisfied are you with your life in general?
2 How satisfied are you with your health?

Similarly, asking:

1 How is your married life?
2 How is your life in general?

will produce different responses from asking these questions in the reverse order of:

1 How is your life in general?
2 How is your married life?

In the above examples, if the question about life in general is asked second, many respondents will exclude consideration of their health (or marriage) from their overall assessment because they have already answered a question about this. Thus the investigator should minimize order effects by placing general questions before specific questions. A systematic review of best practice in surveys of health service staff and patients by McColl *et al.* (2001) confirmed that general questions should precede specific questions.

However, the investigator can only control order effects in interviewer-administered questionnaires. With self-administered instruments respondents can read through the questionnaire or battery of scales and start anywhere they choose to, even if asked not to.

There has been little research on the effects of question ordering, and the order of batteries of measurement scales, in relation to research on health. The issue is of importance because it is increasingly common for investigators to ask respondents to complete both a generic (general) health status scale and a disease-specific scale. It could be hypothesized that if a disease-specific scale or battery is asked before a general health status scale, then the ratings of general health status would be more favourable because the disease-specific health status had already been considered and therefore excluded in replies to the general ratings. Thus Keller and Ware (1996) recommended that the generic Short Form-36 Health Survey Questionnaire (SF-36) and the shorter Short Form-12 version should be presented to respondents before more specific questionnaires about health and disease, and that there is a clear break between batteries of scales (making clear to respondents that they are starting a new module on the questionnaire).

Barry *et al.* (1996) investigated the order effects of the different sequencing of disease-specific and general health status scales among men with benign prostatic hyperplasia. They reported that men's ratings of their general health status, using the SF-36 item health survey (Ware *et al.* 1993) were slightly more favourable when disease-specific modules (on benign prostatic hyperplasia) were administered first, but they were not statistically significant, and they concluded that they could find no significant evidence of order effects. Bowling *et al.* (1999) reported that the Health Survey for England in 1996 broke the rules on order effects and administered the generic SF-36 health survey questionnaire at the end of a lengthy interview about respiratory and other health problems. This might have explained some of the, albeit unexpectedly, poorer SF-36 scores obtained in that survey in comparison with other national and regional surveys using the SF-36.

Question wording

Poor question wording or design leads to inaccurate or uninterpretable responses. When designing questions, items should not be too long, and the questions should be simple, and not contain double-negatives, colloquialisms, acronyms or words which have culture-specific meanings. If complex questions are to be asked within a structured format, then they should be broken up into a series of shorter, simpler, questions which are more easily understood, even though this lengthens the questionnaire. Questions also need to be unambiguous and culturally shared. It cannot be assumed that all people share the same frame of reference and interpret words in the same way. Therefore, it is also important to use short, simple and generally familiar words, and to ensure that any translated questionnaires have been fully assessed by panels of experts and lay people for meaning and cultural equivalence. Questions should also never include two questions in one sentence ('double barrelled') as this will lead to confusion; questions should each be asked separately. Details can always be placed on show cards and handed to respondents (e.g. background information for a question, or a long list of response choices). Questions should be worded as specifically as possible. For example, do not ask 'Do you have a car?' Ask the more meaningful question: 'Is there a car/van available for private use by you or a member of your household?' And instead of asking simply for current age, ask for date of birth – age can then be calculated from date of birth on the computer and is more exact.

Specific questions in relation to the topic of interest are preferable to general questions. It is particularly important to use specific rather than general question wording when assessing satisfaction. The question 'Are you satisfied or dissatisfied with your doctor?' is inadequate, as it does not provide the respondent with a frame of reference, and it will not provide any information on the components of satisfaction or dissatisfaction. It is common for good and poor institutions (e.g. schools, hospitals, neighbourhoods) to receive similarly high satisfaction ratings in surveys. Specific questions about details are more sensitive. It is preferable to ask about the specific, such as 'Are you satisfied or dissatisfied with the personal manner of your GP?'

Question wording can also affect response in several other ways. Questions which do not reflect balance, complex questions and questions containing double negatives can all lead to biased replies. Loading questions (as when assuming behaviour) is a technique which must be carefully used and only in certain situations, such as threatening topics. It is important to avoid using leading questions and to train interviewers not to slip into them. Typical leading questions are 'Don't you agree that . . .?' or 'You haven't got difficulty with X have you?' Leading questions bias respondents' replies: they are reluctant to contradict the interviewer, who appears to know what answer they are looking for, and will agree in order to proceed quickly to the next question. The failure to specify the full range of alternative response choices clearly in the question is, in effect, a form of leading question. With attitude questions it is particularly important to present both sides of a case, as offering no alternative can increase support for the argument offered. Avoid tagging 'or not' on to the end of opinion questions – the inadequate statement of the alternative opinion can be confusing. For example, rather than simply asking 'Do you prefer to see the specialist in the hospital clinic or not?', respondents should be asked 'Do you prefer to see the specialist in the hospital clinic or in your GP's surgery, or do you have no preference?', and a matching range of response categories must be provided.

The way in which the question is framed can also influence the response. For example, providing doctors and patients with information firstly about the benefits and then the risks of a particular medical treatment produces different results on their treatment preferences to the alternative approach of providing them with the information about risks before the benefits (Edwards and Elwyn 2001).

Questions about threatening, sensitive, embarrassing topics, knowledge, behaviour

Sensitive questions (e.g. about sexual behaviour) need careful construction in order to minimize bias (see Bradburn and Sudman 1974). Some questions may lead the respondent to feel embarrassed or threatened by them. This makes the questions difficult to answer and to an under-reporting of the attitude or behaviour in question (i.e. biased response). It should be remembered that people want to present themselves in their best light (social desirability bias). If the questionnaire is administered by an interviewer it will have allowed time for good rapport to be established, and in a self-administered questionnaire if the easy and non-sensitive questions are asked first the interest of the respondent will have been engaged. Further, if sensitive questions are asked towards the end, this does not threaten the completion of the rest of the questionnaire. On the other hand, with self-completion methods, the respondent can read all the questions before completing them, and may not complete the entire questionnaire if they object to any of the questions. In the case of embarrassing questions, one technique is to prefix a personal question with an opinion question on the topic, but opinions and behaviour are not necessarily consistent. Open questions, as well as self-completed questionnaires and alternatives to question-response frames (e.g. card sorting, giving respondents sealed envelopes in which to enclose their response, diaries, sentence completion exercises) are best for eliciting sensitive, embarrassing or undesirable behaviour. While it is a common rule that sensitive, embarrassing or threatening questions obtain more honest responses in postal surveys where there is no interviewer bias and social desirability bias is minimized, there is no good evidence that respondents respond more truthfully to these questions in postal than in face-to-face interview surveys (McColl *et al.* 2001).

Questions measuring respondents' level of knowledge about a topic should only be asked where respondents are likely to possess, or have access to, the information required, and are able to give meaningful replies. No one enjoys admitting ignorance, and respondents will guess the answer rather than do so. Knowledge questions can also appear threatening to respondents if they do not know the answer. There are techniques for reducing the level of threat, such as using phrases such as 'Do you happen to know . . .?' or (offhand) 'Can you recall . . .?', and use of opinion question wording in order to disguise knowledge questions: 'Do you think . . .?' 'Don't know' categories should also be used in order to minimize guessing and to reduce feelings of threat. This reassures respondents that it is acceptable not to know the answer – no one likes feeling foolish or uninformed. With threatening questions, or questions asking about undesirable attitudes or behaviour, loading the question can be appropriate and adopting a casual approach is productive. Assume the behaviour ('everyone does it'): 'Even the calmest parents smack their children sometimes. Did your child(ren) do anything in the past seven days to make you smack them?' In relation to cigarette smoking, where under-reporting is expected, it is preferable to ask 'How many cigarettes do you smoke each day?' rather than prefixing this with the lead-in 'Do you smoke?' (similarly with alcohol intake), or start with questions about past behaviour as this makes the current (sensitive) behaviour in question easier for respondents to admit to (see Box 17.9). These are the only circumstances

> **Box 17.9 Examples of questions on smoking from the British General Household Survey (Walker *et al.* 2001)**
>
> Have you ever smoked a cigarette, a cigar, or a pipe? Yes . . . 1 No . . . 2
>
> Do you smoke cigarettes at all nowadays? Yes . . . 1 No . . . 2
>
> *If Yes (1):*
>
> About how many cigarettes A DAY do you usually smoke on weekends?
>
> About how many cigarettes A DAY do you usually smoke on weekdays?
>
> Do you usually smoke:
>
> Filter-tipped cigarettes . . . 1
>
> Or plain or untipped cigarettes . . . 2
>
> Or hand-rolled cigarettes . . . 3
>
> Which brand of cigarette do you usually smoke . . .?

in which presuming questions are permitted. Otherwise the question should be prefixed with a question to ascertain the behaviour, before asking only those who admit to it for further details (of frequency etc.). There is also the danger of encouraging a positive bias in the results with this technique.

Asking about the actual number of cigarettes smoked per day is preferable to providing pre-coded response categories such as 1–3 cigarettes, 4–6 cigarettes, 7–9 cigarettes 10–21, 21+. This is because pre-coded information is less precise and can group people together inappropriately (e.g. in the above example, people who smoke 21 cigarettes per day and those who smoke 40 or more per day may all be grouped together under '21+'). Also, many people who smoke 21–25 cigarettes per day may not wish to select the last category of 21+ (e.g. on a self-administered instrument) as that places them in the heaviest smoking category, and social desirability bias might then lead them to select a lower frequency code (e.g. 18–20). If pre-coded numerical response categories are provided, care is needed to ensure they are mutually exclusive. A common error is to list numbers more than once in response categories – for example, 'under 5, 5–10, 10–20, 20+'. Because the categories are not mutually exclusive, some people can be coded in more than one category. The responses cannot then be clearly interpreted, and the response choices are irritating to respondents.

The difficulty with asking about any type of behaviour is that the amount (e.g. number of units of alcohol) and also the frequency of the behaviour needs to be recorded, as well as how typical the time period used is of usual behaviour.

Behaviour is difficult to measure precisely as responses are subject to motivation to remember, memory and social desirability bias, as well as random error. The careful use of appropriate reference periods is important in order to optimize recall and obtain information about unbiased behaviour. Questionnaire methods can be supplemented by use of diaries, direct observation and methods of automatic recording where realistic.

Questions about time periods involving memory

Respondent recall (memory) bias is always possible in questions asking about the past. Success in recall depends on the length of the time period asked about. The most reliable information will be obtained by asking respondents about short time periods. Asking about events beyond the past 6 months should be avoided, except on topics of high saliency to respondents (e.g. death, childbirth), where memory is better. The salience, pleasantness or unpleasantness of the topics asked about, the characteristics of the respondent (e.g. their motivation to complete the question-naire as accurately as possible), and question techniques employed during inter-views can all affect recall. If the topic is salient to the respondent (e.g. childbirth, separation, divorce, terminal care) then longer time frames (such as 12 months plus) can be asked about, as they are less prone to recall bias. Recall is generally good for life events such as periods of hospitalization, surgery, experience of major illness and respondents' children's infectious illnesses (e.g. measles) and behaviours such as smoking history, even for periods of a few years. Experiments in psychology have demonstrated that most people date events that objectively occurred longer ago as too recent, and recently occurring events as too old (known as forward telescoping for the earliest dates, and backward telescoping for the more resent ones) (see Tourangeau *et al.* 2000).

More reliable information is also obtained if behaviour within an exact time period is asked about, rather than 'usual' behaviour. Health status and quality of life scales usually ask respondents to rate themselves in relation to the past week (acute conditions), or four weeks to three months (chronic conditions). Some scales have acute and chronic versions with different time frames (e.g. the SF-36; Ware *et al.* 1997). Time frames of between three and seven days are the most valid and reliable periods to use for questions about health status, although investigators will often want to find out about longer time periods (perhaps the past three months). Respondents can be helped to recall events by asking them to check any docu-ments they have, and in some prospective studies a sub-sample can be asked to keep a diary. There are also interviewer techniques to help respondents who seem to have difficulties with precise dates or periods: 'Was it more or less than three months ago?' Wide response codes can also assist here (e.g. 'In the past week/more than a week but less than two weeks ago/two weeks or more ago but less than a month ago etc.). Respondents can also be given lists of likely responses to aid their memory.

There is insufficient space within the confines of one chapter to provide more examples of the rules of asking questions; readers are referred on to Dillman (2000) for techniques of question writing and structuring.

Conclusions

The process of questionnaire and attitude scale development is time-consuming and can be expensive, but the price is ultimately worthwhile: the quality of the data is only as good as the quality of the measurement process. Planning and piloting are essential at the outset of constructing a questionnaire. It is important to keep ques-tion wording simple, meanings should be clear and biases avoided, and only one question should be asked at a time (i.e. not two questions in one). The type of measurement scale, and level of data it yields for analysis, also needs to be considered. It was explained that question form, order and wording can all affect the type of answers received. Human beings are complex to study and there are many biases to minimize. For example, respondents usually want to present themselves in a positive light, they under-report undesirable behaviour, and will more frequently endorse an attitude statement in a scale than disagree with its opposite, and more frequently endorse the right-hand side statements. In sum, while questions should contain simple and familiar words that everyone will understand, underlying their simplicity and presentation is a rigorous set of design rules and procedures for psychometric testing.

Key points

- Question wording should be simple, meanings should be clear and biases avoided, and questions should be piloted.

- Closed questions, with pre-coded response choices, are simpler and quicker to administer and code than open-ended responses, although they risk forcing people's responses into inappropriate categories unless all reasonable alternatives have been included in the response list.

- Open-ended questions are preferable when asking about knowledge, frequency of undesirable behaviour and threatening questions.

- Single-item questions are the least burdensome method of measurement and, if carefully constructed, can have good levels of reliability and validity. But they may not tap a given phenomenon as effectively as a measurement scale containing several carefully designed and tested items, and may be more prone to distortion from biases.

- Psychometric validation is the process by which a measure is assessed for reliability (its degree of reproducibility and consistency) and validity (does it measure what it purports to?). A rigorous set of design rules and procedures for the psychometric testing of measurement instruments exists, which should be followed.

- A scaled response to a question is simply the attachment of a number to a response category (response scale); scaling involves the assignation of numbers to responses following a specified method and set of associated rules. Scaling should be based on existing well-developed methods. The three main methods of unidimensional scaling are Thurstone (equal appearing interval scaling), Likert (summative scaling) and Guttman (cumulative or hierarchical scaling). A three-dimensional concept could be measured using a semantic-differential scale.

- Measures should satisfy other criteria including responsiveness to actual change and precision, and should be assessed for their factor structure.

- There are many potential biases and errors in measurement, including acquiescence bias, interviewer bias, observer bias, random measurement error, reactive effects, recall bias, reporting bias and social desirability bias. The various biases and errors inherent in a study are known as its *systematic error*. The form, order and wording of questions can affect responses; the skill of questionnaire design is to minimize these influences and the subsequent biases in the results.

- The levels of measurement are *nominal* (numbers are used as classifications), *ordinal* (items are in some kind of relation to each other), *interval* (same as ordinal but the distances between any two numbers on the scale are of a known size), and *ratio* (same as interval but the zero point is true).

- There are also rules and techniques which should be followed for asking questions about knowledge, facts, behaviour, threatening, sensitive or embarrassing topics, and questions which rely on the respondent's memory.

References

Bajekal, M., Harries, T., Breman, R. and Woodfield, K. (2004) *Review of Disability Estimates and Definitions*. London: Department of Work and Pensions, in-house report no. 128.

Barry, M.J., Walker-Corkery, E., Chang, Y. *et al.* (1996) Measurement of overall and disease-specific health status: does the order of questionnaires make a difference? *Journal of Health Services Research and Policy*, 1: 20–7.

Bergner, M., Bobbitt, R.A., Carter, W.B. *et al.* (1981) The Sickness Impact Profile: development and final revision of a health status measure, *Medical Care*, 19: 787–805.

Bernhard, J., Sullivan, M., Hürny, C. *et al.* (2001) Clinical relevance of single item quality of life indicators in cancer clinical trials, *British Journal of Cancer*, 84: 1156–65.

Bierman, B.S., Bubolz, T.A., Elliott, A. *et al.* (1999) How well does a single question about health predict the financial health of Medicare managed care plans? *Effective Clinical Practice*, 2: 56–62.

Blanchflower, D.G. and Oswald, A.J. (2001) *Well-being Over Time in Britain and the USA*. Warwick: University of Warwick, research paper no. 616, Department of Economics.

Bland, M. (1995) *An Introduction to Medical Statistics*. Oxford: Oxford University Press.

Bowling (2002) *Research Methods in Health*. Buckingham: Open University Press.

Bowling, A. (2004) *Measuring Health*, 3nd edn. Maidenhead: Open University Press.

Bowling, A. (2005) Just one question: if one question works, why ask several? *Journal of Epidemiology and Community Health 2005*, 59: 342–345.

Bowling, A., Bond, M., Jenkinson, C. and Lamping, D. (1999) Short Form-36 (SF-36) Health Survey Questionnaire: which normative data should be used? Comparisons between the norms provided by the Omnibus Survey in Britain, the Health Survey for England and the Oxford Health and Lifestyle Survey, *Journal of Public Health Medicine*, 21: 255–70.

Bradburn, N.M. (1969) *The Structure of Psychological Well-being*. Chicago: Aldine Publishing.

Bradburn, N.M. and Sudman, S. (1974) *Improving Interview Method and Questionnaire Design*. San Francisco: Jossey Bass.

Cattell, R.B. (ed.) (1966) *Handbook of multivariate experimental psychology*. Chicago: Rand McNally.

Cohen, J. (1968) Weighted Kappa: nominal scale agreement with provision for scaled disagreement or partial credit, *Psychological Bulletin*, 70: 213–20.

Cohen, G., Forbes, J. and Garraway, M. (1996) Can different patient satisfaction survey methods yield consistent results? Comparison of three surveys, *British Medical Journal*, 313: 841–4.

Coste, J., Guillemin, F., Pouchot, J. and Fermanian, J. (1997) Methodological approaches to shortening composite measurement scales, *Journal of Clinical Epidemiology*, 50: 247–52.

Crocker, L. and Algina, J. (1986) *Introduction to Classical and Modern Test Theory*. Austin, TX: Holt, Rinehart & Winston.

Cronbach, L.J. (1951) Coefficient alpha and the internal structure of tests, *Psychometrika*, 22: 293–6.

Crossley, T.F. and Kennedy, S. (2000) *The Stability of Self-assessed Health Status: Social and Economic Dimensions of an Aging Population*, SEDAP research paper no. 26. Canberra: SEDAP, Australian National University.

de Boer, A.G.E.M., van Lanschot, J.J.B., Stalmeier, P.F.M. *et al.* (2004) Is a single item visual analogue scale as valid, reliable and responsive as multi-item scales in measuring quality of life?, *Quality of Life Research*, 13: 311–20.

Dillman, D.A. (2000) *Mail and Internet surveys: The Tailored Design Method*. New York: Wiley.

Edwards, A. and Elwyn, G. (2001) Understanding risk and lessons for clinical risk communication about treatment preferences, *Quality in Health Care*, 10 (suppl. I): i9–13.

Edwards, P., Roberts, I., Clarke, M. *et al.* (2001) *Methods to Influence Response to Postal Questionnaires* (Cochrane Methodology Group), The Cochrane Library, Issue 1. Chichester: Wiley.

Eriksson, I., Undén, A.L. and Elofsson, S. (2001) Self-rated health: comparisons between three different measures. Results from a population study, *International Journal of Epidemiology*, 30: 326–33.

EuroQol Group (1990) EuroQol – a new facility for the measurement of health-related quality of life, *Health Policy*, 16: 199–208.

Fayers, P.M. and Hand, D.J. (2002) Causal variables, indicator variables and measurement scales: an example from quality of life, *Journal of the Royal Statistical Society*, 165: 1–21.

Fayers, P.M. and Machin, D. (2000) *Quality of Life: Assessment, Analysis and Interpretation.* Chichester: Wiley.

Fleiss, J.L. (1981) The measurement of inter-rater agreement, in J.L. Fleiss (ed.) *Statistical Methods for Rates and Proportions.* New York: Wiley.

Gardener, D.G., Cumming, L.L., Durham, R.B. and Pierce, J.L. (1998) Single-item versus multiple-item measurement scales: an empirical comparison, *Education, Psychology, Measurement*, 58: 898–915.

Goldberg, D.P. and Williams, P. (1988) *A User's Guide to the General Health Questionnaire.* Windsor: Nfer-Nelson.

Goldstein, M.S., Siegel, J.M. and Boyer, R. (1984) Predicting changes in perceived health status, *American Journal of Public Health*, 74: 611–15.

Greiner, P.A., Snowdon, D.A. and Greiner, L.H. (1999) Self-rated function, self-rated health, and postmortem evidence of brain infarcts: findings from the Nun study, *Journal of Gerontology (B)*, 54: S219–22.

Guttman, L. (1950) The basis for scalogram analysis, in S.A. Stouffer (ed.) *Measurement and Prediction.* Princeton, NJ: Princeton University Press.

Harries, C., Bowling, A., Forrest, D. and Harvey, N. (2004) *How does a patient's age affect clinical decision making?* Unpublished report. London: Department of Psychology, University College London.

Hays, R.D. and Hadhorn, D. (1992) Responsiveness to change: an aspect of validity, not a separate dimension, *Quality of Life Research*, 1: 73–5.

Helmstater, G.C. (1964) *Principles of Psychological Measurement.* New York: Appleton-Century-Crofts.

Hobart, J.C., Riazi, A., Lamping, D.L. *et al.* (2004) Improving the evaluation of therapeutic interventions in multiple sclerosis: development of a patient-based measure of outcome, *Health Technology Assessment*, 8(9).

Idler, E.I. and Kasl, S.V. (1995) Self-ratings of health: do they also predict change in functional ability?, *Journal of Gerontology (B)*, 50: S344–53.

Jaeschke, R., Singer, J. and Guyatt, G. H. (1990) A comparison of seven-point and visual analogue scales: data from a randomised trial, *Controlled Clinical Trials*, 11: 43–51.

Jenkinson, C., Ziebland, S., Fitzpatrick, R. *et al.* (1991) Sensitivity to change of weighted and unweighted versions of two health status measures, *International Journal of Health Sciences*, 2: 189–94.

Joyce, C.R.B., O'Boyle, C.A. and McGee, H. (1999) *Individual Quality of Life: Approaches to Conceptualisation and Assessment.* The Netherlands: Harwood Academic Publishers.

Kaplan, G. and Baron-Epel, O. (2003) What lies behind the subjective evaluation of health status? *Social Science and Medicine*, 56: 1669–76.

Kaplan, G.A. and Camacho, T. (1983) Perceived health and mortality: a nine-year follow-up of the Human Population Laboratory Cohort, *American Journal of Epidemiology*, 117: 292–8.

Keller, S.D. and Ware, J.E. (1996) Questions and answers about SF-36 and SF-12, *Medical Outcomes Trust Bulletin*, 4: 3.

Kelly, G. (1955) *The Psychology of Personal Constructs.* New York: Norton.

Kessler, R. and Mroczek, D. (1995) Measuring the effects of medical interventions, *Medical Care*, 33: AS109–19.

Kline, P. (1986) *A Handbook of Test Construction*, London: Methuen.

Kubovy, M. and Psotka, J. (1976) The predominance of seven and the apparent spontaneity of numerical choices, *Journal of Experimental Psychology, Human Perception and Performance*, 2: 291–4.

Last, J.M. (1988) *A Dictionary of Epidemilogy.* Oxford: Oxford University Press.

Likert, R. (1952) *A Technique of Measurement for Attitudes.* New York: Columbia University Press.

Manning, W.G., Newhouse, J.P. and Ware, J.E. (1982) The status of health in demand estimation: beyond excellent, good, fair and poor, in V.R. Fuchs (ed.) *Economic Aspects of Health*.
Chicago, IL: University of Chicago Press.

Manor, O., Matthews, S. and Power, C. (2001) Self-rated health and limiting longstanding
illness: inter-relationships with morbidity in early adulthood, *International Journal of
Epidemiology*, 30: 600–7.

McColl, E., Jacoby, A., Thomas, L. *et al.* (2001) Design and use of questionnaires: a review of
best practice applicable to surveys of health service staff and patients, *Health Technology
Assessment*, 5: 31.

McHorney, C.A., Ware, J.E., Rogers, W. *et al.* (1992) The validity and relative precision of
MOS short- and long-form health status scales and Dartmouth COOP charts: results from
the Medical Outcomes Study, *Medical Care*, 30: MS253–65.

Meurer, L.N, Layde P.M. and Guse, C.E. (2001) Self-rated health status: a new vital sign for
primary care? *Wisconsin Medical Journal*, 100: 35–9.

National Heart and Lung Institute (1976) Report of a task group on cardiac rehabilitation, in
Proceedings of the Heart and Lung Institute Working Conference on Health Behaviour. Bethesda,
MD: US Department of Health, Education and Welfare.

Nunnally, J. (1978) *Psychometric Theory*, 2nd edn. New York: McGraw-Hill.

Nunnally, J. and Bernstein, I. (1994) *Psychometric Theory*, 3rd edn. New York: McGraw-Hill.

Oppenheim, A.N. (1992) *Questionnaire Design, Interviewing and Attitude Measurement*, 2nd edn.
London: Pinter Publishers.

Osgood, C.E., Suci, C.J. and Tannanbaum, P.H. (1957) *The Measurement of Meaning*. Urbana,
IL: University of Illinois Press.

Petty, R.E. and Cacioppo, J.T. (1981) *Attitudes and Persuasion: Classic and Contemporary
Approaches*. Dubuque, IA: W.C. Brown.

Roethlisberger, F.J. and Dickson, W.J. (1939) *Management and the Worker*. Cambridge, MA:
Harvard University Press.

Rowe, G., Lambert, N., Bowling, A. *et al.* (2005) Ascertaining patients' preferences for treatment for angina using a modified repertory grid method, *Social Science and Medicine*,
60: 2585–95.

Salomon, J.A., Tandon, A. and Murray, C.J.L. (2004). Comparability of self-rated health:
cross-sectional multi-country survey using anchoring vignettes, *British Medical Journal*, 328:
258.

Scheier, M.F., Carver, C.S. and Bridges, M.W. (1994) Distinguishing optimism from
neuroticism (and trait anxiety, self-mastery, and self-esteem): a reevaluation of the Life
Orientation Test, *Journal of Personality and Social Psychology*, 67: 1063–1078.

Schoenfeld, D.E., Malmrose L.C., Blazer, D.G. *et al.* (1994) Self-rated health and mortality in
the high-functioning elderly – a closer look at healthy individuals: Macarthur field study
of successful ageing, *Journal of Gerontology*, 49: M109–15.

Schuman, H. and Presser, S. (1981) *Questions and Answers in Attitude Surveys*. New York:
Academic Press.

Siegel, M., Bradley, E.H. and Kasl, S.V. (2003) Self-rated life expectancy as a predictor of
mortality: evidence from the HRS and AHEAD surveys, *Gerontology*, 49: 265–71.

Singer, E., Garfinkel, R., Cohen, S.M. *et al.* (1976) Mortality and mental health: evidence
from the midtown Manhattan re-study, *Social Science and Medicine*, 10: 517–21.

Stevens, S.S. (1946) On the theory of scales of measurement, *Science*, 103: 677–80.

Stevens, S.S. (1951) Mathematics, measurement and psychophysics, in S.S. Stevens (ed.)
Handbook of Experimental Psychology. New York: Wiley.

Streiner, D. L. and Norman, G. R. (2003) *Health Measurement Scales: A Practical Guide to their
Development and Use*, 3rd edn. Oxford: Oxford University Press.

Sudman, S. and Bradburn, N.M. (1983) *Asking Questions*. New York: Jossey Bass.

Thurstone, L.L. and Chave, E.J. (1929) *The Measurement of Attitudes*. Chicago: University of
Chicago Press.

Tourangeau, R., Rips, L.J. and Rasinski, K. (2000) *The Psychology of Survey Response*.
Cambridge: Cambridge University Press.

Wagner, E.H., Koepsell, T.D., Anderman, C. *et al.* (1991) The evaluation of the Henry J.
Kaiser family foundation community health promotion grant program: design, *Journal of
Clinical Epidemiology*, 44: 685–99.

Walker, A., Maher, J., Voulthard, M. *et al.* (2001) *Living in Britain: Results from the 2000 General Household Survey*. London: The Stationery Office.

Ware, J.E., Snow, K.K., Kosinski, M. and Gandek, B. (1993) *SF-36 Health Survey: Manual and Interpretation Guide*. Boston, MA: The Health Institute, New England Medical Center.

Ware, J.E., Snow, K.K., Kosinski, M. and Gandek, B. (1997). *SF-36 Health Survey: Manual and Interpretation Guide*, 2nd revised edn. Boston, MA: The Health Institute, New England Medical Center.

White, M. and Elander, G. (1992) Translation of an instrument: the US–Nordic Family Dynamics Nursing Research Project, *Scandinavian Journal of Caring Science*, 6: 161–4.

Measuring health outcomes from the patient's perspective

Ann Bowling

Introduction

There are many definitions of health outcomes. Dictionary definitions of outcome relate to a 'result', 'consequence', 'visible effect' or 'something that follows an action'. In the context of health services, outcomes relate to the effect of service interventions on individuals' previous health status, in relation to the aims of the intervention. But in the broader context of health and illness (regardless of whether services are received), 'outcome' can simply be defined in relation to the individual's goals and priorities. An improvement in health, for example, may not be attributable to services. Whether health outcomes of disease are investigated independently of services, or health outcomes of service interventions are the research issue, the patient's subjective perception of the outcome is of importance.

Purchasers of health care across the world are required to allocate care resources on the basis of the evidence of their effectiveness, and in terms of their health gain in the broadest sense. Measures of the outcome, or consequences, of disease, its treatment or care, which are based on patients' own perspectives ('patient-based') can be used to supplement the medical model of disease with a social model of health and ability. Their use helps to answer the question of whether the treatment leads to a life worth living in social and psychological, as well as physical, terms, by providing a more patient-led baseline against which the effects of the intervention can be evaluated. It is the patient's perceptions of their health, level of functioning and the impact of their health on their lives which are largely responsible for their decisions on whether to seek health or social care, their acceptance of an intervention and whether they consider their needs to have been met. What matters is how the patient feels, rather than how others *think* they feel.

Where a new treatment results in limited gains in survival or cure, it could be deemed preferable to existing treatments if the patient's perceptions of their broader health status and quality of life were improved by using it. Similarly, any gain in therapeutic efficiency needs to be weighed against decreases in these. The increasing emphasis on the patient's perspective during the past three decades has represented a paradigm shift in the approach to the operationalization and measurement of health outcomes (O'Boyle 1997). However, the concepts of broader health status and quality of life (QoL) are not new to clinicians. Many related measures were developed over half a century ago, although they were often crude and limited to single dimensions, such as physical functioning (e.g. Karnofsky *et al.* 1948).

The philosophy of social scientists working in health and social care settings is to listen to what people have to say, and to work within their value systems. They have made a large contribution to knowledge about people's experiences and perceptions, using both qualitative research which provides insight into patients' experiences and perspectives, and quantitative research which has led to the development of a range of measurement scales for patients to complete. These scales are administered in health surveys, and in clinical trials before and after a clinical intervention, alongside clinical indicators, in order to assess the intervention's benefit from the patient's perspective. While there has been an exponential increase in the use of indicators of broader health status and health-related quality of life (HRQoL) over the past two decades, there has been relatively little standardization of measurement instruments (Garrett *et al.* 2002). But most measures of health status, broader health status and HRQoL still take health and life quality as a starting point and measure deviations away from it (deteriorating health and quality of life), rather than also encompassing gradations of healthiness and good QoL. A perspective which captures the positive end of the spectrum is still required in order to create a balance.

In social care, in contrast, the measurement of the effectiveness of services was relatively limited for many years. Attention was on performance and activity indicators (inputs and processes of care), rather than the outcomes for service users. There was also increasing concern that, for example, the number of hours of home care allocated to clients did not indicate how effectively their needs had been met (Nocon and Qureshi 1996). Changes in community care arrangements in the UK during the 1990s led to an increasing emphasis on service monitoring, setting service objectives, measuring people's needs and met needs, and to the broadening of indicators of outcomes to include client's concerns, rather than just, for example, measuring their physical functioning.

Definitions

A patient-based assessment measure, then, is an instrument which aims to measure patients' (or clients') perceptions of their condition, and/or its effects on their lives, and changes in this/these following an intervention (see Bowling 2001; Garratt *et al.* 2002). Measures can relate to the patient's general health status, dimensions of this, generic HRQoL, or disease specific quality of life (DSQoL) (see Box 18.1). Their essential feature is that they are subjective, tapping perceptions. These types of measure are also referred to as 'self-reported' or 'patient-reported' outcome measures (see Fitzpatrick *et al.* 1998). Investigators increasingly aim to tap HRQoL, either generically or in relation to a specific disease, and not just health status.

While the concepts of health status, HRQoL and QoL are often used interchangeably, investigators do not always define their terms. Many state that they aim

---

Box 18.1   Types of patient-based outcome measure

- Generic, or broader, health status (e.g. physical, psychological and social functioning and well-being).
- Single dimensions of health status (e.g. physical functioning).
- HRQoL (the impact of health/and treatment on a patient's life).
- DSQoL (the impact of a specific condition/and its treatment on a patient's life).

to measure QoL, but then misguidedly select a measure of broader health status to tap it, or they implicitly define their terms in relation to the content of the measurement instrument they have selected to apply. This has led to a great deal of conceptual confusion.

What is health and HRQoL?

In health care, where clinical interventions are usually more specific and invasive than in social care, outcome assessment has a long tradition. Thus most existing clinical indicators reflect a traditional 'disease' model. The 'disease' model of health is a medical conception of a state of pathological abnormality which is indicated by signs and symptoms. Health, then, has traditionally been viewed negatively, in terms of 'dis'abilities, and measured accordingly (e.g. with activities of daily living and physical and role functioning scales).

But a person's 'ill health' is indicated by feelings of pain and discomfort or perceptions of change in usual functioning and feeling. Illnesses can be the result of pathological abnormality, but not necessarily so. A person can feel ill without medical science being able to detect disease. The World Health Organization (WHO) (1948) therefore developed a multidimensional definition of health as a 'state of complete physical, mental and social well-being and not merely the absence of disease or infirmity'. WHO (1984) has since added 'autonomy' to this list. Functional theory in sociology regards health more broadly, and in the context of society, as the level of fitness and functioning (social, psychological or physical) which a person requires in order to fulfil expected social roles, based on his or her cultural norms. The social sciences not only focus on people's role functioning and social norms, but other perspectives emphasize people's definitions of health and illness (see Bowling 2002 for overview) and individuals' subjective perceptions of their health (Hunt 1988).

Like health, HRQoL has also been implicitly defined from a sociological functionalist perspective of society which relates to a person's ability to perform activities of daily living and fulfil role obligations (necessary for the functioning of society as a whole). For example, Kaplan (1988) defined it in terms of the impact of disease and treatment on disability and daily functioning. But this overlaps closely with definitions of broader health status; HRQoL is more than this.

In recogniton of the need to define HRQoL more broadly, Bullinger et al. (1993) defined it as the ability to lead a fulfilling life. Others have defined it in terms of social expectations and the gap between desired achievements and actual achievements (Calman 1984). The theoretical framework for HRQoL is increasingly based on a multidimensional perspective of health, derived from the WHO's (1948) multidimensional definition. Greer et al. (1986), for example, defined HRQoL in terms of people's social, emotional and physical well-being. But, again, this definition does not distinguish it sufficiently from health status. HRQoL is a broader concept than this and includes the *perceived effects* of health, disease and treatment on a *wider* range of areas of life, and not simply about states and feelings of healthiness or wellness, or functional ability to perform daily tasks and social roles (which come within definitions of broader health status). It should also be noted that HRQoL is also just one part of QoL, as the latter includes an even broader range of dimensions of relevance to the individual (e.g. outlook on life, social participation and inclusion, neighbourhood social capital, independence and autonomy and financial circumstances) (Bowling et al. 2003; Bowling and Gabriel 2004).

Like health, HRQoL (and broader QoL) should be viewed as a double-sided concept, incorporating positive as well as negative aspects of well-being and life. It is multidimensional, incorporating social, psychological and physical health, and it is also, ultimately, a personal and a dynamic concept, because perspectives change with the onset of major illness. More broadly, HRQoL also needs to be divided into *subjective* and *objective* areas, and should encompass ability and access to society's resources and opportunities as well as well-being. Social psychologists have contributed most to the concept of HRQoL, and broader QoL, in terms of subjective well-being (see Patrick and Erickson 1993).

While HRQoL is often conceptualized crudely to facilitate its operationalization and measurement, the concept, like health and like broader QoL itself, is an abstraction with different meanings to different people. Phenomenological models hold that, unlike matter, humans have a consciousness. They interpret and experience the world in terms of meanings and actively construct an individual social reality. These models in social science focus on the individual's unique perceptions of their circumstances (O'Boyle 1997). In recognition of the importance of the individual's perspective, the WHO Quality of Life Group (WHOQOL) defined QoL in the context of health broadly as the individual's perception of their position in life in the context of the culture and value systems in which they live, and in relation to their goals (WHOQOL Group 1993). Measures of HRQoL should therefore aim to tap a person's *perceptions* of how their mental or physical health status impacts on the different areas of their life.

In sum, there are multiple influences upon patient outcome, and these require broad models of health and HRQoL to incorporate them. Of course, no definition or study can realistically aim to encompass all of these relevant dimensions and factors. The important issue is for the investigator to be clear about the definition of health status or QoL they have decided to use and to select a measuring instrument which clearly operationalizes the chosen definition.

Indicator and predictor variables

There is often an inadequate distinction between variables which are simply indicators of the phenomenon of interest and those which influence or predict it (i.e. causal variables) (Fayers and Hand 2002). Therefore, investigators need to be clear about which of their selected variables, and associated measures, make up health and/or HRQoL, and which actually influence these concepts.

QoL is a good example here with its complex collection of potentially interacting objective and subjective dimensions. Most investigators focus on its multidimensionality. Beckie and Hayduk (1997) argued, however, that multidimensional definitions of QoL confound the dimensionality of the concept with the multiplicity of its causal sources. They argued that QoL could be considered as a unidimensional concept with multiple causes. Thus it is logical for a unidimensional indicator of QoL (e.g. a self-rating global QoL uniscale) to be the dependent variable in analyses. The predictor variables include the range of health, social and psychological factors. The predictor variables in a model of self-evaluated global QoL would, by necessity, have to include a wide range of life domains to mirror how those evaluations were made. In addition, these factors may interact, adding to the complexity of the evaluation. Beckie and Hayduk argued that if the QoL evaluation is greater than the sum of its parts, then this can be problematic for causal analyses, but that the diversity, multiplicity and complexity of sources of the concept warrants treating its measurement in terms of a global assessment.

Similarly, Zissi *et al.* (1998) argued that there is a need for a model of QoL which focuses on the potential link between psychological factors (e.g. self-esteem or self-worth, self-efficacy, perceived control and self-mastery, and autonomy) and subjective evaluations of QoL. Their theoretical model, which was supported by their data on people with mental health problems, focused on how subjectively perceived QoL is *mediated* by several interrelated variables, including self-related constructs and how these perceptions are *influenced* by cognitive mechanisms. Zissi *et al.* pointed to the confusion surrounding the many psychological concepts commonly used to denote QoL, with their potential roles as influences, constituents or mediators of perceived life quality. They argued, then, that perceived QoL is likely to be *mediated* by interrelated, self-related constructs (e.g. self-mastery and self-efficacy, morale and self-esteem, perceived control over life), and these are likely to be influenced by cognitive mechanisms (e.g. expectations of life, social values, beliefs, aspirations and social comparison standards). Although the model is attractive, there is still little empirical data to support or refute the distinction between psychological constructs as *mediating* or *influencing* variables in determining the QoL. These dilemmas are reported here in order to raise awareness of the complexity of investigating multidimensional concepts, and the need for caution in interpretation.

Response shift

Making an overall judgement about the quality of one's life requires the complex assessment of one's experiences and priorities. These priorities can also change over time, perhaps influenced by experience in life, and by changing values in response to life and health events. Measurement scales need to be sensitive to this issue.

Relevant cognitive or affective processes in individuals when faced with changing circumstances include making comparisons of one's situation with others who are better or worse off (e.g. making oneself feel more positive by downward social comparisons, such as 'My health is poor but I'm not as ill as Mrs X'); cognitive dissonance reduction (defensive preference for the circumstances experienced); reordering of goals and values; and response shift. Response shift refers to the process whereby internal standards and values are changed – and hence the perception of one's health status or (health related) QoL may change (Sprangers and Schwartz 1999). Consciously or unconsciously, people may adjust to deteriorating circumstances because they want to feel as good as possible about themselves. The roots of this process are in psychological control theory, with goals of homeostasis.

Albrecht and Devlieger (1999), for example, focused on the issue of why so many people with serious and persistent disabilities report their QoL to be good or excellent, when their lives would be viewed as undesirable by external observers. Their in-depth interviews with people indicated that consideration of QoL is dependent upon not just a single dimension, but on finding a balance between body, mind and self (spirit), and on establishing and maintaining harmonious relationships, supporting the theory of homeostasis.

Investigators need to be aware of these problems and, if possible, test for them. Some investigators of QoL use 'then test' techniques to test for changes in internal standards. With this method, respondents are asked about their perceptions of their situation at baseline (Tn), and then again at follow-up (Tn + 1), along with retrospective questions at follow-up about how they perceive themselves to have been at baseline (then test for Tn). Analysis and comparison of the scores indicates the response shift and the change in QoL (Sprangers *et al.* 1999; Joore *et al.* 2002). However, the reliability and validity of this method has yet to be fully tested.

Choosing a patient-based measure

It is important that the measure selected (e.g. of HRQoL) should include topics relevant to the research question and questions which are considered to be important by the target population themselves (e.g. patients). Thus it should include, but not be totally based on, the existing theoretical and empirical literature or 'expert' views. For example, Hunt and McKenna (1992) developed their Quality of Life in Depression Scale from qualitative interviews with 30 patients who had, or who had recently recovered from, depression, as opposed to 'expert opinion'. When choosing a patient-based measurement scale, the investigator also needs to ensure that it is relevant to the target population, appropriate for the research question and satisfies the principles of measurement (see Box 18.2).

Box 18.2   Features of a measurement scale

Measures should:

- be based on a theoretical model;
- incorporate the perceptions of the target population (i.e. items generated from interviews);
- be directly relevant to, and appropriate for, the research population;
- contain items related to the target population's identified needs and outcomes;
- be reliable, valid, precise and responsive to changes associated with treatment;
- have scale scores which are interpretable (i.e. associated with severity of condition with a guide to cut-off points/ranges);
- minimize respondent and interviewer burden and be acceptable to respondents;
- have alternative forms available (interviewer and self-administration versions);
- have made cultural and language adaptations, in accordance with good practice on obtaining cultural equivalence.

The investigator has to decide whether to use a measure of health status, a broader measure of HRQoL or a measure of DSQoL (see Box 18.1). The choice depends on the aims of the study, the relevant variables identified for assessment and the type of population or intervention studied. There is little point in including a broad generic health status or HRQoL measure if it is unlikely to detect the specific effects of treatment. Specific disease-related QoL scales do exist. Generic measures of broader health status such as the Short Form-36 (SF-36) (Ware *et al.* 1997) are successful at distinguishing between patient types and predicting outcome of treatment, although they will be less specific and sensitive than condition-specific QoL measures. On the other hand, the case for using general, rather than specific, indicators of health status in population surveys has been clearly argued by Kaplan (1988). For example, detailed information about specific disease categories may appear overwhelming to many respondents not suffering from them. Also, the use of disease-specific measures precludes the possibility of comparing the outcomes of services that are directed at different groups suffering from different diseases.

It is not possible within the space of a single chapter to review available measures of health status, HRQoL and DSQoL. Several reviews of these have been published elsewhere (e.g. McDowell and Newell 1996; Spilker 1996; Bowling 2001, 2004;

Haywood *et al.* 2004). Therefore, the following sections, based on the reviews in Bowling (2004) describe just two of the most well-known and best tested measures of broader health status (SF-36) and QoL for use with general and patient populations (World Health Organisation QoL questionnaire: WHOQOL).

The SF-36

The SF-36 was developed at the Rand Corporation in the USA for use in the Health Insurance Study Experiment/Medical Outcomes Study (HIS/MOS) (Stewart and Ware 1992; Ware *et al.* 1993, 1997). It is a concise 36-item health status questionnaire, and its use across the world has escalated since 1990. The authors of the SF-36 aimed to develop a short, generic measure of subjective health status that was psychometrically sound, and that could be applied in a wide range of settings. It was constructed with the aim of satisfying the minimum psychometric standards necessary for making comparisons between groups. It is underpinned by a clearly defined measurement model (Ware 2004). The eight dimensions it includes were selected from the 40 dimensions included in the MOS, and were selected to represent the most frequently measured concepts in health surveys (and those most affected by disease and treatment), and the most psychometrically sound.

Rand distribute, free of charge, the original SF-36, and it is called the Rand 36-item Health Survey. They also distribute a 12-item version. Similar forms of the full instrument, as well as 12- and 8-item versions, are also distributed by the Medical Outcomes (Study) Trust (MOT) of the Health Institute at the New England Medical Center in Boston, where one of the instrument's original developers, John Ware, is based. This full version is known as the SF-36 Health Survey (Ware *et al.* 1993; Ware 2004), and is copyrighted. Users are requested to complete and submit an online licence application to QualityMetric Incorporated (license@qualitymetric.com). A manual is obtainable from the QualityMetric website. A variable fee is now payable for the use of the MOT instrument (US, UK and other versions) (except in cases of unfunded academic research).

The SF-36, and its short forms the SF-12 and SF-8, can be self-, interviewer, telephone or computer administered. The SF-36 takes about five minutes to complete, and population norms for it in many countries have been published (see Ware *et al.* 1993, 1997), including the UK (see Jenkinson *et al.* 1993, 1996, 1999).

In 1996, Version 2.0 of the SF-36 was developed by Ware *et al.* (Ware *et al.* 2000, 2003; Ware 2004), which corrected deficiencies in the first version. In brief, the second version improved the instructions, shortened and simplified some questionnaire items, improved the layout of the self-administered form, increased the comparability of translated and culturally adapted instruments, and improved the response formats.

An early Anglicized version was developed, and a second Anglicized version, compatible with the US Version 2.0, was subsequently developed by Jenkinson *et al.* (1999). The changes in the second version have increased the instrument's reliability, raised the ceiling and lower the floor ends of the scale, and improved its precision (Jenkinson *et al.* 1996, 1999). A manual for the UK version can be purchased (Jenkinson *et al.* 1996).

Content

The SF-36 contains 36 items which measure eight dimensions (sub-scales): physical functioning (10 items), social functioning (2), role limitations due to physical problems (4), role limitations due to emotional problems (3), mental health (5), energy/vitality (4), pain (2) and general health perception (5). There is also a single item about perceptions of health changes over the past 12 months (in effect, providing a ninth domain). It claims to measure positive as well as negative health. Two versions are available with varying time-recall referents (assessments of health over the past four weeks or one week). Examples are shown in Box 18.3.

Box 18.3   Examples from the SF-36

In general, would you say your health is:

Excellent/Very good/Good/Fair/Poor

Health and daily activities. The following questions are about activities you might do during a typical day. Does your health limit you in these activities? If so, how much?

Yes, limited a lot/Yes, limited a little/No, not limited at all
Vigorous activities, such as running, lifting heavy objects, participating in strenuous sports
Moderate activities, such as moving a table, pushing a vacuum, bowling or playing golf
Lifting or carrying groceries
Climbing several flights of stairs
Climbing one flight of stairs
Bending, kneeling or stooping
Walking more than a mile
Walking half a mile
Walking 100 yards
Bathing and dressing yourself

During the past 4 weeks, how much of the time have you had any of the following problems with your work or other regular daily activities as a result of your physical health?

Cut down on the amount of time you spent on work or other activities
Accomplished less than you would like
Were limited in the kind of work or other activities
Had difficulty performing the work or other activities (e.g. it took **extra** effort)

All of the time/Most of the time/Some of the time/A little of the time/None of the time

(*Source:* SF-36 Health Survey, Ware *et al.* 1993. Copyright © Medical Outcomes Trust. All rights reserved. Reproduced with permission of the Medical Outcomes Trust; www.qualitymetric.com)

Scoring

The scaling and scoring assumptions which underpinned the development of the SF-36 were based on long-established, rigorous guidelines used in psychology and education measurement (Ware 2004). The practical implication is an increase in the scale's precision and reduced concentrations of scores at the top and bottom of the scale ('ceiling' and 'floor' effects).

However, as the mix of scaled and dichotomous response formats in the first version of the SF-36 confused respondents and led to some item non-response, the second version changed the dichotomous response formats in the two role-physical and role-mental dimensions to five-level response choices, as well as changing the six-level response format on the mental health dimension to five levels. The coding format requires recoding before each sub-scale can be summed. The scores for each of the eight dimensions are reported. In the original scoring method, the item scores for each of the eight dimensions are summed and transformed, using a scoring algorithm, into a scale from 0 (poor health) to 100 per cent (good health). The original 0–100 scoring algorithms of the SF-36 (based on summated ratings) have been improved on by norm-based scoring (the standardization of mean scores and standard deviations for the SF-36 scales), which has facilitated the speed and ease of interpretation of SF-36 scores. Ware *et al.* (1994) described how linear transformations were performed to transform the scale scores to a mean of 50 and a standard deviation of 10 (in the general US population). With this method, then, each scale is scored to have the same average (50) and the same standard deviation (10). Without the need to refer to norms, scale values below 50 are interpreted as below average, and each point is one-tenth of a standard deviation. The scoring details for the second version have been described by Ware *et al.* (2000).

Two summary scales can also be obtained – the Physical Component Summary Score (PCS-36) and the Mental Component Summary Score (MCS-36), with the advantage of enabling a reduction in the number of statistical comparisons conducted. These two summary scales capture about 85 per cent of the reliable variance in the eight scale SF-36 and yield average scores which closely mirror those in the 36-item scale (Ware *et al.* 1994, 1995; Jenkinson *et al.* 1997; Ware 2004).

Validity

Ware *et al.* (1993), in the manual of the SF-36, reported studies showing that in tests for validity the SF-36 was able to discriminate between groups with physical morbidities. In particular, strong correlations were reported between the physical and mental health sub-scales and their equivalent sub-scales of other commonly used measures of health status (0.51 to 0.85). The International Quality of Life Assessment Project published the psychometric properties of the translated and tested versions of the SF-36 in international use (Gandek and Ware 1998). Ware (2004) summarized much of the pertinent literature on the psychometric properties of the instrument in his updated description.

The results of British studies of the reliability and validity of the SF-36 have been summarized by Jenkinson *et al.* (1996, 1999). In Britain it has been found, in a postal survey, to be more sensitive to gradations in poor health than other well-known instruments (Brazier *et al.* 1992). Bowling *et al.* (1999) compared the various British norms for the SF-36 and critically discussed their variations by mode of administration, survey context and question order. Their conclusions were consistent with those of McHorney *et al.* (1994) and Lyons *et al.* (1999) who found underreporting of health problems using the SF-36 in personal interviews in comparison with postal approaches, especially in relation to emotional and mental health.

Some studies have found that the SF-36 has a higher rate of item non-response among older people in postal surveys (Brazier *et al.* 1992; Sullivan *et al.* 1995), and Anderson *et al.* (1993) suggested that the item codes can be subject to 'ceiling' effects as they appear too crude to detect improvements. The modifications to the item scores in the second version of the SF-36 should alleviate this problem.

Reliability

Brazier *et al.* (1992) reported internal coefficiency correlations for the eight scales, from a UK postal survey, to range from 0.60 to 0.81, with a median of 0.76. High inter-item correlations were reported for the sub-scales. Jenkinson *et al.* (1993) reported that it had high internal consistency between dimensions, with Chronbach's alphas being obtained of between 0.76 and 0.90. Garratt *et al.* (1993), in another British postal study, reported that the internal consistency between the items exceeded 0.80 with Chronbach's alpha, and inter-item correlations ranged from 0.55 to 0.78. Ware *et al.* (1993) and Ware (2004) reviewed US studies which analysed the reliability of the SF-36. The reliability coefficients for internal consistency range from 0.62 to 0.94 for the sub-scales, for test-retest reliability the coefficients range from 0.43 to 0.90, and for alternate form reliability the coefficient was 0.92. In relation to internal consistency, all but 11 coefficients reported in studies in the USA and UK exceeded the 0.70 standard. Reliability estimates for the two summary scores generally exceed 0.90 (Ware *et al.* 1994). Ware *et al.* (1993) also reported the results of a factor analysis of the SF-36, which provided strong evidence for the conceptualization of health underlying the measure, and indicated that some scales principally measure physical health some measure mental health and others measure both. Factor analyses from studies across the world have confirmed the distinct scale dimensions (Garratt *et al.* 1993; Ware *et al.* 1998).

The SF-36 is probably the most widely used and (carefully) translated health status scale across the world (information about translations, as well as an online scoring service, and missing data estimator, is available on www.SF-36.com or on www.qualitymetric.com). This increasing standardization of measurement facilitates comparisons between populations and evaluations of patient outcomes. Shorter versions are available (SF-12, SF-8) with good psychometric properties (Ware *et al.* 1992, 1996a, 1996b, 2002; Ware 2004), although the shorter scales are inevitably less sensitive indicators. Due to its coverage of social, physical and emotional health, many investigators use the SF-36, and short forms, uncritically as a proxy measure of HRQoL. Ware *et al.* (1993) acknowledged the increasing use of the SF-36 as a measure of HRQoL and partly justified it *post hoc* with reference to significant correlations between the SF-36 and a QoL criterion measure comprising a happiness/satisfaction rating of life from the General Psychological Well-Being Index (Dupuy 1984). While the correlations ranged from $r = 0.19$ to 0.60 (median around 0.36), the two concepts only partly overlap.

The WHOQOL

As pointed out earlier the constitution of the WHO (1948) defined health as 'A state of complete physical, mental and social well-being not merely the absence of disease . . .'. Thus it followed that a measure of health outcomes should include not just assessment of clinical changes but also of broader well-being and HRQoL. The WHO, in collaboration with 15 centres worldwide, developed two instruments for measuring QoL – the WHOQOL-100 and the WHOQOL-BREF – which were intended for use in a wide range of cultural settings, enabling different populations to be compared (WHOQOL Group 1994, 1996). While developed for use in clinical practice, clinical and policy research on outcomes, and audit, the WHOQOL instruments were designed broadly to reflect the WHOQOL Group's (1993) definition of QoL as based on individuals' perceptions of their position in the context of their culture and value systems, and in relation to their goals, expectations, standards and concerns. The Group regarded QoL as not confined to domains of health but as broad-ranging and affected by a person's physical health, psychological state, personal beliefs, social relationships and relationship to their environment.

The WHOQOL was developed from statements collected from patients with a range of conditions, professionals, and healthy people, and was initially piloted by expert review and qualitative fieldwork. It was subsequently tested for validity and reliability on 250 patients and 50 healthy respondents in the 15 participating centres. The original instrument contained 300 items, and this was reduced to 100, which form the current instrument – WHOQOL-100. The WHOQOL-BREF, a 26-item version of the WHOQOL-100, was developed using data from the field trials of the parent instrument (WHOQOL Group 1998b). Work is continuing on the psychometric properties of the instruments.

The core WHOQOL instruments assess QoL across situations. Modules were also developed which collect more detailed information from specific groups (e.g. elderly people, refugees, people with specific diseases such as cancer, HIV/ AIDS). The WHOQOL is administered by an interviewer, although the WHOQOL-BREF can be self-administered. The full instrument takes between 10 and 20 minutes of administration time. It is available in over 20 different languages, and each translation was tested for cultural equivalence. A methodology is available for further translations. A manual is also available from the developers. The questionnaires and scoring methods can be accessed on www. who.int/msa/qol.

The original WHOQOL-100 contained six broad *domains* of QoL, 24 *facets* of QoL (four items per facet) and four *general items* covering subjective overall QoL and overall health. These produced 100 items in total. The domains (and facets where they apply) of the WHOQOL-100 initially comprised an overall domain (overall QoL and general health) and six specific domains: (1) physical health (energy and fatigue; pain and discomfort; sleep and rest); (2) psychological (bodily image and appearance; negative feelings; positive feelings; self-esteem; thinking, learning, memory and concentration); (3) level of independence (mobility; activities of daily living; dependence on medicinal substances and medical aids; work capacity); (4) social relations (personal relationships; social support; sexual activity); (5) environment (financial resources; freedom, physical safety and security; health and social care – accessibility and quality; home environment; opportunities for acquiring new information and skills; participation in, and opportunities for, recreation/ leisure; physical environment – pollution/noise/traffic/climate; transport); (6) spirituality/religion/personal beliefs (single facet).

Analyses of the factor structure of the WHOQOL-100 indicated that some domains could be merged, thereby creating four domains of QoL instead of six: physical, psychological, social relationships and environment. These reflect the current grouping and scoring and were supported in cross-cultural studies (WHOQOL Group 1998b; Power *et al.* 1999). All items are rated on a five-point scale. The time reference for the questions is 'in the last two weeks'.

Content

The WHOQOL-100 now contains the above mentioned four broad domains of QoL, 24 facets of QoL (four items per facet), and four general items covering subjective overall QoL and overall health. These produce 100 items in total. The WHOQOL-BREF contains two items for overall QoL and general health and one item from each of the 24 facets in the WHOQOL-100. All items are rated on a five-point scale. The time reference for the questions is 'in the last two weeks'. Examples from the WHOQOL-100 are shown in Box 18.4.

Box 18.4   Examples from the WHOQOL

The following questions ask you to say how satisfied, happy or good you have felt about various aspects of your life over the past two weeks. For example, about your family life or the energy that you have. Decide how satisfied or dissatisfied you are with each aspect of your life and circle the number that best fits how you feel about this. Questions refer to the past two weeks.

How satisfied are you with the quality of your life?
In general, how satisfied are you with your life?
How satisfied are you with your health?
How satisfied are you with the energy you have?
Very dissatisfied/Dissatisfied/Neither satisfied nor dissatisfied/Satisfied/Very satisfied

The following questions ask about **how much** you have experienced certain things in the last two weeks, for example, positive feelings such as happiness or contentment. If you have experienced these things an extreme amount circle the number next to 'An extreme amount'. If you have not experienced these things at all, circle the number next to 'Not at all'. You should circle one of the numbers in between if you wish to indicate your answer lies somewhere between 'Not at all' and 'Extremely'. Questions refer to the last two weeks.

How safe do you feel in your daily life?
Not at all/Slightly/Moderately/Very/Extremely
Do you feel you are living in a safe and secure environment?
Not at all/Slightly/Moderately/Very much/Extremely

How much do you worry about your safety and security?
Not at all/A little/A moderate amount/Very much/An extreme amount
How comfortable is the place where you live?
Not at all/Slightly/Moderately/Very/Extremely
How much do you like it where you live?
Not at all/A little/A moderate amount/Very much/An extreme amount

The next few questions ask about how well you were able to move around in the last two weeks. This refers to your physical ability to move your body in such a way as to allow you to move around and do the things you would like to do, as well as the things that you need to do.

How well are you able to get around?
Very poor/Poor/Neither poor nor good/Good/Very good
How much do any difficulties with mobility bother you?
To what extent do any difficulties in movement affect your way of life?
Not at all/A little/A moderate amount/Very much/An extreme amount
How satisfied are you with your ability to move around?
Very dissatisfied/Dissatisfied/Neither satisfied nor dissatisfied/Satisfied/Very satisfied

Source: WHOQOL www.who.int/msa/qol © World Health Organization.
Reproduced with permission.

Scoring

The WHOQOL-100 produces scores relating to specific facets of QoL, as well as for the main domains measured, a score for overall QoL and a score for general health. The WHOQOL-BREF produces domain but not facet scores. Scores are produced for physical, psychological, social relationships and environment.

Validity

The WHOQOL instruments have been shown to have good discriminant and content validity although work on their validity and reliability is continuing (WHOQOL Group 1998a, 1998b). They appear to be well accepted by respondents. There are too many diverse studies of the psychometric performance of the instruments to report in detail here. The difficulty with reviewing the overall psychometric properties of the instruments is that the studies all relate to different language versions, and different disease or population groups. For example, Pibernik-Okanovic (2001) tested the discriminant validity of the WHOQOL-100 with a small sample of diabetic patients in Croatia and reported that, at two months follow-up, it was sensitive to improvement in condition in patients whose treatment was changed, in comparison with controls. The WHOQOL-100 was reported to have good concurrent validity, greater comprehensiveness and good responsiveness to clinical change in comparison with the SF-36, in a study over 100 outpatients with chronic pain in the UK (Skevington et al. 2001).

Domain scores produced by the WHOQOL-BREF have been reported to correlate highly (0.89) with the four domains of the WHOQOL-100, and this shorter instrument was reported to have good discriminant and content validity, internal consistency and test-retest reliability (WHOQOL Group 1998b). The WHOQOL-BREF was tested by de Girolamo et al. (2000) in over 300 people who were in contact with health services in Italy. They reported that only the physical and psychological domains were able to discriminate between healthy and unhealthy respondents. Although results vary, investigators in various countries have reported that the WHOQOL-100 and WHOQOL-BREF can successfully discriminate between patient groups across a wide range of conditions, and have generally good psychometric properties. It was reported earlier that factor analysis of the WHOQOL-100 supported four domains of QoL instead of six: physical, psychological, social relationships and environment.

Reliability

The WHOQOL Group (1998a) reported on the initial psychometric properties of the WHOQOL-100: both published and unpublished data show that the instrument was shown to have good test-retest and face reliability, and high internal consistency (Power et al. 1999; Skevington 1999). While tests for reliability are ongoing, there are, again, several studies reporting on the initial results for the reliability of the instrument for the different language versions and in different contexts.

Test-retest reliability of the WHOQOL-BREF was tested by de Girolamo et al.'s (2000) study in Italy, and they reported correlations of between 0.76 and 0.93 for the domains. They also reported internal consistency with alphas ranging from 0.65 to 0.80. Leplege et al. (2000), on the basis of their study of over 2000 patients in different types of clinic in France, reported that the homogeneity of the short version was lower than the full instrument, but was still acceptable: item scale correlations was greater than 0.40 for two-thirds of the items and the Cronbach's alphas for all domains on the WHOQOL-BREF were over 0.65. Pibernik-Okanovic's (2001) study of diabetic patients in Croatia found that the WHOQOL-100 produced Cronbach's alphas of 0.76 to 0.95 for the four domains.

While the WHOQOL-100 is lengthy, the advantage is its breadth of scope and applicability in different cultures. The short version also has good psychometric properties, but short forms are always weaker than the fuller versions. The manual, appropriate language version of the instrument, scoring instructions and syntax files for their computation, permission for use and other details of the instruments can be obtained from the relevant national centre (see WHO website: http://www.who.int) or from the WHOQOL Group at the WHO in Geneva.

Conclusions

The aim of including patient-based measures of broader health status and QoL in health outcome assessment is to be responsive to patients' evaluations of their treatment and outcome. There are numerous measures to choose from. Investigators should define the concepts to be measured, and choose a measurement instrument in relation to the aims of the study, the target population and the variables relevant to the study. They should also attempt to separate indicator and predictor variables, especially when using multidimensional measures.

If a measurement scale is to be of value in clinical and population health research, it needs to be conceptually clear, valid, sensitive and responsive to clinically significant change over time, reliable and to have an identified factor structure, and its scoring system needs to be interpretable. It needs to be acceptable to respondents, and population norms should be available for the instrument.

Key points

- The aim of including measures of individuals' perceptions of their health and QoL in outcomes research is to be responsive to patients' evaluations of their treatment and outcome.

- Measures of the outcome, or consequences, of disease, its treatment or care, which are based on patients' own perspectives ('patient-based') can be used to supplement the medical model of disease with a social model of health and ability.

- Measures can be selected which relate to a person's general health status, single dimensions of this, generic HRQoL and/or DSQoL.

- There has been a huge increase in the use of subjective indicators of health status and HRQoL over the past two decades, although there has been relatively little standardization of measurement instruments.

- Investigators need to be clear about which of their selected variables, and associated measures, influences health and/or HRQoL, and which make up these concepts.

- Making an overall judgement about the quality of one's life requires a complex assessment of experiences and priorities. These priorities, and values, can change over time. Measurement scales need to be sensitive to this issue.

- When choosing a measurement scale to assess outcome, investigators need to ensure that it is relevant to the target population, appropriate for the research question and satisfies the principles of measurement, including reliability and validity.

- The SF-36 and its short forms are the most frequently used measures of generic health status across the world.

- The WHO has developed two instruments for measuring quality of life – the WHOQOL-100 and the WHOQOL-BREF – for use in clinical practice, and clinical and policy research on outcomes. They are intended for use in a wide range of cultural settings, enabling different populations to be compared.

References

Albrecht, G.L. and Devlieger, P.J. (1999) The disability paradox: high quality of life against all odds, *Social Science and Medicine*, 48: 977–88.

Anderson, R.T., Aaronson, N.K. and Wilkin, D. (1993) Critical review of the international assessments of health-related quality of life, *Quality of Life Research*, 2: 369–95.

Beckie, T.M. and Hayduk, L.A. (1997) Measuring quality of life, *Social Indicators Research*, 42: 21–39.

Bowling, A. (2001) *Measuring Disease: A Review of Disease Specific Quality of Life Measurement Scales*, 2nd edn. Buckingham: Open University Press.

Bowling, A. (2002) *Research Methods in Health*. Buckingham: Open University Press.

Bowling, A. (2004) *Measuring Health: A Review of Quality of Life Measurement Scales*, 3rd edn. Maidenhead: Open University Press.

Bowling, A. and Gabriel, Z. (2004) An integrational model of quality of life in older age: a comparison of analytic and lay models of quality of life, *Social Indicators Research*, 69: 1–36.

Bowling, A., Bond, M., Jenkinson, C. and Lamping, D. (1999) Short Form-36 (SF-36) Health Survey Questionnaire: which normative data should be used? Comparisons between the norms provided by the Omnibus Survey in Britain, the Health Survey for England and the Oxford Health and Lifestyle Survey, *Journal of Public Health Medicine*, 21: 255–70.

Bowling, A., Gabriel, Z., Dykes, J. et al. (2003). Let's ask them: a national survey, of definitions of quality of life and its enhancement among people aged 65 and over, *International Journal of Aging and Human Development*, 56: 269–306.

Brazier, J.E., Harper, R., Jones, N. et al. (1992) Validating the SF-36 health survey questionnaire: a new outcome measure for primary care, *British Medical Journal*, 305: 160–4.

Bullinger, M., Anderson, R., Cella, D. and Aaronson, N. (1993) Developing and evaluating cross-cultural instruments from minimum requirements to optimal models, *Quality of Life Research*, 2: 451–9.

Calman, K.C. (1984) Quality of life in cancer patients – a hypothesis, *Journal of Medical Ethics*, 10: 124–7.

de Girolamo, G., Rucci, P. and Scocco, P. (2000) Quality of life assessment: validation of the Italian version of the WHOQOL-brief, *Epidemiologia Psichiatria Sociale*, 9: 45–55.

Dupuy, H.J. (1984) The psychological general well-being (PGWB) index, in N.K. Wenger, M.E. Mattson, C.D. Furberg and J. Elinson (eds) *Assessment of Quality of Life in Clinical Trials of Cardiovascular Therapies*. New York: Le Jacq Publishing Company.

Fayers, P.M. and Hand, D.J. (2002) Causal variables, indicator variables and measurement scales: an example from quality of life, *Journal of the Royal Statistical Association*, 165, Part 2: 1–21.

Fitzpatrick, R., Davey, C., Buxton, M.J. and Jones, D.R. (1998) Evaluating patient-based outcome measures for use in clinical trials, *Health Technology Assessment*, 2(14).

Gandek, B. and Ware, J.E. (eds) (1998) Translating functional health and well-being: international quality of life assessment (IQOLA) project studies of the SF-36 Health Survey, *Journal of Clinical Epidemiology*, 51: 891–1214.

Garratt, A.M., Ruta, D.A., Abdalla, M.I. et al. (1993) The SF-36 health survey questionnaire: an outcome measure suitable for routine use within the NHS? *British Medical Journal*, 306: 1440–4.

Garratt, A., Schmidt, L., Mackintosh, A. and Fitzpatrick, R. (2002) Quality of life measurement:

bibliographic study of patient assessed health outcome measures, *British Medical Journal*, 324: 1417.

Greer, D.S., Mor, V., Morris, J.N. *et al.* (1986) An alternative in terminal care: results of the National Hospice Study, *Journal of Chronic Diseases*, 39: 9–26.

Haywood, K.L., Garratt, A.M., Schmidt, L.J. *et al.* (2004) *Health Status and Quality of Life in Older People: A Structured Review of Patient-assessed Health Instruments*. Oxford: Department of Public Health, University of Oxford.

Hunt, S.M. (1988) Subjective health indicators and health promotion, *Health Promotion*, 3: 23–34.

Hunt, S.M. and McKenna, S.P. (1992) British adaptation of the General Well-Being Index: a new tool for clinical research, *British Journal of Medical Economics*, 2: 49–60.

Jenkinson, C., Coulter, A. and Wright, L. (1993) Short Form-36 (SF-36) health survey questionnaire: Normative data for adults of working age. *British Medical Journal*, 306: 1437–40.

Jenkinson, C., Layte, R., Wright, L. and Coulter, A. (1996) *The UK SF-36: An Analysis and Interpretation Manual. A Guide to Health Status Measurement with Particular Reference to the Short Form 36 Health Survey*. Oxford: University of Oxford, Department of Public Health and Primary Care, Health Services Research Unit.

Jenkinson, C., Layte, R. and Lawrence, K. (1997) Development and testing of the SF-36 summary scale scores in the United Kingdom: results from a large scale survey and clinical trial, *Medical Care*, 35: 410–16.

Jenkinson, C., Stewart-Brown, S., Peterson, S. and Paice, C. (1999) Assessment of the SF-36 version 2 in the UK, *Journal of Epidemiology and Community Health*, 53: 46–50.

Joore, M.A., Potjewijd, J., Timmerman, A.A. *et al.* (2002) Response shift in the measurement of quality of life in hearing impaired adults after hearing aid fitting, *Quality of Life Research*, 11: 299–307.

Kaplan, R.M. (1988) New health promotion indicators: the general health policy model, *Health Promotion*, 3: 35–48.

Karnofsky, D.A., Abelmann, W.H., Craver, L.F. *et al.* (1948) The use of nitrogen mustards in the palliative treatment of carcinoma, *Cancer*, I: 634–56.

Leplege, A., Reveilere, C., Ecosse, E. *et al.* (2000) Psychometric properties of a new instrument for evaluating quality of life, the WHOQOL-26, in a population of patients with neuromuscular diseases, *Encephale*, 26: 13–22.

Lyons, R.A., Wareham, K., Lucas, M. *et al.* (1999) SF-36 scores vary by method of administration: implications for study design, *Journal of Public Health Medicine*, 21: 41–5.

McDowell, I. and Newell, C. (1996) *Measuring Health: A Guide to Rating Scales and Questionnaires*, 2nd edn. New York: Oxford University Press.

McHorney, C.A., Kosinski, M. and Ware, J.E. (1994) Comparisons of the costs and quality of norms for the SF-36 Health Survey collected by mail versus telephone interview: results from a national survey, *Medical Care*, 32: 551–67.

Nocon, A. and Qureshi, H. (1996) *Outcomes of Community Care for Users and Carers: A Social Services Perspective*. Buckingham: Open University Press.

O'Boyle C.A. (1997) Measuring the quality of later life, *Philosophy Transactions of the Royal Society of London*, 352: 1871–9.

Patrick, D.L. and Erickson, P. (1993) *Health Status and Health Policy: Quality of Life in Health Care Evaluation and Resource Allocation*. New York: Oxford University Press.

Pibernik-Okanovic, M. (2001) Psychometric properties of the World Health Organization quality of life questionnaire (WHOQOL-100) in diabetic patients in Croatia, *Diabetes Research in Clinical Practice*, 51: 133–43.

Power, M., Harper, A., Bullinger, M. and the WHO Quality of Life Group (1999) The World Health Organization WHOQOL-100: tests of the universality of quality of life in 15 different cultural groups worldwide, *Health Psychology*, 18: 495–505.

Skevington, S.M. (1999) Measuring quality of life in Britain: introducing the WHOQOL-100, *Psychomatic Research*, 47: 449–59.

Skevington, S.M., Carse, M.S. and Williams, de C. (2001) Validation of the WHOQOL-100: pain management improves quality of life for chronic pain patients, *Clinical Journal of Pain*, 17: 264–75.

Spilker, B. (ed.) (1996) *Pharmacoeconomics and Quality of Life in Clinical Trials*, 2nd edn. Philadelphia, PA: Lippincott-Raven.

Sprangers, M.A.G. and Schwartz, C.E. (1999) Integrating response shift into health-related quality of life research: a theoretical model, *Social Science and Medicine*, 48: 1507–15.

Sprangers, M.A.G., Van Dam, F.S.A.M., Broersen, J. *et al.* (1999) Revealing response shift in longitudinal research on fatigue: the use of the then test approach, *Acta Oncologica*, 38: 709–18.

Stewart, A.L. and Ware, J.E. (1992) *Measuring Functioning and Well-being: The Medical Outcomes Study Approach*. Durham, NC: Duke University Press.

Sullivan, M., Karlsson, J. and Ware, J.R. (1995) The Swedish SF-36 Health Survey – 1. Evaluation of data quality, scaling assumptions, reliability and construct validity across general populations in Sweden, *Social Science and Medicine*, 10: 1349–58.

Ware, J.E. (2004). SF-36 Health Survey update, in M. Maruish (ed.) The use of psychological testing for treatment planning and outcome assessment. Mahwah, NJ: Lawrence Erlbaum Associates.

Ware, J.E., Sherbourne, C.D. and Davies, A.R. (1992) Developing and testing the MOS 20-item Short Form Health Survey: a general population application, in A.L. Stewart and J.E. Ware (eds) *Measuring Functioning and Well-being: The Medical Outcomes Study Approach*. Durham, NC: Duke University Press.

Ware, J.E., Snow, K.K., Kosinski, M. and Gandek, B. (1993) *SF-36 Health Survey*. Boston, MA: New England Medical Centre.

Ware, J.E., Kosinski, M. and Keller, S.D. (1994) *SF-36 Physical and Mental Health Summary Scales: A User's Manual*. Boston, MA: The Health Institute, New England Medical Center.

Ware, J.E., Kosinski, M. and Keller, S.D. (1995) *How to Score the SF-12 Physical and Mental Health Summary Scales*, 2nd edn. Boston, MA: The Health Institute, New England Medical Center.

Ware, J.E., Kosinski, M. and Keller, S.D. (1996a) SF-12: An even shorter health survey, *Medical Outcomes Trust Bulletin*, 4: 2.

Ware, J.E., Kosinski, M. and Keller, S.D. (1996b) A 12-item short-form health survey: construction of scales and preliminary tests of reliability and validity, *Medical Care*, 34: 220–33.

Ware, J.E., Snow, K.K., Kosinski, M. and Gandek, B. (1997) *SF-36 Health Survey: Manual and Interpretation Guide*. Boston, MA: The Health Institute, New England Medical Center.

Ware, J.E., Kosinski, M., Gandek, B. *et al.* (1998) The factor structure of the SF-36 Health Survey in 10 countries: results from the International Quality of Life Assessment (IQOLA) Project, *Journal of Clinical Epidemiology*, 51: 1159–65.

Ware, J.E., Kosinski, M. and Dewey, J.E. (2000). *How to Score Version Two of the SF-36 Health Survey*. Lincoln, RI: QualityMetric.

Ware, J.E., Kosinski, M., Turner-Bowker, D.M. and Gandek, B. (2002) *How to Score Version 2 of the SF-12 Health Survey* (with a supplement documenting version 1). Lincoln, RI: QualityMetric.

Ware, J.E., Kosinski, M. and Dewey, J.E. (2003) *Version Two of the SF-36 Health Survey*. Lincoln, RI: QualityMetric.

WHO (World Health Organization) (1948) *Preamble to the Constitution of the World Health Organization* as adopted by The International Health Conference, New York, 19–22 June 1946. Geneva: World Health Organization.

WHOQOL Group (1993) *Measuring Quality of Life: The Development of the World Health Organization Quality of Life Instrument (WHOQOL)*. Geneva: WHO.

WHOQOL Group (1994) The development of the WHO Quality of Life assessment instrument (the WHOQOL), in J. Orley and W. Kuyken (eds) *International Quality of Life Assessment in Health Care Settings*. Heidelberg: Springer-Verlag.

WHOQOL Group (1996) The World Health Organization Quality of Life (WHOQOL) assessment instrument, in B. Spilker (ed.) *Quality of Life and Pharmacoeconomics in Clinical Trials*, 2nd edn. Hagerstown, MD: Lipincott-Raven.

WHOQOL Group (1998a) The World Health Organization Quality of Life Assessment (WHOQOL): development and general psychometric properties, *Social Science and Medicine*, 46: 1569–85.

WHOQOL Group (1998b) Development of the World Health Organization WHOQOL-BREF Quality of Life assessment, *Psychological Medicine*, 28: 551–8.

WHO (World Health Organization) (1984) *Uses of Epidemiology in Aging: Report of a Scientific Group, 1983*. Technical report series no. 706. Geneva: WHO.

Zizzi, A., Barry, M.M. and Cochrane, R. (1998) A mediational model of quality of life for individuals with severe mental health problems, *Psychological Medicine*, 28: 1221–30.

19 Genetics, health and population genetics research

Sarah J. Lewis, George Davey Smith and Shah Ebrahim

Introduction

It is now widely accepted that almost all human disease has some genetic basis – even susceptibility to infectious diseases is determined by an individual's genetic make-up. Some rare diseases are the result of a single mutation in a single gene, whereas others occur as a result of complex interactions between many genes and environmental factors. For most complex diseases, we are still a long way from completely understanding the role played by genetic factors; however, progress is rapid. Just over 50 years ago the structure of deoxyribonucleic acid (DNA), the molecule which holds the genetic code, was defined by Watson and Crick (1953). Since then many genes, which may play a role in disease, have been identified, and the whole human genome has been sequenced to provide a blueprint for life. Research in genetics is transforming our understanding of health and disease. Until recently genetics in health care had centred around the identification of rare disorders caused by a single gene, and incorporation of this knowledge into disease prevention through pre-pregnancy or antenatal genetic counselling. However, the identification of common gene variants associated with common chronic diseases such as coronary heart disease, diabetes, psychiatric disease and cancers may lead to clinical testing for increased disease susceptibility, which will allow health professionals to offer prevention options or lifestyle advice. Furthermore, it is widely believed that genetic testing for drug responsiveness will be used to provide individualized treatments.

This chapter aims to give a brief overview of the physical aspects of genetic material including how this is replicated and translated into proteins, followed by an outline of how the genetic component of a given disease may be identified. The chapter then deals with population-based studies of genetic factors for complex diseases, and how genes can be used as tools in the identification of environmental causes of disease. Finally we have outlined some examples of genetic models of disease, screening for genetic susceptibility to disease and individualized medicine.

An introduction to the genome

DNA

The genetic information of all animals is contained within DNA which provides the code to make proteins which are essential for all the functions of the body. A DNA molecule consists of two helical chains coiled around the same axis. The chains consist of many thousands of nucleotides held together by phosphodiester bonds, each nucleotide comprising a phosphate group, a five-carbon sugar (2-deoxyribose) and a cyclic nitrogen-containing compound called a base. There are four different bases which appear in DNA: adenine, guanine, thymine and cytosine. Adenine and guanine are double-ringed bases and are called purines; cytosine and thymine are single-ringed and called pyrimidines. The combination of bases along a chain of DNA gives the molecule its unique code. Hydrogen bonding between purine and pyrimidine bases on opposite chains holds the double helix together. Since adenine is always paired with thymine and guanine with cytosine, one chain is always complementary to the other, so if the sequence of bases on one chain is known, the sequence on the other can be inferred. The specific pairing also provides a copying mechanism for the genetic material. Before cells divide, DNA is replicated, the double-stranded DNA molecular unwinds and the separated strands serve as templates for the alignment of incoming nucleoside triphosphates, which are bonded together to form new strands complementary to the parental strands. The DNA sequence is identical in each cell of the body.

Chromosomes

Within the genome, DNA is sub-divided into chromosomes of variable size. Normal human cells contain 23 chromosome pairs, 22 autosome pairs (numbered 1–22) and one sex chromosome pair which is denoted either XX for a female or XY for a male. These are called diploid cells. Sperm and unfertilized egg cells, which are haploid cells, contain one copy of each chromosome and one sex chromosome. During cell division it is possible to observe stained chromosomes under a light microscope and to identify each chromosome by its characteristic banding pattern. From this, one can photograph the chromosomes and produce a karyogram in which chromosomes are ordered in pairs from the largest chromosome to the smallest, followed by the sex chromosomes (see Figure 19.1). This is useful in identifying extra or lost chromosomes (aneuploidy) or regions of chromosomes which have been deleted, inverted or translocated to another chromosome. One common example of aneuploidy is Down's syndrome in which affected individuals inherit three copies of chromosome 21.

Genes and gene expression

It is estimated that there are around 30,000 genes held on chromosomes in the human genome. A typical gene contains between 1 and 200 kilobases (a kilobase is 1000 A–T or C–G base pairs), although some are much larger. Only a small proportion of the sequence codes for proteins, this is spread across small sequence blocks called exons, which are interspersed between introns (see Figure 19.2). In order for a gene to be expressed the sequence of DNA, which defines a gene, must firstly be transcribed into messenger ribonucleic acid (mRNA). mRNA is similar in structure to DNA except that it is much shorter, single-stranded, the sugar is ribose rather deoxyribose and uracil replaces the base thymine. An mRNA molecule is translated

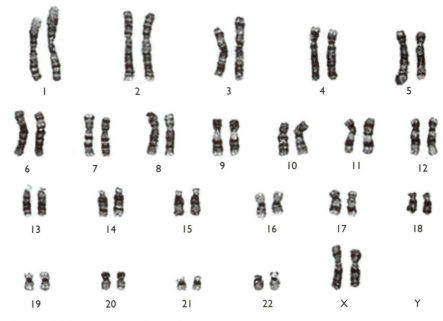

Figure 19.1 A human female karyogram

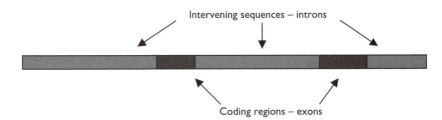

Figure 19.2 A simplified example of a human gene, showing exons and introns

into a series of amino acids according to the sequence of bases it contains, and these amino acids transcribe proteins.

Cell division

The cell cycle refers to the process which occurs between a new cell being formed and that cell dividing into two. The cell cycle consists of four phases: G1, S, G2 and mitosis (in most cells of the body), or meiosis (in germ cells). During G1, chromosomes are diffuse, and transcription of DNA can occur to produce proteins so that the cell can function. The S phase is the time when DNA replication occurs to produce identical copies of the DNA molecules. After replication the cells enter the G2 phase which is a brief period of cell growth, before entering into mitosis or meiosis.

Mitosis

During mitosis the chromosomes become compact, as represented on a karyogram, and are visible under the light microscope (see Figure 19.1). The newly-replicated chromosome is attached to the original chromosome at this point, and these are referred to as sister chromatids. During mitosis the sister chromatids separate, and migrate to opposite poles of the cell. The cell divides at the centre into two identical daughter cells each containing identical genetic material.

Meiosis

Meiosis only occurs in germ cells and results in the production of haploid cells, which contain just one copy of each chromosome from the parent cell. The difference between the first part of meiosis and mitosis is that prior to cell division, rather than sister chromatids separating, chromosome pairs separate. Therefore the resultant cell contains just one copy of each chromosome, each containing two genetically identical sister chromatids (see Figure 19.3). During the segregation of chromosome pairs, maternal and paternal homologues (i.e. chromosomes inherited from the mother and father) can assort independently of other chromosomes so that each new cell will contain a random assortment of the 23 chromosomes. This means

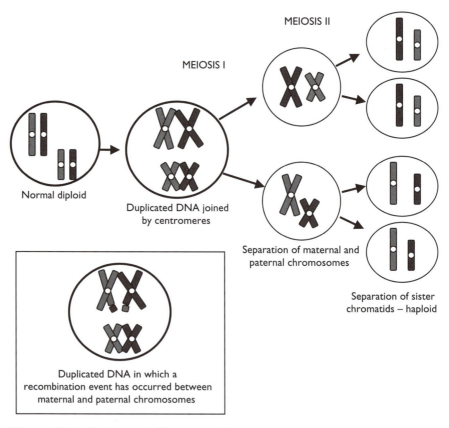

MEIOSIS II

MEIOSIS I

Normal diploid

Duplicated DNA joined
by centromeres

Separation of maternal and
paternal chromosomes

Separation of sister
chromatids – haploid

Duplicated DNA in which a
recombination event has occurred between
maternal and paternal chromosomes

Figure 19.3   A schematic illustration of meiosis

that at least 2^{23} (i.e. over 8 million) possible types of sperm or ova can be produced by one individual. Meiosis II then occurs in an identical manner to mitosis and results in division into two cells.

Recombination

In the process of separation during meiosis I, the two chromosomes may cross over at a point – a chiasma – and some material from one may become transferred to the other. This is called recombination (see Figure 19.4). Two positions in a DNA sequence – known as loci – separated by a single crossover event will appear as a recombinant, meaning that the offspring will possess a different sequence of alleles (see below), than either of their parents at the two loci. The number of recombinants gives an indication of the distance between two alleles on a chromosome, and this concept is exploited in linkage analysis.

Mutations and polymorphisms

The term mutation is used in two ways, firstly to refer to the process by which DNA is modified and new variants of a gene arise, and second to describe a rare variant of a gene – a gene mutation. A mutation resulting in a change in DNA sequence can occur naturally during DNA replication, or can occur as a result of an 'insult' from an environmental agent or mutagen – for example, tobacco smoke. Highly deleterious mutations are usually rare but cause severe disease phenotypes such as cystic fibrosis; very deleterious mutations are not compatible with survival. However, many mutations do not have dangerous consequences and exist as common variations in DNA (present in at least 1 per cent of individuals), and these are conventionally referred to as polymorphisms. Common polymorphisms do not cause monogenic disease, but may play a role in multifactorial diseases (see Box 19.1). Alternative DNA sequences found at polymorphic loci are called alleles. There are several types of polymorphism: single nucleotide polymorphisms (SNPs, called 'snips'), frameshift mutations and variable number tandem repeats. SNPs occur when a single nucleotide in a DNA molecule is substituted for another nucleotide: the substitution of a purine for another purine or a pyrimidine for another pyrimidine is called

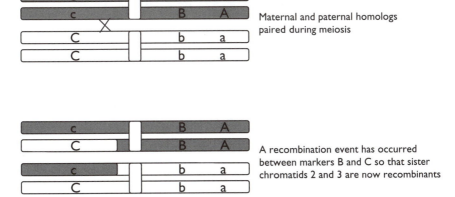

Figure 19.4   An illustration of recombination during meiosis

> ### Box 19.1   Monogenic, oligogenic, polygenic and multifactorial traits
>
> - **Monogenic:** a trait which arises due to mutation at a single locus, and which is inherited in a Mendelian manner.
> - **Oligogenic:** a trait which arises due to variation at a few different genetic loci.
> - **Polygenic:** a trait which arises due to variation at many different genetic loci.
> - **Multifactorial/complex:** a trait which arises due to variation at one or more genetic loci, plus environmental factors.

a transition, and the substitution of a purine for a pyrimidine or vice versa is known as a translation. When a SNP occurs in a coding region, it can be classified as synonymous (silent) or non-synonymous, depending on whether or not it changes the amino acid sequence of the resultant protein. Frameshift mutations arise from an insertion or deletion of one or more base pairs into the DNA molecule, which disrupts the reading frame within a gene. Variable number tandem repeats are short sequences of DNA that are repeated many times in succession with the number of repeats varying between individuals, as a result of misalignment of the repeated unit during DNA replication.

The subject is complex, so we have listed some key terms in Box 19.2.

> ### Box 19.2   Some useful genetic terms
>
> - **Allele:** one of the alternative versions of DNA sequence at a given locus.
> - **Genotype:** the composition of alleles present in an individual at a given locus.
> - **Phenotype:** the characteristic which is observable in individuals.
> - **Heterozygote:** an individual who carries two different alleles at the locus of interest.
> - **Homozygote:** an individual who carries two identical alleles at the locus of interest.

Identifying the genetic component of disease

Ideally it would be useful to have some estimate of the genetic contribution to a particular disease before embarking on a search for specific susceptibility genes. It is often claimed that a disease or a characteristic, such as obesity, has a given genetic component. Such information may come from studies of familial aggregation of the disease or characteristic, twin studies, adoption studies, segregation analysis and animal models.

Familial aggregation of disease

Diseases that appear to cluster in families may indicate that a genetic component exists. The level of familial clustering can be expressed as λ_R, which is the risk to relative 'R' of being affected by the disease of interest compared with the population risk. The magnitude of λ_R is related to the degree of concordance for the disease of interest. When $\lambda_R = 1$ there is no familial aggregation of the disease, values greater than 1 indicating familial clustering. However, estimates of λ_R can be greater than 1 due to shared environmental or behavioural factors within families, as well as a shared genetic component. λ_R, as a measure of the genetic component of a disease, is affected by the biological relationship between the proband (affected individual) and relative, R. The proportion of shared genes is on average 0.5 for parents and offspring, 0.5 for siblings, 0.25 for grandparents and their grandchildren, 0.125 for first cousins, 0 for unrelated spouses and 0 for adoptees and their adoptive parents. Diseases that show greater λ_R among more closely related family members are therefore more likely to have a strong underlying genetic component, whereas those that show a similar distribution of λ_R among closely and less closely related family members tend to indicate that the observed familial aggregation of the disease (or characteristic) is due to shared environmental factors. The risk to siblings of an affected individual λ_S is ≈ 500 for cystic fibrosis, 15 for Type I diabetes, 8.6 for schizophrenia and 3.5 for Type II diabetes (Lander and Schork 1994). The risks of schizophrenia and epilepsy, for example, for less closely related individuals, such as first and second cousins, drop markedly compared with siblings, making a strong genetic component very likely.

Age of onset

Some multifactorial diseases, which do not typically show strong familial clustering, show larger familial risk among relatives of cases with a young age of onset. A twin study of coronary heart disease carried out in Sweden showed that the magnitude of relative risk decreased as the age at which the co-twin had died of heart disease increased. Among women whose monozygotic co-twin had died before 65 years, the relative risk of coronary heart disease was 15.0, but this fell to 1.2 among women whose co-twin had died of coronary heart disease at 86 years or older (Marenberg *et al.* 1994). Similar results have been found for prostate, breast, colorectal and many other cancers (Risch 2001). Such findings demonstrate that the genetic component of a disease will depend on the extent to which other environmental factors are able to operate – with increasing age the effects of dietary fats and smoking will, inevitably, prove to be stronger causal factors than at younger ages. However, given that heart disease and cancer are more common among the elderly and early onset cases are rare, it could be argued that despite a smaller relative component of genetics with increasing age, the population risk which can be attributed to genetics at advanced ages is still considerable.

Segregation analysis and Mendelian inheritance

In 1865 Gregor Mendel carried out a series of breeding experiments on pea plants, and, although he was not aware of the terms 'genes', 'chromosome' and 'alleles', he came up with two basic principles of inheritance based on differentiating characteristics of the plants. In the context of current knowledge, the first principle was that each individual carries two copies of each gene. One is inherited from each parent, and alleles at a given locus are inherited randomly and with equal probability in the offspring. This principle is known as segregation of alleles. The second law of independent assortment stated that alleles of different genes are transmitted independently of each other. We now know that the second principle only holds true if the two genes are not located close together on the same chromosome.

Mendel's work informs our current understanding of the inheritance of genetic

> ### Box 19.3   Dominance
>
> - **Dominant:** a single copy of the 'at risk' allele is sufficient to produce an increased disease risk and this increase in risk is no greater among individuals with two copies of the 'at risk' allele.
> - **Recessive:** two copies of the 'at risk' allele are required to increase disease risk.
> - **Codominant:** all possible genotypes have different effects on disease risk; usually the risk among heterozygotes is intermediate between the two homozygotes.

disease and allows prediction of models of inheritance based on how a disease appears to be segregating within families. Once it is established that the disease of interest clusters in families, the next step is often to determine whether the disease follows a Mendelian pattern of inheritance, and hence whether a major gene is segregating within families to cause the disease. Segregation analysis involves collecting data on the families of probands (affected individuals) and ascertaining the presence of the disease or phenotype, ideally within each member of the family. Typically, an extended family tree is plotted, with affected individuals identified. The concept of dominance (see Box 19.3) is important in defining the genetic basis of disease, and it is often also possible, by looking at pedigrees, to determine whether the disease is segregating mainly in males and if the underlying variant is therefore likely to be present on the X chromosome (sex-linked).

Models of Mendelian inheritance are as follows.

Autosomal dominant

All affected individuals must have at least one affected parent, so the disease will occur in all generations, approximately equal numbers of males and females will be affected, and both sexes will transmit the disease to their offspring. Examples are familial hypercholesterolaemia (raised blood cholesterol) and Huntington's disease (a degenerative disease of the central nervous system). In Huntington's disease, both parents appear normal initially because of the late age of manifestation of the disease.

Autosomal recessive

Most affected individuals have two normal parents, so the disease appears to skip generations. The disease is expressed and transmitted by both sexes, on average a quarter of offspring produced by two heterozygote parents will be affected. Studies of familial aggregation will show greater relative risks among siblings than among parents and their offspring. Matings between affected and normal individuals will yield normal offspring who are carriers (carry one copy of the disease allele) for the disease. All offspring of two affected individuals will have the disease. Examples include cystic fibrosis and phenylketonuria.

Sex-linked inheritance

Males have only one X chromosome whereas females have two, therefore for genes carried on the X chromosome a sex-specific pattern of inheritance can be seen, which will depend on whether the father or the mother was the mutation carrier, the sex of the offspring and whether the disease exhibits a dominant or a recessive mode of inheritance. The Y chromosome, which denotes maleness, has little replicating DNA, but it does contain 'pseudoautosomal' regions and there is a possibility of Y chromosome-related traits.

Dominant sex-linked

If the mother is affected she will pass on the allele to half of her offspring regardless of gender, and those who inherit the allele will develop the disease. If the father is affected he will pass on the X chromosome to all of his daughters, and they will all be affected, but not his sons.

Recessive sex-linked

If the mother is the carrier, she will pass on the allele to half of her offspring: the females inheriting the allele will be carriers, but the males will be affected. If the father is affected he will pass on the mutation to his daughters and they will be carriers, but not affected.

Segregation analysis is a useful method for selecting the model which best fits the observed data for monogenic diseases, but can become very complicated for multi-factorial diseases. However, segregation analysis was used to show that a dominantly acting rare allele was responsible for a small proportion of breast cancer cases (Claus *et al.* 1991).

Heritability

Reports of family clustering of a disease or trait can give some evidence of a possible genetic component for complex diseases, and segregation analysis is useful to identify genetic models. However, in order to distinguish between the relative contribution of shared environmental and genetic factors for complex diseases, further investigations are required. Heritability (h^2) can be estimated for multifactorial diseases using comparisons of disease risk among different family members, monozygotic and dizygotic twins and adopted and biological siblings. These methods examine departure from the null hypothesis of no genetic contribution by taking into account the expected level of genetic sharing, shared and unshared environmental factors. For instance, siblings reared apart will share on average 50 per cent of their genes, but will have no environmental sharing, hence any increased sibling risk is likely to be due solely to genetic factors. Heritability is the proportion of the total phenotypic variance of a particular trait which is due to genetic factors. However, it should be noted that heritability estimates are limited to the population in which they are measured and are subject to temporal trends in environmental exposure. Adult height can be used to illustrate this point: in an unfavourable environment, where malnutrition is common, childhood diet and infections will probably be the overriding factors determining height. In a favourable environment where food is plentiful, genetics will play a more important role. Consequently, heritability estimates tend to decrease with greater environmental heterogeneity. Korpelainen (2000) looked at lifespan among nineteenth-century Finns, who were historically a population of large socioeconomic inequality. She found that rural Finns possessed a distinctly lower level of heritability of lifespan compared with aristocratic Finns. Among rural Finns, poverty was an overriding factor determining lifespan, whereas among the aristocrats environmental conditions were optimized and genetics played a larger role.

Twin studies

Monozygotic twins are genetically identical and dizygotic twins share, on average, 50 per cent of their genes. This difference in the genetic make-up between monozygotic and dizygotic twins makes it possible to compare segregation of diseases or traits and estimate the magnitude of genetic and environmental contributions to a particular disease or trait. An important assumption in twin studies is that the degree of environmental sharing is the same for monozygotic and dizygotic twin pairs; this assumption is likely to inflate estimates of the genetic contribution. Nevertheless, twin studies can be used to give some indication of how important genetics is for the disease in question, but should be regarded as potential overestimates.

Twin studies have estimated that around two-thirds of the variance in obesity is genetic in origin. However, when we consider trends in obesity in recent years, we see that the prevalence has increased worldwide (in the USA, for example, obesity rates have increased from 12 per cent in 1991 to 19 per cent in 1999). These dramatic and rapid changes clearly indicate the influence of changing environmental factors, since it is impossible for the genetic make-up of a population to change over such short periods. Similar findings of a high apparent genetic component coupled with rapid changes in disease prevalence over time have been seen for diabetes. There are several reasons for these discrepancies. Firstly, the statistical models used to generate heritability estimates may be misleading: they can make untenable assumptions about equal similarity of the environment of monozygotic and dizygotic twins, ignore intrauterine exposures and, most importantly, ignore gene-environment and gene-gene interactions. Secondly, with shifts in the population to a higher energy intake/energy expenditure ratio, the variance between individuals can remain strongly genetically based, but overriding environmental factors will influence the population prevalence of obesity (Davey Smith and Ebrahim 2001).

Identifying candidate genes in humans

Linkage analysis

Linkage analysis can be used to determine the approximate chromosomal location of a gene by analysing whether the allele of interest is inherited with other marker alleles of known location. If two loci are situated close together on the same chromosome they are likely to be inherited together, and are said to be linked. Linkage analysis is a way of measuring how close together two loci are, since widely spaced loci on the same chromosome will not be inherited together any more often than one would expect by chance. Widely spaced markers scattered throughout the genome can be used in initial linkage analysis to identify a candidate region – this is referred to as a genome scan. This process is typically followed by linkage analysis using denser scanning of a candidate region with markers which are closer together. Affected sibling pairs are often used in linkage analysis and the hypothesis tested is that these pairs are more likely to share marker alleles which are close to the disease locus than are randomly selected unaffected sibling pairs. However, many studies of affected sibling pairs will have only affected individuals, therefore markers are tested for sharing against an expected 50 per cent of allele sharing between siblings.

Once a set of markers close to the disease susceptibility locus have been identified, the region is sequenced to look for mutations and polymorphisms which might be causing the disease of interest. This process is very labour-intensive if the region is large, so the closer the markers are to the disease region the better. Linkage analysis and sequencing were used to pinpoint the breast cancer susceptibility genes

BRCA1 and BRCA2 to specific regions on chromosomes 17 and 13 respectively, and to identify mutations causing the increased breast cancer risk.

Identification of candidate genes from functionality data

Now that the human genome has been fully sequenced and many genes have been characterized, it is possible to select candidate genes for a disease of interest by identifying those which contribute to biological pathways leading to disease. Once candidate genes have been identified it is sometimes possible to then identify polymorphisms in these genes posted on the internet, or later published in scientific journals, and to carry out association studies to determine whether certain polymorphisms are more common among individuals with the disease. There are many databases, such as those provided by the National Center for Biotechnology Information (www.ncbi.nlm.nih.gov), which can serve as tools in this process. Alternatively, novel polymorphisms may also be detected by direct sequencing of the gene in the laboratory.

Population-based studies of genetic factors for complex diseases

For complex diseases or phenotypes, although there may be evidence of familial aggregation, they do not segregate in a Mendelian manner and individual alleles are neither necessary nor sufficient for the disease of interest. In these circumstances identification of causative genes has been problematic (Keaveney 2002). Epidemiological studies of the association between polymorphic loci and disease have been widely used in an attempt to identify variants, which confer susceptibility to complex diseases. If an allele is causal, the frequency of this allele will be greater among those who develop the disease than among the general population. The design of such studies is essentially the same as any aetiological epidemiological study (see Chapter 6). Genetic polymorphisms are simply substituted for environmental factors. DNA for use in these studies can be obtained from blood, tissue, saliva, urine or other biological material.

Types of study

Cohort

An outline of the cohort design can be found in Chapter 6. The cohort design has not been as widely used to look for genes for complex diseases as the case-control design. The main reason for this is that it is necessary to collect biological samples from several thousand individuals and follow them for a long period of time (typically decades) until cases have developed. This is often viewed as inefficient, and it is difficult to ascertain enough cases for sufficient power to observe the modest genetic effects which are typical in complex diseases. However, there are now some large cohort studies in existence, which stored biological samples several years ago. Because genotypes do not change over time, retrospective assessment of genotype by disease status is now possible.

Case-control

A case-control design is much more efficient for assessing gene-disease associations than a cohort disease (Clayton and McKeigue 2001). However there are several drawbacks with this design including survivor bias and selection of controls. If the allele of interest is associated with disease survival, then retrospective selection of cases could lead to an underestimation of the effect of the allele in disease pathology. Also, because of the possibility of confounding by ethnicity (population stratification), controls must be selected from the source population of the cases. Finding a representative control group is difficult because there is likely to be variation in allele frequencies even within ethnic groups, depending on ancestral origin, but this may not be apparent in the recruitment phase of a study.

Case-sibling

To overcome the potential problem of population stratification, discordant sibling pairs can be used as controls. However, because most complex diseases are age-dependent, an eligible sibling should have reached the age at which the case developed the disease, which will restrict the sample to twins or older siblings. The use of older siblings can be problematic in the analysis of gene-environment interactions if there are secular changes in exposure levels. Also, because cases and their siblings are more likely to share genotypes than two random members of the general population, the use of sibling controls is approximately half as efficient as the use of population controls. It may also be difficult to find a sufficient number of case-sibling pairs if the disease is rare.

Case-parent trios

In the case-parent design, cases and their parents are genotyped, but the parents themselves are not the controls. Instead, hypothetical pseudo-siblings are constructed using the other three genotypes, which could have been transmitted from the parents to the case, but were not. The case-pseudo siblings are then analysed as a 1:3 case-control design. This design does not suffer from loss of efficiency as does the case-sibling design, but it does require that DNA is available from both parents for genotyping, which may be a problem when looking at diseases of middle and old age.

Case-only

Case-only studies can be used to investigate gene-environment interactions if the genetic variant and the environmental exposure are unrelated in the source population. If an association exists between a polymorphism and an environmental exposure among cases, this suggests that there is a gene-environment interaction on the multiplicative scale. The simplest scenario is if an environmental factor only influences disease risk among individuals with a particular genotype. The advantage of using a case-only design is that it removes the problem of recruiting a control group, which is representative of the general population, and hence the problem of population stratification. A case-only study is also more efficient than a case-control study because the statistical uncertainty within the control group is removed from the equation. However, case-only studies cannot be used to look at the main effects of genes.

What does an association between a polymorphism and disease mean?

Many positive associations of polymorphisms and disease can now be found in the literature, but a large proportion of these findings are not consistently replicated. To explore why this is so it is important to understand why a positive association

> **Box 19.4   Reasons for finding a positive association between a polymorphism and disease (Colhoun et *al.* 2003)**
>
> * The genetic variant is on the causal pathway for the disease
> * The genetic variant is in linkage disequilibrium with the disease-causing allele.
> * Confounding by population admixture (population stratification) has occurred.
> * The association is a false positive due to chance.

between a genetic marker and a disease may arise (Colhoun *et al.* 2003) (see Box 19.4).

The genetic variant is on the causal pathway for the disease

When carrying out genetic association studies one would ideally like to have some criteria to determine whether the association detected is causal. Bradford Hill presented guidelines to assess causality in epidemiology in 1965. These were: strength; consistency; specificity; temporality; biological gradient; biological plausibility; coherence with previous knowledge; experimental evidence; and reasoning by analogy. While these guidelines were not written with genetic studies in mind and cannot be applied strictly to genetic association studies (Page *et al.* 2003), they do go some way in helping us to understand whether a particular genetic variant is causal.

Strength

Many genes, which confer susceptibility to complex diseases, play a minor role individually. For example, the odds ratio for lung cancer among individuals who carry a deletion in the glutathione S-transferase carcinogen detoxification gene is around 1.17 (95 per cent confidence interval = 1.07–1.27) compared to individuals who do not have this deletion (Benhamou *et al.* 2002). Hence, for complex diseases one would not necessarily expect the strength of association to be large for individual genes, but the strength of the association in a sufficiently large study may give some indication of the importance of the gene in that particular disease.

Consistency

Many genetic associations found in the literature are not consistently replicated (Hirschhorn *et al.* 2002). One way to test for replication and examine heterogeneity between studies is to carry out a systematic review or meta-analysis of the available studies. The Human Genome Epidemiology Network database is one site where published reviews may be found (www.cdc.gov/genomics/hugenet/reviews.htm), and provides guidelines for individuals wishing to carry out a review in this field.

Specificity

For monogenic disorders such as cystic fibrosis, it is possible to show that the candidate gene is specific for the disease in question. However, as mentioned previously, for complex diseases genetic variants are often neither necessary nor sufficient. Many genes have a key role in several biological pathways and may therefore be implicated in a lot of different diseases. Also it is often interactions between many genes and environmental factors within several different biological pathways which ultimately lead to disease.

Temporality

Temporality as defined by Bradford Hill (1965) does not apply to genetic factors. He was referring to the presence of the risk factor prior to the manifestation of disease, to control for the possibility of reverse causation. Since an individual's genotype is defined at birth this must always be the case when looking at genes as risk factors.

Biological gradient

Where the disease model is a co-dominant one, a greater disease risk should be observed among individuals who are homozygous for the 'at risk' allele versus heterozygotes. For example, individuals who are heterozygous for the factor V Leiden mutation have a 3–8 fold increased risk for venous thrombosis, but this rises to a 30–140 fold increased risk for homozygous individuals (Vandenbroucke *et al.* 1996) A biological gradient may also be seen by severity of mutation. For example, muscular dystrophies range from the severe Duchenne muscular dystrophy to the milder Becker muscular dystrophy. Mapping and molecular genetic studies indicate that they are the result of different mutations in the dystrophin gene, where Duchenne muscular dystrophy mutations are more severe and usually result in a severely truncated protein (Koenig *et al.* 1989).

Biological plausibility

Genes which are known to be involved in biological pathways important for the disease of interest are good candidates for assessing genetic susceptibility. Within these genes, polymorphisms which confer some functional change to the biological pathway of interest are more likely to be causal. Functional variants are usually in the coding (exons) or promoter region of the gene where they lead to a change in the resultant protein which has a demonstrable effect on the intermediate phenotype and tend to be conserved cross-species.

Coherence with previous knowledge, experimental evidence and reasoning by analogy

These criteria refer to collecting prior knowledge, which relates to the gene-disease association of interest, and determining whether the association found is consistent with this knowledge. Such information may be available from a range of sources: mechanistic studies using animals, cell lines or tissue culture, epidemiological studies, collection of spatial and temporal data etc. In short, all information available on the disease pathway and polymorphism of interest can be used to determine whether an association is causal.

Prior to concluding that there is a causal relationship between the gene of interest and disease, even in light of the above, one should consider the three other possible explanations for finding an association, as follows.

The genetic variant is in linkage disequilibrium with the disease-causing allele

Linkage disequilibrium is the non-random association between the alleles at two genetic loci. In biological terms it implies that the two loci are close together on the same chromosome and thus segregate together more often than one would predict by chance. In an association study, if the studied allele is in linkage disequilibrium with the causal allele, an association between the studied allele and disease may arise, because the alleles are co-segregating. However, this can still be informative with respect to the eventual identification of the causal allele.

Confounding by population admixture (population stratification)

Allele frequencies can differ widely by population, as does disease incidence and prevalence, hence cohort and case-control studies using unrelated individuals as controls may be confounded by ethnicity (Cardon and Palmer 2003). This phenomenon is known as population stratification. Since there are often large differences in allele frequencies within broad racial groupings which are used to define populations in genetic studies, population stratification may be an important problem. However, in order for substantial bias to arise in the study due to population stratification, there must be variation in the frequency of the allele being considered across ethnic groups and variation in disease risk, which is unrelated to the allele of interest. The use of family controls may overcome this problem, although such studies may experience other problems such as selection bias and reduced efficiency. Other methods to overcome population stratification include carrying out genome-wide analysis using methods such as genomic control and structured association (see Box 19.5).

Box 19.5   Laboratory methods for detecting population admixture (Devlin et al. 2001)

- **Genomic control** tests multiple polymorphisms throughout the genome, only some of which are pertinent to the disease of interest. The degree of overdispersion generated by population sub-structure can be estimated and taken into account.
- **Structured association** assumes that the sampled population, while heterogeneous, is composed of sub-populations that are themselves homogeneous. By using multiple polymorphisms throughout the genome, sampled individuals are probabilistically assigned to these latent sub-populations.

The association is a false positive due to chance

There are estimated to be more than 15 million single nucleotide polymorphisms, with a frequency of greater than 1 per cent in at least one population, in the human genome. There are also a large number of potential outcomes including sub-categories of disease, plus there are a large number of potential sub-group stratifications one could use to explore the data. All of this gives rise to many thousands of potential gene-disease or gene-phenotype associations that could be tested in a single study. Given the fact that most studies published to date are extremely small (less than 200 cases), false positives are inevitable. To overcome this problem, increased statistical stringency is recommended and larger studies are being set up, collaborative efforts between investigators of several different studies are being established, and meta-analyses are appearing in the literature.

Mendelian randomization

While most genetic association studies are set up to look at whether genetic variants cause the disease of interest, genes can also be used as a tool in epidemiology to determine whether a particular environmental exposure is a risk factor for disease, to elucidate mechanistic pathways between an environmental exposure and disease, and to improve exposure-disease estimates.

Associations between modifiable exposures and disease seen in observational epidemiological studies are often confounded and thus yield misleading inferences. This is particularly true of lifestyle factors, because components are highly inter-correlated and socially patterned. However, Mendelian randomization provides one method for assessing the causal nature of some environmental exposures, through investigating genetic variant-disease associations that are not generally susceptible to the reverse causation or confounding which may distort interpretations of conventional observational studies (Davey Smith and Ebrahim 2003, 2004). The concept is based on the fact that the inheritance of a genetic trait is independent of the inheritance of other traits, with the exception of genes which are in linkage disequibrium. Genetic variants exist which either influence the level of, or mirror the biological effects of, modifiable environmental exposures, which in turn alter disease risk. These variants should therefore themselves be related to disease to the extent predicted by their influence on exposure. Common polymorphisms that have a well-characterized biological function can therefore be used to study the effect of a suspected exposure on disease risk. Thus Mendelian randomization provides new opportunities to test causality, and demonstrates how investment in the human genome project may contribute to understanding and preventing the adverse effects on human health of modifiable exposures.

Examples of Mendelian randomization

Agricultural workers exposed to sheep dips containing organophosphates attribute a variety of symptoms of poor health to this exposure but there have been claims that such attribution is false and may reflect secondary gain from compensation or paid early retirement on health grounds. Thus it is difficult to obtain reliable evidence in this area, and randomized controlled trials are not feasible. People who become cases in studies of health-related outcomes of organophosphate exposure generally know that the exposure is hypothesized to cause health problems, and it is thus difficult, if not impossible, to conduct unbiased case-control studies. The enzyme, paraoxonase, deactivates a potentially toxic component found in many sheep dips. There is a polymorphism in the gene encoding this enzyme which results in different isoforms with differing biological activity. A study was carried out to determine whether the component of sheep dip that is detoxified by paraoxonase does cause symptoms of ill health among people exposed to sheep dip (Cherry et al. 2002). Among a group of people, all of whom had been exposed to sheep dip, a higher proportion of those reporting symptoms were found to be poor detoxifiers. Since it is unlikely that genotype is related to potential confounding factors, to the tendency to report symptoms differentially, or to a desire for compensation or early retirement, these findings provide evidence that there is a causal effect of the sheep dip exposure on health outcomes.

Another example of the use of genetic studies to elucidate mechanistic pathways between exposure and disease is illustrated by looking at alcohol intake, the ALDH2 gene polymorphism and esophageal cancer. Alcohol drinking is an established risk factor for oesophageal cancer, and exposure to high levels of acetaldehyde, the principle metabolite of alcohol, is hypothesized to be responsible for the increased cancer risk. The major enzyme responsible for the elimination of acetaldehyde is ALDH2. In some populations, including Japanese and Chinese, the ALDH2 gene is polymorphic and an individual's genotype at this locus determines blood acetaldehyde concentrations after drinking. A single point mutation in the ALDH2 gene has resulted in the ALDH2*2 allele. The resultant protein has an amino acid substitution, an inactive sub-unit and an inability to metabolize acetaldehyde. Individuals who are homozygous for the ALDH2*2 allele are characterized by a facial flushing and other unpleasant symptoms after consumption of alcohol which prevents them from heavy drinking. Along with heavy alcohol intake, smoking is also a known risk factor for oesphageal cancer, and as these factors tend to co-segregate in individuals, in that heavy drinkers tend to smoke and vice versa, it is therefore difficult to obtain an accurate, unconfounded, estimate of risk associated with alcohol intake. However, the ALDH2 genotype, while influencing alcohol intake, is not associated with smoking and hence this can be used as a surrogate for alcohol drinking to assess the independent importance of this factor. There is strong evidence that the ALDH2 heterozygote genotype increases oesophageal cancer risk, at a given alcohol intake level, and this is due to markedly increased acetaldehyde levels among ALDH2 heterozygotes compared with ALDH2*1, thus supporting the hypothesis that acetaldehyde plays an important role in oesophageal carcinogenesis. However, ALDH2*2 homozygotes are protected against oesophageal cancer, because these individuals do not drink.

Some genetic disease models and screening for genetic disease

Monogenic diseases

There are several hundred rare diseases caused by mutations at single gene loci, which collectively account for a significant proportion of infant mortality and morbidity in the developed world. About 5 per cent of live births are expected to carry a single-gene disorder or a condition with an important genetic component, and about 3 per cent will have a major birth defect with some genetic component (Botto and Mastroiacovo 2000). These individuals will have a high incidence of premature death and hospitalization, and account for a high proportion of health care costs. Collectively, genetic abnormalities cause about 10 per cent of all childhood mortality in Britain.

Genetic conditions are no less prevalent among infants born in developing countries, although the relative contribution of genetics to infant mortality is less because of the high incidence of diseases caused by poverty, infections and malnutrition. The infrastructure for surveillance of genetic disease is generally also poor. However, the prevalence of specific diseases does differ between distinct populations due to founder effects, environmental selection, consanguinity and migration, which are discussed below. In northern European Caucasian populations, phenylketonuria and cystic fibrosis are prevalent at high frequencies relative to other populations (see Table 19.1) whereas haemoglobin diseases and thalassaemia are common in sub-Saharan Africa, where carrier status offers some protection against malaria.

Consanguinity

Consanguinity occurs when two parents have one or more recent ancestors in common, and arises from marriage between relatives. In some regions and cultures consanguineous marriages are common; in Southern India, for example, 25–60 per cent of all marriages are consanguineous and this practice contributes to economic

Table 19.1   Population frequency of some monogenic diseases in the UK

Disease	Gene	Prevalence in UK population	Genetic model
Cystic fibrosis	CFTR	1/2500	Autosomal recessive, fully penetrant
Huntington's disease	IT15	1/15,000	Autosomal dominant, fully penetrant, disease manifest in adulthood
Fragile X	FMR-1	1/4000 males and 1/8000 females	X-linked, fully penetrant in males, approx. 50% penetrance in females
Phenylketonuria	PKU	1/12,000	Autosomal recessive, fully penetrant
Muscular dystrophy	Dystrophin	1/5600 males (Duchenne) 1/18000 males (Becker)	X-linked, recessive condition, fully penetrant

and family stability. However, marriage between relatives increases the likelihood of two copies of rare autosomal recessive alleles being inherited in the offspring and is associated with stillbirth, infant death and severe congenital abnormalities.

Founder effects

In populations which were founded by a small number of individuals and which have experienced restricted mobility for many generations, there are often clusters of monogenic diseases. An example of this is the high incidence of Tay-Sachs and Gauchers disease among Ashkenazi Jews.

Multifactorial/complex diseases

Unlike the disease models above, which arise from the segregation of alleles at a single locus, multifactorial diseases are the result of a combination of environmental and genetic factors. Such diseases – for example, coronary heart disease and many cancers – are the major causes of human morbidity and mortality, and while genetic models for these diseases are complex and currently limited, genes nevertheless are still likely to play an important role (see Table 19.2).

Allelic structure of common disease

Diseases which are largely multifactorial can be caused by severe mutations in a small sub-set of cases, and analysis of the families of these cases will identify a monogenic model. For example, familial Alzheimer's disease is caused by one of

Table 19.2   Population prevalence and heritability of some common multifactorial diseases in the UK

Disease	Heritability	Lifetime risk
Alzheimer's disease	0.74	10–12%
Breast cancer	0.27	8% in women
Colorectal cancer	0.35	4%
Coronary heart disease	0.57 among males 0.38 among females	12%

several rare mutations in one of three genes, and a small proportion of breast and colorectal cases have a strong family history due to a genetic mutations segregating within the family. Familial hypercholesterolaemia, with an autosomal dominant inheritance, greatly increases the risk of premature coronary heart disease. But, essentially, several genes are involved in the causal pathways of multifactorial diseases. There are in fact two extreme models which are usually outlined for complex disease traits, and these relate to the number of disease-causing variants (Smith and Lusis 2002).

Model 1 is referred to as the common disease/common variant (CD/CV) approach, which stipulates that common polymorphisms at a handful of loci cause disease. One example of this is the increased risk of heart disease, which is associated with a common allele of the MTHFR gene present at around 30 per cent in most populations (Kim and Becker 2003).

Model 2 is the common disease/rare variant (CD/RV) approach, in which one of many rare mutations at different loci, either within a single gene or within many genes, causes the disease. In the small proportion of breast cancer patients with a strong family history, there are many different disease-causing mutations, such that mutations are almost family-specific.

These models are very important for screening and individualized medicine. If a few alleles at a small number of loci are responsible for disease, then detection will be easy, whereas if a large number of alleles are responsible then screening will be very laborious and expensive. However, as in the breast cancer example, it is likely that most complex diseases are the result of a mixture of the two extreme models.

Genetic screening for disease

For many diseases with a strong genetic component there is still no cure despite recent progress in gene therapy techniques. Prenatal testing is therefore the only possibility of preventing these diseases. For classic monogenic diseases inherited in a Mendelian manner, risk can be predicted based on inheritance within the family. High-risk families are referred to a genetic councillor whose role is to advise individuals of the likely risk to themselves or their offspring, and to outline the alternatives for disease prevention. It is however possible to screen for genetic mutations using DNA samples. Most genetic testing carried out to date has been for single-gene variants which cause disease in high-risk families, such as cystic fibrosis. This is often in the form of prenatal or preconceptual testing for couples who want to have a child but have some history of genetic disease in their family. Newborn screening programmes also test babies for congenital disorders such as phenyl-ketonuria, galactosemia and hypothyroidism, which can be treated if detected before the onset of the disease. It is however also possible to screen individuals for mutations associated with adult disease long before the onset of any symptoms, such as Huntington's disease and breast cancer.

Criteria for population genetic risk screening

Due to the emerging wealth of data on genetic susceptibility to disease and to the development of tests for detecting high-risk individuals, the subject of genetic screening has received a great deal of attention. An unfavourable result from a genetic test can have a considerable impact on an individual's well-being even if they are asymptomatic for the disease in question. Certain factors should be considered prior to the implementation of genetic testing (see Box 19.6).

> **Box 19.6   The implementation of genetic testing in a population**
>
> - **The likelihood of the individual having the disease genotype or being carrier for the disease:**
>   informed by the population prevalence of disease and the disease allele and the individual's family history of the disease
> - **The severity of the disease/trait**
>   prenatal testing for sex of fetus is highly questionable
> - **Knowledge of the genetic model**
>   number of genes involved
>   dominance and penetrance
>   well characterized, disease-causing mutations identified
> - **Cost-effectiveness of testing**
>   population prevalence of the mutation and the disease
>   cost of treatment for the disease or caring for an individual with the disease
> - **Penetrance**
>   degree to which the presence of the genetic variant predicts disease
> - **The natural history of the disease**
>   age on onset and progression predicted by the genetic variant should be well understood
> - **Treatments available**
>   must be an effective and acceptable intervention
> - **Harm associated with genetic testing**
>   potential for psychological harm to an individual knowing their genetic status
> - **Infrastructure for pre- and post-test education**
>   investment in genetic medical services
>   possible role for primary care services

Case studies: to screen or not to screen?

Preconceptual carrier status screening

Cystic fibrosis

Cystic fibrosis (CF) is the most common autosomal recessive condition in the UK, and 1 in 25 individuals carry a mutation in the CF gene. It is a serious and progressive disease with no cure, although treatment has improved in recent years and has increased the average life expectancy to over 30 years. The disease is characterized by severe respiratory problems, inadequate pancreatic function (caused by accumulation of mucus) and elevated levels of chloride in the sweat, and most males with CF are sterile. Four common mutations have been show to account for around 90 per cent of all cystic fibrosis cases. Screening for cystic fibrosis is therefore possible. In the UK, neonatal screening for CF began throughout Scotland at the start of February 2003, and although coverage in England is currently only around 20 per cent of the country, there are plans to introduce this programme throughout England. The rationale for neonatal screening is that very early detection and treatment may improve outcomes for children with CF, although there is some controversy over this. However, neonatal screening for CF is considered cost-effective compared to traditional diagnosis of CF. Carrier screening at the population level is also feasible, and would go some way to preventing the occurrence of the disease. The aim of carrier screening is to identify women and their partners who are both carriers. These couples have a one in four chance of having an infant with the disease, and can be referred to a genetic councillor who can advise them of their options for disease prevention, including in-vitro fertilization and pre-implantation screening of the resulting embryos. At the moment, CF screening is not offered on a population level in the UK, but individuals who have a family history of the disease can opt for screening.

Newborn screening

Phenylketonuria (PKU)

Phenylketonuria is characterized by a deficiency of phenylalanine hydroxylase, due to a mutation in the gene encoding this enzyme. This leads to high blood levels of phenylalanine which are toxic to the developing brain. Chronic exposure to phenylalanine leads to microcephaly, learning difficulties and epilepsy. Phenylalanine is an essential amino acid, but dietary restriction can lower levels and markedly improve the outcome. While the incidence of this condition in the UK is rare, the severity of the disease and the fact treatment can be very effective, provided it is given from birth, have led to screening of all newborns by taking a blood spot from a heel prick, and measuring the phenotype associated with disease. Screening for phenylketonuria was introduced in the UK over 30 years ago.

Screening adults

Breast cancer

For at least 95 per cent of breast cancer there is not a clear inherited genetic susceptibility, although genetic factors have been shown to play a role. However, about 5 per cent of breast cancer sufferers have a strong hereditary predisposition to the disease, with multiple family members affected, often at an early age. Inherited mutations in one of two genes, BRCA1 and BRCA2, are responsible for the strong breast cancer susceptibility in most of these 'breast cancer families'. BRCA1 mutations account for about 40–50 per cent and BRCA2 for 20–30 per cent. Carriers of these mutations are also at increased risk for several other cancers, particularly ovarian cancer. The cancer susceptibility caused by mutations in the BRCA1 and BRCA2 genes is inherited in a dominant fashion. BRCA gene mutations are highly penetrant, although this appears to be dependent on family history, and is probably a consequence of the severity of the mutation. In families with multiple affected members (who often develop disease at an early age), women carrying BRCA1 or BRCA2 mutations have an approximately 80 per cent chance of developing breast cancer by the age of 70 (normal risk about 8 per cent); the lifetime risk of ovarian cancer in BRCA1 carriers is around 50 per cent and in BRCA2 carriers around 30 per cent (population risk 1–2 per cent). Population-based studies suggest that the risks to mutation carriers without a strong family history are lower (breast cancer risk about 65 per cent for BRCA1 mutation carriers and 45 per cent for BRCA2; ovarian cancer risk about 40 per cent for BRCA1 and 10 per cent for BRCA2). Because of this difference in penetrance among carriers of BRCA1/2 mutations, it is difficult to predict lifetime risk, and hence to offer informed interventions. Studies have found that among carriers opting for prophylactic mastectomy, the number of life years gained compared to those who opted for surveillance alone was just 2.9 years among those with a low penetrance mutation (Griffith *et al.* 2004). This raises the question of the value of screening for BRCA1/2 mutations over close surveillance of individuals with a familiy history. A further problem is that there are so many mutations in BRCA1 and BRCA2, screening is almost family specific, and in most cases it is necessary to sequence the genes rather than looking for common SNPs, which makes screening very expensive.

Factor V Leiden

The factor V Leiden mutation is a risk factor for deep vein thrombosis, present at a frequency of around 5 per cent among white individuals, although frequencies vary widely between populations. Factor V is a blood clotting (coagulation) factor; the mutation, a single G (guanine) to A (adenine) base substitution (G1691A), causes a change in amino acid from arginine to glutamine at position 506 (Arg506Gln) in the factor V protein. This mutation prevents the inactivation of factor V by activated protein C (APC), a component of the anticoagulant system. The anticoagulant system functions to limit blood clotting; dysfunction of the system can result in excess clotting, which in turn can lead to venous thromboembolism. Heterozygous individuals have a 3–8 fold increased risk for venous thrombosis, but this rises to a 30–140 fold increased risk for homozygous individuals. However, the risk increases still further among users of oral contraceptives.

Vandenbroucke *et al.* (1996) estimated that the incidence of deep vein thrombosis in the legs among women in the Netherlands who did not use contraceptives and did not have the mutation was 0.8 per 10,000 women years, increasing to 3 per 10,000 among oral contraceptive users and to 5.7 per 10,000 among carriers of the factor V Leiden mutation. However, among women who were both oral contraceptive users and carriers of the mutation the incidence was 28.5 per 10,000 women years. Some controversy has therefore arisen over whether or not women should be screened prior to being given oral contraceptives. The main objections are that screening may deny oral contraception to around 5 per cent of women, which may led to other problems such as unwanted pregnancies. Also, because death from pulmonary embolus is rare, a large number of women would have to be screened to prevent one death, which would be very expensive (see Table 19.3).

Huntington's disease

Huntington's disease is an incurable neurodegenerative disease, which is manifest in middle age. The disease is autosomal dominant and is caused by a tri-nucleotide repeat expansion in the IT15 gene. While it is possible to screen for this disease, knowledge of the fact that one is going to develop an incurable and severe disease later in life is likely to cause psychological damage and has led to suicide in some cases. There is a 50 per cent risk to any offspring if one parent is found to be

Table 19.3 Risk of venous thromboembolism among women with the factor V Leiden mutation and by oral contraceptive use

Factor V Leiden	Oral contraceptives	Relative risk	Incidence of venous thromboembolism[a]
–	–	1.0	0.8
–	+	3.7	3.0
+	–	6.9	5.7
+	+	34.7	28.5

[a]Incidence per 10,000 women per year.
Source: Vandenbroucke *et al.* (1996)

affected, or a 25 per cent risk if one of their grandparents is affected. Prenatal testing can prevent the disease in any future offspring. However, because the parents' genetic status can be inferred from prenatal testing in the offspring, this can cause conflict among high-risk individuals and their partners, who are planning a family (Tassicker *et al.* 2003).

Individualized medicine

As well as predicting disease risk, polymorphisms can affect the way an individual metabolizes drugs and responds to treatment. These include polymorphisms in genes which code for proteins that bind to a drug and deliver it to its target tissue, or enzymes which activate or detoxify a drug, or receptors which are the target sites for the drug, or components of the immune system which control drug tolerance. All may influence an individual's response to drug treatments.

These polymorphisms lead to differences in the dose of drugs required to evoke a similar response between individuals. For example, warfarin is a widely used anticoagulant metabolized by the P450 enzyme CYP2C9. A small proportion of individuals have variant alleles which reduce the enzyme's efficiency and its ability to clear warfarin from the body. These individuals, if treated with warfarin at the standard dose, can suffer from severe bleeding.

It is thought that most serious adverse drug reactions are caused by common polymorphisms in genes of metabolic enzymes. Drug companies are therefore now developing kits to screen for polymorphisms prior to treatment. The idea of tailor-made treatments, which limit side-effects and depend on an individual's genotype, offers a seductive promise of better treatments, and would provide a more tangible expression of the benefits of the human genome project and the associated genetic research than simply detecting polymorphisms with low disease predictability. Individualized medicine is, not surprisingly, a fast-growing area of research (Collins and McKusic 2001; Abbot 2003).

The example of the Bcr-Ab1 gene that causes Philadelphia chromosome-positive chronic myeloid leukaemia (CML) is widely cited as an example of the advent of personalized medicine, as in this case, the drug Imatinib – a Bcr-Ab1 tyrosine-kinase signal-transduction inhibitor – has proved effective in treating CML (Kantarjian *et al.* 2002). However, it might be more appropriate to consider this as an example of the application of genomics to diagnosis, and assign the appriopriate treatment to an aetiological and pathologically distinct type of leukaemias. A wide range of currently poorly phenotyped conditions may turn out to be better characterized by exploiting genetic variation.

Including genetic polymorphisms in coronary risk scores has been promoted as providing better prediction of coronary risk than existing scores based on conventional risk factors (Topol and Lauer 2003). However, it is highly improbable that genetic polymorphisms, despite being causally associated with cardiovascular disease, will be useful in risk scores as the associations that are being found are very weak and have negligible predictive power for an individual (Haga *et al.* 2003).

In the case of statin treatment to lower blood cholesterol and thereby prevent coronary heart disease, two variant forms of the HMG-CoA reductase gene have been discovered that are associated with differential response to statin treatment (Chasman *et al.* 2004). Large reductions in blood cholesterol of 21 and 26 per cent in LDL-cholesterol in those with and without these variants were found, which would be expected to give substantial protection against coronary heart disease. Commentators on this work interpreted these findings as constituting statin 'non-responder' status (Haga and Burke 2004), and hailed these findings as strong clinical evidence that there may be promise in personalized medicine.

These examples illustrate the 'hype' that surrounds so much of the post-human genome attempt to maintain interest in and funding for the enterprise. One of the key roles of public health and health service researchers is to attempt to separate this inevitable enthusiasm from attempts to promote new genetic tests on individuals and populations without sufficiently rigorous evaluation.

Conclusions

Genetics is an area of research which is rapidly developing, and discoveries are informing our understanding, not only of rare diseases caused by mutations in single genes, but also common complex diseases such as coronary heart disease and many cancers, which have a significant genetic component. Many genes causing monogenic diseases have now been identified via family studies and characterized, which has meant that preconceptual and prenatal screening is possible. In the future it is expected that technology will advance such that it will be possible to correct defective genes at the cellular level. However, the greatest impact on population health is likely to come from the identification of genes which are involved in complex diseases. Population-based epidemiological studies of candidate genes are now widely used to detect genes which confer susceptibility to disease, and it is also possible to use genes as a tool to identify environmental causes and elucidate biological mechanisms of multifactorial disease. Although these studies are not without problems, it is likely that large, better-designed studies will in future offer invaluable insights which will lead to the improved health of individuals and populations.

Key points

- Multifactorial diseases are the result of a combination of many environmental and genetic factors. Such diseases, including heart disease and cancer, are the major causes of human morbidity and mortality.

- The degree of familial clustering is often the first indicator as to whether a disease has a strong genetic component.

- It is possible to select candidate genes for a disease of interest by identifying those which contribute to biological pathways leading to disease and to carry out association studies to determine whether certain polymorphisms of these genes are more common among individuals with the disease.

- Many positive associations of polymorphisms and disease can now be found in the literature, but a large proportion of these findings are not consistently replicated.

- A positive association between a genetic marker and a disease may arise due to the genetic variant being a cause of the disease; the variant being in linkage disequilibrium with the disease-causing variant; population stratification; or chance.

- Common polymorphisms that have a well-characterized biological function can be used to study the effect of an environmental exposure on disease risk – 'Mendelian randomization'.

- Most serious adverse drug reactions are likely to be caused by common polymorphisms in genes of metabolic enzymes, and characterization of these genes will lead to individualized treatments in the future.

- Genetic testing has traditionally been restricted to monogenic diseases where the disease model is well understood, but this is has been extended to individuals at high risk of multifactorial diseases such as breast cancer.

- Certain factors should be considered prior to the implementation of genetic testing, including likely risk; severity of the disease; understanding of the genetic model; penetrance of the gene; and potential harm to the patient.

Further reading

Khoury, M.J., Burke, W. and Thomson, E.J. (eds) (2000) *Genetics and Public Health in the 21st Century*. Oxford: Oxford University Press.

Khoury, M.J., Little, J. and Burke, W. (eds) (2003) *Human Genome Epidemiology*. Oxford: Oxford University Press.

Lewin, B. (1997) *Genes*. Oxford: Oxford University Press.

Thomas, D.C. (2004) *Statistical Methods in Genetic Epidemiology*. Oxford: Oxford University Press.

References

Abbot, A. (2003) With your genes? Take one of these, three times a day, *Nature*, 425: 760–2.

Benhamou, S., Lee, W.J. and Alexandrie, A.K. (2002) Meta- and pooled analyses of the effects of glutathione S-transferase M1 polymorphisms and smoking on lung cancer risk, *Carcinogenesis*, 23: 1343–50.

Botto, L.D. and Mastroiacovo, P. (2000) Surveillance for birth defects and genetic disease, in M.J. Khoury, W. Burke and E.J. Thomson (eds) *Genetics and Public Health in the 21st Century*. Oxford: Oxford University Press.

Cardon, L.R. and Palmer, L. (2003) Population stratification and spurious allelic association, *Lancet*, 361: 598–604.

Chasman, D.I., Posada, D., Subrahmanyan, L. *et al.* (2004) Pharmacogenetic study of statin therapy and cholesterol reduction, *Journal of the American Medical Association*, 291: 2821–7.

Cherry, N., Mackness, M., Durrington, P. *et al.* (2002) Paraoxonase (PON1) polymorphisms in farmers attributing ill health to sheep dip, *Lancet*, 359: 763–4.

Claus, E.B., Risch, N. and Thompson, W.D. (1991) Genetic analysis of breast cancer in the cancer and steroid hormone study, *American Journal of Human Genetics*, 48: 232–42.

Clayton, D. and McKeigue, P.M. (2001) Epidemiological methods for studying genes and environmental factors in complex diseases, *Lancet*, 358: 1356–60.

Colhoun, H.M., McKeigue, P.M. and Davey Smith, G. (2003) Problems of reporting genetic associations with complex outcomes, *Lancet*, 361: 865–72.

Collins, F.S. and McKusick, V.A. (2001) Implications of the human genome project for medical science, *Journal of the American Medical Association*, 285: 540–4.

Davey Smith, G. and Ebrahim, S. (2001) Epidemiology – is it time to call it a day?, *International Journal of Epidemiology*, 30: 1–11.

Davey Smith, G. and Ebrahim, S. (2003) Mendelian randomization: can genetic epidemiology contribute to understanding environmental determinants of disease?, *International Journal of Epidemiology*, 32: 1–22.

Davey Smith, G. and Ebrahim, S. (2004) Mendelian randomization: prospects, potentials, and limitations, *International Journal of Epidemiology*, 33: 30–42.

Devlin, B., Roeder, K. and Wasserman, L. (2001) Genomic control: a new approach to genetic-based association studies, *Theoretical Population Biology*, 60: 155–66.

Griffith, G.L., Edwards, R.T. and Gray, J. (2004) Cancer genetics services: a systematic review of the economic evidence and issues, *British Journal of Cancer*, 90: 1697–703.

Haga, S.B. and Burke, W. (2004) Using pharmacogenetics to improve drug safety and efficacy, *Journal of the American Medical Association*, 291: 2869–71.

Haga, S.B., Khoury, M.J. and Burke, W. (2003) Genomic profiling to promote a healthy lifestyle: not ready for prime time, *Nature Genetics*, 34: 347–50.

Hill, A.B. (1965) The environment and disease: association of causation? *Proceedings of the Royal Society of Medicine*, 58: 295–300.

Hirschhorn, J.N., Lohmueller, K., Byrne, E. and Hirschhorn, K. (2002) A comprehensive review of genetic association studies, *Genetics in Medicine*, 4: 45–61.

Kantarjian, H., Sawyers, C., Hochhaus, A. *et al.* (for the International STI571 CML Study Group) (2002) Hematologic and cytogenetic responses to imatinib mesylate in chronic myelogenous leukemia, *New England Journal of Medicine*, 346: 645–52.

Keaveney, B. (2002) Genetic epidemiological studies of coronary heart disease, *International Journal of Epidemiology*, 31: 730–6.

Kim, R.J. and Becker, R.C. (2003) Association between factor V Leiden, prothrombin G20210A, and methylenetetrahydrofolate reductase C677T mutations and events of the arterial circulatory system: a meta-analysis of published studies, *American Heart Journal*, 146: 948–57.

Koenig, M., Beggs, A.H., Moyer, M. *et al.* (1989) The molecular basis for Duchenne versus Becker muscular dystrophy: correlation of severity with type of deletion, *American Journal of Human Genetics*, 45: 498–506.

Korpelainen, H. (2000) Variation in the heritability and evolvability of human lifespan, *Naturwissenschaften*, 87: 566–8.

Lander, E.S. and Schork, N.J. (1994) Genetic dissection of complex traits, *Science*, 265: 2037–48.

Marenberg, M.E., Risch, N., Berkman, L.F. *et al.* (2004) Genetic susceptibility to death from coronary heart disease in a study of twins, *New England Journal of Medicine*, 330: 1041–6.

Page, G.P., George, V., Go, R.C. *et al.* (2003) 'Are we there yet?': deciding when one has demonstrated specific genetic causation in complex diseases and quantitative traits, *American Journal of Human Genetics*, 73: 711–19

Risch, N. (2001) The genetic epidemiology of cancer: interpreting family and twin studies and their implication for molecular genetic approaches, *Cancer Epidemiology Biomarkers and Prevention*, 10: 733–41.

Smith, D.J. and Lusis, A.J. (2002) The allelic structure of common disease, *Human Molecular Genetics*, 11: 2455–61.

Tassicker, R., Savulescu, J., Skene, L. *et al.* (2003) Prenatal diagnosis requests for Huntington's disease when the father is at risk and does not want to know his genetic status: clinical, legal and ethical viewpoints, *British Medical Journal*, 326: 331–3.

Topol, E.J. and Lauer, M.S. (2003) The rudimentary phase of personalised medicine: coronary risk scores, *Lancet*, 362: 1776–7

Vandenbroucke, J.P., van der Meer, F.J.M., Helmerhost, F.M. and Rosendal, F.R. (1996) Factor V Leiden: should we screen oral contraceptive users and pregnant women? *British Medical Journal*, 313: 1127–30.

Watson, J.D. and Crick, F.H.D. (1953) Structure for deoxyribose nucleic acid, *Nature*, 171: 737.

20 Tools of psychosocial biology in health care research

Andrew Steptoe

Introduction

Much health care research involves measurement of biological function. This chapter is concerned with the assessment of biological function in psychosocial research on health. The psychosocial factors studied in health care research include features of the individual's sociodemographic position (age, gender, ethnicity, socio-economic status etc.), aspects of social experience (such as social networks and social support), exposure to different types of adversity (e.g. work stress, life events, informal care-giving), family and neighbourhood factors (such as family conflict and neighbourhood social cohesion), and psychological parameters (such as depression, anxiety and hostility). Psychosocial studies in health care research are concerned with the contribution of these factors to disease causation, progression and prognosis, and the impact of psychosocial interventions on disease status and quality of life. The biological measures assessed in psychosocial research fall into three categories:

1 Biological indicators of disease states, such as blood pressure in hypertension, or airways resistance in bronchial asthma. The biological measures in this category are direct markers of the physiological dysfunction constituting the disease state, and are used in research on the role of psychosocial factors in the aetiology or prognosis of disease states, and in studies evaluating the impact of psychosocial interventions.
2 Biological markers of processes involved in the aetiology of disease. Examples include measures of vascular endothelial function, fibrinogen and C-reactive protein in the study of coronary heart disease, the concentration of CD4 lymphocytes in the study of HIV/AIDS, and the measurement of metabolites of corticosteroids and catecholamines in the investigation of obesity and insulin resistance. The biological parameters assessed in such studies are more distal to disease states than those assessed in Category 1, but nevertheless provide objective information concerning the impact of psychosocial factors on precursors of disease or on underlying physiological dysfunctions.
3 Non-specific biological markers of stress-related activation or resistance to disease. Biological measures in this category include heart rate, blood pressure, sweat gland activity, the stress hormones cortisol, adrenaline and noradrenaline, circulating lymphocyte numbers and activity, and concentrations of inflammatory cytokines and immunoglobulins. These biological variables are not assessed as

markers of specific disease states, but as more general indicators of psycho-biological activation and resistance.

Biological measures are used extensively in animal research on psychosocial factors, but this chapter will be limited to work on humans. Biological measures are assessed in three types of psychosocial study: epidemiological surveys, naturalistic monitoring studies and experimental studies. Each of these applications will be described, along with their strengths and limitations. I also discuss issues of practical measurement and interpretation for several common measures. This chapter is not exhaustive, since different areas of health care research can involve complex and sophisticated biological assessments related to specific medical conditions (Cacioppo *et al.* 2000).

I have also not included discussion of biological correlates or indicators of health behaviours in this chapter. Examples include the measurement of cotinine or exhaled carbon monoxide in the study of smoking, the use of accelerometers for assessing physical activity and the monitoring of biomarkers for alcohol intake and specific dietary nutrients. The purpose of such measures is to provide more objective information about health-related activities than is available with self-report assessments. These measures are all important, but give rise to issues of validity and reliability that go beyond psychosocial research.

Theoretical foundations of psychosocial biology

Biological processes underpin all actions and behaviours, ensuring appropriate supplies of energy to working muscle, brain and other tissues, and the maintenance of bodily functions. The body's defence mechanisms are continuously active, providing physical and chemical barriers against pathogens and invading micro-organisms, and responding to potential dangers. The foundations of psychosocial biology lie in the disturbance of these regulatory processes, and in the notion that psychosocial factors influence bodily functions and thereby lead to increased or decreased risk of illness. These influences are mediated through psychobiological pathways: the pathways through which central nervous system function activates the autonomic nervous system, neuroendocrine and immunological responses (Steptoe 1998).

There is a substantial research literature on the relationship between psychosocial factors and biological function, much of which derives from the study of the effects of acute and chronic stress (Weiner 1992; Fink 2000; Ader *et al.* 2001). Biological stress responses occur both under conditions of extreme psychosocial adversity (such as a natural disaster or assault), and when longer-term but lower-level demands exceed the individual's capacity to cope (Steptoe and Ayers 2004). Physiological stress responses encompass most of the main organ systems and regulatory processes of the body, including respiration and cardiovascular function, water balance, glucose metabolism and energy supply, blood clotting, inflammation and immune defences. These multiple components are controlled through the autonomic nervous system and neuroendocrine circuitry. During stressful encounters, the sympathetic branch of the autonomic nervous system is activated in concert with catecholamines such as adrenaline released from the medulla of the adrenal glands. The opposing parasympathetic branch of the autonomic nervous system becomes more active under conditions of conservation or behavioural withdrawal. The hypothalamic-pituitary-adrenocortical (HPA) axis is the most important neuroendocrine pathway in stress responses, although other neurotransmitters and hormone systems are also involved. Activation of the HPA axis leads to the release of cortisol in humans (corticosterone in rodents) from the adrenal cortex. The sympathoadrenal and HPA axes are interdependent, and are controlled by complex feedback loops involving the central nervous system (Sapolsky *et al.* 2000). Even short-term stressors can trigger gene expression of enzymes regulating neuroendocrine function (Sabban and Kvetnansky 2001).

The acute activation of biological variables elicited by stress is adapted for the support of vigorous physical activity and defence (fight or flight). Risk to health arises for two reasons. First, the circumstances in everyday life that provoke psychobiological responses are typically not ones in which vigorous activity is required; having an abrasive interaction with family members, or being frustrated at work by equipment breakdown do not call for high levels of energy expenditure. Consequently, the intense mobilization of biological responses is inappropriate. Second, the psychosocial factors that elicit biological responses are ubiquitous in people's lives, so repeated activation is common. In many areas of health care research it is low level, repeated, or chronic disturbance of function that is more significant than large reactions to severe but rare stressful events.

In recent years, the concept of allostatic load has become influential in understanding the chronic dysregulation of biological responses caused by psychosocial factors. This construct was introduced by Sterling and subsequently developed by McEwen (1998; McEwen and Wingfield 2003). It refers to the cumulative cost to the body of the process of achieving stability of physiological systems in the face of environmental challenge. Central to allostatic load is alteration in the activity of mediators such as the HPA axis and the sympathoadrenal system, resulting in imbalances that can increase risk to health.

A very simplified schematic description of possible manifestations of disturbed psychobiological function is shown in Figure 20.1. The graph on the left represents the normal pattern of response, with a biological system such as blood pressure or cortisol increasing in the face of challenge, then decreasing back to reference levels following termination of the stimulus. The graphs on the right summarize three types of disturbance to this response pattern (illustrated with the dotted line). In graph A, the response is heightened above normal levels, perhaps as a consequence of concurrent psychosocial adversity. For example, our group has shown that people reporting low control at work produce heightened fibrinogen responses to demanding behavioural tasks (Steptoe *et al.* 2003a), and relationships between neuroendocrine responses and social support have been described (Uchino *et al.* 1996). Heightened responsivity may in turn be associated with disease risk. Thus it has been found that high blood pressure stress reactivity, coupled with exposure to elevated life stress or work demands, predicts increased risk of hypertension and progression of subclinical atherosclerosis (Everson *et al.* 1997; Light *et al.* 1999). High levels of cortisol promote increased concentration of lipids in the circulation, accumulation of abdominal fat, impaired fertility and decalcification of bone (Weiner 1992).

In graph B, the magnitude of responses is not altered, but restitution of homoeostasis is impaired. This leads to prolongation of responses and delays in post-stress recovery. An example of this pattern comes from a study of men and women recruited from the Whitehall II epidemiological cohort to investigate the psychobiological concomitants of low socioeconomic position. The magnitude of biological responses to behavioural tasks did not differ with socioeconomic position defined by a grade of employment. However, post-stress recovery in blood pressure and in heart rate variability was impaired in lower socioeconomic status participants (Steptoe *et al.* 2002). Additionally, lower-status individuals showed prolonged increases in prothrombotic factors (plasma viscosity and Factor VIII) following termination of the behavioural challenge (Steptoe *et al.* 2003b). Recovery in cortisol and catecholamines can be delayed for several hours after stressful work (Sluiter

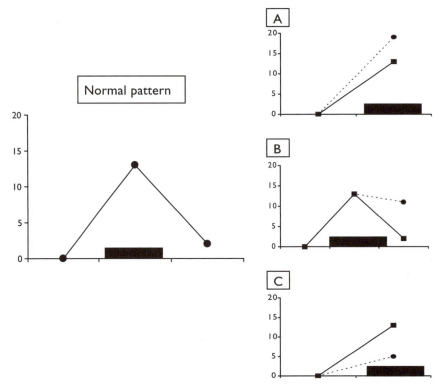

Figure 20.1 Schematic outline of patterns of biological response to behavioural or social challenge. The left panel shows the normal response pattern, and on the right three types of disturbed response are illustrated, as described in the text. The vertical axis scale is arbitrary, and could refer to a variety of responses (blood pressure, cortisol, muscle tension, immune reaction, etc.). The solid bar in each schematic illustrates the period of exposure to challenge.

et al. 2000). Heightened or prolonged cortisol responses may also lead to downregulation of immune function, rendering the individual more vulnerable to infection (Vedhara *et al.* 1999a).

Graph C illustrates a third manifestation of allostatic load, with reduced responsivity in the biological parameter, due either to changes in receptor sensitivity or depletion of physiological mediators. The best studied example is hypocortisolism, or suppressed cortisol output and responsivity (Heim *et al.* 2000a). Several clinical conditions appear to be associated with low levels of cortisol including chronic fatigue syndrome, bronchial asthma and rheumatoid arthritis. Since cortisol suppresses inflammatory responses, low levels can lead to overactivity of the immune system in autoimmune disease. The circumstances in which these different disturbances of psychobiological responses are elicited depend on a combination of the nature and duration of the challenge, and the life stage of the individual (McEwen and Wingfield 2003). Low cortisol has also been recorded in several studies of post-traumatic stress disorder (Yehuda 2002), although this pattern has not been replicated in some population-based studies (Young *et al.* 2004).

Research paradigms

There is no single 'ideal' feasible study of psychosocial biology that can definitively prove or falsify the involvement of psychobiological dysfunctions in a particular health outcome. Instead, the case depends on the convergence and aggregation of data from different types of study, each with its strengths and limitations.

Epidemiological studies

Epidemiological studies provide the core method of establishing the contribution of psychosocial factors to the development of disease, and are also used to identify the biological mediators of these associations. For example, lower socioeconomic status is associated with heightened fibrinogen, vascular inflammation and incidence of the metabolic syndrome, which in turn increase risk of coronary heart disease (Brunner et al. 1997; Hemingway et al. 2003). High levels of anger and hostility have been related to blood pressure in population studies, and may increase risk of hypertension (Jorgensen et al. 1996; Yan et al. 2003). Biological and psychosocial measures from large samples can be obtained at relatively low cost, prospective study designs can be employed and potential confounders can be taken into account statistically. However, the biological measures in epidemiological studies are generally recorded on a single occasion under resting conditions (in a clinic or medical office) that are not typical of everyday life. Such studies can provide limited information about the dynamics of biological response, or the consequences of biological activation. Factors such as time of day and nutritional state affect many measures used in psychosocial biology, and may need to be recorded to permit accurate interpretation.

Naturalistic monitoring studies

The second kind of study in psychosocial biology involves the sampling of biological variables during everyday life. Such studies take many forms, from recordings during challenging tasks such as parachuting or speaking in public, to repeated measures of blood pressure or salivary cortisol over an ordinary day. Some of these techniques are extensions of methods used in clinical investigation, such as 'Holter' monitoring of the electrocardiogram in patients with coronary disease, and the use of ambulatory blood pressure monitors for evaluating hypertension. The purpose of these methods in psychosocial research is to assess biological activity under natural conditions and to examine the covariation between everyday activities, emotions and biology. For example, one study of people with bronchial asthma and non-asthmatic controls involved repeated spirometric measurements and mood assessments several times a day for three weeks (Ritz and Steptoe 2000). Negative mood states were associated with reduced forced expiratory volume in asthmatic participants but not in controls. Multiple samples of saliva have been obtained to measure the profile of cortisol release over the day, showing that cortisol increases in response to stressful daily events (Van Eck et al. 1996). Measurements of muscle tension from surface electrodes have been made in supermarket cashiers, and have shown heightened trapezius muscle tension during work that is associated with complaints of neck and shoulder pain (Lundberg et al. 1999).

Naturalistic monitoring methods have the advantage of ecological validity, evaluating biological activity in real life rather than the artificial conditions of a laboratory or clinic. Associations between psychosocial factors and biological responses may be observed that are not detectable when single measures are taken under clinical conditions. But naturalistic methods also have limitations. First, the range of biological markers that can be assessed is relatively small in comparison with the more sophisticated possibilities available in the clinic. Second, the measurement techniques need to be relatively unobtrusive, so as not to interfere with ongoing activities. There have been some heroic developments in naturalistic monitoring, such as the development of portable radioactivity detectors focused over the heart, and mounted in vest-like garments, that have been used to assess the impact of mental stress on cardiac function in patients with coronary artery disease (Burg *et al.* 1993). Much of the data on circadian rhythms of cortisol secretion have involved venepuncture every two hours for 24 hours, or the periodic withdrawal of blood from an indwelling catheter (Van Cauter *et al.* 2000). There is a danger that such methods are so stressful in themselves that they will obscure any association between psychosocial factors and biological responses, and certainly they can cause sleep disturbance (Jarrett *et al.* 1984). Measures of hormones such as cortisol, dehydroepian-drosterone (DHEA), testosterone, prolactin and estrogen in saliva overcome many of these problems. Third, there are several extrinsic factors that influence biological function that need to be taken into account, including cigarette smoking, food and caffeine intake, sleep and physical activity. These factors have to be monitored in naturalistic studies and taken into account statistically in analysis. Multilevel modelling has become the method of choice in analyses of these data (Schwartz and Stone 1998).

Mental stress testing

The third research method involves monitoring biological responses to standardized psychological or social stimuli. A wide range of mental stress tests are employed, including cognitive and problem solving tasks, simulated public speaking, upsetting films and interpersonal conflict tasks. Mental stress testing is typically carried out in a laboratory or clinic, but similar methods have been applied in home settings, particularly with children and elderly groups. A mental stress testing session involves a period of rest so that baseline levels of physiological function can be established, followed by a stress or challenge period that may last anything from five minutes to three hours. Further biological measures are obtained during the challenge period and for some time afterwards, depending on the dynamics of the measure under investigation. For example, blood pressure and heart rate respond within 1–2 minutes of onset of stress, while cortisol in saliva and blood may not peak for 30 minutes, and inflammatory cytokines such as interleukin (IL) 6 continued to rise for at least two hours. It is possible to obtain measures from several people simultaneously, if equipment is available. An important series of studies by Kiecolt-Glaser *et al.* involved measurement of cardiovascular, endocrine and immune function from couples during discussion of areas of conflict. Hostile and negative behaviours elicited heightened biological responses in both men and women, and there were also striking differences in the response patterns of husbands and wives (Kiecolt-Glaser and Newton 2001). Interestingly, the magnitude of adrenaline and noradrenaline responses during the conflict task were found to predict troubled marriages and divorce ten years later (Kiecolt-Glaser *et al.* 2003a).

The value of mental stress testing is that responses to psychosocial stimuli can be monitored under environmentally controlled conditions, reducing many of the sources of bias and individual difference that might otherwise be present. Experimental designs can be used with randomization to different conditions (such as low and high stress controllability), and sophisticated biological measures are possible. There are two major limitations. The first is that the stimuli used are often arbitrary and divorced from everyday life; few people spend much of their lives carrying out mental arithmetic or problem-solving under time pressure. Studies using more ecologically valid challenges such as interpersonal conflict tasks remain in the minority. Second, the stimuli used are brief, so that only acute biological responses are recorded. Chronic challenges may elicit different response patterns because of habituation and adaptation. The generalizability of biological adjustments therefore remains uncertain in many cases.

Intervention studies

One of the principal methods of determining causality in biomedical research is to modify putative causal pathways and assess impact on outcome. Biological measures are used extensively in intervention studies to assess the impact of lifestyle or cognitive-behavioural treatments on disease processes (e.g. Tuomilehto *et al.* 2001). It is also known that psychological treatments such as relaxation training have effects on neuroendocrine activity, muscle tension and blood pressure that are opposite to those induced by stress (Antoni 2003). However, intervention methods have not been extensively used to test causal models, for instance by evaluating the effects of changes in putative biological mediators of psychosocial influence. Such an approach has been used to test mechanisms in animal research, applying beta-adrenergic pharmacological blockade to demonstrate that sympathetic activation mediates the impact of social stress on atherosclerosis in primates (Kaplan *et al.* 1991). But intervention approaches have yet to be exploited fully in psychobiological research in many health care settings.

Combinations of methods

I have described the main research methods in psychosocial biology, but there is an increasing trend towards combining the different methods. For example, naturalistic monitoring of salivary cortisol has been included in epidemiological population studies such as the CARDIA (Coronary Artery Risk Development in Young Adults) and Whitehall II surveys. Mental stress testing has been extended into the epidemiological framework, allowing the impact of individual differences in stress responsivity on disease progression to be evaluated (Everson *et al.* 1997; Carroll *et al.* 2003). Mental stress testing and naturalistic monitoring have been combined to evaluate the extent to which individual differences in acute blood pressure stress reactivity generalize to everyday life situations (Kamarck *et al.* 2000). This trend is very welcome, and is likely to grow with advances in instrumentation of technology and biological assay of techniques.

Measurement and interpretation of biological variables

This section provides an overview of some of the principle biological variables measured in psychosocial studies. Space prevents detailed evaluation of all the methods available, so the aim is to focus on general measures of neuroendocrine function cardiovascular activity, inflammatory processes, immune function and musculoskeletal activity. For each set of measures, I outline why they are assessed, how they are collected and processed, and what factors need to be taken in account in health care research settings to ensure accurate interpretation.

Neuroendocrine factors

Cortisol

Cortisol is a steroid glucocorticoid hormone produced by the adrenal cortex under the control of adrenocorticotropic hormone (ACTH) and the HPA axis. It acts on almost all the nucleated cells in the body. It is implicated in a variety of conditions studied in health care research including depression, disturbances of cognitive function, obesity (particularly abdominal or central obesity), inhibition of growth and fertility, hypertension, Type II diabetes, inflammatory, and autoimmune conditions (McEwen *et al.* 1997; Lupien *et al.* 1999; Bjorntorp 2001; Wolf 2003). There are changes in cortisol with age which may have implications for the maintenance of memory function, particularly in old age (Lupien and Lepage 2001). Low socio-economic status has been associated with heightened cortisol levels both in adults and children (Lupien *et al.* 2000; Steptoe *et al.* 2003c). Many aspects of the ways in which cortisol dysfunction affects disease risk are still poorly understood. The biological actions of cortisol depend not only on output, but on the ability of cortisol to bind to glucocorticoid receptors. The relative importance of changes in secretion as opposed to alterations in uptake and tissue clearance is unclear, and impaired signalling may prove critical in many situations (Raison and Miller 2003).

Cortisol can be assessed in blood, urine and saliva. For many years, urine was the preferred vehicle for non-invasive assessments, and it provides an integrated measure of the secretion of cortisol and its metabolites over several hours. For example, increased secretion of urinary cortisol metabolites collected over a 24-hour period was recently observed in individuals with the metabolic syndrome (Brunner *et al.* 2002). But salivary cortisol has become the method of choice in much psycho-biological research for a number of reasons (Kirschbaum and Hellhammer 2000):

- First, the method of collection is less complicated and embarrassing than for urinary measurement. The individual spits into a test tube, or gently chews a dental roll for a couple of minutes until it is saturated with saliva.
- Second, samples are stable over several days at room temperature and can be sent through the post. This means that samples can be collected by people in their own homes or at work over several days without an investigator being involved.
- Third, levels in saliva respond quickly, and are more sensitive to psychosocial experience than are integrated urinary assessments. For example, several studies have failed to show that urinary cortisol is higher on work than leisure days, and this has cast doubt on the impact of work stress on neuroendocrine function (e.g. Pollard *et al.* 1996). But salivary measures indicate higher levels on work days, with differences in the magnitude of secretions associated with work stress factors such as low job control (Kunz-Ebrecht *et al.* 2004a, 2004b).
- Fourth, methods of analysis are relatively straightforward and inexpensive, with established techniques using enzyme-linked immunosorbent assay (ELISA), radioimmunoassay, and immunofluorescence being available in many laboratories. The level of free cortisol in saliva is only a fraction of that in blood, but it nevertheless correlates highly with plasma and serum concentrations.

Cortisol shows a pronounced circadian rhythm. Figure 20.2 summarizes data averaged from 163 middle-aged men and women over a working day. Cortisol levels are high early in the morning, and decline over the day, with a small peak associated with eating lunch. Data can be analysed using point comparisons, averages, or by calculating the slope of decline across the day (Stone *et al.* 2001). Additionally, there is typically an increase in cortisol over the first 20–30 minutes after waking. The cortisol waking response is of great interest in itself, since it has been associated with several psychosocial factors (Clow *et al.* 2004). In particular, it has been shown to be larger in more depressed individuals, those experiencing chronic life stress, and in more lonely people (Pruessner *et al.* 2003; Steptoe *et al.* 2004). It is inversely associated with socioeconomic position, and positively with work stress (Kunz-Ebrecht *et al.* 2004a). The evidence is inconsistent about whether it is associated with time of waking or quality of sleep. Cortisol levels can be affected by

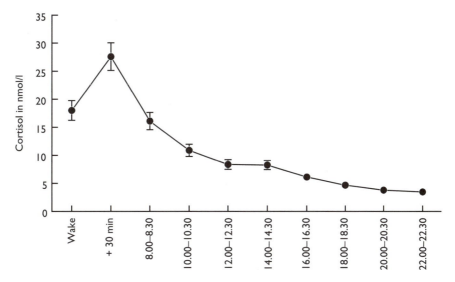

Figure 20.2   Mean levels of free cortisol sampled in saliva from 163 middle-aged men and women over a working day and evening. Timing of samples is indicated along the horizontal axis. Error bars are 95 per cent confidence intervals.

Source: Steptoe *et al.* (2003c)

smoking, medication, use of oral contraceptives, food consumption and body mass index, so these factors need to be controlled. The assessment of cortisol is compromised in people taking corticosteroid medication.

Experimental studies of acute stress responses have shown increases in cortisol following demanding tasks such as simulated public speaking (Biondi and Picardi 1999). However, it is striking that cortisol increases are frequently not observed with behavioural challenges that elicit responses in blood pressure and other variables. The reason may be that stimulation needs to be quite intense to produce reliable cortisol responses. The time course of cortisol increases is also longer than that of many biological variables, so that peak increases may not emerge until 20–40 minutes following the onset of stimulation. Increased cortisol responsivity to laboratory stress has been positively correlated with waist/hip ratio (Epel *et al.* 2000) and with the experience of chronic stress (Biondi and Picardi 1999), though some studies have described attenuated responses in stressed groups (Kristenson *et al.* 1998). Evidence from animal research indicates that adversity in early life promotes corticosteroid stress responsivity in adult animals (Meaney 2001), but evidence in humans is limited to date (Heim *et al.* 2000b). In contrast, lower than normal salivary cortisol responses to challenging tasks have been recorded from children with autoimmune conditions such as atopic dermatitis (Buske-Kirschbaum *et al.* 1997).

DHEA and DHEA sulphate

DHEA and its sulphate are the most abundant steroid hormones in the human circulation. They have marked effects on the central nervous system, having an antiglucocorticoid function, and an impact on memory and emotional behaviour in animal studies (Wolf and Kirschbaum, 1999). Animal studies also indicate that

DHEA administration reduces body fat and risk of diabetes mellitus and coronary heart disease, while enhancing immune function (Herbert 1995). The concentration of DHEA and DHEA sulphate increases during adolescence, reaching a peak between ages 20 and 30. It then declines markedly with age, such that levels in people aged 70–80 years are less than 20 per cent of those in young adults. There are, however, important individual differences in this age-related decline, and people with smaller decrements have less deterioration in memory and functional capacity in old age (Berkman *et al.* 1993). Low DHEA predicted increased mortality in the Rancho Bernardo study and in a French cohort of men, but not women (Mazat *et al.* 2001). Some investigators argue that the ratio of cortisol to DHEA is crucial. Low DHEA and an elevated cortisol/DHEA ratio has been reported in depressed patients (Young et al. 2002). Research by Goodyer *et al.* (2001) has shown that depressive disorder in adolescence is associated with high cortisol and low DHEA, and that these hormones predict subsequent depression in high-risk individuals independently of life events, long-term difficulties and premorbid symptom levels. Low DHEA is a component of allostatic load, which has been shown to predict mortality and functional decline in the MacArthur studies of successful ageing (Seeman *et al.* 2001). All these findings might suggest that DHEA administration would reverse age-related decline in function. Unfortunately, trails of DHEA supplementation in old age have yet to demonstrate that effects of low levels can be reversed (Huppert and Van Niekerk 2001).

DHEA and its sulphate can be measured in blood and saliva. There is a diurnal rhythm in output, but this is less marked than for cortisol. Many of the same factors that are relevant for cortisol collection and interpretation apply to DHEA.

Catecholamines

The catecholamines noradrenaline (norepinephrine), adrenaline (epinephrine) and dopamine are released from nerve terminals and the adrenal glands into the blood, urine and cerebrospinal fluid. Most noradrenaline is produced by sympathetic nerves and activates adrenergic receptors locally, so only a small fraction enters the bloodstream. Adrenaline by contrast is produced by the adrenal medulla and acts as a hormone, being distributed by the bloodstream to adrenergic receptors in many areas. Catecholamines are measured as indices of sympathoadrenal activity in psychosocial biology, and can be assessed at present in blood and urine but not in saliva.

Urinary measures of catecholamines and their metabolites can be used to provide an indication of sympthoadrenal activity, and have demonstrated associations with psychosocial factors such as work stress (Frankenhaeuser *et al.* 1989), and with precursors of disease such as the metabolic syndrome (Brunner *et al.* 2002). Urinary concentrations of adrenaline and noradrenaline collected over 12 hours were components of the index of allostatic load used to predict functional decline in the MacArthur studies of successful ageing (Karlamangla *et al.* 2002). But studies of responsivity to psychosocial stimuli require measures that change over shorter time periods.

Plasma noradrenaline and adrenaline are often measured for this purpose, yet face several technical and conceptual problems. The most accurate assessments are carried out with high-pressure liquid chromatography, but reproducibility and sensitivity is far from perfect. A more important point is that the noradrenaline concentration measured in venous blood samples is strongly determined by overflow from local tissues (Hjemdahl 1993). Thus about half of the catecholamine extracted from blood samples taken from the forearm is derived from the muscles of the arm itself. Sympathetic nervous system activity is highly differentiated, particularly under stressful conditions, with levels of activity in different tissues varying widely. This means that venous samples are not good indicators of general 'sympathetic tone'. This problem has yet to be resolved. More precise measures of sympathetic activity include direct microneurographic assessments from nerves, and measures of radio-actively-labelled noradrenaline. For example, Esler *et al.* (1989) showed that mental stress elicited no change in venous noradrenaline, while radiotracer techniques demonstrated large increases in noradrenergic activity in the heart and kidney. Unfortunately, these are technically demanding methods that cannot be widely used in health care research at present (Grassi and Esler 1999).

Other hormones

Insulin-like growth factor-1 (IGF-1) is produced in response to growth hormone released by the pituitary gland. IGF-1 has a variety of effects in the central nervous system, being involved in the differentiation of neurons, the release of neuro-transmitters and stimulation of dendritic growth (Schneider *et al.* 2003). The decrease in hippocampal neurogenesis with advancing age is mediated by reduced IGF-1 among other factors. Both cross-sectional and prospective studies have shown positive associations between IGF-1 and cognitive function. Age-related declines in IGF-1 are associated with deleterious changes in body composition, while studies of growth hormone administration in older adults have documented rises in IGF-1 together with increased bone mineral density content and reduced fat mass (Lamberts *et al.* 1997). But effects on disease are poorly understood. Numerous studies have shown adverse effects of IGF-1 on atherosclerosis, glucose metabolism and diabetic vascular lesions, and high IGF-1 is associated with increased risk of some cancers (Hankinson *et al.* 1998; Sandhu *et al.* 2002). On the other hand, low rather than high circulating IGF-1 has been related prospectively with the incidence of coronary heart disease (Juul *et al.* 2002).

The gonadal hormones testosterone and oestrogen have also been studied in human psychosocial research. There is ample evidence from animal studies that stressful conditions and social adversity impair gonadal function and reproductive viability. Testosterone levels have been positively related to aggression and violent behaviour in some but not all investigations, and sustained production of testosterone in older men is associated with maintenance of muscle strength and functional well-being (Lamberts *et al.* 1997; Charney 2004). There is evidence that oestrogen blunts HPA axis and catecholamine stress responses in perimenopausal women (Komesaroff *et al.* 1999), and effects on mood have been described (McEwen 2002). Additionally, Taylor *et al.* (2000) have proposed that oxytocin is released as part of the stress response in women, and may mediate sex-specific coping behaviours in the face of adversity.

Cardiovascular measures

Blood pressure

The need for rigour in the measurement procedure and standardization of conditions when measuring blood pressure cannot be overemphasized. At the least, two readings should be obtained, preferably with a validated electronic blood pressure monitor, after the person has been seated quietly in a chair for five minutes, with feet on the floor and arm supported at heart level. An important issue for psychosocial studies is the 'white coat' effect, or the tendency of some people to have higher blood pressure when measured by a physician in the clinic than at home. White coat hypertension, where the blood pressure is sufficiently elevated when measured clinically to warrant a diagnosis, is thought to occur in at least 20 per cent of patients (Pickering *et al.* 1988). There is little evidence for white coat effects being associated with particular physiological profiles, and exaggerated responsivity to other stimuli is often not present. It is possible that white coat effects are specific conditioned responses, with the negative emotional concomitants of measurement in the clinic leading to a classically conditioned response in some individuals. One way of overcoming this difficulty in psychosocial studies is to carry out self-monitoring or ambulatory blood pressure monitoring, as described below.

There is an extensive literature concerning blood pressure responses to mental stress testing, and the use of this method to investigate the role of psychological stress in the development of essential hypertension and coronary heart disease (Steptoe 1997). This has stimulated detailed methodological examinations of such issues as the duration of baselines, the blood pressure measurement technique, the control of physical activity and the effects of smoking and hormonal status, that go well beyond the scope of this chapter (Schneiderman *et al.* 1989). The clinical significance of acute blood pressure stress responses has been a particular concern, and has led to the gradual accumulation of prospective data that tend to confirm that heightened stress responsivity predicts future hypertension and cardiovascular disease risk (Steptoe and Willemson 2002). New technologies, such as the Finapres instrument which assesses blood pressure on a beat by beat basis from the finger, are providing more refined insights into the ways in which psychosocial factors affect the cardiovascular system.

Ambulatory blood pressure and self-measurement

Ambulatory monitoring devices consist of an arm cuff, a signal detection device and a portable pump. They work in the same way as standard blood pressure monitors, except that the equipment is miniaturized and portable, and can be worn beneath clothing. The cuff is programmed to inflate periodically, with intervals of 15–60 minutes being used in different studies, so that a profile of blood pressure over the day can be built up. Ambulatory monitors are often used at night as well, and provide useful information about blood pressure 'dipping' and subsequent morning surges (Kario *et al.* 2003).

Clinically, the use of ambulatory monitors has increased because of the evidence that they provide better risk assessments than do conventional methods (Pickering 2002). In psychosocial studies, ambulatory devices allow the impact of daily life experience to be measured, and effects are frequently observed that are not detectable with conventional methods. A good example is in the study of work stress. The relationship between clinical blood pressure and work stress is very inconsistent, but it has now been found in several investigations that work stress is associated with small elevations in blood pressure recorded over the working day (Steenland *et al.* 2000). Figure 20.3 illustrates results from a recent investigation of 200 male and female participants in the Whitehall II study who carried out ambulatory blood pressure monitoring every 20 minutes over a working day. Low control at work was associated with higher systolic and diastolic blood pressure both during the day and in the evening after work, and these effects were independent of age, gender, socioeconomic position, smoking, body mass, and physical activity (Steptoe and Willemsen 2004). Ambulatory blood pressure has been related to many other psychosocial factors as well, including marital conflict, social support, hostility and mood (Schwartz *et al.* 1994; Baker *et al.* 1999). Care has to be taken in the interpretation of ambulatory results, since physical activity, smoking, consumption of coffee and alcohol can all affect blood pressure values. Multilevel modelling has been introduced into the analysis of ambulatory blood pressure in order to tease out the independent contribution of psychosocial factors (Schwartz *et al.* 1994).

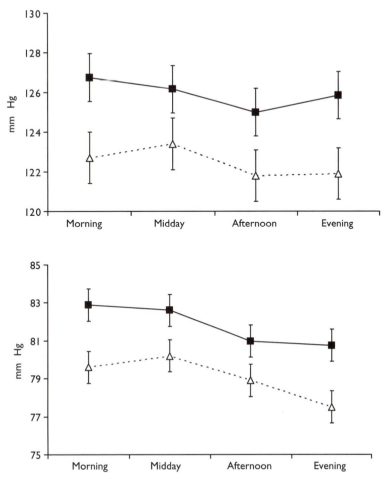

Figure 20.3   Mean systolic pressure (upper graph) and diastolic pressure (lower graph) in men and women reporting low job control (solid lines) and high job control (dotted lines), over the working day. Data are averaged into four time periods over the day, and are adjusted for gender, employment grade, age, body mass index, smoking status and concomitant physical activity. Error bars are standard error of the mean.

Source: Steptoe and Willemson (2004)

Self-measurement of blood pressure is a less expensive method, and has increased greatly in popularity with the availability of reliable instruments. It has been endorsed in the guidelines of the respected Joint National Committee on prevention, detection, evaluation and treatment of high blood pressure as an aid to management (Chobanian *et al.* 2003), and can equally well be used in psychosocial studies. For example, Evans and Steptoe (2001) carried out a study in which nurses and accountants performed self-measurement of blood pressure and heart rate on work and leisure days. Blood pressure was typically lower on leisure days, while heart rates were reduced in people who had high social support.

Heart rate variability

Heart rate variability has become an important indicator of autonomic nervous system control over the heart. The heart rate varies naturally with the breathing cycle and other modulators. Variability can be assessed in the time domain by measuring the difference between short and long interbeat intervals, or in the frequency domain with power spectrum analysis. Low heart rate variability is a marker of reduced parasympathetic and high sympathetic control, and is a predictor of all cause mortality, and the prognosis of coronary heart disease and diabetes (Bigger *et al.* 1993; Dekker *et al.* 2000). Heart rate variability decreases with age, and the maintenance of higher heart rate variability may be an indicator of successful ageing. Studies in healthy populations have shown that heart rate variability is reduced during acute stress, and is associated with factors such as social isolation and psychological distress (Hemingway *et al.* 2001). It has been postulated that reduced heart rate variability partly mediates the association between depression and acute myocardial infarction (Carney *et al.* 2001), and low heart rate variability has also been observed in the metabolic syndrome (Brunner *et al.* 2002). It should, however, be pointed out that heart rate and heart rate variability are typically inversely correlated. It is unclear in some psychosocial studies whether the more complicated variability measures provide sufficient additional information over and above that obtained with heart rate assessments to warrant the extra work required.

Measures of inflammation

Inflammatory markers have been introduced into psychosocial studies only in recent years. The measures assessed include C-reactive protein, fibrinogen and the proinflammatory cytokines IL-6 and tumour necrosis factor α (TNFα). Inflammation is involved in many of the diseases studied in health care research, including coronary heart disease, hypertension, diabetes, some cancers, rheumatoid conditions, osteoporosis, multiple sclerosis and periodontal disease. Inflammatory markers have been associated with all cause mortality and death from cardiovascular disease in several cohort studies (Danesh *et al.* 1998; Ridker *et al.* 2000). Proinflammatory cytokines regulate the major drivers of postnatal growth, namely growth hormone and IGF-1. They are also relevant to ageing and overproduction of IL-6 is associated with frailty and functional decline in old age. Cytokines play a major role in inducing sickness behaviour (Dantzer 2001), and may be responsible for the multiple symptoms associated with certain treatments for cancer (Cleeland *et al.* 2003).

There is growing evidence for an influence of psychosocial factors on inflammatory processes. Fibrinogen concentration is inversely associated with socioeconomic status, and has also been related to low control at work, effort–reward imbalance, social isolation and hostility (Brunner *et al.* 1996; Wamala *et al.* 1999). Chronic stressors such as caring for a dementing relative stimulate more rapid increases in IL-6 with age (Kiecolt-Glaser *et al.* 2003b). Clinical depression and non-clinical depressed mood have been associated with higher IL-6, TNFα and C-reactive protein concentrations (Penninx *et al.* 2003). The magnitude of IL-6 and C-reactive protein responses to the acute stress of surgery is inversely related to rate of recovery, while chronic stress has been found to predict the magnitude of local inflammation in wounds (Glaser *et al.* 1999). Several other forms of stress such as academic examination stimulate heightened inflammatory cytokines and C-reactive protein, and the IL-6 response to acute mental stress is greater in people of lower socioeconomic status (Brydon *et al.* 2004). Inflammatory processes are also affected by body weight, smoking, physical activity and alcohol consumption, and interactions between adiposity and depression in the prediction of IL-6 have been described (Miller *et al.* 2003).

Inflammatory markers are assessed with relatively standard biochemical assays of blood samples, and commercial kits are available. In the quantification of C-reactive protein, so-called high sensitivity assays are required. Plasma or serum levels of these substances are typically measured, but in addition, inflammatory cytokines can be quantified by stimulating the mononuclear cells with the mitogen lipopolysac-charide. This procedure requires culturing cells and incubation of samples, so is more complicated than the assessment of plasma levels.

Immunological measures

The interdisciplinary field of psychoneuroimmunology has become very promin-ent over the last 25 years (Ader *et al.* 2001). Much of this research is focused on basic physiology, the regulation of the immune system, and on the interplay between the brain and immune responses. But psychoneuroimmunology is also relevant to health care research for a number of reasons. First, the evidence indicates that psychosocial factors can modulate immune defences against pathogens such as bacteria, fungi and viruses, and can therefore increase or reduce resistance to disease (Kiecolt-Glaser *et al.* 2002). Second, there are disorders in which disturb-ances of immune function are a central feature, notably HIV/AIDS. Psychological characteristics and social factors are thought to be responsible in part for the large variations in the rate of progression of HIV in different individuals, and these influences may be mediated by central nervous system factors (Antoni 2003). Third, variations in clinical status, exacerbations of control, or flares in conditions such as rheumatoid arthritis, diabetes mellitus and systemic lupus erythematosus are associated with psychosocial factors (Da Costa *et al.* 1999; Zautra *et al.* 1999). Psychoneuroimmunological pathways may be responsible for these effects.

Measurement of immune function

The measurement of immune function in psychosocial research is complicated, and only a brief summary is given here (Vedhara *et al.* 1999b; Ader *et al.* 2001). Perhaps the most basic method is to count white blood cells and sub-sets of lymphocytes in the circulation. This is done using flow cytometry, with specific antigens detecting cluster designation (CD) markers on different immune cells. For example, cells marked with CD4+ are T helper cells, CD8+ are cytotoxic T cells, CD19+ is a B cell marker and CD16/CD56 designates natural killer cells. Lymphocyte counts are modified by acute and chronic stress, and in conditions such as depression (Zorrilla *et al.* 2001). A limitation to this method is that cell numbers do not necessarily correlate with cell function. Various functional assays are therefore used. These include measures of cytotoxicity, in which the ability of natural killer cells or T cells to destroy target cells is measured. Another functional measure is the assessment of lymphocyte proliferation in response to stimuli such as the lectin phytohemag-glutinin, where greater proliferation implies that the lymphocytes are more respon-sive to the presence of potentially dangerous substances. An early finding in psychoneuroimmunology was that proliferative responses were impaired in people who had recently suffered a personal bereavement, a group that is known to be at raised risk for various illnesses (Bartrop *et al.* 1977). Natural killer cell cytotoxicity has been shown to be impaired in a range of stressful conditions, but to be positively associated with social support (Uchino *et al.* 1996; Zorrilla *et al.* 2001).

A different set of assays are used to quantify humoral immunity and levels of immunoglobulin. Antibodies are produced by B cells in response to exposure to antigens, and are grouped in major classes such as immunoglobulin A (IgA), which is secreted in saliva and tears and protects mucosal surfaces, and immunoglobulin E (IgE) which is involved in the release of histamine and is implicated in conditions such as bronchial asthma. Immunoglobulins can be assayed from blood or saliva using ELISA techniques, and levels have been found to vary with psychosocial factors such as mood and daily stressors. However, the interpretation of responses can be problematic. Some investigators assess total immunoglobulin levels, but these values are only moderately associated with specific antibody responses. Antibody titres in response to specific antigens are more precise, but depend on recent exposure to the antigen.

Other methods assess immune function *in vivo*, rather than through processing of blood or saliva samples in the laboratory. Administration of live virus has been used in experimental research on upper respiratory infection. In a series of studies, Cohen *et al.* (1991, 1997) demonstrated that stress increases the likelihood that a moderate dose of experimentally administered coronavirus will lead to infection and a clinical cold, while social networks have a protective effect. Another model involves measurement of antibody responses to attenuated viruses such as those used in influenza vaccination. It has been shown in some studies that antibody responses to vaccination are impaired in individuals experiencing chronic life stress, and this may be indicative of weakened immune defences (Vedhara *et al.* 1999a).

Musculoskeletal measures

There is substantial evidence linking psychosocial aspects of work with upper extremity musculoskeletal problems (Sauter and Moon 1996). Factors such as low autonomy, lack of role clarity, low job satisfaction and high work pressure have been associated with pain in the neck and shoulder regions, and with hand or wrist problems. A recent systematic review confirmed these observations, but also pointed to evidence relating upper extremity problems with psychosocial factors outside work such as low social support and general stress (Bongers *et al.* 2002). Work-related upper extremity disorders are particularly common in jobs with a static load involving monotonous and repetitive tasks, even when physical demands are only low or moderate. Computer data entry, cashier work in supermarkets and other outlets, routine scientific bench work and traditional assembly line work all have these characteristics, and musculoskeletal problems are particularly common among women (Klumb and Lampert 2004).

Much research on musculoskeletal disorders is based on self-report or physical examination. However, direct measurement of muscle tension using surface electromyography (EMG) provides valuable additional information. Miniaturized transducers and telemetric equipment are available that allow readings to be obtained from free-moving individuals. Positive correlations have been reported between objectively assessed muscle tension and feelings of stress and exhaustion during work, but correlations with pain are often not obtained (e.g. Rissen *et al.* 2000). Studies of this kind indicate that the perception and appraisal of muscle tension may be important as well as objective differences in tension. Work with chronic back pain patients has identified problems in the accuracy of discrimination of EMG levels recorded from back muscles, and a tendency to overestimate muscle tension by some individuals (Flor *et al.* 1999). Surface electromyography is also used extensively in headache research, with monitoring of muscles of the neck, back and forehead. A meta-analysis of studies of frontal (forehead) EMG indicated that patients with tension-type headache do have higher muscle tension than controls on average, but with wide variability (Wittrock 1997). This suggests that a combined assessment of subjective and objective measures may be valuable in the investigation of these problems.

Conclusions

There are many applications of biological measures in health care research. Their use in psychosocial studies is particularly appealing, since they provide objective evidence for the influence of psychological and social processes on pathophysiology and the biological mechanisms underlying disease states. There is sometimes scepticism about whether psychosocial factors are associated with genuine health outcomes, or only with symptom complaints and illness behaviour (Watson and Pennebaker 1989). The evidence that alterations in neuroendocrine function, inflammatory responses, viral antibodies or cardiovascular activity take place allows effects to be verified objectively. The field of psychosocial biology is continually expanding, with recent research on phenomena such as vascular endothelial dysfunction, cytokine gene expression and glucocorticoid receptor sensitivity supplementing the more established measures described here. Great care needs to be taken in the measurement and interpretation of biological measures, and their inclusion in a health care research project may call for additional standardization, both of the setting and timing of assessments. However, the gain in understanding of psychosocial influences can be considerable, so the extra costs and effort required for including biological measures is well worthwhile.

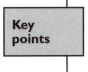

Key points

- The biological measures assessed in psychosocial research are: biological indicators of disease states; biological markers of processes involved in the aetiology of disease; and non-specific biological markers of stress-related activation or resistance to disease.

- There is a substantial amount of research on the relationship between psychosocial factors and biological function.

- Epidemiological studies provide the core method of establishing the contribution of psychosocial factors to the development of disease, and are also used to identify the biological mediators of these associations. However, biological measures in epidemiological studies have the limitation that they are generally recorded on a single occasion, under resting conditions that are not typical of everyday life.

- Naturalistic monitoring studies involve sampling biological variables during everyday life, from recordings during challenging tasks to repeated measures (e.g. of blood pressure over an ordinary day).

- Naturalistic monitoring methods have the advantage of ecological validity, although the range of biological markers that can be assessed is relatively small, and need to be relatively unobtrusive.

- Another method is mental stress testing, involving monitoring biological responses to standardized psychological or social stimuli. A wide range of mental stress tests are employed, and experimental designs can be used. Limitations are that the stimuli in mental stress testing are often divorced from everyday life and are brief, so only acute biological responses are recorded.

- Biological measures are frequently used in intervention studies to assess the impact of lifestyle or cognitive-behavioural treatments on disease processes, although intervention methods have not been extensively used to test causal models.

- Some of the principal biological variables measured in psychosocial studies include neuroendocrine function, cardiovascular activity, inflammatory processes, immune function and musculoskeletal activity.

- Care needs to be taken in the measurement and interpretation of biological measures, and in the design of the overall study.

References

Ader, R., Felten, D.L. and Cohen, N. (eds) (2001) *Psychoneuroimmunology*, 3rd edn, 2 vols. San Diego, CA: Academic Press.

Antoni, M.H. (2003) Stress management effects on psychological, endocrinological, and immune functioning in men with HIV infection: empirical support for a psychoneuroimmunological model, *Stress*, 6: 173–88.

Baker, B., Helmers, K., O'Kelly, B. *et al.* (1999) Marital cohesion and ambulatory blood pressure in early hypertension, *American Journal of Hypertension*, 12: 227–30.

Bartrop, R.W., Luckhurst, E., Lazarus, L., Kiloh, L.G. and Penny, R. (1977) Depressed lymphocyte function after bereavement, *Lancet*, 1: 834–6.

Berkman, L.F., Seeman, T.E., Albert, M. *et al.* (1993) High, usual and impaired functioning in community-dwelling older men and women: findings from the MacArthur Foundation Research Network on Successful Aging, *Journal of Clinical Epidemiology*, 46: 1129–40.

Bigger, J.T., Fleiss, J.L., Rolnitzky, L.M. and Steinman, R.C. (1993) The ability of several short-term measures of RR variability to predict mortality after myocardial infarction, *Circulation*, 88: 927–34.

Biondi, M. and Picardi, A. (1999) Psychological stress and neuroendocrine function in humans: the last two decades of research, *Psychotherapy Psychosomatics*, 68: 114–50.

Bjorntorp, P. (2001) Do stress reactions cause abdominal obesity and comorbidities?, *Obesity Review*, 2: 73–86.

Bongers, P.M., Kremer, A.M. and ter Laak, J. (2002) Are psychosocial factors risk factors for symptoms and signs of the shoulder, elbow, or hand/wrist?: a review of the epidemiological literature, *American Journal of Industrial Medicine*, 41: 315–42.

Brunner, E., Davey Smith, G., Marmot, M. *et al.* (1996) Childhood social circumstances and psychosocial and behavioural factors as determinants of plasma fibrinogen, *Lancet*, 347: 1008–13.

Brunner, E.J., Marmot, M.G., Nanchahal, K. *et al.* (1997) Social inequality in coronary risk: central obesity and the metabolic syndrome: evidence from the Whitehall II study, *Diabetologia*, 40: 1341–9.

Brunner, E.J., Hemingway, H., Walker, B.R. *et al.* (2002) Adrenocortical, autonomic, and inflammatory causes of the metabolic syndrome: nested case-control study, *Circulation*, 106: 2659–65.

Brydon, L., Edwards, S., Mohamed-Ali, V. and Steptoe, A. (2004) Socioeconomic status and stress-induced increases in interleukin-6, *Brain, Behavior and Immunity*, 18: 281–90.

Burg, M.M., Jain, D., Soufer, R., Kerns, R.D. and Zaret, B.L. (1993) Role of behavioral and psychological factors in mental stress-induced silent left ventricular dysfunction in coronary artery disease, *Journal of the American College of Cardiology*, 22: 440–8.

Buske-Kirschbaum, A., Jobst, S., Wustmans, A. *et al.* (1997) Attenuated free cortisol response to psychosocial stress in children with atopic dermatitis, *Psychosomatic Medicine*, 59: 419–26.

Cacioppo, J.T., Tassinary, L.G. and Berntson, G. (eds) (2000) *Handbook of Psychophysiology*, 2nd edn. New York: Cambridge University Press.

Carney, R.M., Blumenthal, J.A., Stein, P.K. *et al.* (2001) Depression, heart rate variability, and acute myocardial infarction, *Circulation*, 104: 2024–8.

Carroll, D., Ring, C., Hunt, K. *et al.* (2003) Blood pressure reactions to stress and the prediction of future blood pressure: effects of sex, age, and socioeconomic position, *Psychosomatic Medicine*, 65: 1058–64.

Charney, D.S. (2004) Psychobiological mechanisms of resilience and vulnerability: implications for successful adaptation to extreme stress, *American Journal of Psychiatry*, 161: 195–216.

Chobanian, A.V., Bakris, G.L., Black, H.R. *et al.* (2003) The Seventh Report of the Joint National Committee on Prevention, Detection, Evaluation, and Treatment of High Blood Pressure: the JNC 7 report, *Journal of the American Medical Association*, 289: 2560–72.

Cleeland, C.S., Bennett, G.J., Dantzer, R. *et al.* (2003) Are the symptoms of cancer and cancer treatment due to a shared biologic mechanism? A cytokine-immunologic model of cancer symptoms, *Cancer*, 97: 2919–25.

Clow, A., Thorn, L., Evans, P. and Hucklebridge, F. (2004) The awakening cortisol response: methodological issues and significance, *Stress*, 7: 29–37.

Cohen, S., Tyrrell, D.A.J. and Smith, A.P. (1991) Psychosocial stress and susceptibility to the common cold, *New England Journal of Medicine*, 325: 606–12.

Cohen, S., Doyle, W.J., Skoner, D.P., Rabin, B.S. and Gwaltney, J.M. (1997) Social ties and susceptibility to the common cold, *Journal of the American Medical Association*, 277: 1940–4.

Da Costa, D., Dobkin, P.L., Pinard, L. *et al.* (1999) The role of stress in functional disability among women with systemic lupus erythematosus: a prospective study, *Arthritis Care Research*, 12: 112–19.

Danesh, J., Collins, R., Appleby, P. and Peto, R. (1998) Association of fibrinogen, C-reactive protein, albumin, or leukocyte count with coronary heart disease: meta-analyses of prospective studies, *Journal of the American Medical Association*, 279: 1477–82.

Dantzer, R. (2001) Cytokine-induced sickness behavior: mechanisms and implications, *Annals of the New York Academy of Sciences*, 933: 222–34.

Dekker, J.M., Crow, R.S., Folsom, A.R. *et al.* (2000) Low heart rate variability in a 2-minute rhythm strip predicts risk of coronary heart disease and mortality from several causes: the ARIC Study – atherosclerosis risk in communities, *Circulation*, 102: 1239–44.

Epel, E.S., McEwen, B., Seeman, T. *et al.* (2000) Stress and body shape: stress-induced cortisol secretion is consistently greater among women with central fat, *Psychosomatic Medicine*, 62: 623–32.

Esler, M., Jennings, G. and Lambert, G. (1989) Measurement of overall and cardiac norepinephrine release into plasma during cognitive challenge, *Psychoneuroendocrinology*, 14: 477–81.

Evans, O. and Steptoe, A. (2001) Social support at work, heart rate, and cortisol: a self-monitoring study, *Journal of Occupational Health Psychology*, 6: 361–70.

Everson, S.A., Lynch, J.W., Chesney, M.A. *et al.* (1997) Interaction of workplace demands and cardiovascular reactivity in progression of carotid atherosclerosis: population-based study, *British Medical Journal*, 314: 553–8.

Fink, G. (ed.) (2000) *Encyclopedia of Stress*, 3 vols. San Diego, CA: Academic Press.

Flor, H., Furst, M. and Birbaumer, N. (1999) Deficient discrimination of EMG levels and overestimation of perceived tension in chronic pain patients, *Applied Psychophysiology and Biofeedback*, 24: 55–66.

Frankenhaeuser, M., Lundberg, U., Fredrikson, M. *et al.* (1989) Stress on and off the job as related to sex and occupational stress in white-collar workers, *Journal of Organizational Behavior*, 10: 321–46.

Glaser, R., Kiecolt-Glaser, J.K., Marucha, P.T. *et al.* (1999) Stress-related changes in proinflammatory cytokine production in wounds, *Archives of General Psychiatry*, 56: 450–6.

Goodyer, I.M., Park, R.J., Netherton, C.M. and Herbert, J. (2001) Possible role of cortisol and dehydroepiandrosterone in human development and psychopathology, *British Journal of Psychiatry*, 179: 243–9.

Grassi, G. and Esler, M. (1999) How to assess sympathetic activity in humans, *Journal of Hypertension*, 17: 719–34.

Hankinson, S.E., Willett, W.C., Colditz, G.A. *et al.* (1998) Circulating concentrations of insulin-like growth factor-I and risk of breast cancer, *Lancet*, 351: 1393–6.

Heim, C., Ehlert, U. and Hellhammer, D.H. (2000a) The potential role of hypocortisolism in the pathophysiology of stress-related bodily disorders, *Psychoneuroendocrinology*, 25: 1–35.

Heim, C., Newport, D.J., Heit, S. *et al.* (2000b) Pituitary-adrenal and autonomic responses to stress in women after sexual and physical abuse in childhood, *Journal of the American Medical Association*, 284: 592–7.

Hemingway, H., Malik, M. and Marmot, M. (2001) Social and psychosocial influences on sudden cardiac death, ventricular arrhythmia and cardiac autonomic function, *European Heart Journal*, 22: 1082–1101.

Hemingway, H., Shipley, M., Mullen, M.J. *et al.* (2003) Social and psychosocial influences on inflammatory markers and vascular function in civil servants (the Whitehall II study), *American Journal of Cardiololgy*, 92: 984–7.

Herbert, J. (1995) The age of dehydroepiandrosterone, *Lancet*, 345: 1193–4.

Hjemdahl, P. (1993) Plasma catecholamines: analytical challenges and physiological limitations, *Baillieres Clinical Endocrinology Metabolism*, 7: 307–53.

Huppert, F.A. and Van Niekerk, J.K. (2001) Dehydroepiandrosterone (DHEA) supplementation for cognitive function, *Cochrane Database Systematic Reviews*: CD000304.

Jarrett, D.B., Greenhouse, J.B., Thompson, S.B. *et al.* (1984) Effect of nocturnal intravenous cannulation upon sleep-EEG measures, *Biological Psychiatry*, 19: 1537–50.

Jorgensen, R.S., Johnson, B.T., Schreer, G.E. and Kolodziej, M.E. (1996) Elevated blood pressure and personality: a meta-analytic review, *Psychological Bulletin*, 120: 293–320.

Juul, A., Scheike, T., Davidsen, M. *et al.* (2002) Low serum insulin-like growth factor I is associated with increased risk of ischemic heart disease: a population-based case-control study, *Circulation*, 106: 939–44.

Kamarck, T.W., Debski, T.T. and Manuck, S.B. (2000) Enhancing the laboratory-to-life generalizability of cardiovascular reactivity using multiple occasions of measurement, *Psychophysiology*, 37: 533–42.

Kaplan, J.R., Pettersson, K., Manuck, S.B. and Olsson, G. (1991) Role of sympathoadrenal medullary activation in the initiation and progression of atherosclerosis, *Circulation*, 84: VI23–32.

Kario, K., Pickering, T.G., Umeda, Y. *et al.* (2003) Morning surge in blood pressure as a predictor of silent and clinical cerebrovascular disease in elderly hypertensives: a prospective study, *Circulation*, 107: 1401–6.

Karlamangla, A.S., Singer, B.H., McEwen, B.S. *et al.* (2002) Allostatic load as a predictor of functional decline: MacArthur studies of successful aging, *Journal of Clinical Epidemiology*, 55: 696–710.

Kiecolt-Glaser, J.K. and Newton, T.L. (2001) Marriage and health: his and hers, *Psychology Bulletin*, 127: 472–503.

Kiecolt-Glaser, J.K., McGuire, L., Robles, T.F. and Glaser, R. (2002) Emotions, morbidity, and mortality: new perspectives from psychoneuroimmunology, *Annual Review of Psychology*, 53: 83–107.

Kiecolt-Glaser, J.K., Bane, C., Glaser, R. and Malarkey, W.B. (2003a) Love, marriage, and divorce: newlyweds' stress hormones foreshadow relationship changes, *Journal of Consulting and Clinical Psychology*, 71: 176–88.

Kiecolt-Glaser, J.K., Preacher, K.J., MacCallum, R.C. *et al.* (2003b) Chronic stress and age-related increases in the proinflammatory cytokine IL-6, *Proceedings of the National Academy of Sciences of the USA*, 100: 9090–5.

Kirschbaum, C. and Hellhammer, D.H. (2000) Salivary cortisol, in G. Fink (ed.) *Encyclopedia of Stress*, vol. 3. San Diego, CA: Academic Press.

Klumb, P.L. and Lampert, T. (2004) Women, work, and well-being 1950–2000: a review and methodological critique, *Social Science and Medicine*, 58: 1007–24.

Komesaroff, P.A., Esler, M.D. and Sudhir, K. (1999) Estrogen supplementation attenuates glucocorticoid and catecholamine responses to mental stress in perimenopausal women, *Journal of Clinical Endocrinolgy Metabolism*, 84: 606–10.

Kristenson, M., Orth-Gomer, K., Kucinskiene, Z. *et al.* (1998) Attenuated cortisol response to a standardized stress test in Lithuanian versus Swedish men: the LiVicordia study, *International Journal of Behavioral Medicine*, 5: 17–30.

Kunz-Ebrecht, S.R., Kirschbaum, C., Marmot, M. and Steptoe, A. (2004a) Differences in cortisol awakening response on work days and weekends in women and men from the Whitehall II cohort, *Psychoneuroendocrinology*, 29: 516–28.

Kunz-Ebrecht, S.R., Kirschbaum, C. and Steptoe, A. (2004b) Work stress, socioeconomic status, and neuroendocrine activation over the working day, *Social Science and Medicine*, 58: 1523–30.

Lamberts, S.W., van den Beld, A.W. and van der Lely, A.J. (1997) The endocrinology of aging, *Science*, 278: 419–24.

Light, K.C., Girdler, S.S., Sherwood, A. *et al.* (1999) High stress responsivity predicts later blood pressure only in combination with positive family history and high life stress, *Hypertension*, 33: 1458–64.

Lundberg, U., Dohns, I.E., Melin, B. *et al.* (1999) Psychophysiological stress responses, muscle tension, and neck and shoulder pain among supermarket cashiers, *Journal of Occupational Health Psychology*, 4: 245–55.

Lupien, S.J. and Lepage, M. (2001) Stress, memory, and the hippocampus: can't live with it, can't live without it, *Behavioural Brain Research*, 127: 137–58.

Lupien, S.J., Nair, N.P., Briere, S. *et al.* (1999) Increased cortisol levels and impaired cognition in human aging: implication for depression and dementia in later life, *Reviews in Neuroscience*, 10: 117–39.

Lupien, S.J., King, S., Meaney, M.J. and McEwen, B.S. (2000) Child's stress hormone levels correlate with mother's socioeconomic status and depressive state, *Biological Psychiatry*, 48: 976–80.

Mazat, L., Lafont, S., Berr, C. *et al.* (2001) Prospective measurements of dehydroepiandrosterone sulphate in a cohort of elderly subjects: relationship to gender, subjective health, smoking habits, and 10-year mortality, *Proceedings of the National Academy of Science, USA*, 98: 8145–50.

McEwen, B. (2002) Estrogen actions throughout the brain, *Recent Progress in Hormone Research*, 57: 357–84.

McEwen, B.S. (1998) Protective and damaging effects of stress mediators, *New England Journal of Medicine*, 338: 171–9.

McEwen, B.S. and Wingfield, J.C. (2003) The concept of allostasis in biology and biomedicine, *Hormones and Behavior*, 43: 2–15.

McEwen, B.S., Biron, C.A., Brunson, K.W. *et al.* (1997) The role of adrenocorticoids as modulators of immune function in health and disease: neural, endocrine and immune interactions, *Brain Research Review*, 23: 79–133.

Meaney, M.J. (2001) Maternal care, gene expression, and the transmission of individual differences in stress reactivity across generations, *Annual Review of Neuroscience*, 24: 1161–92.

Miller, G.E., Freedland, K.E., Carney, R.M., Stetler, C.A. and Banks, W.A. (2003) Pathways linking depression, adiposity, and inflammatory markers in healthy young adults, *Brain, Behavior and Immunity*, 17: 276–85.

Penninx, B.W., Kritchevsky, S.B., Yaffe, K. *et al.* (2003) Inflammatory markers and depressed mood in older persons: results from the Health, Aging and Body Composition study, *Biological Psychiatry*, 54: 566–72.

Pickering, T. (2002) Future developments in ambulatory blood pressure monitoring and self-blood pressure monitoring in clinical practice, *Blood Pressure Monitor*, 7: 21–5.

Pickering, T.G., James, G.D., Boddie, C. *et al.* (1988) How common is white coat hypertension? *Journal of the American Medical Association*, 259: 225–8.

Pollard, T.M., Ungpakorn, G., Harrison, G.A. and Parkes, K.R. (1996) Epinephrine and cortisol responses to work: a test of the models of Frankenhaeuser and Karasek, *Annals of Behavioral Medicine*, 18: 229–37.

Pruessner, M., Hellhammer, D.H., Pruessner, J.C. and Lupien, S.J. (2003) Self-reported depressive symptoms and stress levels in healthy young men: associations with the cortisol response to awakening, *Psychosomatic Medicine*, 65: 92–9.

Raison, C.L. and Miller, A.H. (2003) When not enough is too much: the role of insufficient glucocorticoid signaling in the pathophysiology of stress-related disorders, *American Journal of Psychiatry*, 160: 1554–65.

Ridker, P.M., Rifai, N., Stampfer, M.J. and Hennekens, C.H. (2000) Plasma concentration of interleukin–6 and the risk of future myocardial infarction among apparently healthy men, *Circulation*, 101: 1767–72.

Rissen, D., Melin, B., Sandsjo, L. *et al.* (2000) Surface EMG and psychophysiological stress reactions in women during repetitive work, *European Journal of Applied Physiology*, 83: 215–22.

Ritz, T. and Steptoe, A. (2000) Emotion and pulmonary function in asthma: reactivity in the field and relationship with laboratory induction of emotion, *Psychosomatic Medicine*, 62: 808–15.

Sabban, E.L. and Kvetnansky, R. (2001) Stress-triggered activation of gene expression in catecholaminergic systems: dynamics of transcriptional events, *Trends in Neurosciences*, 24: 91–8.

Sandhu, M.S., Heald, A.H., Gibson, J.M. *et al.* (2002) Circulating concentrations of insulin-like growth factor-I and development of glucose intolerance: a prospective observational study, *Lancet*, 359: 1740–5.

Sapolsky, R.M., Romero, L.M. and Munck, A.U. (2000) How do glucocorticoids influence stress responses? Integrating permissive, suppressive, stimulatory, and preparative actions, *Endocrine Reviews*, 21: 55–89.

Sauter, S.L. and Moon, S.D. (eds) (1996) *Beyond Biomechanics: Psychosocial Factors and Musculo-skeletal Disorders in Office Work*. New York: Taylor & Francis.

Schneider, H.J., Pagotto, U. and Stalla, G.K. (2003) Central effects of the somatotropic system, *European Journal of Endocrinology*, 149: 377–92.

Schneiderman, N., Weiss, S.M. and Kaufman, P.G. (eds) (1989) *Handbook of Research Methods in Cardiovascular Behavioral Medicine*. New York: Plenum.

Schwartz, J.E. and Stone, A.A. (1998) Strategies for analyzing ecological momentary assessment data, *Health Psychology*, 17: 6–16.

Schwartz, J.E., Warren, K. and Pickering, T.G. (1994) Mood, location and physical position as predictors of ambulatory blood pressure and heart rate: application of a multi-level random effects model, *Annals of Behavioral Medicine*, 16: 210–20.

Seeman, T.E., McEwen, B.S., Rowe, J.W. and Singer, B.H. (2001) Allostatic load as a marker of cumulative biological risk: MacArthur studies of successful aging, *Proceedings of the National Academy of Sicence, USA*, 98: 4770–5.

Sluiter, J.K., Frings-Dresen, M.H., Meijman, T.F. and van der Beek, A.J. (2000) Reactivity and recovery from different types of work measured by catecholamines and cortisol: a systematic literature overview, *Occupational and Environmental Medicine*, 57: 298–315.

Steenland, K., Fine, L., Belkic, K. *et al.* (2000) Research findings linking workplace factors to CVD outcomes, *Occupational Medicine*, 15: 7–68.

Steptoe, A. (1997) Behavior and blood pressure: implications for hypertension, in A. Zanchetti and G. Mancia (eds) *Handbook of Hypertension – Pathophysiology of Hypertension*. Amsterdam: Elsevier Science.

Steptoe, A. (1998) Psychophysiological bases of disease, in M. Johnston and D. Johnston (eds) *Comprehensive Clinical Psychology Volume 8: Health Psychology*. New York: Elsevier Science.

Steptoe, A. and Ayers, S. (2004) Stress, health and illness, in S. Sutton, A. Baum and M. Johnston (eds) *Sage Handbook of Health Psychology*. London: Sage.

Steptoe, A. and Willemsen, G. (2002) Psychophysiological responsivity in coronary heart disease, in S.A. Stansfeld and M.G. Marmot (eds) *Stress and the Heart*. London: BMJ Books.

Steptoe, A. and Willemsen, G. (2004) The influence of low job control on ambulatory blood pressure and perceived stress over the working day in men and women from the Whitehall II cohort, *Journal of Hypertension*, 22: 915–920.

Steptoe, A., Feldman, P.M., Kunz, S. *et al.* (2002) Stress responsivity and socioeconomic status: a mechanism for increased cardiovascular disease risk?, *European Heart Journal*, 23: 1757–63.

Steptoe, A., Kunz-Ebrecht, S., Owen, N. *et al.* (2003a) Influence of socioeconomic status and job control on plasma fibrinogen responses to acute mental stress, *Psychosomatic Medicine*, 65: 137–44.

Steptoe, A., Kunz-Ebrecht, S., Rumley, A. and Lowe, G.D. (2003b) Prolonged elevations in haemostatic and rheological responses following psychological stress in low socioeconomic status men and women, *Thrombosis and Haemostasis*, 89: 83–90.

Steptoe, A., Kunz-Ebrecht, S., Owen, N. *et al.* (2003c) Socioeconomic status and stress-related biological responses over the working day, *Psychosomatic Medicine*, 65: 461–70.

Steptoe, A., Owen, N., Kunz-Ebrecht, S. and Brydon, L. (2004) Loneliness and neuroendo-crine, cardiovascular, and inflammatory stress responses in middle-aged men and women, *Psychoneuroendocrinology*, 29: 593–611.

Stone, A.A., Schwartz, J.E., Smyth, J. *et al.* (2001) Individual differences in the diurnal cycle of salivary free cortisol: a replication of flattened cycles for some individuals, *Psychoneuroendo-crinology*, 26: 295–306.

Taylor, S.E., Klein, L.C., Lewis, B.P. *et al.* (2000) Biobehavioral responses to stress in females: tend-and-befriend, not fight-or-flight, *Psychological Review*, 107: 411–29.

Tuomilehto, J., Lindstrom, J., Eriksson, J.G. *et al.* (2001) Prevention of type 2 diabetes mellitus by changes in lifestyle among subjects with impaired glucose tolerance, *New England Journal of Medicine*, 344: 1343–50.

Uchino, B.N., Cacioppo, J.T. and Kiecolt-Glaser, J.K. (1996) The relationship between social support and physiological processes: a review with emphasis on underlying mechanisms and implications for health, *Psychological Bulletin*, 119: 488–531.

Van Cauter, E., Leproult, R. and Plat, L. (2000) Age-related changes in slow wave sleep and REM sleep and relationship with growth hormone and cortisol levels in healthy men, *Journal of the American Medical Association*, 284: 861–8.

Van Eck, M., Berkhof, H., Nicolson, N. and Sulon, J. (1996) The effects of perceived stress, traits, mood states, and stressful daily events on salivary cortisol, *Psychosomatic Medicine*, 58: 447–58.

Vedhara, K., Cox, N.K.M., Wilcock, G.K. *et al.* (1999a) Chronic stress in elderly carers of dementia patients and antibody response to influenza vaccination, *Lancet*, 353: 627–31.

Vedhara, K., Fox, J.D. and Wang, E.C. (1999b) The measurement of stress-related immune dysfunction in psychoneuroimmunology, *Neuroscience and Biobehavioral Reviews*, 23: 699–715.

Wamala, S.P., Murray, M.A., Horsten, M. *et al.* (1999) Socioeconomic status and determinants of hemostatic function in healthy women, *Arteriosclerosis, Thrombosis and Vascular Biology*, 19: 485–92.

Watson, D. and Pennebaker, J.W. (1989) Health complaints, stress, and distress: exploring the central role of negative affectivity, *Psychological Review*, 96: 234–54.

Weiner, H. (1992) *Perturbing the Organism: The Biology of Stressful Experience*. Chicago: University of Chicago Press.

Wittrock, D.A. (1997) The comparison of individuals with tension-type headache and headache-free controls on frontal EMG levels: a meta-analysis, *Headache*, 37: 424–32.

Wolf, O.T. (2003) HPA axis and memory, *Best Practice in Research Clinical Endocrinology of Metabolism*, 17: 287–99.

Wolf, O.T. and Kirschbaum, C. (1999) Actions of dehydroepiandrosterone and its sulfate in the central nervous system: effects on cognition and emotion in animals and humans, *Brain Research Reviews*, 30: 264–88.

Yan, L.L., Liu, K., Matthews, K.A. *et al.* (2003) Psychosocial factors and risk of hypertension: the Coronary Artery Risk Development in Young Adults (CARDIA) study, *Journal of the American Medical Association*, 290: 2138–48.

Yehuda, R. (2002) Current status of cortisol findings in post-traumatic stress disorder, *Psychiatric Clinics of North America*, 25: 341–68.

Young, A.H., Gallagher, P. and Porter, R.J. (2002) Elevation of the cortisol-dehydroepiandrosterone ratio in drug-free depressed patients, *American Journal of Psychiatry*, 159: 1237–9.

Young, E.A., Tolman, R., Witkowski, K. and Kaplan, G. (2004) Salivary cortisol and posttraumatic stress disorder in a low-income community sample of women, *Biological Psychiatry*, 55: 621–6.

Zautra, A.J., Hamilton, N.A., Potter, P. and Smith, B. (1999) Field research on the relationship between stress and disease activity in rheumatoid arthritis, *Annals of the New York Academy of Science*, 876: 397–412.

Zorrilla, E.P., Luborsky, L., McKay, J.R. *et al.* (2001) The relationship of depression and stressors to immunological assays: a meta-analytic review, *Brain, Behavior and Immunity*, 15: 199–226.

Part 4
Data analysis

21

Key issues in the statistical analysis of quantitative data in research on health and health services

Kate Tilling, Tim Peters and Jonathan Sterne

Introduction

The field of medical statistics has grown rapidly, with increasingly sophisticated methods available to researchers. In this chapter, we focus on the basic concepts underlying the reporting of statistical analyses, and on regression methods, which are used for most analyses of data from health services research. We will discuss particular issues in the analysis of randomized controlled trials (RCTs) and other study designs in health services research, and briefly outline methods that can be used when assumptions underlying standard methods are not valid.

Interpreting the results of statistical analyses

The purpose of statistical reasoning is to use the data collected in a sample to make inferences about the population from which the sample came. This is done by using the data to estimate *parameters*, which represent quantities of interest in the population. For example, we might estimate:

- the *mean* cholesterol in a group of overweight patients attending primary care for dietary advice;
- the *mean difference* in blood pressure when comparing patients randomized to a low salt diet with patients randomized to usual diet;
- the *odds ratio* comparing the odds of a first myocardial infarction (MI) in patients randomized to primary prevention with statins compared to patients randomized to placebo.

The aim is usually to examine the relationship between an *outcome* (e.g. mean blood pressure) and an *exposure* (e.g. high-salt diet). Statistical analyses are done when the results of interventions or exposures (also called *risk factors*) are unpredictable. For example, some patients randomized to primary prevention of MI using statins will nonetheless experience MI, while some patients randomized to the

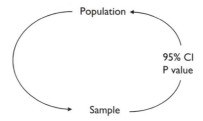

Figure 21.1   Use of confidence intervals and P values to make inferences about the population from a sample

placebo will not experience MI. This unpredictability means that our parameter estimate will not precisely equal the value of the parameter in the population. We will now describe how *confidence intervals* (CIs) and *P values* are used to quantify this uncertainty and hence to make inferences about the value of the parameter in the population, as shown in Figure 21.1.

Confidence intervals (CIs)

If the distribution of a numerical variable is normal (i.e. follows the well-known bell-shaped curve) then 95 per cent of observations lie within 1.96 standard deviations of the mean. An important finding from mathematical statistics (the 'central limit theorem') states that, providing the sample size is large enough, the sampling distribution of a mean will be normal even if the distribution of individual observations is not. It follows that in 95 per cent of samples, the interval:

$$\bar{x} - 1.96 \times \text{s.e.}(\bar{x}) \text{ to } \bar{x} + 1.96 \times \text{s.e.}(\bar{x})$$

where $\bar{x}$ is the sample mean and s.e.$(\bar{x})$ is its standard error, contains the (unknown) population mean. This interval is called a 95 per cent CI. Note that, as explained in more detail in the description of Figure 21.2, the population mean is a fixed unknown number: it is the CI that will vary between samples.

For example, in a study of 100 hypertensive patients, mean systolic blood pressure was 160mmHg. The standard deviation was 18mmHg and so the standard error of the mean is $18/\sqrt{100} = 18/10 = 1.8$. The 95 per cent CI for the population mean is thus from 156.5mmHg to 163.5mmHg. The interpretation of this interval is that, with 95 per cent confidence, the mean systolic blood pressure in the population of hypertensive adults lies between 156.5 and 163.5mmHg.

In health services research, we are usually interested in comparing two or more groups. For example, in an RCT we might be interested in the difference in mean blood pressure comparing two different anti-hypertensive treatments. Because the sampling distribution of the difference between two means is also normal, a 95 per cent CI for the difference between the population means can be calculated in the same way as above from the difference between the two sample means $(\bar{x}_1 - \bar{x}_2)$ and the standard error of this difference (s.e.$(\bar{x}_1 - \bar{x}_2)$) (Kirkwood and Sterne 2003). The confidence interval for the difference is:

$$(\bar{x}_1 - \bar{x}_2) - 1.96 \times \text{s.e.}(\bar{x}_1 - \bar{x}_2) \text{ to } (\bar{x}_1 - \bar{x}_2) + 1.96 \times \text{s.e.}(\bar{x}_1 - \bar{x}_2)$$

Provided the sample size is large enough, the sampling distribution of most parameter estimates is approximately normal. Therefore 95 per cent CIs for other statistics of interest, such as proportions or the difference between two proportions, or a 95 per cent CI for a regression coefficient (see p. 506) are calculated in exactly

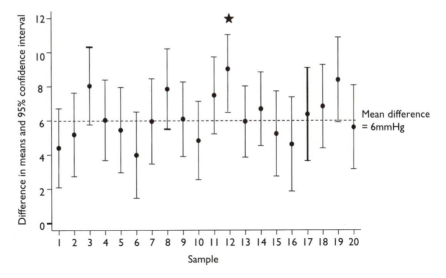

Figure 21.2 CIs for the difference in mean systolic blood pressure six months after treatment between hypertensive adults prescribed current drug C and hypertensive adults prescribed new drug N

the same way. The 95 per cent CI for a statistic S with sample (observed) value s, and standard error s.e.(s) is from (Kirkwood and Sterne 2003):

$$s - 1.96 \times \text{s.e.}(s) \text{ to } s + 1.96 \times \text{s.e.}(s)$$

Example 1

Figure 21.2 shows CIs for the difference in mean systolic blood pressure six months after treatment between hypertensive adults prescribed current drug C and hypertensive adults prescribed new drug N. A CI is presented for each of 20 random samples of size 100, from a population of hypertensive adults where the true difference in means was 6mmHg. The differences in the sample means vary around the population value of 6mmHg. One of the twenty 95 per cent CIs does not contain the true population difference in means. Note that when we do statistical analyses in practice our inference will be based on the CI from just one sample.

P values and hypothesis testing

Suppose we believe that everybody who lives to age 90 or more is a non-smoker. We could investigate this hypothesis in two ways:

- *prove* the hypothesis by finding every single person aged 90 or over and checking that they are all non-smokers;
- *disprove* the hypothesis by finding just one person aged 90 or over who is a smoker.

It is much easier to find evidence *against* the hypothesis than to prove it to be correct. Statistical methods formalize this idea by using relevant data to look for evidence against a *null hypothesis*. Usually these are statements that there is no association between an exposure or intervention and the outcome. For example:

- MMR vaccination does not affect a child's subsequent risk of autism;
- birth weight is not associated with subsequent IQ;
- living close to power lines does not change children's risk of leukaemia.

We examine the evidence against the null hypothesis by calculating a *P value* (also known as a *significance level*). This is the probability of observing a difference (magnitude of association) at least as far from the null hypothesis as that observed in our study, if the null hypothesis were really true. The smaller the P value, the lower the chance of getting a difference as big as the one observed if the null hypothesis is true. Therefore the smaller the P value, the stronger the evidence against the null hypothesis (see Figure 21.3). Details of the calculation of P values will not be given here, but can be found in any standard statistical text (e.g. Altman 1991; Kirkwood and Sterne 2003).

Example 2

In an RCT, systolic blood pressure in hypertensive adults after six months treatment with new drug N was on average 6mmHg lower than in adults treated with control drug C. We need to know whether this provides evidence against the null hypothesis that drugs N and C have equal effects on systolic blood pressure. The 95 per cent CI for the difference in mean blood pressure between C and N was from 4.2 to 8.2mmHg, P = 0.001.

The P value calculated here is the probability of observing a difference in systolic blood pressure at least this big, if the average systolic blood pressure in the populations are really the same. The *smaller* is the P value, the *stronger* is the evidence against

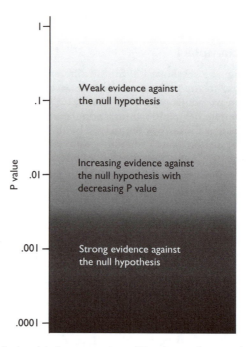

Figure 21.3   Relationship between size of P value and strength of evidence against the null hypothesis

the null hypothesis that among hypertensive adults drugs N and C have equal effects on systolic blood pressure six months after treatment.

Use of thresholds to determine 'statistical significance'

The difficulty in obtaining precise P values in the days before widespread use of computers led to the use of the arbitrary cut-off of 0.05 to divide 'significant' from 'non-significant' results. However, this concept is outdated (Sterne and Davey Smith 2001) and, as discussed below, can lead to misinterpretation of results. Instead, the precise P value should be quoted and interpreted as a continuum of evidence against the null hypothesis (as in Figure 21.3).

Use and mis-use of P values and CIs

Three common errors arise from the use of the 'significance' threshold (Sterne and Davey Smith 2001; Kirkwood and Sterne 2003):

* Potentially clinically important differences observed in small studies, for which P > 0.05 are denoted as 'non-significant' and ignored. We can protect ourselves against this error if we always examine the CI as well as the P value. In small studies, in which the standard error of the difference will be large, the CI will often be wide, indicating that the results are consistent with a wide range of differences in the population.
* 'Statistically significant' (P < 0.05) findings are assumed to result from real treatment effects. By definition, 1 in 20 comparisons in which the null hypothesis is true will result in P < 0.05. Sterne and Davey Smith (2001) show that, in circumstances typical of medical research, this implies that P < 0.05 does not constitute strong evidence against the null hypothesis.
* 'Statistically significant' (P < 0.05) findings are assumed to be of clinical importance. Given a large sample size, even a small (clinically unimportant) difference will be 'statistically significantly' different from zero. Again, we must always examine the *magnitude* of the difference as well as the P value.

Sub-group analyses

A common example of misinterpretation of statistical significance occurs when significance tests are performed separately in sub-groups, and the P values within each sub-group are used rather than a formal test of interaction (Brookes *et al.* 2004).

Example 3

A randomized trial of treatment in stroke units or general medical wards with stroke team support was carried out in 457 acute stroke patients (Evans *et al.* 2002). Fewer patients in the stroke unit arm than the general medical ward arm of the trial were dead or in an institution at 12 months (21/152 [14%] vs. 45/149 [30%], odds ratio = 0.37 [95% CI 0.20 to 0.67], P < 0.001). The authors carried out separate analyses for 164 patients with large vessel infarcts and 103 with lacunar infarcts, and concluded that 'Stroke units improve the outcome in patients with large-vessel infarcts but not lacunar infarcts'. The results presented for mortality and institutionalization in the stroke unit compared to the general medical ward arm of the trial were:

Large vessel infarcts: OR 0.36 (95% CI 0.16 to 0.77), P = 0.01

Lacunar infarcts: OR 0.20 (95% CI 0.04 to 1.11), P = 0.06

If we judge results solely according to statistical significance at the conventional level of 0.05, then we are misled into believing that there is a beneficial effect of stroke units only for large-vessel infarcts. However, the estimated effect of stroke unit care is in fact *greater* in the lacunar than the large vessel group, although the CI is wider because of the smaller numbers in the lacunar group. Note also that subgroups should never be compared based on their separate P values. Rather, the size of effect in each group should be compared and, more formally, P values derived for *interaction* (these test the null hypothesis that the size of the difference is the same in each group) (Brookes *et al.* 2004). This is discussed further in the section on regression (see p. 508).

Bayesian methods

P values and CIs are derived using the *frequentist framework* for statistical inference. In this framework, we assume that there is a true (fixed) population value for the parameter that we are trying to estimate. For example, we may assume that there is a true value for the odds ratio comparing the odds of death if the entire population of stroke patients were treated in a stroke unit with the odds of death if the entire population were treated in a general medical ward. The frequentist approach is to use data (e.g. odds of death up to 1 year post-stroke for people admitted to a stroke unit and those admitted to a general medical ward) to draw conclusions about this 'true' value, using P values and CIs. For example, given a set of data, we might conclude that the odds ratio for death if treated in a stroke unit compared to a general medical ward is 0.5, with a 95 per cent CI from 0.37 to 0.67. Thus we are 95 per cent confident that the true odds of death if treated in a stroke unit are between 0.37 and 0.67 times the odds if treated in a general medical ward.

In contrast, the *Bayesian approach* starts with a *prior belief* (expressed as a probability distribution) about the likely values of the parameters, and then uses the observed data to modify this belief. We will denote this prior belief by prob(parameters). Bayes' formula provides the mechanism to update this belief in the light of the data:

Prob (model parameters given data) =

$$\frac{\text{prob (data given model parameters)} \times \text{prob (parameters)}}{\text{prob (data)}}$$

The probability distribution of the model parameters given the data and the prior belief is known as the *posterior distribution*. Using this, we can derive a 95 per cent *credible interval*, within which there is 95 per cent probability that the parameter lies.

The stronger the prior opinion about the parameter to be estimated, the more the posterior probability will be influenced by this prior belief compared to the influence of the observed data. If the prior opinion about the parameter is very vague (we consider a very wide range of values to be equally likely) then the results of a frequentist analysis will be very similar to the results of a Bayesian analysis. Table 21.1 compares the Bayesian and frequentist approaches to statistical inference.

Confounding

A variable that is related both to the outcome variable and to the exposure of interest, and that is not a part of the causal pathway between them, is called a *confounding variable*. Ignoring the effects of confounding variables may lead to bias in

Table 21.1   Comparison of frequentist and Bayesian approaches to statistical inference about a risk ratio

Frequentist statistics	Bayesian statistics
We use the data to make inferences about the true (but unknown) population value of the risk ratio.	We start with our *prior* opinion about the risk ratio, expressed as a probability distribution. We use the data to modify that opinion (we derive the *posterior* probability distribution for the risk ratio based on the data *and* the prior distribution).
The 95% CI gives us a range of values for the population risk ratio that is consistent with the data. 95 per cent of the times we derive such a range it will contain the true (but unknown) population value.	A 95% *credible interval* is one that has a 95 per cent chance of containing the population risk ratio.
The P value is the probability of getting an estimate at least as far from the null value as the one found in our study; if the null hypothesis is true.	The posterior distribution can be used to derive direct probability statements about the risk ratio, e.g. the probability that the drug *increases* the risk of death.

Source: Sterne and Davey Smith (2001)

the estimate of the exposure-outcome association. Confounding is a fundamental problem in the analysis of observational (non-experimental) studies and in the analysis of experimental studies that are not randomized, as the groups being compared may differ with regard to prognostic variables.

As a general rule, variables that are known *a priori* to be important confounders based on previous work should be controlled for in the analysis of observational and non-randomized studies. In addition, other possible confounders may be selected as a result of exploratory analysis. The choice of confounding factors to include in the models should be based on both the data being analysed and external knowledge (e.g. from the results of other studies or biological knowledge). Careful consideration is needed of the likely direction of association between the exposure E, the outcome D and the confounder C to decide whether it is appropriate to control for C in estimating the E-D association. Causal diagrams (Greenland and Brumback 2002; Hernan *et al.* 2002), which link exposure, outcome and other variables by arrows representing direct causal effects, are useful in identifying variables which should and should not be included as confounders. For example, Figure 21.4(a) shows an example where the confounder C is causally related to both exposure E and outcome D. Figure 21.4(b) shows an example where the exposure E occurs before the confounder C, which occurs before the outcome D. In cases like this, where the confounder may be an intermediate on the causal pathway between exposure and disease, the confounder should not be adjusted for in analyses of the exposure-disease association.

Example 4

Hernan *et al.* (2002) present data from a case-control study on folic acid supplementation and risk of neural tube defects. The odds ratio adjusted for whether the pregnancy ended in stillbirth/induced abortion was 0.80 (95 per cent CI: 0.62, 1.21). However, consideration of causal diagrams (e.g. Figure 21.5) suggested that this variable should not be included as a confounder (because the event occurs after the exposure), and that therefore the crude odds ratio of 0.65 (95 per cent CI: 0.46, 0.94) should be used.

(a) C is a confounder for the relationship between E and D

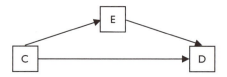

(b) C is on the causal pathway for the relationship between E and D

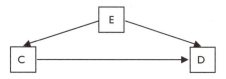

Figure 21.4   Causal diagrams showing possible relationships between confounder C, exposure E and outcome D

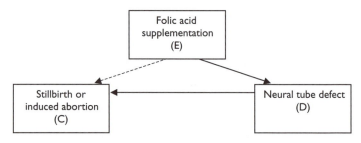

Figure 21.5   Causal diagram showing one possible relationship between folic acid supplementation and neural tube defects in pregnancy

Regression models

Regression models are often used to estimate exposure–disease associations controlled for the confounding effects of a number of different variables. Only a basic outline of regression models will be given here – further details are available in several statistical and epidemiological texts (e.g. Szklo and Nieto 1999; Kirkwood and Sterne 2003).

Simple linear regression

We firstly consider *simple linear regression* in which only one numerical exposure variable is considered. The mathematical equation for a straight line is:

$$y = \beta_0 + \beta_1 x$$

We say that β_0 and β_1 are the *parameters* of the linear regression: β_1 is the slope of the line, and β_0 is the point where the line intercepts with the y axis. Thus, β_1 represents the average change in the outcome (y) associated with a unit change in the exposure

(x), and β_0 represents the average value of y when $x = 0$. The best-fitting line is derived using the method of *least squares* (Kirkwood and Sterne 2003).

Example 5

A study of 200 middle-aged men measured weight (in kg) and height (in cm). Table 21.2 shows the regression coefficients for a regression of weight on height. The regression coefficient for height is the estimate of the gradient of the line (β_1) while the regression coefficient labelled 'constant' is to the estimate of the intercept (β_0). Therefore, the regression line that best describes the relationship between weight and height in middle-aged men is:

weight (kg) = −64.6 + 0.85 × height (cm)

So the average increase in weight associated with a 1cm increase in height is 0.85kg. The intercept, −64.6 kg, technically represents the weight for a man of height 0cm but, in practice, this is meaningless.

   In fact it is often the case in practical medical statistics that the intercept is of little interest; we are usually more interested in the slope of the regression line since this tells us about the magnitude of the association between the exposure and the outcome. The intercept can be made more interpretable by 'centring' the exposure variable – for example by creating a new variable by subtracting the mean height for this population (168cm) from the height variable. In a regression of weight on this 'centred' height, the intercept is 77.5kg (95 per cent CI, 75.5 to 79.5kg), while the slope of the regression line is unchanged (0.85kg/cm). In this case, the intercept is the mean weight at the mean height in the population.

Assumptions involved in regression analyses

There are four main assumptions underlying linear regression: that the observations are independent (see the section on clustered data, p. 510); that, for any value of x, y is normally distributed; that the magnitude of the scatter of the points about the line is the same throughout the length of the line; and that the relationship between x and y is linear. These assumptions should be investigated. Some techniques that may be used when these assumptions are not satisfied are discussed in the last section of this chapter (see p. 511).

Linear regression when the exposure variable is binary

Simple linear regression is used to relate two numerical variables (e.g. height and weight). However, often the exposure of interest is a binary variable – for example in an RCT, the exposure is a binary indicator for the two arms of the trial. Linear regression simplifies to include binary exposures as follows:

$y = \beta_0 + \beta_1 x$

Table 21.2 Regression coefficients for the relationship between weight and height in middle-aged men

Weight (kg)	Coefficient	95% CI	P > t
Height (cm)	0.85	0.62 to 1.07	< 0.001
Constant	−64.6	−102.0 to −27.1	0.001

where x (the binary exposure) is a 0 for individuals in the control group and 1 for individuals in the intervention group. The regression coefficient β_1 represents the estimated difference in mean outcome (y) between the two arms of the trial. The 95 per cent CI for the estimated difference in mean outcome between the two arms of the trial is given by the 95 per cent CI for the regression coefficient. The intercept represents the mean outcome in the control group.

Linear regression of a numerical outcome on a binary exposure is equivalent to performing a t-test, giving the same estimate, 95 per cent CI and P value. This is one example of regression providing a general means of carrying out statistical analyses which are often seen as distinct procedures.

Regression when the outcome is not numerical

The outcome of interest may not be numerical – for example in a trial of stroke unit care, one outcome of interest is the binary outcome of death by one year post-stroke. The probability of death by one year cannot be modelled directly using linear regression because it is constrained to lie between 0 and 1. Instead, it is transformed to an unconstrained quantity. For a binary outcome, the most common transformation used is the log of the odds of the outcome. Here, we use the log of the odds of death (also called the *logit* of the probability of death), that is:

$$\log(\textit{odds of death}) = \log\!\left(\frac{p(\textit{death})}{1 - p(\textit{death})}\right)$$

where $p(\textit{death})$ is the probability of death by 1 year. We can then relate this to the exposure variable x (which may be numerical or binary), exactly as in simple linear regression:

$$\log(\textit{odds of death}) = \beta_0 + \beta_1 x$$

If the exposure is numerical, then the regression coefficient is the estimated increase in the log of the odds of death associated with a one unit increase in the exposure. If the exposure is binary, the regression coefficient is the *log odds ratio*: the difference between the log of the odds of death in the group for which $x = 1$ and the log of odds of death in the group for which $x = 0$. It is common to exponentiate these coefficients before presenting them, giving *odds ratios*. This type of regression model is referred to as *logistic regression* (see Table 21.3).

Different regression models, not covered in detail here, are available for unordered and ordered categorical outcomes and time-to-event outcomes (e.g. Agresti 1996; Szklo and Nieto 1999; Agresti 2002; Kirkwood and Sterne 2003). These are summarized in Table 21.3.

Table 21.3　Summary of the main regression models

Type of outcome variable (y)	Type of regression model	Measure of exposure effect	Model format
Numerical	Linear	Difference in means	$y = \beta_0 + \beta_1 x$
Binary	Logistic	Odds ratio	$\log(\text{odds of } y) = \beta_0 + \beta_1 x$
Matched binary	Conditional logistic	Odds ratio	$\log(\text{odds of } y) = \beta_0 + \beta_1 x$
Ordered categorical	Ordinal logistic	Odds ratio	$\log(\text{odds of } y) = \beta_0 + \beta_1 x$*
Time to binary event	Poisson	Rate ratio	$\log(\text{rate of } y) = \beta_0 + \beta_1 x$
Time to binary event	Cox	Hazard ratio	$\log(\text{hazard of } y) = \beta_0 + \beta_1 x$

* Comparing any division of the categories of y into an upper and lower group.

It is often the case that we have a choice of which regression model to use, depending on how the outcome variable is expressed (Kirkwood and Sterne 2003). For example, blood pressure may be expressed as a numerical, binary or ordered categorical variable, in which case we would use linear, logistic or ordinal logistic regression respectively. It is desirable to choose the regression model that uses as much of the information in the data as possible. In the blood pressure example, this would favour using linear regression with blood pressure as a numerical variable, since categorizing or dichotomizing it would discard some of the information collected. However, it is often sensible to use simpler models before proceeding to more complex ones and to assess whether the gain in precision of the estimates obtained justifies the extra complexity and potential loss of ease of interpretation and clinical relevance.

Multiple regression

Regression models with a single exposure variable can be extended to the situation where we want to look at the relationship between the outcome variable and not one but several exposure variables simultaneously. For example, where there are p exposure variables (x_1 to x_p), the multiple linear regression equation for outcome y on these exposures is:

$$y = \beta_0 + \beta_1 x_1 + \beta_2 x_2 + \ldots + \beta_p x_p$$

Regression models for binary and other non-numerical outcomes can be extended to include more than one exposure variable in exactly the same way. For example, a logistic model relating p exposure variables (x_1 to x_p) to the binary outcome y has the form:

$$\log(odds\ of\ y) = \beta_0 + \beta_1 x_1 + \beta_2 x_2 + \ldots + \beta_p x_p$$

Regression models can deal with many exposure variables, which may be categorical or numerical. A categorical exposure with k categories would be included in the regression equation as $k-1$ *dummy* (also known as *indicator*) variables, each representing one category of exposure. It is usual to choose the category containing the highest proportion of subjects as the *reference* (or baseline) category, and then include dummy variables for the other categories, unless there are *a priori* reasons for choosing a different category as the reference. For example, suppose exposure is age, grouped in three categories: 0–20, 20–40 and 40–60, with 40 per cent of participants falling in the 20–40 age group and 30 per cent in each of the others. The 20–40 age group would be chosen as the reference category, and two exposure variables x_1 and x_2 chosen such that:

$x_1 = 1$ when age = 0–20, and 0 otherwise

$x_2 = 1$ when age = 40–60, and 0 otherwise

In a linear regression model, regression coefficient for x_1 then represents the mean difference in outcome between those aged 0–20 and those aged 20–40.

When reading a report of any observational study, it is vital to consider whether the authors have accounted adequately for the effects of confounding factors in their analyses (see earlier section on confounding, p. 502). Therefore it is usual to display both the *crude association* and the association *controlling* or *adjusting* for potential confounders.

Interactions

The regression models presented assume that each of the exposure variables included acts independently. For example, in a model relating stroke outcome at one year (alive or dead) to age (grouped as < 80 or 80) and whether the patient was treated in a stroke unit, it would be assumed that the effect of being treated in a stroke unit was the same for those aged under 80 as those aged over 80. The logistic regression model for this would be:

$$\log(odds\ of\ death) = \beta_0 + \beta_1\ (\text{age}) + \beta_2\ (\text{stroke unit})$$

However, it may be that stroke unit care was more effective for those aged under 80 than for those aged over 80. In this case, the model would include an *interaction term:*

$$\log(odds\ of\ death) = \beta_0 + \beta_1\ (\text{age}) + \beta_2\ (\text{stroke unit}) + \beta_3\ (\text{age} \times \text{stroke unit})$$

The interaction term β_3 represents the difference in effect of stroke unit on outcome between those aged under and over 80. The null hypothesis that this interaction term is 0 can be tested using the P value corresponding to the regression coefficient.

One common use for the interaction test is in a sub-group analysis (see p. 00). For example, in an RCT of stroke unit and general medical ward care for stroke patients, a planned sub-group analysis might be to investigate whether the intervention (stroke unit care) has different effects in different sub-types (see Example 3, p. 00) (Evans *et al.* 2002). This would involve fitting an interaction term between stroke unit care and stroke sub-type, and examining the strength of the evidence against the null hypothesis of no interaction effect. Studies are often underpowered with respect to tests for interactions (Brookes *et al.* 2004).

Strategies for analysis

It is essential to plan and conduct statistical analyses in a way that maximizes the quality and interpretability of the findings. In a typical study, data are collected on a large number of variables and it can be difficult to decide which methods to use and in what order. The following list provides a brief summary of what should be considered (Kirkwood and Sterne 2003).

- Formulate an analysis plan in advance (see Chapter 5). This will be more specific for a randomized trial than for an observational study.
- Careful checking and editing of the dataset for errors is essential before statistical analysis commences.
- Descriptive analysis: the distributions of each of the variables should be examined.
- Data reduction: it may be necessary to derive new variables by grouping the values of some of the original variables – *never* overwrite the original variables.
- Univariable analyses: look at crude associations between outcome and exposure to familiarize with the dataset and possible associations – later analyses controlling for the effects of other variables will supersede this stage.
- Allow for confounding.
- Analyse for interactions where they are of specific interest.
- Make analyses reproducible by keeping a record of all new variables created and analyses performed.

Issues in analysis of RCTs

RCTs provide the best evidence on the effectiveness of treatments and health care interventions. Their key design features (see Chapter 5) ensure that the intervention groups do not differ systematically with respect to either known or unknown prognostic factors, and hence that such factors do not confound the estimated effect of the intervention. It is for this reason that RCTs allow us to make causal inferences about the effect of intervention. Here, we discuss two important issues in the analysis of RCTs: intention to treat and adjustment for baseline covariates.

Intention to treat analysis

The primary analysis of an RCT should always be an 'intention to treat' analysis, in which participants are analysed according to the intervention group to which they were randomly assigned, whether or not they actually accepted, received or adhered to this intervention. The reason that the primary analysis should be intention to treat is that only the groups to which patients were randomized are guaranteed not to differ systematically according to prognostic factors. That is, characteristics of patients that predict whether they accept, receive or adhere to their randomized intervention may also be associated with patients' prognosis.

Analyses based on the actual intervention received, or with patients excluded if they did not adhere to their prescribed treatment, are known as 'per protocol' analyses. For the reasons explained above, a per protocol analysis can produce seriously biased estimates of the effect of an intervention. For example, consider a placebo-controlled trial of a new drug with unpleasant side-effects. If the most ill patients are unable to take the new drug they may withdraw from the assigned treatment. Such problems will not affect the placebo group, and therefore a per protocol analysis would overestimate the effect of the drug by comparing less sick patients in the drug group with all patients in the placebo group.

Use of the CONSORT guidelines (see Chapter 5) ensures that the number of withdrawals from treatment allocations, and the reasons for withdrawals, are reported. Comparison of those who did and did not adhere to their allocated treatment allows some assessment of the bias in a per protocol analysis. Analytical methods validly allowing for non-adherence are available (e.g. White *et al.* 2002; Walker *et al.* 2004), but should be used only with expert advice.

Adjusting for baseline covariates

When the outcome of a trial is numerical (and assumed to be normally distributed), adjustment for baseline covariates may be desirable in order to minimize bias and maximize statistical efficiency (Pocock *et al.* 2002). The choice of the baseline variables that should be included in the regression model depends on the magnitude of the association between the baseline covariate and the outcome. If an outcome variable (e.g. blood pressure six months after treatment) is also measured at baseline (e.g. at the randomization appointment) then the baseline value of the variable should be included in a regression model for the final outcome, as correlations between baseline and outcome variable are likely to be high (Pocock *et al.* 2002). A variable that is known *a priori* to be strongly related to outcome ought to be included in a regression model for final outcome, regardless of whether there is imbalance in this variable between the two arms of a particular trial. The analysis plan should specify covariates to be included in the regression model for final outcome. In practice, a review showed that unadjusted and covariate-adjusted analyses tend to give similar results (Assmann *et al.* 2000).

Where the outcome is binary, adjustment for baseline covariates that are strongly related to the outcome does not result in more precise estimates, but does result in estimates that are further from the null value. Adjustment for a covariate that is strongly related to the outcome also leads to increased statistical power (Pocock *et al.* 2002).

Issues in analysis of health services research data

Clustered data

In most health services research studies, the unit of intervention/exposure (and hence of analysis) is the individual. However, in some cases, the intervention is applied to groups of people (e.g. a cluster randomized trial, see Chapter 5) or groups of people undergo the same exposure (e.g. each member of the family experiences the same household diet). In such studies, the groups are commonly called 'clusters'. Because people from the same cluster may be more similar to each other than people from different clusters (e.g. due to shared genes, socioeconomic background, access to health care, etc.), any clustering must be taken into account in the analysis. This can be done in four main ways (Kirkwood and Sterne 2003; Peters *et al.* 2003):

- Make comparisons at the cluster level data – for example, calculate a mean outcome for each cluster, and then use these means as the data for analysis. This method does not take account of the varying precision with which the outcome may be measured within each cluster (e.g. because of varying sample sizes). However, this problem can be overcome by weighting the analysis by the precision for each cluster.
- Analyse the data as if the individuals were not clustered, then use robust standard errors to adjust the standard errors for the clustering.
- Use generalized estimating equations (GEE), which adjust the estimates and standard errors for clustering but treat the clustering itself as a nuisance parameter (so no estimates of between–cluster variation are obtained).
- Use a random effects model to allow for variation between clusters in addition to variation between individuals within clusters. This adjusts estimates and standard errors for clustering, and also models the degree of similarity between and within clusters.

Missing data

One issue which occurs in most studies in health services research is that of missing data. There are three different ways in which data can be 'missing' (Little and Rubin 1987):

- *Missing completely at random (MCAR)*: the probability that a particular observation is missing does not depend on the value of any observable variable(s). For example, missing blood pressure measurements due to breakdown of an automatic sphygmomanometer might reasonably be assumed MCAR, since the fact that a measurement could not be obtained depends neither on the missing value itself nor (probably) on other observed values for those subjects with missing values.
- *Missing at random (MAR)*: conditional on the observed data, the probability that observations are missing is independent of the true values of the missing data. For example, suppose that younger people are less likely to return to the clinic to have their blood pressures measured, but that the probability that a blood pressure

measurement is missing is unrelated to actual blood pressure at the time the measurement would have been taken, after taking age into account. In this case the missing blood pressure measurement would be MAR in models including age. If age were omitted from the analysis, however, these missing values would no longer be MAR.

*   *Missing not at random (MNAR)*: the probability that observations are missing is not independent of the true outcome, even after taking the other measured variables into account. For example, if highly stressed people are less likely to return to a clinic for a blood pressure measurement, *even after taking account of all measured variables such as age, height, weight, social class etc.* then missing blood pressure measurements will be MNAR. When data are MNAR it is not possible to perform valid inferences without making (untestable) assumptions about the missing data mechanism.

It is important to realize that the data can help to distinguish between MCAR and MAR, but cannot distinguish between MAR and MNAR, because to demonstrate MNAR would require knowledge of the missing data. The most common way to deal with missing data in statistical analyses, and the default in most statistical software packages, is to restrict analyses to individuals with no missing values in any variable. However, this causes loss of efficiency even when the data are MCAR. Standard analytical methods will give biased estimates unless the data are MCAR. If data on *outcome* are MAR, then standard analytical methods (e.g. regression models relating outcome to exposures), including the variables relating to the missing data mechanism, will give unbiased estimates. However, if data on *exposures* are MAR, standard analytical methods may still be biased.

One approach that can generate unbiased and efficient estimates in the presence of missing data is the method of *multiple imputation* followed by complete data analyses. Here, we generate multiple complete datasets based on a model for the missing values given the observed data that incorporates the uncertainty in predicting the missing values. Each of the datasets may then be analysed using standard methods, and will give a different set of parameter estimates and their standard errors. Valid inferences may be obtained by using the average of these parameter estimates as the overall estimate of the parameter of interest. The overall standard error is a combination of the standard error of the parameter estimates and the average of the imputed standard errors (Little and Rubin 1987).

Methods to use when regression model assumptions are violated

In standard regression models, the precision of the estimated associations between disease and exposure is quantified by the standard error of the regression coefficient. For example, logistic regression might be used to estimate an odds ratio for death or institutionalization at 12 months for stroke unit compared to general medical ward care. The standard error of the log of the odds ratio would be used to derive a CI for this estimate. However, this CI depends on the assumption that the log of the odds ratio is normally distributed, as will be the case when model assumptions are satisfied and the sample size is sufficiently large.

The following three methods (bootstrap, jackknife and robust standard errors) avoid making assumptions about the distribution of the parameter of interest, and are thus useful to validate the assumption of normality (e.g. when using small datasets), and to avoid bias where this assumption is not satisfied.

Bootstrap

There are two bootstrap methods, parametric and non-parametric, as described in Carpenter and Bithell (2000). The principle behind the bootstrap is to obtain information on the sampling distribution of the parameter of interest by examining the relationship between the parameter estimate from the observed dataset and the value(s) estimated from *resampled* datasets.

Resampling is usually done by *sampling with replacement* from the observed dataset (the non-parametric bootstrap). Suppose we have a dataset consisting of N individuals. Sampling with replacement would mean creating a new data set also of N individuals. To choose the first individual for the new dataset, an individual would be selected at random from the N in the original dataset. The second individual would be chosen the same way – so, by chance, the same individual could appear as both the first and second individual in the new dataset. This process would continue until N individuals had been chosen for the new dataset. One or more individuals from the original dataset will appear more than once in the new dataset while other individuals will not appear in the new dataset.

The resampling could alternatively be performed by sampling from the distribution function of the parameter estimate from the observed dataset (the parametric bootstrap). Further details are available in Carpenter and Bithell (2000).

Jackknife

The jackknife is similar to the bootstrap method, but instead of resampling from the whole distribution (with replacement), one measurement in turn is removed for each 'resampling'. The jackknife has now been superseded by the bootstrap for general use, as bootstrap estimators tend to be less biased and have lower variance than jackknife estimators. The jackknife also does not work well for non-smooth parameters (such as the median), where removal of one data point can cause a large change in the parameter estimate (Efron 1981). The main uses of the jackknife are to detect influential observations, or to test the predictive power of prognostic models (Zheng and Agresti 2000).

Robust standard errors

The method of robust standard errors, which was suggested independently by Huber (1967) and White (1980), uses the variability in the data, rather than the variability predicted by the model, to estimate the standard errors (Kirkwood and Sterne 2003; Peters *et al.* 2003). The formula to derive robust standard errors is based on the residuals, that is, the difference between the observed outcome for each individual and that predicted by the regression model. With sufficiently large sample sizes, robust standard errors will be correct (providing that the regression model relating mean outcome to covariates is correct) even if the probability model for the outcome variables is wrong. Robust standard errors can thus be used when numerical outcomes are not normally distributed. They are also often used in the analysis of clustered data (see p. 510) (Peters *et al.* 2003).

Conclusions

The number of medical journals, and hence the amount of information published on health services research, has increased over the past decade. However, the quality of statistical analyses in published reports has remained of concern. An editorial in

1994 reported on the 'scandal of poor medical research', discussing common errors such as misuse of statistical techniques (Altman 1994). Almost a decade later, a commentary reported that, in the area of randomized trials, 'poor methodology and reporting are widespread', and that other study designs also suffer from error in analysis and reporting (Altman 2002). Correct conduct and interpretation of analyses is essential to ensure that the evidence base for medicine is robust.

<table>
<tr>
<td>

Key points

</td>
<td>

- The purpose of statistical analysis is to use the data collected in a sample to make inferences about the population from which the sample came.

- Confidence intervals are used to derive a plausible range for the value of a parameter of interest in the population.

- It is easier to find evidence against a hypothesis than to prove it to be correct; statistical methods formalize this by using the data to look for evidence against a null hypothesis. The evidence against the null hypothesis is examined by calculating a P value.

- It is better to present the precise P value than to declare results as 'statistically significant' or not.

- A common misinterpretation of 'statistical significance' occurs when significance tests are performed separately in sub-groups, and the P values within each sub-group are used to determine whether the association of interest differs between the sub-groups. Such differences should be examined using tests for interaction.

- P values and confidence intervals are usually derived using the 'frequentist' framework for statistical inference, in which it is assumed there is a true (fixed) population value for the parameter that we are trying to estimate. This contrasts with the Bayesian approach in which a prior belief (expressed as a probability distribution) about the likely values of the parameters is modified by the observed data to give a posterior distribution.

- A variable that is related to both the outcome variable and to the exposure of interest, and that is not a part of a causal pathway between them, is called a confounding variable.

- Regression models are often used to estimate exposure-disease associations controlled for the confounding effects of a number of different variables.

- The primary analysis of an RCT should be an 'intention to treat' analysis, in which participants are analysed according to the intervention group to which they were randomly assigned, whether or not they actually accepted, received or adhered to this intervention.

- In most health services research, the unit of intervention/exposure (and hence analysis) is the individual. When individuals within groups (clusters) tend to be more similar to each other than to other individuals in the sample, standard statistical methods are not valid. This situation occurs when interventions are assigned to groups rather than individuals. Methods to deal with clustering are available.

- Bias can be introduced by missing data, and methods to deal with this have recently become available.

</td>
</tr>
</table>

- When the assumptions underlying a regression model are violated, the standard errors may not be valid. In such situations 'bootstrap' standard errors or 'robust' standard errors may be used.

References

Agresti, A. (1996) *An Introduction to Categorical Data Analysis.* New York: Wiley.

Agresti, A. (2002) *Categorical Data Analysis,* 2nd edn. New York: Wiley.

Altman, D.G. (1991) *Practical Statistics for Medical Research.* London: Chapman & Hall.

Altman, D.G. (1994) The scandal of poor medical research, *British Medical Journal,* 308: 283–4.

Altman, D.G. (2002) Poor-quality medical research: what can journals do?, *Journal of the American Medical Association,* 287: 2765–7.

Assmann, S.F., Pocock, S.J., Enos, L.E. and Kasten, L.E. (2000) Subgroup analysis and other (mis)uses of baseline data in clinical trials, *Lancet,* 355: 1064–9.

Brookes, S.T., Whitely, E., Egger, M. *et al.* (2004) Subgroup analyses in randomized trials: risks of subgroup-specific analyses; power and sample size for the interaction test, *Journal of Clinical Epidemiology,* 57: 229–36.

Carpenter, J. and Bithell, J. (2000) Bootstrap confidence intervals: when, which, what? A practical guide for medical statisticians, *Statistics in Medicine,* 19: 1141–64.

Efron, B. (1981) Nonparametric estimates of standard error – the jackknife, the bootstrap and other methods, *Biometrika,* 68: 589–99.

Evans, A., Harraf, F., Donaldson, N. and Kalra, L. (2002) Randomized controlled study of stroke unit care versus stroke team care in different stroke subtypes, *Stroke,* 33: 449–55.

Greenland, S. and Brumback, B. (2002) An overview of relations among causal modelling methods, *International Journal of Epidemiology,* 31: 1030–7.

Hernan, M.A., Hernandez-Diaz, S., Werler, M.M. and Mitchell, A.A. (2002) Causal knowledge as a prerequisite for confounding evaluation: an application to birth defects epidemiology, *American Journal of Epidemiology,* 155: 176–84.

Huber, P.J. (1967) The behaviour of maximum likelihood estimates under non-standard conditions, in *Proceedings of the Fifth Berkeley Symposium on Mathematical Statistics and Probability.* Berkeley, CA: University of California.

Kirkwood, B.R. and Sterne, J.A.C. (2003) *Essential Medical Statistics,* 2nd edn. Oxford: Blackwell.

Little, R.J.A. and Rubin, D.B. (1987) *Statistical Analysis with Missing Data.* New York: Wiley.

Peters, T.J., Richards, S.H., Bankhead, C.R. *et al.* (2003) Comparison of methods for analysing cluster randomized trials: an example involving a factorial design, *International Journal of Epidemiology,* 32: 840–6.

Pocock, S.J., Assmann, S.E., Enos, L.E. and Kasten, L.E. (2002) Subgroup analysis, covariate adjustment and baseline comparisons in clinical trial reporting: current practice and problems, *Statistics in Medicine,* 21: 2917–30.

Sterne, J.A. and Davey Smith, G. (2001) Sifting the evidence – what's wrong with significance tests?, *British Medical Journal,* 322: 226–31.

Szklo, M. and Nieto, F.J. (1999) *Epidemiology: Beyond the Basics.* Gaithersburg, MD: Aspen Publishers.

Walker, A.S., White, I.R. and Babiker, A.G. (2004) Parametric randomization-based methods for correcting for treatment changes in the assessment of the causal effect of treatment, *Statistics in Medicine,* 23(4): 571–90.

White, H. (1980) A Heteroskedasticity-consistent covariance-matrix estimator and a direct test for heteroskedasticity, *Econometrica,* 48: 817–38.

White, I.R., Walker, S. and Babiker, A.G. (2002) strbee: randomization-based efficacy estimator, *Stata Journal,* 2: 140–50.

Zheng, B.Y. and Agresti, A. (2000) Summarizing the predictive power of a generalized linear model, *Statistics in Medicine,* 19: 1771–81.

22

Key issues in the analysis of qualitative data in health services research

Jenny Donovan and Caroline Sanders

Introduction

Qualitative research methods are being increasingly employed in multidisciplinary research on health and health services. In most cases, such methods – including in-depth interviews, focus group interviews and observational techniques – are included as one set of research methods alongside others, such as questionnaires, epidemiological, statistical or economic evaluations. Some qualitative research may be undertaken independently, often in health services research (HSR) as a precursor to quantitative research. Within HSR, qualitative research can be anywhere along a scale from a simple summary description of an open text field in a questionnaire survey, to a complex ethnography of a health system, and there are many methods and degrees of complexity in between. Methods of data analysis may similarly span a continuum from basic description (content analysis) to longitudinal grounded theory. Whatever the method of data collection and analysis, key characteristics of qualitative research include the interrelationship, and often iterative process, between data collection and analysis. In this chapter, while the focus is on methods of data analysis, attention will be drawn to the type of data collected and the methods involved at all stages of the research.

When multidisciplinary research is being undertaken, there are often tensions between the disciplines and research designs as researchers strive to implement each of the methods with rigour. In multi-disciplinary HSR, qualitative research is often 'bolted' or 'tacked' onto projects employing primarily quantitative designs, such as a survey or randomized controlled trial. The demands of HSR are often to produce results within a set time frame (which is usually underestimated), to satisfy a particular policy or commissioning brief. In such cases, a major tension often emerges between the need for the research to be undertaken quickly to facilitate the conduct of the quantitative research, and the wish on the part of the qualitative researcher to conduct a piece of work according to sociological or anthropological tradition, requiring time and immersion to produce high quality insights. This tension, and the tendency for qualitative research (and researchers) to be the junior partner in multidisciplinary studies, has led to much qualitative HSR becoming synonymous with small numbers of interviews analysed descriptively to assist the quantitative research – for example, in the development of quantitative measures, refining hypotheses or understanding the perspectives of patients involved in the research. Little of this research is published as it fails to satisfy either epidemiological or social science audiences. It also underutilizes qualitative research as there are many other qualitative research methods and analytical techniques that provide opportunities for multi- and interdisciplinary research and development in HSR.

A key dilemma for qualitative research in HSR is to find the right balance between the highly rigorous, traditional sociological/anthropological approaches and the need to work quickly and in narrow, applied fields to satisfy research commissioners and principal investigators. In the sections that follow, a number of approaches to qualitative research are described with reference to their relevance and suitability for HSR. The chapter then moves on to discuss a number of theoretical and practical issues for qualitative data analysis, and then considers the future for qualitative research in HSR.

Approaches to qualitative data collection

A number of methods of data collection and analysis come within the umbrella of qualitative research, and a plethora of (sometimes competing) theoretical approaches inform such methods (Gubrium and Holstein 1997). Many approaches have their roots in anthropology and interpretive sociology and draw on the epistemologies of phenomenology, ethnomethodology and symbolic interactionism (see e.g. Cuff *et al.* 1990). What they all have in common is a theoretical concern with meaning and action in social life and this is reflected in the qualitative methods used to study such phenomena. Gubrium and Holstein (1997) provide a useful overview of some of the common threads applicable to research in multidisciplinary health contexts:

- First, they mention a *'working scepticism'* of conventional (especially quantitative) assessments that fail to appreciate the nuances of the social world.
- Second, there is a *'commitment to close scrutiny'* of social phenomena to see what other types of inquiry may have missed.
- Third, there is a *'search for the "qualities" of social life'* by studying the taken for granted as meaningful substance.
- Fourth, there is a *'focus on process'* – on the ways in which the subjects of research actively and reflexively constitute and shape social life.
- Next they mention an *'appreciation for subjectivity'*, and the way in which a world comprised of meanings, interaction and so on must be scrutinized on its own terms.
- Finally, they mention a *'tolerance for complexity'*, particularly the complexities of people's views, experiences and the social context of subjective action.

There are very many approaches to qualitative data collection, but the major types of relevance to HSR are described next.

Interviews

Although interviews are very commonly used in studies about health, illness and health services, styles of interviewing vary widely. Interviewing is not one single method, but rather a collection of techniques (Arksey and Knight 1999). Types of interview range from the highly structured survey interview where responses can be categorized and analysed quantifiably, to the in-depth and unstructured 'long' interview (McCracken 1988). Interviews themselves have various terms, depending on the degree of control exerted by the researcher:

- *structured*;
- *unstructured*;
- or, the most common, *semi-structured*.

Interviews can be with individuals (most commonly), or with groups of people (focus groups). The basic techniques are similar but various texts have been written to provide help in conducting focus groups. The theoretical underpinnings of interviews can also be seen to span a paradigmatic range from positivism to the interpretative stance of qualitative methodology – which is probably a major reason why they have been taken up so enthusiastically in (quantitative dominated) HSR.

Arksey and Knight (1999) likened the interviewer in qualitative interviews to a jazz musician in a jam session: 'the key may have been set and there is an initial theme: thereafter it is improvisation. Your ability to "jam" is crucial to the success of these interviews'. Initial questions do set the key, but from then on the direction and content of conversation tends to vary. The ordering of questions in practice should flow naturally, as one topic of discussion leads to another related topic. Sometimes the researcher needs to move the conversation on to another related area; and sometimes respondents move the conversation on.

Methods for analysing interview data are many. A researcher may view interviews as 'speech events' (see Mishler 1986), which are mutually constituted and socially constructed via interaction between the interviewer and the interviewee, and then might use conversation or discourse analytic techniques (see below). Alternatively, a researcher who believes it is possible to capture the 'real' experience of those they are researching via interviews, and takes conversation at 'face value' may carry out a basic content analysis of the same data (Weber 1990) (see below). Interview data also provide rich stories for narrative analysis or various forms of interpretive, thematic analysis (see below). The theoretical range is wide: from relativism to realism, with the majority of researchers somewhere in the middle (Hammersley 1990; Kelle 1997).

Observation

Some researchers have pointed out the limitations of relying solely on interview data for qualitative research, and recommend (where possible) studying natural settings via observational work (e.g. Dingwall 1997; Silverman 1997a; Lambert and McKevitt 2002). As many researchers have shown, people's actions are not always consistent with what they say in response to questions (Dingwall 1997; Silverman 1997a; Arksey and Knight 1999). Observation of settings in their natural state requires considerable time commitment, and so these methods are rather underused in HSR. Observation (also known as field research or ethnography) can be undertaken on a continuum from full-participant/observer to non-participant/observer, depending on the researcher's role and access to the site (Burgess 1982). It requires the researcher to examine all apparently taken-for-granted action and the minutiae of behaviour, with the aim of gaining a full understanding of the operation of that particular segment of the social world. Interviews are usually undertaken as an integral part of the research, with opportunities taken to interview participants at any time and often in an unstructured way, rather than the more formal arrangements made for interview studies. Detailed notes are taken, often arranged as substantive or interpretive, and these form the raw material for analysis (see below). Tape-recordings may also be made, particularly of interactions, which can then be subjected to the range of qualitative data analysis techniques (see below). While the practical constraints of many studies in HSR make observational work difficult, these techniques are used much less frequently than they could be.

Other methods of data collection

Qualitative data can also be extracted from texts, including, for example, the media. Qualitative research methods are also being used flexibly and in combination with other research methods to explore topics in HSR. For example, case vignettes – hypothetical but socially situated stories – can be used to explore general beliefs, understandings and attitudes towards often sensitive issues (Finch 1987; Miles 1990; Hughes 1998). They have been used particularly within questionnaires, but can provide useful qualitative data in interviews (Adamson *et al.* 2004). A common criticism of vignettes is that they relate only to hypothetical issues which can be divorced from reality (Finch 1987; Hughes 1998). While this can be true, particularly when vignettes are used in questionnaire surveys, the flexibility of the in-depth interview means that the relevance of particular vignettes to individuals can be explored. Another method that has recently been suggested has been termed 'questerviews' – the use of in-depth interviewing to explore responses to standardized/structured self-completion questionnaires (Adamson *et al.* 2004). A mixture of observational, conversation analytic and interviewing has been used to understand recruitment to a randomized controlled trial (Donovan *et al.* 2002). It is likely that increasing varieties of methods will be suggested to exploit the flexibility of qualitative research methods in multidisciplinary contexts.

'Action' research

This approach also has particular relevance for applied areas and provides a method for evaluating change. It has been termed 'cooperative enquiry' (Reason and Bradbury 2001). The aim here is to use various qualitative research methods (interviews, observation, field notes, as appropriate) to evaluate the impact of a service as it happens, and sometimes to inform developments in a service (Entwistle *et al.* 1998). It can allow the evaluation of a service alongside its introduction, and proponents would advocate that the qualitative methods can indicate impact and essential changes, whereas others would claim that it allows services to be introduced without a formal evaluation that might have suggested alternatives. It may have more to offer HSR, and it is increasingly being used, although not necessarily under that banner. The embedding of a randomized trial within qualitative research methods and repeated changes to information could be construed as a piece of 'action research', although the authors do not suggest this (Donovan *et al.* 2002).

Approaches to qualitative data analysis

The wide range of methods of data collection for qualitative research is also reflected in the many and varied approaches to data analysis. Many texts exploring qualitative research methods provide the theoretical background to data analysis, and the major approaches are described below.

Ethnographic/observational approaches

Traditionally, anthropological and sociological research using qualitative research methods have been undertaken over a prolonged time-period. A full-scale ethnographic study should properly take years to undertake and would typically be written up in the form of a long book or monograph. Ethnographic research requires full immersion in the topic under study, and the use of a range of methods, usually including observation and interviewing, with varying degrees of participation from full participant/observer to non-participant/observer (Burgess 1982). Data are collected by field notes, supplemented sometimes with audio tape recordings. The study should proceed over a long period of time to facilitate understanding of taken-for-granted processes within the particular setting and ensure 'saturation' (when no new findings emerge). Few details have ever been provided by researchers about how exactly data analysis is undertaken, but it involves systematic scrutiny of notes, derivation of understandings and exploration of theories with further data collection.

An ethnographic approach has been employed successfully in many health-related settings, notably to understand medical training (Becker *et al.* 1961) and the process of dying (Strauss and Glaser 1977). It has clear relevance for the understanding of the contexts studied in HSR, but its prolonged timeframe does not fit with typical HSR deadlines and so mitigates against its use. In addition, while the practical methods of analysis are not clearly specified, researchers who have undertaken such studies have much to offer HSR, as many of the observational and interviewing techniques, and allied methods of analysis, can provide extremely relevant insights when applied to HSR topics.

Grounded theory/thematic approaches

The grounded theory approach was first described by Glaser and Strauss (1967) as an attempt to provide a detailed methods handbook for ethnographic researchers. It has its roots in symbolic interactionism and the work of G.H. Mead (Gerhardt 1989). According to the interactionist standpoint, individuals give meanings to their behaviour via interaction with others (Blumer 1969). These meanings are then organized in 'definitions of the situation' which then structure the actors' understanding of the social world, and can be viewed as a process of negotiation (Gerhardt 1989). The aim of grounded theory was to reveal interactive reality that is 'grounded' in 'definitions of the situation' (Gerhardt 1989). The main premise of the approach is that theory emerges from, and is grounded in, data. The key to allowing such emergence is by means of the method termed 'constant comparison', in which data collection and analysis are a cyclical process in which attempts are made to compare data segments with each other:

- data are collected in batches, so that each batch is compared with data collected previously and informs data collected subsequently;
- from these comparisons, themes emerge which summarize the phenomena under study, and then theory is generated inductively from these themes;
- this is facilitated by the derivation of conceptual categories to explain relationships in the data.

The honing of theory by constant comparison has been referred to as a process of 'theoretical sensitivity' and the idea was that this process would continue until a level of 'saturation' was reached (Glaser 1978). At this point, nothing new would emerge from the data, merely repetitions of the theoretical relationships which had already been discovered.

The proper conduct of grounded theory is a time-consuming enterprise, requiring the implementation of an iterative approach to data collection and analysis over an extended period of time. It requires close attention to sampling, with techniques such as 'maximum variation' (i.e. inclusion of individuals covering the widest range of characteristics), and theoretical/purposive/purposeful sampling (using data analysis to determine types of individuals to be selected). Further, there should be attempts to find 'negative' cases – individuals who do not fit emerging theory –

to allow further interrogation of the data to refine or change the developing theory. These issues are discussed further below.

There is considerable controversy over what really constitutes 'grounded theory', and indeed the original authors have famously disputed the nuances of the approach (Glaser 1992). In the 1970s and 1980s it became fashionable to claim the production of grounded theory, often without providing details of the methods of analysis in the reporting of work (Coffey *et al.* 1996; Green 1998). Similarly, 'grounded theory' came to be used as an 'approving bumper sticker' to denote academic respectability (Bryman and Burgess 1994). The grounded theory approach has clear relevance to HSR, as indicated above for ethnographic approaches. Of particular relevance to HSR, however, is the concept of thematic analysis and the specific method known as 'constant comparison'. The process originally outlined (vaguely) by Glaser and Strauss has been refined, adapted and developed by many others so that it is now probably the most commonly used interpretative analytical technique. The method of 'constant comparison' emphasizes the need for repeated comparison of sections of text with other sections, which requires coding, reorganizing of text, the derivation of themes and various methods of displaying and synthesizing data to form a conceptual scheme or pattern (see also below).

Narrative approaches

Narrative analysis gives primacy to story-telling in the context of research, and it is a general assumption that telling stories is one of the significant ways in which individuals construct and express meaning (Mishler 1986; Riessman 1993). This approach has also been developed from a concern with social action and interaction and a phenomenological concern to study the meanings behind taken-for-granted aspects of everyday life. As Riessman (1993) stated: 'The story is being told to particular people; it might have taken a different form if someone else were the listener . . . In telling about an experience, I am creating a new self – how I might want to be known by them'.

Story-telling is seen to function as a social performance, in which individuals present themselves in particular ways (Reissman 1990). Unstructured interviews are the most common source of data collection, and such an approach advocates allowing subjects to 'hold the floor'. Thus, in conducting interviews, researchers would try to minimize interruptions, and facilitate extended talk from respondents. At the stage of analysis, narrative approaches are generally presented as the polar opposite to those involving coding and thematic segmentation of the data (Bury 2001). In narrative analysis, the interview is taken as a whole story (or series of stories) in order to preserve the context in which it is (they are) told. Instead of coding into discrete categories, longer stretches of talk are presented as a means of displaying elements of the story (stories) and abstracting meanings pertaining to the worlds of respondents (Mishler 1986; Riessman 1993).

The use of narrative approaches is increasing, but it is not without controversy, as some have made clear the problems and limitations, as well as the potential, of this approach (Atkinson 1997; Bury 2001). Coffey and Atkinson (1996) pointed out that there are various ways of dealing with stories in text. On the one hand, a formal narrative analysis involves identifying structural elements of stories and the role of the interviewer in the production of the story, with a close scrutiny of the linguistic structure of the text to examine, for example, the temporal ordering of clauses that form a plot describing action and interaction (Mattingly 1998). On the other hand, other formal approaches involve detailed coding in order to classify clauses within the story – see, for example, Labov's classification scheme (1972). A further way of dealing with stories is to draw attention to their forms and functions. They may, for example, take the form of 'moral tales' or a chronicling of events, and may have a performative function (Reissman 1993). Examining the various forms and functions of stories can facilitate relating individual stories to a broader social and cultural context (Coffey and Atkinson 1996; Atkinson 1997).

It is clear, however, that increasing attention is being given to narrative approaches in HSR (Garro 1994; Frank 1995; Greenhalgh and Hurwitz 1998, 1999; Mattingly 1998; Greenhalgh 1999; Keshavjee *et al.* 2001). While it is sometimes suggested that narrative and grounded theory approaches are conflicting because they advocate the use of different analytical techniques, there are actually many points of overlap. For example, Charmaz (1990) claimed to have used a social constructionist version and application of grounded theory with a 'phenomenological cast' – a method that appears different to the original authors and more in common with the theoretical stance of narrative analysts such as Riessman (1993). Similarly, approaches to narrative analysis that emphasize the forms and functions of stories in their social context, rather than as private stories of isolated actors, have much in common with the social interactionist emphasis in grounded theory. In HSR, a combination of these approaches to data analysis may be beneficial. As Coffey and Atkinson (1996) suggest, 'complementary strategies' that are responsive to the data themselves are often best, particularly in multidisciplinary applied contexts such as HSR.

Content (descriptive) analysis

Content analysis is the simplest method for producing descriptions of qualitative data. It is essentially the first stage of the thematic and framework approaches, and requires the identification of codes to begin the early categorization of data. It can be used to analyse free text in questionnaires as well as data from individual or group interviews, and is also a way of beginning to make sense of detailed observational field notes. The method essentially derives from phenomenology, and in HSR usually relates to simple cross-sectional data from interviews or questionnaires. After the application of codes to interview data, descriptive accounts can be produced using the codes as a framework. It is increasingly used as a method in its own right for analysing interview data in HSR, although if this is all that is undertaken, it produces somewhat superficial findings. If the researcher uses it as the first stage of an iterative process of data collection and analysis, the analytic process becomes more akin to the 'constant comparison/thematic' approach described above.

Analysis of talk and interaction

Qualitative research often focuses on the use of language, and several methods have been developed to address specifically issues involved in interaction and talk. It is increasingly recognized that language is the medium through which social interaction takes place, and should thus be considered central (Silverman 1993b). A developing area for HSR is the investigation of interactions, particularly between patients and clinicians, and so these methods are being increasingly used.

Discourse analysis

The discourse analysis approach emphasizes the socially constructed nature of language and is associated with poststructuralist philosophy. The aim of discourse analysis is to deconstruct the hidden meanings within various texts and the social constitution of interactions (see e.g. Stainton Rogers 1991; Pierret 1993; Radley and Billig 1995). It can be useful for the investigation of interactions, but also in interviews to focus on how language is used to establish meaning, and how events and beliefs are presented, sometimes in contradictory ways.

Conversation analysis

Conversation analysis lends itself to a more specific focus on the working of inter-actions and provides techniques for understanding patterns in talk, particularly in organized settings (such as medicine). Underlying it are three fundamental assump-tions: that talk exhibits stable, organized patterns; that there is a sequential organiza-tion to talk that requires reference to its immediate context; and that analysis has to be undertaken with interactions transcribed accurately and in considerable detail (Silverman 1993b). Conversation analysis is derived from work by Harvey Sacks (1984) that showed that people talk one at a time and that interesting things happen when conversation passes from one speaker to another – turn-taking. Conversation analysis has been used to examine 'ordinary' talk, but has particular relevance for talk in institutional settings, such a doctor-patient interactions (Strong 1979; Sil-verman 1997b). The analysis tends to be very focused, often on very short passages in transcripts of appointments. Those undertaking conversation analysis are very careful to ensure that extremely detailed and accurate transcripts are provided (see below). Conversation analysis has produced some interesting analyses of interactions in, for example, HIV counselling, paediatrics and oncology settings (Silverman 1993, 1997b).

Framework approach

This is an analytical approach to qualitative data analysis developed for applied policy research contexts (Ritchie and Spencer 1994) and which is increasingly being used in HSR. The approach is geared particularly to the tight timeframes for applied research and the need to work in teams. The framework approach provides a clearly defined procedure which aims to be transparent, thus allowing policy-makers access to the process, and to allow researchers to work together and meet tight deadlines. Data collection is targeted towards the issue under scrutiny, and is usually undertaken through interviews (individual or group), sometimes with some observation. In most cases, data collection is completed before analysis commences. There are five stages to the framework method of analysis (Ritchie and Spencer 1994):

1 *Familiarization*: overview of issues, immersion in data, identification of recurrent themes.
2 *Identification of the thematic (coding) framework*: identification of key concepts and themes to be indexed, derived from aims of the research and emerging from data.
3 *Indexing*: systematic application of the coding framework.
4 *Charting*: abstraction of themes, using headings from the framework, across cases or cross-sectional; production of a 'picture' of the data that can be viewed by others and shows the themes and links.
5 *Mapping and interpretation*: description of the findings, comprising typologies, concepts, associations and explanations relevant for policy-makers.

Ritchie and Spencer (1994) emphasized that this is just one method for the analysis of qualitative data – one that is particularly helpful for policy-relevant research. It clearly has relevance for HSR, particularly as it provides a rapid method for the analysis of qualitative data. It provides a quick and relatively easy method for producing results, but it can be criticized for constraining what can be studied and suppressing complexity. It also removes several of the key aspects of traditional qualitative research: induction of themes, flexibility in design and sampling, and, most significant, an iterative approach to data collection and analysis.

As indicated above, most of the texts about qualitative data analysis are long on theoretical approaches, but rather thin on practical advice and detail, particularly for research in multidisciplinary contexts, such as HSR. There are several key issues in undertaking qualitative data analysis in HSR, most of which relate to the dilemma of how to balance the wish to carry out rigorous traditional qualitative research versus the time and resource constraints exerted by time-limited and multidisciplinary HSR. In the section that follows, a method of data analysis suitable for HSR is suggested, followed by discussion of the key dilemma that follows: how we can be assured of the rigour of qualitative research in HSR?

Qualitative data analysis in HSR: a way forward?

As the most common form of data collection in HSR is through interviews (individual or group), the method that follows is applicable most directly to audiotaped data, although it could also be applied to material from observational field notes or textual material from documents. The framework method is one that could be applied in HSR, but this does not allow two key aspects associated with traditional qualitative research: a flexible, iterative approach to data collection and analysis and the induction of findings from the data gathered. The method suggested here draws heavily on the principles of 'constant comparison' and applies these to particular health and health care related topics.

The process of analysis in qualitative research is not always well described or transparent. It will vary according to the particular methods employed, the training of the researcher and the question being considered. Those following the anthropological and ethnographic research traditions tend to produce lengthy textual description of data (Geertz 1999; Hammersley 1999). Such descriptions are not easily accessible to HSR audiences, and so various methods of coding and data reduction are used. The 'framework' approach provides a relatively clear method but is targeted and can be too focused, failing to allow findings to emerge. Perhaps the most detailed text to explore practical methods of data analysis is by Miles and Huberman, who describe three main stages of qualitative data analysis: data reduction, data display and conclusion drawing (Miles and Huberman 1994). Researchers following different analytic traditions will vary in their approach, but it is likely that those engaged in the most common method, constant comparison, will follow these broad stages. For example, the grounded theory approach (as outlined in the work of Strauss and Corbin) echoes these three stages with *open coding* (data reduction), *axial coding* (data display) and *selective coding* (conclusion drawing) (Strauss and Corbin 1990). First, however, data have to be in a format for analysis.

Transcription

Many qualitative research projects rely on recorded talk. Part of the analytic process is the repeated listening to recordings (Silverman 1993b). Further analysis requires the conversion of the data into written transcripts. There is considerable debate about optimum methods of transcription. Traditionally, it was seen to be important for the researcher who undertook the interviews to also transcribe them – since they would be able to ensure an accurate representation. However, increasing demands on researchers in HSR mean that often specialist audio-typists are employed. Researchers then lose the opportunity to absorb the data, and need later to check to ensure that the transcriptions are accurate. Some authors advocate selective transcription (Strauss and Corbin 1990), while others state the importance of detailed transcription of everything as a necessary prerequisite to valid analysis and interpretation (Mishler 1986; Poland 1999). Techniques such as conversation analysis have very detailed rules and instructions for how transcripts should be produced, including a large number of symbols and marks to indicate pauses, overlaps, changes of tone etc. (Silverman 1993b). However, such detail is not required for simple interview studies, although the presence of pauses and other non-verbal clues can be helpful for interpretation. Ultimately, the level of detail of transcription and the use of all or some transcripts must depend on the aims of the study (Mishler 1986) – although this then becomes a matter of judgement.

Data reduction: coding and processing

A key difficulty with transcribed qualitative data relates to its volume. One way of dealing with the quantity of data produced is to reduce its quantity and complexity by assigning labels or codes. A basic requirement in qualitative data analysis is the reading and rereading of transcripts or notes. This detailed scrutiny or 'constant comparison' cannot be avoided, although various computer packages may allow for the searching and assigning of codes. Traditionally, researchers manually appended codes to sections of transcript, using a variety of coloured pens/pencils, and physically cut sections of coded text and placed them in new files or documents. Such methods have largely been replaced by word processors and various computer packages, although the basic process remains the same. Essentially, the code is a label that identifies the segment of text in terms of its meaning or property.

Coding may be carried out in an open way, deriving the codes from the content of the transcripts, or in a more formal way by deriving a coding scheme and applying it (as suggested by the framework approach, above). Commonly in HSR, a combination of these approaches is employed as the research is usually targeted at a particular issue or group, and so data collection will have been driven by that agenda, but with the flexibility to allow new issues to emerge through inductive codes. In the framework approach, the coding framework will be devised and then applied; with constant comparison techniques, the coding framework will be derived as coding proceeds and will develop as each new piece of data is added.

Data display: reorganizing and re-presenting

The process of coding makes it possible to display and examine the data in a new format. While it is essential to retain transcripts in their original form and return to these to understand the context of utterances, the use of codes allows the easier comparison of similar text units. The scrutiny of sections from various transcripts with the same codes allows basic descriptive data analysis (sometimes referred to as content analysis) and the production of summaries of the similarities and differences relating to codes (descriptive accounts of themes). Miles and Huberman (1994) recommend a range of tables, charts, matrices and networks to display the content of coded data and thus facilitate comparison.

There is a temptation to write up these initial themes and present them as the results of the qualitative inquiry. At this stage, it is possible only to produce thematic description, which may be all that is required. Repeating the process and adding new data from different sources will, however, produce richer insights and be closer to the aims of constant comparison/thematic/ethnographic research.

Conclusion-drawing: further analysis and theorizing

The need for flexibility in qualitative data analysis means that it is difficult to describe or be prescriptive about the final stages of analysis. The aim in qualitative research is to understand the perspectives of those being studied and/or their social world, and so the process is essentially inductive and determined by the data gathered and the research participants (researcher and researched). Most qualitative researchers strive to reach 'data saturation' – the point at which no new insights can be gained from further data collection or analysis. Thus, qualitative research requires a cyclical and iterative process of analysis followed by data collection driven by the findings of analysis, and then further analysis. A key aspect is to investigate 'negative' cases – examples that do not seem to accord with the majority views or findings (Strauss and Corbin 1990; Mays and Pope 1995; Popay *et al.* 1998). Understanding negative cases usually requires a return to the original transcripts or tapes to examine the context of the emergence of the negative case, and may then generate further data collection to substantiate or refute its finding. This is essentially how theory develops from qualitative data analysis, as the findings are synthesized and explained, and theoretically salient insights emerge.

Iterative approach

An iterative approach is characteristic of most traditional qualitative research, including grounded theory but not, for example, of the framework approach. Although HSR is always constrained in terms of time and resources, it is beneficial to retain an iterative approach, both because it provides a simple and relatively rapid way to deal with the data and produce some early descriptive findings, and because it allows flexibility and the development of rich insights and theory generation. This is achieved by gathering data and analysing it in batches. The size of batches can vary according to the experience of the researcher and the complexity of the gathered data. First, between three and five interviews are undertaken and then these transcripts are coded and analysed, with the production of a descriptive account. The findings are used to determine the next interviews to be undertaken, and then a second batch of three or five is undertaken and analysed, with the production of another descriptive account. This process continues until the researcher is reasonably sure that no new themes are emerging (sometimes termed 'saturation'), and then a combined descriptive account is produced. In order to produce theory and deepen and contextualize the findings, further interviews may be undertaken, or other data collection, or the re-analysis of the material in cases (case-study approach), or attending to the significance of stories (narrative approach).

The production of useful insights and theory may require considerable time and further data collection or different patterns of analysis. The process of breaking up data into segments and then reassembling it has been criticized for stripping data of its context and removing the essential richness of stories. This is another key dilemma in qualitative research analysis – the need to make sense of large quantities of complex data by simplifying it with codes and themes, and the contrasting need to understand the context of the data and retain its richness and complexity. Narrative analysis provides the rationale for studying stories in their original form, but this may make cross-sectional insights difficult. For well-rounded HSR, it is probably necessary to ensure that several types of analysis are included as well as various types of data collection.

However the data are collected and analysed, a key question that is always posed is: 'how rigorous and reliable is the research?'

Rigour and quality in qualitative research

Determining rigour and reliability in qualitative research is a vexed and contested area. In HSR, the question is usually posed in terms of the validity and reliability of the research, using the criteria which apply to quantitative methods. Indeed, a degree of resistance to accepting interpretive work as legitimate knowledge has been manifested in the terminology used to describe it (Ceci *et al.* 2002). Such descriptions incorporate terms such as 'soft', 'journalistic' (Denzin and Lincoln 1994), 'sloppy' and 'merely subjective' (Lincoln and Guba 1999). Within the realm of qualitative research, there has been much discussion and debate about means of verifying research findings, with a wish to use rules developed out of the interpretative paradigm. Specifically in the sphere of HSR, there has been a recent expansion in the number of texts and checklists drawn up to establish criteria for judging the quality of findings for the purposes of peer review (Mays and Pope 1995, 2000; Seale and Silverman 1997; Dingwall *et al.* 1998; Popay *et al.* 1998; Malterud 2001). Such guides have sometimes been criticized for creating a cookbook method of doing qualitative research (Harding and Gantley 1998) and for advocating certain technical procedures merely as a means of making it more acceptable to traditional scientific conventions, and thus more acceptable to HSR audiences. Some have argued that focusing on such techniques can detract from the substance of qualitative research and can in the end compromise quality (Barbour 2001; Lambert and McKevitt 2002). This is thought to be a particular issue in the presentation of qualitative findings in clinical journals when presentation must be brief.

Qualitative researchers seem broadly agreed that the quality and rigour of qualitative research must be judged on its own terms, rather than measured against the benchmarks of positivism (Popay *et al.* 1998; Lincoln and Guba 1999; Mays and Pope 2000). This has four major implications.

Plausibility

In qualitative research, there is usually considerable emphasis on the need to establish the 'trustworthiness' (Lincoln and Guba 1999) or 'plausibility' of the research, rather than 'truth' or 'validity'. The idea is that different research perspectives make different kinds of knowledge claims, and the criteria for significant knowledge can vary accordingly – 'different strokes for different folks' (Lincoln and Guba 1999). Plausibility is very much an interpretive judgement. It can be enhanced by triangulation – the use of multiple research methods in the study of the same phenomenon. This might mix quantitative and qualitative methods, or involve several qualitative methods (such as observation, interviews and field notes, often used together in ethnography). Triangulation can be used to confirm findings from one method with another, or to enhance understanding of phenomena. There can be difficulties when different methods produce different findings (Bloor 1997). Arksey and Knight (1999) claim that triangulation has potential merits, 'especially if it is conceived less as a strategy for confirmation and more as one for in-depth understanding and completeness'.

Plausibility may also be enhanced by reference to previous research or the views of others in the field. It is sometimes recommended that the findings should be relayed to those who were participants in the research to check – so-called 'member validation'. Again there is considerable debate about the usefulness of this strategy. It may be helpful to ensure that findings reflect the views of participants but it may present a burden to them. It may also be that individuals would not agree with a general presentation of findings, particularly if they were a 'negative case'. It is not clear what use can be made of participants' views on findings, particularly if they conflict in any way. This remains a contested and actively debated area.

Generalizability

The non-probabilistic basis of sampling in qualitative research means that it cannot claim statistical generalizability (nor would it want to). In the strictest sense, the findings of qualitative research are generalizable only to the small sample investigated. However, if the findings have clear plausibility, then they are likely to be generalizable more widely. Again, this is a contested area that relies heavily on judgement.

Reliability

In HSR, it is considered essential that the research process (including data collection and analysis) should be made readily transparent (Mays and Pope 2000). It is suggested that there should be an 'audit trail' available for scrutiny (Lincoln and Guba 1999). This is closely allied to 'reliability' in quantitative research. For qualitative research, this can be achieved by carefully documenting the research process, including who collected and analysed the data and in what ways. Reliability can be improved by ensuring that the same questions are asked of all informants and in the same basic ways, while also allowing development and flexibility. The process of analysis can also be described clearly and applied methodically and systematically. The processes can be checked or open to scrutiny, for example, with coding carried out by more than one person independently to allow coding categories or coded text segments to be compared and checked. Independent coding of material by multiple researchers can be used to calculate (quantitatively) the level of inter-rater reliability. More qualitatively, it can be a useful method of discussing and refining coding frames and categories (Barbour 2001). This is insisted upon by journals such as the *British Medical Journal*, although there is no evidence to indicate that it affects coding strategies or improves the quality of data analysis. Our own experience of this, for what it is worth, is that the background and research interests of the 'coder' will affect to some degree what they see and how they code it, although if it is a cohesive research team, there will be considerable overlaps in descriptions of codes and themes. In our group, for example, the two sociologists (CS and JD) identified almost identical code names and coded segments, whereas Paul Dieppe (rheumatologist) tended to identify and name codes that were related to the clinical presentation. Descriptive accounts can also be 'checked' by others for relevance to the topic or clinic area.

The introduction of the concept of reliability into qualitative research is tending to make researchers more consistent and systematic in their work, and this is being reflected in the clearer description of the methods in journals. Increasingly, checklists are being employed to ensure that researchers have complied with reliability criteria. It seems intuitively logical that qualitative research, particularly in an HSR context where it is judged alongside quantitative research, would do well to be more systematic and transparent about its processes of data collection and analysis. There is, however, little or no evidence to indicate that this is a beneficial strategy for the coherence and quality of the research itself. Indeed, there is some evidence from recent qualitative syntheses (which attempt to bring together the findings of qualitative studies in the same area using interpretative techniques) that qualitative research is becoming more uniform *but* that it is also becoming less rich and insightful (Campbell *et al.* 2003, forthcoming).

Reflexivity

The concept of reflexivity is unique and integral to qualitative research. As qualitative research is a process that is part of social action and the social world, qualitative researchers appreciate that the researcher plays a part that should be considered and taken into account. Thus, while it is the intention in quantitative research for the researcher to be neutral and uninvolved (Van Maanen 1988), reflection on the role of the qualitative researcher and the methods and analyses is considered an important component of high-quality qualitative research (Hammersley 1987; Atkinson 1990; Mays and Pope 2000). Reflexivity is often achieved in traditional qualitative research by the presentation of a biography of the researcher and discussion of the potential influence of these characteristics on the research and research participants. There is often insufficient space for such deliberation in HSR journals, and it is not expected for audiences dominated by quantitative approaches. Interestingly, the concept has much to offer quantitative and qualitative research in terms of understanding findings. An important qualitative analysis of the findings of quantitative HSR might be to understand the origin of the findings and the process of their emergence.

Conclusions

A method of analysis for qualitative research in HSR has been proposed above that seeks to retain key aspects to ensure the high quality of the research, while being practical enough to allow it to be undertaken successfully in the context of applied and time-constrained HSR. Qualitative research in HSR is a developing area, and one in which changes are likely to occur into the future. In the past, its contribution to HSR has been in a 'handmaiden' role, providing data to refine hypotheses or develop quantitative outcome measures, or to understand the process of implementation of an intervention. More recently, it has been shown that qualitative research can lead and drive the agenda for HSR – a randomized trial of treatments for localized prostate cancer was effectively embedded within a qualitative investigation of the feasibility of undertaking such a study (Donovan *et al.* 2002). The qualitative research allowed an understanding of the process of recruitment and randomization from the perspectives of patients and clinicians, and changes made to the presentation of information increased the recruitment rate to a level that allowed the full-scale randomized trial to be launched (Donovan *et al.* 2002). There have been few such opportunities for qualitative research to really show what it can offer HSR, but it seems likely that its influence will improve and increase.

There are a number of tensions that exist for qualitative researchers working in an HSR context, particularly the demands for data on particular issues in rapid time. Such demands conflict with the need for immersion, reflexivity and flexible, iterative data collection and analysis – the hallmarks of high-quality qualitative research. Methods of data collection and analysis are always subject to trends of popularity (Coffey *et al.* 1996; Atkinson 1997). The advantage for HSR in utilizing qualitative techniques, however, is that the choice of method should always be pragmatic as well as contingent on the aims of research (Silverman 1993a, 1997a). In situations where the qualitative research can reach parity with quantitative research, the combination of the two should produce additional insights and exciting collaborations. What is essential is that qualitative research should not be judged by the rules of quantitative research, and that researchers must not be distracted from carrying out the fundamental aspects of the qualitative design. Qualitative research in HSR has tended to homogenize into a morass of phenomenology, often consisting of a relatively small number of interviews subjected to simple content analysis and producing a commentary or description of a restricted field. This is the 'poor relation' of qualitative research, and ignores the rich insights and theoretical development that can emerge from the use of other qualitative techniques, such as observation, conversation analysis, constant comparison, grounded theory, and a process of iterative, flexible and reflexive data collection and analysis.

Key points

- A key dilemma for qualitative research in HSR is to find the right balance between the highly rigorous, traditional sociological/anthropological approaches and the need to work quickly and in narrow, applied HSR.

- The major qualitative approaches in HSR share a theoretical concern with meaning and action in social life and include interview methods (individual and group), observation, document research (including the media), conversation and discourse analysis, and, more recently, 'questerviews' (the use of in-depth interviewing to explore responses to standardized/structured self-completion questionnaires).

- The main premise of grounded theory is that theory emerges from, and is grounded in, the data collected. Data collection and analysis are iterative – i.e. batches of data are collected and analysed by 'constant comparison', with the findings used to determine the next data to be collected. This process is repeated until the researcher is confident that no new themes are emerging (saturation). Grounded theory approaches are time-consuming because of their detailed and cyclical approaches, but they produce rich insights.

- In HSR it is common to use the 'constant comparison' methods of grounded theory, often without the immersion or long timescales needed for traditional grounded theory.

- Narrative analysis gives primacy to storytelling in the context of research; the interview is taken as a whole story (or series of stories) in order to preserve context. Instead of coding into categories, longer stretches of talk are presented as a means of displaying elements of the story and abstracting meanings pertaining to respondents' worlds.

- Content analysis requires the identification and application of codes to interview data; then, descriptive accounts can be produced using the codes as a framework.

- The framework approach is a rapid, targeted method that is increasingly used in applied policy research such as HSR. Data collection is targeted towards the issue under scrutiny, and the method provides a clearly defined procedure which aims to be transparent, with data collection usually completed before analysis commences – i.e. the iterative approach is not used.

- Qualitative researchers are broadly agreed that the quality and rigour of their research must be judged on its own terms, rather than measured against the benchmarks of quantitative research (positivism). A number of checklists of criteria for judging the quality of qualitative research have emerged in recent years, but none has been universally accepted. The quality of such research remains a judgement based on the rigour and transparency of methods of data collection and analysis and, most crucially, the plausibility of the findings.

References

Adamson, J., Woolhead, G., Gooberman-Hill, R. and Donovan, J.L. (2004) 'Questerviews' – a new mixed method approach for health services research, *Journal of Health Services Research and Policy*, 9(3): 139–45.

Arksey, H. and Knight P. (1999) *Interviewing for Social Scientists*. London: Sage.

Atkinson, P. (1990) *The Ethnographic Imagination*. London: Routledge.

Atkinson, P. (1997) Narrative turn or blind alley?, *Qualitative Health Research*, 7: 325–44.

Barbour, R.S. (2001) Checklists for improving rigour in qualitative research: a case of the tail wagging the dog?, *British Medical Journal*, 322: 1115–17.

Becker, H.S., Geer, B., Hughes, E.C. and Strauss A.L. (1961) *Boys in White: Student Culture in Medical School*. Chicago: University of Chicago Press.

Bloor, M. (1997) Techniques of validation in qualitative research: a critical commentary, in G. Miller and R. Dingwall (eds) *Context and Method in Qualitative Research*. London: Sage.

Blumer, H.S. (1969) *Symbolic Interactionism: Perspective and Method*. Englewood Cliffs, NJ: Prentice-Hall.

Bryman, A. and Burgess, R.G. (1994) *Analysing Qualitative Data*. London: Routledge.

Burgess, R.G. (1982) The unstructured interview as a conversation, in R.G. Burgess (ed.) *Field Research: A Sourcebook and Field Manual*. London: Routledge.

Bury, M. (2001) Illness narratives: fact or fiction?, *Sociology of Health and Illness*, 23: 263–85.

Campbell, R., Pound, P., Pope, C. *et al.* (2003) Evaluating meta-ethnography: a synthesis of qualitative research on lay experiences of diabetes and diabetes care, *Social Science and Medicine*, 56: 671–84.

Campbell, R., Pound, P., Daker-White, G., Pope, C. *et al.* (forthcoming) Meta-ethnography in health services research: report of HTA project, *Health Technology Assessment*.

Ceci, C., Houger Limacher, L. and McLeod, D.L. (2002) Language and power: ascribing legitimacy to interpretive research, *Qualitative Health Research*, 12: 713–20.

Charmaz, K. (1990) Discovering chronic illness: using grounded theory, *Social Science and Medicine*, 30: 1161–72.

Coffey, A. and Atkinson, P. (1996) *Making Sense of Qualitative Data: Complementary Research Strategies*. London: Sage.

Coffey, A., Holbrook, B. and Atkinson, P. (1996) Qualitative data analysis: technologies and representations, *Sociological Research Online*, 1: 1–16.

Cuff, E.C., Sharrock, W.W. and Francis, D.W. (1990) *Perspectives in Sociology*. London: Unwin Hyman.

Denzin, N.K. and Lincoln, Y. (1994) *Handbook of Qualitative Research*. Thousand Oaks, CA: Sage.

Dingwall, R. (1997) Accounts, interviews and observations, in G. Miller and R. Dingwall (eds) *Context and Method in Qualitative Research*. London Sage.

Dingwall, R., Murphy, E., Watson, P. *et al.* (1998) Catching goldfish: quality in qualitative research, *Journal of Health Services Research and Policy*, 3: 167–72.

Donovan, J.L., Mills, N., Smith, M., *et al.* (2002) Improving the design and conduct of randomised trials by embedding them in qualitative research: the ProtecT study, *British Medical Journal*, 325: 766–70.

Entwistle, V.A., Renfrew, M.J., Yearley, S. *et al* (1998) Lay perspectives: advantages for health research, *British Medical Journal*, 316: 463–6.

Finch, J. (1987) The vignette technique in survey research, *Sociology*, 21(1): 105–14.

Frank, A.W. (1995) *The Wounded Storyteller: Body, Illness, and Ethics*. Chicago: University of Chicago Press.

Garro, L.C. (1994) Narrative representations of chronic illness experience: cultural models of illness, mind, and body in stories concerning the temporomandibular joint (TMJ), *Social Science and Medicine*, 38: 775–88.

Geertz, C. (1999) Thick description: toward an interpretive theory of culture, in A. Bryman and R.G. Burgess (eds) *Qualitative Research*. London: Sage.

Gerhardt, U. (1989) *Ideas About Illness – An Intellectual and Political History of Medical Sociology*. New York: New York University Press.

Glaser, B.G. (1978) *Advances in the Methodology of Grounded Theory: Theoretical Sensitivity*. Mill Valley, CA: The Sociology Press.

Glaser, B.G. (1992) *Basics of Grounded Theory Analysis: Emergence vs Forcing*. Mill Valley, CA: The Sociology Press.

Glaser, B.G. and Strauss, A.L. (1967) *The Discovery of Grounded Theory*. Chicago: Aldine.

Green, J. (1998) Commentary: grounded theory and the constant comparative method, *British Medical Journal*, 316: 1064–5.

Greenhalgh T. (1999) Narrative-based medicine in an evidence-based world, *British Medical Journal*, 318: 323–5.

Greenhalgh, T. and Hurwitz, B. (1998) *Narrative Based Medicine: Dialogue and Discourse in Medical Practice*. London: BMJ Books.

Greenhalgh, T. and Hurwitz, B. (1999) Why study narrative? *British Medical Journal*, 318: 48–50.

Gubrium, J.F. and Holstein J.A. (1997) *The New Language of Qualitative Method*. Oxford: Oxford University Press.

Hammersley, M. (1987) *What's Wrong with Ethnography? Methodological Explorations*. London: Routledge.

Hammersley, M. (1990) *Reading Ethnographic Research*. New York: Longman.

Hammersley, M. (1999) What's wrong with ethnography? The myth of theoretical description, in A. Bryman and R.G. Burgess (eds) *Qualitative Research*. London: Sage.

Harding, G. and Gantley, M. (1998) Qualitative methods: beyond the cookbook. *Family Practice*, 15: 76–9.

Hughes, R. (1998) Considering the vignette technique and its application to a study of drug injecting and HIV risk and safer behaviour, *Sociology of Health and Illness*, 20(3): 381–400.

Kelle, U. (1997) Theory building in qualitative research and computer programs for the management of textual data, *Sociological Research Online*, 2.

Keshavjee, S., Weiser, S. and Kleinman, A. (2001) Medicine betrayed: hemophilia patients and HIV in the US, *Social Science and Medicine*, 53: 1081–94.

Labov, W. (1972) The transformation of experience in narrative syntax, in W. Labov (ed.) *Language in the Inner City: Studies in the Black English Vernacular*. Philadelphia, PA: University of Philadelphia.

Lambert, H. and McKevitt, C. (2002) Anthropology in health research: from qualitative methods to multidisciplinarity, *British Medical Journal*, 325: 210–13.

Lincoln, Y. and Guba, E.G. (1999) Establishing trustworthiness, in A. Bryman and R.G. Burgess (eds) *Qualitative Research*. London: Sage.

Malterud, K. (2001) Qualitative research: standards, challenges, and guidelines, *Lancet*, 358: 483–8.

Mattingly, C. (1998) *Healing Dramas and Clinical Plots: The Narrative Structure of Experience*. Cambridge: Cambridge University Press.

Mays, N. and Pope, C. (1995) Rigour and qualitative research, *British Medical Journal*, 311: 109–12.

Mays, N. and Pope, C. (2000) Assessing quality in qualitative research, *British Medical Journal*, 320: 50–2.

McCracken, G. (1988) *The Long Interview*. London: Sage.

Miles, M. (1990) New methods for qualitative data collection and analysis: vignettes and pre-structured cases, *Qualitative Studies in Education*, 3: 37–51.

Miles, M.B. and Huberman, A.M. (1994) *Qualitative Data Analysis*. London: Sage.

Mishler, E. (1986) *Research Interviewing: Context and Narrative*. London: Harvard University Press.

Pierret, J. (1993) Constructing discourses about health and their social determinants, in A. Radley (ed.) *Worlds of Illness: Biographical and Cultural Perspectives on Health and Discourse*. London: Routledge.

Poland, B.D. (1999) Transcript quality as an aspect of rigor in qualitative research, in A. Bryman and R.G. Burgess (eds) *Qualitative Research*. London: Sage.

Popay J., Rogers, A. and Williams, G. (1998) Rationale and standards for the systematic review of qualitative literature in health services research, *Qualitative Health Research*, 8: 341–51.

Radley, A. and Billig, M. (1996) Accounts of health and illness: dilemmas and representations, *Sociology of Health and Illness*, 18(2): 220–40.

Reason, P. and Bradbury, H. (eds) (2001) *Handbook of Action Research: Participative Inquiry and Practice*. London: Sage.

Riessman, C.K. (1990) Strategic uses of narrative in the presentation of self and illness: a research note, *Social Science and Medicine*, 30: 1195–200.

Riessman, C.K. (1993) *Narrative Analysis*. London: Sage.

Ritchie, J. and Spencer, E. (1994) Qualitative data analysis for applied policy research, in A. Bryman and R.G. Burgess (eds) *Analysing Qualitative Data*. London: Routledge.

Sacks, H. (1984). On doing 'being ordinary', in J.M. Atkinson and J. Heritage (eds) *Structures of Social Action: Studies in Conversation Analysis*. Cambridge: Cambridge University Press.

Seale, C. and Silverman, D. (1997) Ensuring rigour in qualitiative research, *European Journal of Public Health*, 7: 379–84.

Silverman, D. (1993a) *Interpreting Qualitative Data: Methods for Analysing Talk, Text and Interaction*. London: Sage.

Silverman, D. (1993b) *Analysing Qualitative Data*. London: Sage.

Silverman, D. (1997a) Validity and credibility in qualitative research, in G. Miller and R. Dingwall (eds) *Context and Method in Qualitative Research*. London: Sage.

Silverman, D. (1997b) *Discourses of Counselling: HIV Counselling as Social Interaction*. London: Sage.

Stainton Rogeas, W. (1991) *Explaining Health and Illness: An Exploration of Diversity*. Herefordshire: Harvester Wheatsheaf.

Strauss, A.L. and Corbin, J. (1990) *Basics of Qualitative Research: Grounded Theory Procedures and Techniques*. London: Sage.

Strauss, A.L. and Glaser, B.G. (1977) *Anguish: A Case History of a Dying Trajectory*. London: Martin Robertson.

Strong, P. (1979) *The Ceremonial Order of the Clinic: Parents, Doctors and Medical Bureaucracies*. London: Routledge.

Van Maanen, J. (1988.) *Tales of the Field: On Writing Ethnography*. Chicago: University of Chicago Press.

Weber, R.P. (1990) *Basic Content Analysis*. London: Sage.

Part 5
Essential issues to consider when conducting research

<table>
<tr><td>23</td></tr>
</table>

23 Involving service users in health services research

Vikki Entwistle

Introduction

Health services research has been led, for the most part, by health care professionals (especially medical doctors) and academic researchers. Although most have sought to generate knowledge that can be used to improve health services, they have not always been aware of service users' views of what would constitute improvements, and the focus of their efforts has often been strongly influenced by their professional interests and by the concerns of the various commercial, public and voluntary sector organizations that fund their work.

In recent decades, consumer advocacy groups have increasingly sought greater influence over the research agenda, and a growing number of researchers have recognized that there are compelling reasons for involving service users and other 'lay' people in various aspects of the health services research enterprise (Oliver 1995; Entwistle *et al.* 1998; Boote *et al.* 2002). National research agencies and influential policy groups in several countries have endorsed and made commitments to service user involvement in research (see examples in Box 23.1), others are developing policy in this area, and a number of research funding organizations now encourage or require some form of service user involvement in research projects (O'Donnell and Entwistle 2004).

This chapter is written primarily for clinical and academic health service researchers and research managers. It aims to help you to consider possibilities for working with service users in ways that allow them to influence the research agenda. (In this chapter, the term 'service users' is used as a convenient general label, but the groups of people whose involvement is discussed are not all strictly service users, and some would prefer to be described by other terms. There is no single term that all groups find acceptable to describe themselves – Hanley *et al.* 2004.) The chapter is basically about engaging the people with the health conditions you study, the people who have experienced or might receive the health care interventions you evaluate, or the people who have a stake as users in the health services you investigate, in the processes of determining what health services research is done, how it is conducted and how its findings are interpreted and used.

The chapter has adopted a fairly inclusive approach to the topic of service user involvement, considering the involvement of any of a broad range of people (see Box 23.2) who are, or who represent people who:

- may be affected by the processes of research (potential or actual research participants);
- may be affected by the findings and uses made of the research (users and potential users of health services);
- belong to broader communities with an interest in health services research as it is conducted for the common good and who are given, in some way, some kind of a say about any aspect of health services research.

In the following sections, the chapter outlines the context in which interest in service user involvement in research has arisen and the main rationales for promoting it. It explores some key concepts and theoretical dimensions of service user involvement, then illustrates a number of ways in which service users have been (and might be) involved in practice in the activities of research funding organizations, research centres and networks, and specific research projects. The chapter concludes by suggesting some preliminary questions that researchers need to ask when developing service user involvement in their work. The further reading section at the end of the chapter identifies some sources of more detailed practical advice.

Box 23.1   National agencies encourage service user involvement in research

As the users of health and medical services, consumers can provide valuable input to health and medical research. If such research is to continue to provide high quality outcomes, it is important that consumer involvement in research and its ongoing development is facilitated. This includes participation by consumers as equal partners in the development of research goals, questions, strategies, methodologies and information dissemination.

(National Health and Medical Research Council and Consumers' Health Forum of Australia 2001)

Participants or their representatives should be involved wherever possible in the design, conduct, analysis and reporting of research.

(Department of Health 2001)

The Agency for Healthcare Research and Quality (AHRQ) has published a new brochure that offers recommendations on how to increase the use of community-based participatory research (CBPR) in the United States ... The recommendations call on community leaders and research funding organizations, as well as colleges and universities, to build and maintain mutually beneficial, trusting relationships and make use of powerful community-based organizations and other grassroots groups in the design and conduct of studies. The recommendations also urge researchers to involve community leaders in the grant-making process and encourage community leaders to serve on university institutional review boards.   (AHRQ 2003a)

Box 23.2   People whom it might be appropriate to involve in health services research

- People who currently have or have previously experienced health conditions or disabilities.
- People who engage in particular health-related behaviours.
- People who face or have faced particular decisions about health care.
- People who have used particular health care interventions (or who have *not* used them although they might have benefited from them).
- Past, current or potential, new or long-term, occasional or regular users of particular health services.
- Family members and informal carers of the above people.
- Members of particular social or cultural groups (e.g. people from particular age, gender, ethnic, occupational or religious groups, people with a particular educational, family or socioeconomic status).
- People living in a particular geographic area.
- People who have identified a need for, or offered suggestions about, research, perhaps because they believe they have been harmed by something, or denied a health care intervention that they think would be beneficial.
- Leaders and representatives of voluntary support groups for people with particular health concerns.
- Leaders and representatives of other community or interest groups.
- Volunteers and staff of organizations that support (educate, inform, advise, advocate for, provide resources for) people with particular health concerns.

Background to the growth of interest in service user involvement in health services research

Interest in involving people other than health care professionals and professional researchers in health services research is consistent with a number of trends in health policy and with broader social and political developments, including:

- A growing acceptance that the responsiveness or patient-centredness of health services is an important aspect of health care quality (Murray and Frank 2000; Institute of Medicine 2001).
- Movements or aspirations towards greater involvement of patients and clients in the design and delivery of health and social care services, and in decision-making about their own care (Department of Health 1999).
- The exposure of examples of unethical treatment of patients and research participants (Goodare and Smith 1995).
- Concerns about levels of public confidence in, and support for, research (Institute of Medicine 1998; Medical Research Council 2003).
- Moves towards greater openness and accountability in health care and other service industries, especially in the public sector.
- A growing enthusiasm for action and participatory research, both of which require researchers to work closely with local communities or groups affected by issues and to ensure that those communities or groups influence or drive development and research. While these approaches may reflect different

priorities to the more traditional health services research, much may be learned from them (Cornwall and Jewkes 1995; Gray *et al.* 2000; Morrison and Lilford 2001).

- A general trend towards a closer interaction between science and society, and the development of more contextualized research that involves a broader range of people in the processes of defining problems and setting research priorities, that draws upon socially distributed expertise, and that is oriented to the production of socially robust knowledge. (Nowotny *et al.* 2001).

Rationales for involving service users and the public in research

There are a number of aguments for involving service users in health services research, but most have the following underlying premises in common:

- Service users have different perspectives on health services and research than do health care professionals and professional health services researchers.
- These perspectives are valid and important for health services research, because the acceptability of research processes should be judged at least in part from the perspective of research participants and because the purpose of health services research is to generate knowledge to inform improvements to health services, and what constitutes an improvement to health services is ultimately best judged from the perspective of service users.
- Many service users have experiential insights and expertise that could make valuable contributions to health services research.

Some proponents of service user involvement regard it as important because it is in accordance with an ethical or political principle. They might say, for example, that the people who will be asked to participate in research studies should (have a right to) have a say or be represented in the design of those studies, or that people who have a stake as users of health services should have a say or be represented in decisions about research that might shape the future of those services.

Other people advocate involvement primarily because they believe it will be instrumental in securing benefits such as better quality research, greater public confidence in research and enhanced uptake of research findings in practice. Some of the hoped-for benefits, and the mechanisms by which they might be achieved, are outlined here.

Involvement may enhance the relevance of health services research

The relevance of research can be considered on several levels and using various criteria. Arguments that service user involvement might enhance the relevance of the questions asked by health services research have tended to focus on:

- the overall distribution of health services research activity (which topics are investigated, which questions asked) and how well this maps onto the health needs of populations;
- the way in which particular research questions and projects are construed, and how appropriate and important they seem to the people whose health and health care they relate most closely to.

There is some evidence that the distribution of health service research activity does not reflect the priorities of the groups whose decision-making and health care may be affected by that research. For example, an investigation of research relating to treatments for osteoarthritis of the knee found that the pattern of published research studies did not reflect the research priorities identified by people with that condition or the health professionals who treated them. The treatments investigated in published studies were predominantly drug evaluations (reflecting commercial interests and regulatory requirements), while patients and health professionals thought more research was needed into surgical interventions (especially knee replacement), education and advice, and physical therapy (Tallon *et al.* 2000).

It is not a straightforward matter to determine an ideal distribution of health services research for a population and health service, and a number of factors need to be considered (Institute of Medicine 1998; Fleurence and Torgerson in press). However, if the purpose of health services research is to generate knowledge to inform improvements to health services, and if what constitutes an improvement is ultimately best judged from the perspective of service users, then it seems reasonable to argue that closer attention to service users' perspectives could enhance the overall relevance of the research agenda. This might be achieved by, among other things, research funding organizations being able to receive and consider suggestions from service users, and including service users in decision-making about the prioritization of possible research topics.

At the level of particular research projects, it has been noted that evaluations of interventions and services have often not addressed questions that matter to service users, and have thus not been able to inform decision-making about health care as well as they might. Attention to service users', as well as others' concerns and perspectives when formulating research questions might shift the focus of data collection and enhance the relevance of studies conducted (Oliver 1997).

Involvement may improve the acceptability of research processes

Research projects might be less likely to adopt procedures that are unacceptable or harmful to participants if members or representatives of the groups who will be invited to participate in a research study are involved in its design, and particularly in the development of procedures for inviting participation and collecting data from people. The involvement of service users in these activities may help to ensure participants' experiences are as positive as possible and more generally increase confidence that the interests of research participants are being protected and promoted.

Open engagement and dialogue with research participants, consumer representatives and community members might help reduce suspicion about the kinds of research decisions that are made behind closed doors and help research teams to be more accountable for what they do.

Involvement may increase the quantity and quality of data collected

There are several mechanisms by which different forms of involvement might improve the rates of recruitment to research studies that collect data from service users. Voluntary associations of people with particular conditions might contribute directly by helping to identify eligible people, bringing a study to their attention, and more generally raising public awareness about research. Members of communities that tend to be excluded from mainstream society or might otherwise be wary of health services research might help secure access to people whom researchers would otherwise struggle to identify and reach.

Less directly, if service user involvement improves the relevance and acceptability of research studies, it might help ensure that more people make an informed decision to take part, in research, and that participants contribute 'full' or rich datasets – for example, by taking time to complete a whole questionnaire, or being comfortable talking openly with an interviewer about a sensitive topic.

Involvement may promote appropriate interpretations of findings

The inclusion of a broader range of perspectives during discussions about the interpretation of research findings is likely to enhance the social robustness of the conclusions reached and the thoroughness with which potential implications are considered (Entwistle *et al.* 1998).

Involvement may enhance the impact of research findings

Service user representatives who have worked to ensure that research is relevant to their communities' needs and have been involved in the generation of research findings might be particularly committed to help ensure that the findings are appropriately disseminated and acted upon. Voluntary health associations might communicate findings to members and use research evidence to help lobby for changes in policy and practice. Input from service users can also help ensure that research findings are clearly incorporated in research-based information materials to help people make appropriate decisions about their health care (Oliver *et al.* 2002).

Involvement may empower and otherwise benefit service users

The involvement of service user representatives who can recognize and speak up about the concerns that participants might have about research projects has the potential to help avoid the possibility that the research process is disempowering for participants. For disadvantaged groups in particular, it may be important to avoid the possibility that being 'researched on' by others further increases a sense of marginalization or stigmatization (Hanley *et al.* 2004). More positively, service user involvement might encourage the active empowerment of the people involved and of the broader pool of research participants.

Research activity is one of the arenas in which disadvantaged communities might be enabled to develop skills and channel resources to help address problems that concern them – in the context of a particular project and beyond. Health services research does not always have direct developmental or health benefits, or community empowerment, as its primary goal, but these are emphasized in action and participatory research initiatives (Cornwall and Jewkes 1995; Macaulay *et al.* 1999; AHRQ 2003b; O'Toole *et al.* 2003), and may be valued secondary benefits in the context of social and political concerns about groups that are particularly disadvantaged and excluded from mainstream activities.

Involvement may enhance the public profile of health services research

Public perceptions of the relevance of research may be enhanced if people see groups they recognize as working in their interests involved in research activities and/or supporting particular projects. Service user involvement in discussions about individual projects may also help to lay a foundation for broader and more meaningful public debate about issues relating to health services research by increasing the number of people who become familiar with health services research and recognize that they can contribute to discussions about it.

A few comments about the above rationales

Several points should be noted about the above list of potential benefits. First, the various rationales refer to the involvement of different types of people in several aspects of the research enterprise. 'Service user involvement in research' encompasses a range of activities, and it may not always be appropriate to consider them as a homogenous group. Particular forms of involvement may be more or less appropriate if different goals of involvement are emphasized, and may be more or less feasible and useful in different contexts. For example, the potential benefits of service user involvement may be more limited in health services research projects that do not collect data from service users. Service users might have less of an impact if clinical and academic researchers are already well attuned to their perspectives.

Second, although it seems highly plausible that service user involvement may have the benefits outlined above, and a growing number of examples demonstrate that some forms of service user involvement have, in particular circumstances, had valued consequences for the research undertaken and the people involved (Oliver and Bastian 1999), service user involvement in research has not been systematically evaluated, and there are many variables that may affect its outcomes (Boote *et al.* 2002).

Third, the theoretical potential for benefit from service user involvement does not guarantee that such involvement will be easy to achieve in practice, nor that it will actually yield the hoped-for results. A number of researchers have reported tensions and concerns that have arisen during their efforts to work with service users (see e.g. Gray *et al.* 2000; Elliott *et al.* 2002; Triveldi and Wykes 2002). Several issues will need careful attention, including the capacity of service users to participate and researchers to support them, and the possibility of conflicts between professional researchers and service users in terms of their goals, preferred processes and interpretations. The potential for certain approaches to involvement to lead some types of service user to be excluded from involvement processes also needs to be considered (Jewkes and Murcott 1998). At this stage, it is not possible to make confident generalizations about the likely effects of different forms of such involvement in particular research contexts.

Key concepts and theoretical considerations

The theory of service user involvement in health services research is still at a relatively early stage of development (Boote *et al.* 2002). The concept is a complex one, both in the sense mentioned above that a wide range of activities might 'count' as service user involvement, and in the sense that any one example of service user involvement in a research activity has a number of dimensions. These dimensions have not been clearly defined, but the questions listed in Box 23.3 start to suggest the range of features that might be used to characterize different forms.

There has been some interest in describing different 'levels' of service user involvement in research, and various categorizations have been offered. For example, Hanley *et al.* (2004) outlined three levels of involvement, envisaged as lying along a continuum:

- *Consultation*: researchers ask service users about their views, use their views to inform decision-making, but do not make a commitment to act on them.
- *Collaboration*: researchers develop an active, ongoing partnership with service users in the research process.
- *User-controlled research*: service users rather than professional researchers hold the power and are the main locus of decision-making in the research.

Box 23.3   Some dimensions of service user involvement in health services research

Who is involved? Who is not involved?
Have any groups who might have important interests been excluded?

In (or by) what organizational structures or groupings within the research enterprise?
For example, research funding organizations, research ethics committees, research networks, project steering groups, operational project teams.

Which clinical and academic disciplines and which other interest groups are involved?

In what research activities (stages of research)?

What are service user representatives' relationships with formal research organizational structures or groupings?
For example, occasional adviser, voting members on a committee.

What is the quality of their relationships with the other people in these organizational structures or groupings?
For example, what attitudes do they hold towards each other?

Who are they representing and how do they relate to their constituencies?
For example, do service user representatives receive input from and account back to a broader group?

What are their particular interests and biases?
How and by whom else might their views be influenced?

On what matters are their information and opinions sought or given?

How are their voices elicited and heard?
For example, via focus group discussions, directly during committee meetings.

How and to what extent do they influence decision-making?
For example, do they engage in negotiations, have a formal vote?

How do they (and the other parties) experience and view the process of their involvement?

How do they (and the other parties) value their contributions?

The National Health and Medical Research Council and Consumers' Health Forum of Australia (2001) developed a categorization based on five levels of participation identified by Bastian (1996):

- None.
- *Manipulation*: consumers are 'educated' about research or given tokenistic representation on a committee to serve the interests of others.
- *Restricted scope*: consumers may be consulted in a limited way.
- *Open involvement*: consumer representatives serve on project steering committees, but without having been involved in deciding the priority for that project, and with little consultation with broader consumer groups.

- *Wide participation*: research is led and conducted by service users, or a range of strategies are used to maximize the consideration of service users' views (e.g. a combination of consumer representation on steering committees, consultation with broader groups of service users and the use of research literature describing people's experiences).

The concept of 'levels' of involvement incorporates notions of lesser and greater amounts of involvement and seems to imply that 'more' involvement (at the higher levels) is always 'better'. However, the levels of service user involvement may be misleading as indicators of the quality of consumer involvement for several reasons. It may be difficult to categorize examples of involvement appropriately on particular levels because the classification rubrics are not exhaustive and involvement is a dynamic process. The levels do not reflect all the dimensions of involvement that might be important, and they do not address the outcomes of involvement. Also, the fact that user-controlled research appears in the highest levels reflects an emphasis on empowerment that originated in the community development literature. This emphasis might not be appropriate in the context of health services research for which community empowerment is not the primary goal.

The question of what constitutes quality in service user involvement in research is a complex and contested one. Answers will vary according to what respondents perceive to be the main rationales for involvement, and how much weight they attach to the different processes and possible outcomes of involvement.

Examples of involvement and practical considerations

In this section we consider examples of service user involvement in the activities of research funding organizations, research networks and centres, and particular research projects. The examples illustrate a number of different approaches, but do not exhaust the range of possibilities. They are not necessarily 'ideal' exemplars, and some will be more appropriate models for particular contexts and types of research activity than others.

Involvement in the activities of research-funding organizations

Research funding organizations may be particularly well placed to facilitate service user input into the generation of ideas for the research agenda, the prioritization of research topics, the development of research strategy and the oversight of research activities (Entwistle and O'Donnell 2003). Their policies also influence the practice of service user involvement in research projects (O'Donnell and Entwistle 2004). Funding organizations have adopted various approaches to service user involvement. For example, the National Cancer Institute, one of America's National Institutes of Health, has an Office of Liaison Activities that 'supports the Institute's research by fostering strong communications and relationships with the cancer advocacy community' and other groups. This office runs two main programmes that facilitate service user involvement. The Director's Consumer Liaison Group is an all-consumer committee that advises the director on a variety of issues, including research priorities, from a consumer advocacy perspective. The Consumer Advocates in Research and Related Activities programme recruits and trains consumer advocates to participate in a range of activities, including the work of progress review groups (which set research priorities in particular areas), the peer review of research grant applications and the review of educational materials for patients (National Cancer Institute 2004).

The Alzheimer's Society is a membership charity in the UK that works to support patients with dementia and their carers and has an active research programme. The Society established a trained panel of members (the Quality Research in Dementia network) who volunteer to help the charity prioritize which topics should be researched and to review project proposals to inform funding decisions. Network members also serve on the steering groups of particular projects, provide independent progress reports back to the funding organization and contribute to the dissemination of research findings (Alzheimers Society 2004).

The Health Technology Assessment Programme, which is part of the National Health Service Research and Development Programme in the UK, includes two consumer representatives on each of the committees that prioritize and commission research. Consumer representatives also comment on drafts of research commissioning briefs, review research applications (using a specially designed form), and comment on project reports before they are finalized for publication. The Programme is also considering ways of more proactively seeking service user input into its process for identifying potential topics for research (Health Technology Assessment Programme 2004).

Involvement in research networks and centres

Although much of the discussion relating to service user involvement has focused on either the research agenda-setting and prioritization activities of research funders or the activities associated with individual research projects, there may be important opportunities for researchers to develop working relationships with service users at the level of research networks, centres or groups. Research teams may find it easier to involve service users and members of the public at an early stage in the development of particular projects if they have been engaging them in dialogue about their broad area of research interest and potential ideas. For examples, a regional cancer research network in England that sought to develop an infrastructure and way of working that ensured effective involvement of people with cancer in their activities at both network and project level. It used three main strategies:

- Open days that aimed to increase awareness of research among users of cancer services and to encourage open discussion of research ideas.
- The inclusion of people with cancer on the committee that took a strategic overview of the research conducted within the network and determined which research ideas should be developed and funded.
- The establishment of a consumer research panel, comprising people with experience of cancer as either patients or carers, who could be approached by network members to provide a considered consumer perspective, or invited to sit on committees or research project steering groups.

The network sought to maximize the range of people with cancer who were involved in the development and delivery of its research strategy, so in addition to working with established consumer support groups, it advertised widely in the local media and health and community centres, and encouraged clinical staff to suggest to patients and carers that they might participate. The network provided a two-day introductory training session for people who volunteered to join the consumer research panel, and offered ongoing support via a mentoring arrangement. Resources were set aside to pay people for the time they contributed to the network's research activities (Stevens *et al.* 2003).

A further example is SURE (the Service User Research Enterprise), a university-based unit that aims to involve service users in all aspects of mental health research. SURE employs researchers who are also (or have also been) users of mental health services, and is building capacity among service user researchers by encouraging them to register for research degrees. SURE researchers work in collaboration with clinical academics, include broader groups of service users in their own work and support the involvement of service users in other aspects of the research enterprise (Institute of Psychiatry 2004). For example, they support regular service user involvement in the research and development steering group of the local health care provider institution by convening a group of service users who meet monthly, receive and discuss all the papers from the steering group and identify issues that are important to them. This group sends two delegates to the steering group meeting, supported by a SURE employee, to represent their views and then feed back to them at their next meeting (Rose 2003).

Involvement in particular projects

There are numerous examples of service users being involved in various ways in different aspects of research projects. Some researchers and research funding organizations have tried to ensure that there is some form of service user involvement throughout the course of a project. They have done this by including one or more representatives as co-applicants on funding proposals or as members of an active project steering group or advisory committee, by forming a reference group of service users that might feed into the project in several ways, and by assigning one or more service user 'buddies' or partners who are in contact with research teams for the duration of the project.

A review of consumer involvement in a series of nine large trials of coordinated care in Australia found that several models had been adopted:

- One or two consumers were involved on trial management groups.
- A consumer reference group met to discuss issues relating to the trial and provided input via:
  - the group chair participating on the main trial operational committee;
  - group representatives participating on trial steering committees and working parties;
  - the trial manager serving on the consumer reference group;
  - the group taking issues to trial staff.

In considering the advantages and disadvantages of these models, the review noted that consumer reference groups were valued because they allowed service users to talk through issues and support each other, and that consumer representation on trial committees helped to ensure that input from a service user perspective could be made before rather than after decisions were taken (Consumers Health Forum of Australia 2000).

Service user involvement might be emphasized at particular stages in the research process. The examples below illustrate some of the ways in which service users might be involved in different types of project activity.

Involvement in the formulation of research questions

People who are experientially familiar with health problems and the limitations of current service provision may identify problems and potential solutions, and be motivated to see them investigated further. There are currently few formal structures for 'connecting' people with ideas to researchers with the interests and skills to investigate them, but there are some examples of such connections having been made. It is not clear how fruitful it will be for individual research teams to actively solicit research ideas from service users. 'Ordinary' service users may be aware of problems but not know what research has been or could be done to address them, and may struggle to articulate the problems they perceive as research questions, especially if asked in a relatively unstructured one-off consultation exercise (Ong and Hooper 2003).

Nonetheless, researchers developing project ideas might usefully engage in discussions with health service users and other community constituencies, as well as with those who treat them and/or are responsible for organizing and managing services, to ensure they can appreciate the problems they are proposing to tackle from a number of perspectives, and to gauge how important their work may be to those whom it is intended to benefit.

For example, research teams submitting review protocols to the Cochrane Collaboration are likely to have them reviewed by consumer representatives as well as clinical colleagues and experts in systematic review methods. Consumer representatives who review protocols for the pregnancy and childbirth group have tended to encourage researchers to pay more attention than they had previously done to the potential risks of interventions to mothers and babies, to mothers' experiences of and attitudes towards interventions, to the implications of interventions for family relationships, and to long-term outcomes (Cochrane Consumer Network 2004).

Involvement in the design of research studies

There are numerous examples of study designs being influenced by input from service users – either 'experienced' representatives who serve as project advisers or on project steering groups or teams, or 'ordinary' members of the groups who might be asked to participate in the study or who might benefit from it, who are consulted in a 'market research' type way about design ideas.

There is much potential for service user involvement to inform the ways in which approaches will be made to likely service user participants, the content and presentation of study information materials, and the methods of eliciting information from participants. For intervention studies, there may be scope for service users to inform decisions about the precise nature of the intervention, about what would constitute an appropriate comparison intervention, and about which outcomes should be assessed.

A survey of trial centres in the UK found that the involvement of consumers in randomized controlled trials was relatively rare in the 1990s (Hanley et al. 2001). However, there have been an increasing number of reports of service user involvement in the design of such trials, especially when proposed trials are recognized to be controversial. For example, a team seeking to design a trial of thrombolysis treatment for people within three hours of the onset of acute ischemic stroke used a number of approaches to involve senior citizens, stroke patients and carers in discussions about the design of the trial. Clinical researchers were concerned about the ethics and feasibility of mounting such a trial because, while there was some evidence that the treatment might be beneficial, it was also known to carry a risk of fatal intracranial haemorrhage. The elicitation of meaningful informed consent for participation in the trial was likely to be difficult because people are often not in a position to evaluate and discuss their treatment options within three hours of stroke onset.

The researchers discussed these issues with several groups of senior citizens and found that a high proportion of these people said they would be willing to enter a trial of thrombolysis for acute stroke. They then held focus groups comprising volunteers from the initial discussions and from another older people's project, to further discuss the ethical dilemmas of securing consent for participation in stroke trials and to comment on initial drafts of an information leaflet summarizing the trial for potential participants. The participants suggested and considered a number of potential solutions to the ethical dilemmas involved in obtaining informed consent, and expressed some preferences about the way risks should be explained in information material. The researchers then revised the consent procedure and information material in the light of the comments obtained, and discussed the revised procedures and materials with stroke patients and their carers on a rehabilitation ward. They made some further revisions following these discussions, and the resulting recruitment procedure was approved by a multicentre research ethics committee (Koops and Lindley 2002).

In another example, the possibility of a randomized controlled trial of hormone replacement therapy (HRT) in women with breast cancer with symptoms of oestrogen deficiency was contentious because, although women with breast cancer were requesting help with oestrogen deficiency symptoms, most breast cancers are known to be oestrogen dependent. However, a trial was designed in three stages by a collaboration of clinician-researchers, members of a cancer care centre with experience of patient–health professional collaborations in cancer research, and the Consumers' Advisory Group for Clinical Trials (a patient–professional group that aims to improve the quality of breast cancer research). The first stage of the process was a consultation exercise in which nine focus groups of women with breast cancer were asked about their attitudes to the menopause, HRT and a proposed trial of HRT in breast cancer patients. In the second stage, representatives of the three stakeholder groups and six women who had participated in the focus group discussions met to discuss the proposed trial. With the help of an external facilitator, they considered a report of the focus group findings, which included a number of recommendations about the design of the trial. In the third stage, a trial steering committee was convened to finalize a plan for the trial. The committee included the clinician researchers, a (service user) representative from each of the other two stakeholder groups, and two of the original focus group participants. The resulting trial design included several features developed specifically in response to concerns raised in the focus groups (Marsden and Bradburn 2004).

The involvement of service users in the design of a study may facilitate their involvement at subsequent stages of a project. Triveldi and Wykes (2002) describe how a service user group that was approached by a research team with a trial design already prepared initially refused to be involved because of concerns about the outcome measures used.

Researchers need to be aware that power and status differentials between themselves and the service users they seek to involve may make service users reluctant to disagree with their suggestions about study design. For example, reflecting on a participatory research project that investigated the health benefits, strengths and limitations of self-help groups, a group of professional researchers described how, despite their best efforts to design a study that was mutually acceptable to themselves and the self-help groups, the representatives of the groups agreed 'too readily' with the researchers' plan to ask new group members to complete a self-report questionnaire. It was only when the researchers were investigating why the questionnaire was not being distributed that they discovered the group members were 'uncomfortable with, and thus resisting, the procedure to which they had agreed' (Gray *et al.* 2000).

Researchers may also need to consider how best to provide service users with adequate information to enable them to consider issues of study design fully but to avoid inappropriately (even if inadvertently) persuading them to adopt a particular point of view.

Involvement in recruitment and data-collection processes

A number of voluntary organizations have helped with the recruitment of potential participants to trials. For example, the National Association for the Relief of Paget's Disease (NARPD), which is primarily a support group for people affected by this disease, was involved in a number of ways in a multi-centre trial in the UK to compare different treatment strategies. Having contributed to the planning, funding, and protocol development for the trial, NARPD helped to recruit clinical collaborators and distributed information about the trial to people with Paget's disease via patient days, newsletters and flyers to new members. A number of people who had not been invited to participate in the trial by their clinicians actively requested participation after learning about it from NARPD sources (Langston *et al*. 2005).

A number of research teams have employed people from the groups who are the focus of research to identify and recruit potential participants and, sometimes, to collect data from them, either by distributing questionnaires or by serving as 'peer' interviewers. These forms of service user involvement are most commonly used in situations in which it is difficult for 'traditional' researchers to identify, meet, communicate with or discuss the topic of interest with the intended research participants, and in projects which aim to help empower a disadvantaged group. For example, Elliott *et al*. (2002) recruited stable and former drug users to identify and interview parents who use illegal drugs, and Kai and Hedges (1999) recruited and trained people of Bangladeshi and Pakistani origin who were living in the UK to interview members of their local community to explore their views of psychological distress and the services available to help them with such problems.

These forms of involvement, perhaps more obviously than other forms of involvement at a project level, ask service users to take on a task of work for which they need particular research skills. Research teams need to pay careful attention to training, support, ongoing liaison and reimbursement issues. Community politics and the possible exposure of service users to potentially difficult situations need to be taken seriously.

Also, while the use of peer interviewers may facilitate access to certain groups of people, and may help ensure that interviewers understand the subtleties of what is being said when there are cultural gaps between the research team and the researched, it may not be the best approach in all circumstances (Gray *et al*. 2000; Elliott *et al*. 2002).

Involvement in the interpretation of results

Service users have contributed to both the analysis of data (especially in qualitative studies, which are more open to the influence of researchers' perspectives), and to the broader interpretation of study findings, identification of implications and development of recommendations. For example, an American research team conducted a study that aimed to develop patient-focused typologies of medical errors and associated harms in primary care settings. They used in-depth individual interviews to collect narrative accounts from patients, asking them to describe preventable incidents that had resulted in harm. The researchers conducted a preliminary analysis of the narrative accounts and generated an initial typology of errors and harms. They then shared interview excerpts and their preliminary analyses with three reactor panels comprising groups of six to ten patients from similar backgrounds to those who had been interviewed. The research team had envisaged that the reactor panels would either expand the lists of types of errors and harms or would reassure them that they had reached saturation with their data (Kuzel *et al*.

2003). In practice, the reactor panels validated the researchers' tentative typology. They also confirmed that they thought the preventable psychological harms that had been identified from the narrative accounts were important (these types of harms have not been emphasized in work that has investigated medical errors from health professionals' perspectives). The reactor panels additionally suggested that seemingly trivial errors (such as insults) and near misses (errors that were intercepted before they harmed the patient) could lead to more serious problems and a diminished trust in health services (Kuzel *et al.* 2004).

The reactor panels in the above example could be viewed simply as an additional stage of data collection, but they did serve to allow some input by service users into the interpretation of findings. They reflected a commitment on the part of the researchers to ensure that their typology reflected what was important to people who used primary care services. They also provided the research team with an opportunity to raise awareness of the study and the issues it was addressing among the communities from which participants were drawn and which might ultimately benefit from the learning the study generated.

Service user representatives on project teams and steering groups are also sometimes encouraged to contribute to or comment on the analysis of research findings, but researchers need to be aware that their capacity and willingness to do this may vary (Gray *et al.* 2000).

Involvement in the dissemination and application of research results

Service users have contributed in numerous ways to the dissemination and application of research results. For example, people who have been involved with projects have helped to write project reports, journal papers, newsletter articles and information sheets that summarize the study findings (the involvement of service users is often said to help ensure that these are written in an accessible language and style). They have also presented the findings at various conferences and meetings, included articles about the findings in their newsletters and on their websites, and used the findings to lobby for desired changes in policy and practice. More generally, service user representatives are increasingly asked to serve on committees that use research to inform the development of clinical practice guidelines, service protocols and performance standards, and they bring their particular perspectives to bear on the interpretation of findings in those contexts (National Quality Forum 2003; National Institute for Clinical Excellence 2004; SIGN 2004).

Although this chapter is not primarily about the involvement of service users as study participants, it seems appropriate to mention the possibility of offering to provide an accessible summary of the findings to all consenting study participants. This might be done via presentations at meetings or in written form. It can communicate acknowledgement of and thanks for their contribution, and should help raise awareness of the findings among a potentially interested group. It might encourage participants to feel more involved in the study, and may help avoid the possibility that they wonder what was made of their contribution, see nothing about it, and become disillusioned with health services research and less inclined to participate in future studies.

Service user representatives may be particularly helpful in developing summaries of the research that are accessible and useful to participants and the broader audience of people who might be affected by the findings, especially if people have particular communication needs. For example, the National Patient Safety Agency for England and Wales sought to examine the patient safety risks specific to people with learning difficulties as they used health services. They commissioned a self-advocacy charity to interview people with learning difficulties and their family members about their experiences and views. The charity, which was based on a partnership between people with learning difficulties and non-disabled people, helped to prepare a summary of their findings, and a report of the broader scoping exercise, in an accessible format using short words and sentences and informative pictures (National Patient Safety Agency 2004).

It is important to note that academic researchers and service user representatives may have differing priorities relating to the dissemination of project findings. Several teams have agreed to develop multiple outputs to meet their various requirements (Gray *et al.* 2000; Triveldi and Wykes 2002).

Planning and preparing to involve service users

There is no simple prescription or recipe for 'appropriate' or successful involvement – and what constitutes successful involvement has yet to be agreed. Different forms of involvement will be appropriate for different types of project and in different circumstances. Guidance from both the UK and Australia suggests that what is best might depend on a number of factors, and that researchers should strive to develop a contextually appropriate approach (National Health and Medical Research Council and Consumers' Health Forum of Australia 2001; Hanley *et al.* 2004).

An incipient project team of clinical and academic researchers that is considering whether and how to involve service users needs to be aware of:

- possible reasons for involving particular types of service user in this project;
- the policies of the relevant funding organizations, research ethics and governance committees, and their own institutions regarding service user involvement;
- the financial and human resources they can justify and have or might be able to obtain to support user involvement activities.

They need to consider, and to negotiate with the service users they approach about possible involvement:

- the extent to which they are willing to be flexible about their project aims and initial ideas about study design, and thus the scope of influence they are willing to offer;
- the types of people it might be appropriate to involve and the ways in which it might be appropriate to involve them;
- the capacity and willingness of those people to take on particular roles, and any special needs that should be addressed to facilitate their involvement.

It might be appropriate to develop information material for people who will be invited to contribute to the project via consultation exercises, and role descriptions and statements of agreement about ways of working with service users who will be formal partners and members of project teams or reference groups (including payment policies and procedures for dealing with differences of opinion).

Research teams could usefully consider how they might contribute to the development of knowledge, practice and policy relating to service user involvement in health services research by reflecting critically on their own experiences, and reporting their perceptions of the processes and consequences of service user involvement, perhaps via an independent evaluation of their collaborative efforts.

Conclusions

Service user involvement in health services research embraces a diverse range of activities but is basically about enabling people who have relevant perspectives and a stake as research participants and health service users to influence what research is done and how. There are several ethical, political and scientific rationales for involving service users in various aspects of health services research, including beliefs that these people have a right to representation and hopes that their involvement will improve the quality and impact of the research.

Various possible approaches to service user involvement exist. Some are better geared to achieve particular purposes than others. However, the feasibility and value of particular forms of service user involvement in particular contexts are currently poorly understood. Researchers considering how to involve service users in their work need to consider their own goals, operating constraints and resources, and the capacities, needs and preferences of the various people it might be appropriate to involve. Research teams might usefully contribute to the development of knowledge and practice relating to service user involvement in health services research by reflecting critically on their own experiences, and reporting their perceptions of the processes and consequences of such involvement.

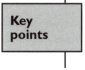

Key points

- Researchers are encouraged to engage with people with the health conditions under investigation, and involve service users in research projects.

- There is growing acceptance that the patient–centeredness of health services is an important aspect of health care quality.

- Service users have different perspectives than health care professionals and researchers, and these should be included in judgements of the acceptability of research processes, and of what constitutes an improvement of health services.

- Involvement of service users may enhance the relevance of health services research and the acceptability of research processes. It may also increase the quantity and quality of data collected, and promote appropriate interpretation of findings and their impact.

- Involvement of service users may also empower and otherwise benefit those users, and enhance the public profile of the research.

- The question of what constitutes quality in service user involvement in research is complex and contested.

Further reading

Hanley, B., Bradburn, J., Barnes, M. *et al.* (2004) *Involving the Public in NHS, Public Health and Social Care Research: Briefing Notes for Researchers*, 2nd edn. Eastleigh: INVOLVE. An introductory document intended for researchers with no previous experience of involving members of the public. Contains numerous examples of involvement and includes helpful checklists for people considering involving members of the public in committees and working groups, plus examples of job descriptions for consumer representatives.

National Health and Medical Reseach Council and Consumers' Health Forum of Australia (2001) *Statement on Consumer and Community Participation in Health and Medical Research.*

Canberra: AusInfo. A thoughtful statement of principle and a practical guide to collaborative working that was developed after wide consultation with consumers and researchers.

Oliver, S. (1997) Exploring lay perspectives on questions of effectiveness, in A. Maynard and I. Chalmers (eds) *Non-random Reflections on Health Services Research*. London: BMJ Publishing. An accessible discussion with many examples that illustrate how the differences of perspective between service users and health professionals can lead to the formulation of different questions for evaluative health services research.

Williamson, C. (2001) What does involving consumers in research mean?, *Quarterly Journal of Medicine*, 94: 661–4. An accessible reflection on some key issues.

Resources

INVOLVE: promoting public involvement in NHS, public health and social care research. www.invo.org.uk/index.htm (accessed 27 March 2004). Wesbite offers information and practical advice about involving people in health-related research.

National Resource Centre for Consumer Participation in Health. www.participateinhealth.org.au/ (accessed 27 March 2004). Website offers information and practical advice about consumer participation in all aspects of health care, health policy and research.

References

AHRQ (2003a) www.ahrq.gov/research/aug03/0803ra25.htm (accessed 14 March 2004). AHRQ publishes recommendations on community based research.

AHRQ (2003b) *Creating Partnerships, Improving Health: The Role of Community-based Participatory Research*. Washington: US Department of Health and Human Services.

Alzheimer's Society (2004) Quality research in dementia advisory network, www.qrd.alzheimers.org.uk/qrd_advisory_network.htm (accessed 24 March 2004).

Bastian, H. (1996) Raising the standard: practice guidelines and consumer participation. *International Journal for Quality in Health Care*, 8: 485–90.

Boote, J., Telford, R. and Cooper, C. (2002) Consumer involvement in health research: a review and research agenda, *Health Policy*, 61: 213–36.

Cochrane Consumer Network (2004) The pregnancy and childbirth group: consumers identify outcomes of importance to women. www.cochrane.no/consumers/Docs.aspx?wfID=34&lid=1&wdID=84 (accessed 27 March 2004).

Consumers' Health Forum of Australia (2000) *Consumer Involvement in the Co-ordinated Care Trials: Consultation Report*. Australian Capital Territory: Consumers' Health Forum of Australia Inc.

Cornwall, A. and Jewkes, R. (1995) What is participatory research?, *Social Science and Medicine*, 41: 1667–76.

Department of Health (1999) *Patient and Public Involvement in the NHS*. London: Department of Health.

Department of Health (2001) *Research Governance Framework for Health and Social Care*. London: Department of Health.

Elliott, E., Watson, A.J. and Harries, U. (2002) Harnessing expertise: involving peer interviewers in qualitative research with hard-to-reach populations. *Health Expectations*, 5: 172–8.

Entwistle, V.A. and O'Donnell, M. (2003) Research funding organisations and consumer involvement, *Journal of Health Services Research and Policy*, 8: 129–31.

Entwistle, V.A., Renfrew, M., Yearley, S. *et al.* (1998) Lay perspectives: advantages for health research, *British Medical Journal*, 316: 463–6.

Fleurence, R.L. and Torgerson, D.J. (in press) Setting priorities for research, *Health Policy*.

Goodare, H. and Smith, R. (1995) The rights of patients in research: patients must come first in research, *British Medical Journal*, 310: 1315–18.

Gray, R.E., Fitch, M., Davis, C. and Phillips, C. (2000) Challenges of participatory research: reflections on a study with breast cancer self-help groups, *Health Expectations*, 3: 243–52.

Hanley, B., Bradburn, J., Barnes, M. *et al.* (2004) *Involving the Public in NHS, Public Health and Social Care Research: Briefing Notes for Researchers*, 2nd edn. Eastleigh: INVOLVE.

Health Technology Assessment Programme (2004). Information sheet 7: the involvement of consumers in the HTA programme, www.hta.nhsweb.nhs.uk/sundry/consumers.rtf (accessed 27 March 2004).

Institute of Medicine (1998) *Scientific Opportunities and Public Needs*. Washington: National Academy Press.

Institute of Medicine (2001) *Crossing the Quality Chasm: A New Health System for the 21st century*. Washington: National Academy Press.

Institute of Psychiatry (2004) *Service User Research Enterprise* (SURE), www.iop.kcl.ac.uk/iopweb/departments/home/default.aspx?locator=300 (accessed 24 March 2004).

Jewkes, R. and Murcott, A. (1998) Community representatives: representing the 'community'? *Social Science and Medicine*, 46: 843–58.

Kai, J. and Hedges, C. (1999) Minority ethnic community participation in needs assessment and service development in primary care: perceptions of Bangladeshi and Pakistani people about psychological distress, *Health Expectations*, 2: 7–20.

Koops, L. and Lindley, R.I. (2002) Thrombolysis for acute ischaemic stroke: consumer involvement in design of new randomised controlled trial, *British Medical Journal*, 325: 415–19.

Kuzel, A.J., Woolf, S.H., Engel, J.D. *et al.* (2003). Making the case for a qualitative study of medical errors in primary care, *Qualitative Health Research*, 13: 743–80.

Kuzel, A.J., Woolf, S.H., Gilchrist, V.J. *et al.* (2004) Patient reports of preventable problems and harms in primary health care. *Annals of Family Medicine*, 2: 333–40.

Langston, A.L., McCallum, M., Campbell, M.K. *et al.* (2005) An integrated approach to consumer representation and involvement in a multicentre randomised controlled trial, *Clinical Trials*, 2: 1–8.

Macaulay, A.C., Command, L.E., Freeman, W.L. *et al.* (1999) Participatory research maximises community and lay involvement, *British Medical Journal*, 319: 774–8.

Marsden, J. and Bradburn, J. (2004) (on behalf of the Consumers Advisory Group for Clinical Trials and the Lynda Jackson Macmillan Centre) Patient and clinician collaboration in the design of a national randomised breast cancer trial, *Health Expectations*, 7: 6–17.

Medical Research Council (2003) *A Vision for the Future*. London: Medical Research Council.

Morrison, B. and Lilford, R. (2001) How can action research apply to health services?, *Qualitative Health Research*, 11: 436–49.

Murray, C.J.L. and Frank, J.A. (2000) A framework for assessing the performance of health systems, *Bulletin of the World Health Organization*, 717–31.

National Cancer Institute (2004) *About the Office of Liaison Activities*, http://la.cancer.gov/about.html (accessed 25 March 2004).

National Health and Medical Reseach Council and Consumers' Health Forum of Australia (2001) *Statement on Consumer and Community Participation in Health and Medical Research*. Canberra: AusInfo.

National Institute for Clinical Excellence (2004) *The Guideline Development Process: An Overview for Stakeholders, the Public and the NHS*. London: NICE.

National Patient Safety Agency (2004) *Understanding the Patient Safety Issues for People with Learning Disabilities*. London: National Patient Safety Agency.

National Quality Forum (2003) *The National Quality Forum's Consensus Development Process*. Washington: National Quality Forum.

Nowotny, H., Scott, P. and Gibbons, M. (2001) *Re-thinking Science: Knowledge and the Public in an Age of Uncertainty*. Cambridge: Polity Press.

O'Donnell, M. and Entwistle, V. (2004) Consumer involvement in research projects: the activities of research funders. *Health Policy*, 69: 229–38.

O'Toole, T.P., Aaron, K.F., Chin, M.H. *et al.* (2003). Community-based participatory research: opportunities, challenges and the need for a common language, *Journal of General Internal Medicine*, 18: 592–4.

Oliver, S. (1995) How can health service users contribute to the NHS research and development programme?, *British Medical Journal*, 310: 1318–20.

Oliver, S. (1997) Exploring lay perspectives on questions of effectiveness, in A. Maynard and I. Chalmers (eds) *Non-random Reflections on Health Services Research*. London: BMJ Publishing.

Oliver, S. and Bastian, H. (1999) Has involving consumers (patients) in research made any difference to what is researched and how?, *Journal of Health Services & Research Policy*, 4: 127–8.

Oliver, S., Entwistle, V. and Hodnett, E. (2002) Roles for lay people in the implementation of healthcare research, in A. Haines and A. Donald (eds) *Getting Research Findings into Practice*, (2nd edn). London: BMJ Publishing.

Ong, B.N. and Hooper, H. (2003) Involving users in low back pain research, *Health Expectations*, 6: 332–41.

Rose, D. (2003) Collaborative research between users and professionals: peaks and pitfalls, *Psychiatric Bulletin*, 27: 404–6.

SIGN (2004) *Patient Involvement in Guideline Development*, www.sign.ac.uk/patients/index.html (accessed 28 March 2004).

Stevens, T., Wilde, D., Hunt, J. and Ahmedzai, S.H. (2003) Overcoming the challenges to consumer involvement in cancer research, *Health Expectations*, 4: 81–8.

Tallon, D., Chard, J. and Dieppe, P. (2000) Relation between agendas of the research community and the research consumer, *Lancet*, 355: 2037–40.

Triveldi, P. and Wykes, T. (2002) From passive subjects to equal partners: qualitative review of user involvement in research, *British Journal of Psychiatry*, 181: 468–72.

24

Ethical and political issues in the conduct of research

Geraldine Barrett and Michel P. Coleman

Introduction

Health researchers work under an increasingly wide range of laws, regulations and professional codes of practice, all designed to protect the rights and interests of the human subjects of their research. Revulsion at the abuse of human subjects of medical research during the Second World War led to a consensus on ethical standards for experimental research on humans. In the last 30 years or so, codification of the ethics and standards of research practice has increased. More recently, the pace of such codification and regulation has been so rapid that even researchers who have only been working a few years will have experienced substantial changes in the regulations, processes and procedures by which they must abide.

In this chapter, we outline the key regulations and codes of which researchers must be aware in the design and conduct of their research. We start with the Declaration of Helsinki and other international codes. We then discuss ethics committees and the impact of national regulations. In the last part of the chapter, we focus on the current debate about the use of 'identifiable data' in research in health and health care. Research with human subjects involves both experimental and non-experimental studies. The distinction has profound ethical and practical implications, yet most statutes, regulations and codes are based on the clinical encounter and the experimental paradigm. This focus of regulatory activity reflects the origin of the Declaration of Helsinki, but some regulations have, wittingly or otherwise, threatened the viability of non-experimental research and public health surveillance. The debate centres on the balance between individual autonomy and the public interest. We discuss some of the profound implications of how this balance is struck for the future of public health and health services research.

International codes and regulations relating to research

The *Declaration of Helsinki*

The first major international code of ethical principles in medical research was the *Declaration of Helsinki*, produced by the World Medical Association in 1964. The World Medical Association is an international organization set up at the end of the Second World War to represent doctors, and funded by national medical associations. The *Declaration of Helsinki* has its roots in the Nuremberg Code, which arose from the 1946–7 'Doctors' Trial' relating to Nazi atrocities (Human and Fluss 2001). The *Declaration* has been revised five times since 1964 and the last major revision was in 2000. A note of clarification was added in 2002 (World Medical Association 2002a). Extracts from the *Declaration* are shown in Box 24.1, with links to the full *Declaration* on the web.

The *Declaration of Helsinki* has been hugely influential in setting ethical standards for medical research (Human and Fluss 2001), but the latest revision has aroused criticism. Disagreement surfaced over Clauses 29 and 30 in particular (see Box 24.1), and the debate about Clause 29 led to the note of clarification in 2002. These clauses have given rise to concern about actual or potential exploitation of research subjects in developing countries by researchers from developed countries (Guenter *et al.* 2000; Nuffield Council on Bioethics 2002; UNAIDS 2002). The clauses have been criticized as being too crude and too absolute. It has been argued that they may even damage the interests of those whom they are intended to protect by inadvertently limiting research enterprise in those countries (Hirsch and Guess 2001; Tollman 2001).

The current version of the *Declaration* has also been criticized for its expanded scope, which now includes all forms of medical research (Bastian 2001; Doll 2001). For example, its designation has changed 'from "recommendations" for doctors, to "ethical principles" for everybody involved in research' (Bastian 2001). Medical research in the twenty-first century is a multidisciplinary enterprise comprising clinical trials, basic scientific research, epidemiological research, health services research and clinical audit, but some of these types of research are either inadequately conceptualized or not addressed at all in the *Declaration of Helsinki*. The focus of the *Declaration* was originally, and still is, the *conduct of human experiments*: the frequent use of the term 'experimentation' in the current version of the *Declaration* is just one manifestation of this. Doll (2001) argues that the *Declaration* only properly applies to 'research in which patients are required to take drugs or have invasive procedures' but that 'even here, however, some of the principles show a lack of understanding of what their effects would be if rigidly applied'

CIOMS guidelines

The Council for International Organizations of Medical Sciences (CIOMS), an international organization established by the World Health Organization (WHO) and the United Nations Educational, Scientific and Cultural Organization (UNESCO) in 1949, has also provided international guidelines for biomedical research involving human subjects. The guidelines, first produced in 1982, with two revisions in 1993 and 2002 (CIOMS 2002), are intended to assist countries in defining national policies on the ethics of biomedical research involving human subjects. The CIOMS guidelines have at their core the *Declaration of Helsinki* (although they incorporate a slightly different view on Clause 29) but they are much more detailed. 'Research' is classified as any 'class of activity designed to develop or contribute to generalizable knowledge' and 'biomedical research' is defined broadly, thereby including studies of physiological, biochemical and pathological processes, clinical trials and various forms of research on human health and health-related behaviour (CIOMS 2002). The preoccupation with clinical intervention studies, however, remains. CIOMS also published separate guidelines for epidemiological studies in 1991 (CIOMS 1991): these are now under revision. According to the epidemiology core working group responsible for the revision, the aim is to bring the new guidelines up to date (e.g. to address globalization aspects,

Box 24.1   Extracts from the *Declaration of Helsinki* (2002)

1   The World Medical Association has developed the Declaration of Helsinki as a statement of ethical principles to provide guidance to physicians and other participants in medical research involving human subjects. Medical research involving human subjects includes research on identifiable human material or identifiable data.

5   In medical research on human subjects, considerations related to the well-being of the human subject should take precedence over the interests of science and society.

7   In current medical practice and in medical research, most prophylactic, diagnostic and therapeutic procedures involve risks and burdens.

10 It is the duty of the physician in medical research to protect the life, health, privacy and dignity of the human subject.

11 Medical research involving human subjects must conform to generally accepted scientific principles, be based on a thorough knowledge of the scientific literature, other relevant sources of information, and on adequate laboratory and, where appropriate, animal experimentation.

13 The design and performance of each experimental procedure involving human subjects should be clearly formulated in an experimental protocol. This protocol should be submitted for consideration, comment, guidance, and where appropriate, approval to a specially appointed ethical review committee, which must be independent of the investigator, the sponsor or any other kind of undue influence. This independent committee should be in conformity with the laws and regulations of the country in which the research experiment is performed.

15 Medical research involving human subjects should be conducted only by scientifically qualified persons and under the supervision of a clinically competent medical person. The responsibility for the human subject must always rest with a medically qualified person and never rest on the subject of the research, even though the subject has given consent.

24 For a research subject who is legally incompetent, physically or mentally incapable of giving consent or is a legally incompetent minor, the investigator must obtain informed consent from the legally authorized representative in accordance with applicable law. These groups should not be included in research unless the research is necessary to promote the health of the population represented and this research cannot instead be performed on legally competent persons.

29 The benefits, risks, burdens and effectiveness of a new method should be tested against those of the best current prophylactic, diagnostic and therapeutic methods. This does not exclude the use of placebo, or no treatment, in studies where no proven prophylactic, diagnostic or therapeutic methods exist.

30 At the conclusion of a study, every patient entered into the study should be assured of access to the best proven prophylactic, diagnostic and therapeutic methods identified by the study.

The full Declaration of Helsinki: www.wma.net/e/policy/b3.htm

Documents related to the Declaration of Helsinki: www.wma.net/e/ethicsunit/helsinki.htm

biobanks, privacy and confidentiality, etc.) and to ensure complementarity with the main CIOMS guidelines (see Box 24.2).

Other international regulations

In 2003, the Council of Europe drafted an additional protocol to the *Convention on Human Rights and Biomedicine*, relating to biomedical research (Council of Europe 2003a). Although the original *Convention on Human Rights and Biomedicine* did partly address medical research (Council of Europe 1997), the new protocol is entirely focused on research (see links in Box 24.2). The *Declaration of Helsinki* and

> **Box 24.3   Extracts from the Council of Europe's draft additional protocol on biomedical research**
>
> - **Article 1 – object and purpose:** parties to this Protocol shall protect the dignity and identity of all human beings and guarantee everyone, without discrimination, respect for their integrity and other rights and fundamental freedoms with regard to any research involving interventions on human beings in the field of biomedicine.
> - **Article 2 – scope:** this Protocol covers the full range of research activities in the health field involving interventions on human beings . . . the term 'intervention' includes i) a physical intervention, and ii) any other intervention in so far as it involves a risk to the psychological health of the person concerned.
> - **Article 3 – primacy of the human being:** the interests and welfare of the human being participating in research shall prevail over the sole interest of society or science.
> - **Article 7 – approval:** research may only be undertaken if the research project has been approved by the competent body after independent examination of its scientific merit, including assessment of the importance of the aim of the research, and multidisciplinary review of its ethical acceptability.
> - **Article 14 – consent:** no research on a person may be carried out, subject to the provisions of both Chapter V and Article 19, without the informed, free, express, specific and documented consent of the person. Such consent may be freely withdrawn by the person at any phase of the research.
> - **Article 15 – protection of persons not able to consent to research:** (*detailed conditions given*).

the language of human rights both feature strongly in this document (see Box 24.3). The draft protocol relates to research involving 'interventions', but Article 2 and the accompanying explanatory document lay stress on the breadth of this term:

> The term 'intervention' must be understood here in a broad sense; in the context of this Protocol it involves all medical acts and interactions relating to the health or well being of persons in the framework of health care systems and any other setting for scientific research purposes . . . Questionnaires, interviews and observational research taking place in the context of a biomedical research protocol constitute interventions when they involve a risk to the psychological health of the person concerned . . . It should not be forgotten that even observation, questions or interviews could be profoundly troubling to a patient if they address a sensitive sphere of that person's private life, such as a previous or current illness.
>
> (Council of Europe 2003b)

The protocol was in advanced draft at the time of writing and is likely to be ratified unchanged.

In the area of clinical trials there have been strong moves towards international harmonization in the past ten years, and many countries have changed their regulations. Publications by the World Health Organization (1995) and the International Conference on Harmonization of Technical Requirements for Registration of Pharmaceuticals for Human Use (1996) were instrumental in this process, and the ICH requirements were accepted by Europe, Japan and the USA. The European

Union (EU) (2001) subsequently approved a directive on good clinical practice in trials in April 2001. The *Good Clinical Practice Directive* became law in all member states in May 2004. In the UK, the Medicines and Healthcare Products Regulatory Agency (MHRA) was responsible for drafting the legislation to implement the *Directive* (see links in Box 24.4). Although the *Directive* codifies established good practice in the conduct of clinical trials, there is great concern that the regulatory apparatus put in place to monitor the *Directive* is potentially punitive and overly bureaucratic, to the particular detriment of trials that are not commercially funded (Crawley 2004; Gaw and Mungall 2004; Woods 2004). In early 2004, clinical researchers published widespread concerns about the impact of the *Directive* on

---

Box 24.4   European directives and UK legislation

The Clinical Trials Directive
The text of Directive 2001/20/EC is available at:
http://europa.eu.int/eur-lex/pri/en/oj/dat/2001/l_121/l_12120010501en00340044.pdf

UK Statutory Instrument: http://www.mhra.gov.uk/news/2004/ctregsdraft.pdf
Medicines and Healthcare Products Regulatory Agency (MHRA): www.mhra.gov.uk

The MRC/DH joint project on clinical trials: www.ncchta.org/eudirective/index.asp

The Save European Research Petition: http://saveeuropeanresearch.org/

The Data Protection Directive
Further information: http://europa.eu.int/comm/internal_market/privacy/index_en.htm
The text of Directive 95/46/EC (in two parts):
http:dReuropa.eu.int/comm/internal_market/privacy/docs/95–46-ce/dir1995–46_part1_en.pdf
http://europa.eu.int/comm/internal_market/privacy/docs/95–46-ce/dir1995–46_part2_en.pdf

Forerunners to the Data Protection Directive:
Council of Europe, 1981, *Convention for the Protection of Individuals with Regard to Automatic Processing of Personal Data:*
http://conventions.coe.int/Treaty/Commun/
QueVoulezVous.asp?NT=108&CM=8&CL=ENG

OECD summary of guidelines from 1980s:
http://www1.oecd.org/publications/e-book/9302011E.PDF

UK 1998 Data Protection Act:
Text of the Act: http://www.hmso.gov.uk/acts/acts1998/19980029.htm
The Data Protection (Processing of Sensitive Data) Order 2000:
www.hmso.gov.uk/si/si2000/20000417.htm
Other information about the Act, including legal guidance, is available from the Information Commissioner's office: www.informationcommissioner.gov.uk

EU-US Safe Harbour Agreement:
US site: http://www.export.gov/safeharbor/
EU site, including information on agreements:
http://europa.eu.int/comm/internal_market/privacy/adequacy_en.htm

clinical research with the 'Save European Research' petition (see Box 24.4). Concern has also been expressed that the *Directive* actually weakens the protection of 'legally incompetent' persons (i.e. those not in a position to give valid consent) by allowing some forms of proxy consent (Cave and Holm 2002; Corrigan and Williams-Jones 2003; Pincock 2004). Since the *Directive* was intended to be a product of international consensus and incorporates the *Declaration of Helsinki*, this is an interesting criticism.

Researchers must also be aware of the EU directive relating to data protection (European Union 1995) (see Box 24.4), although its scope is broader than just research. This directive developed from a set of principles for handling personal data that were laid out by the Council of Europe and the Organization for Economic Cooperation and Development (OECD) in the early 1980s (Council of Europe 1981; OECD 2001). This directive was translated into UK statute law by the Data Protection Act of 1998. The eight principles of the Act are shown in Box 24.5 (note that health data are considered to be 'sensitive data'). The text of Section 33, commonly known as the 'research exemption', is shown in Box 24.6. Schedule 3 of the Act permits processing of personal data without an individual's consent in a number of situations, including if:

> The processing is necessary for medical purposes (including the purposes of preventative medicine, medical diagnosis, medical research, the provision of care and treatment and the management of healthcare services) and is

---

Box 24.5 The eight principles of the Data Protection Act 1998

1 Personal data shall be processed fairly and lawfully and, in particular, shall not be processed unless:

- at least one of the conditions in Schedule 2 is met, and
- in the case of sensitive personal data, at least one of the conditions in Schedule 3 is also met.

2 Personal data shall be obtained only for one or more specified and lawful purposes, and shall not be further processed in any manner incompatible with that purpose or those purposes.

3 Personal data shall be adequate, relevant and not excessive in relation to the purposes for which they are processed.

4 Personal data shall be accurate and, where necessary, kept up to date.

5 Personal data processed for any purpose or purposes shall not be kept for longer than is necessary for that purpose or those purposes.

6 Personal data shall be processed in accordance with the rights of data subjects under this Act.

7 Appropriate technical and organizational measures shall be taken against unauthorised or unlawful processing of personal data and against accidental loss or destruction of, or damage to, personal data.

8 Personal data shall not be transferred to a country or territory outside the European Economic Area, unless that country or territory ensures an adequate level of protection for the rights and freedoms of data subjects in relation to the processing of personal data.

Box 24.6   Data Protection Act 1998: Section 33 – Research, history and statistics

1   In this section:
    'research purposes' includes statistical or historical purposes;
    'the relevant conditions', in relation to any processing of personal data, means
    the conditions –

    a that the data are not processed to support measures or decisions with
       respect to particular individuals, and
    b that the data are not processed in such a way that substantial damage or
       substantial distress is, or is likely to be, caused to any data subject.

2   For the purposes of the second data protection principle, the further processing
    of personal data only for research purposes in compliance with the relevant
    conditions is not to be regarded as incompatible with the purposes for which
    they were obtained.
3   Personal data which are processed only for research purposes in compliance
    with the relevant conditions may, notwithstanding the fifth data protection
    principle, be kept indefinitely.
4   Personal data which are processed only for research purposes are exempt from
    Section 7 if –

    a they are processed in compliance with the relevant conditions, and
    b the results of the research or any resulting statistics are not made available in a
       form which identifies data subjects or any of them.

5   For the purposes of subsections (2) to (4) personal data are not to be treated as
    processed otherwise than for research purposes merely because the data are
    disclosed –

    (a) to any person, for research purposes only,
    (b) to the data subject or a person acting on his behalf,
    (c) at the request, or with the consent, of the data subject or a person acting on
        his behalf, or
    (d) in circumstances in which the person making the disclosure has reasonable
        grounds for believing that the disclosure falls within paragraph (a), (b) or (c)

undertaken by – a) a health professional; or b) a person who owes a duty of confidentiality which is equivalent to that which would arise if that person were a health professional.

(Data Protection Act 1998, Schedule 3, paragraph 8)

A Data Protection Order, published in 2000, defines further situations in which sensitive data may be processed (see Box 24.4). The directive has regularized data handling in the EU, and the EU has reciprocal arrangements with some non-EU countries, including a 'safe harbour agreement' with the USA (see Box 24.4). We will discuss some of the implications of this directive for health research later in the chapter.

Ethics committees

Ethics committees have become a feature of health research over the past 40 years. The 1975 version of the *Declaration of Helsinki* first suggested that ethics committees be created to review proposed research (Edwards *et al.* 2004) and this recommendation has been strengthened in subsequent revisions. All the international guidelines relating to health research now advocate ethical review, and ethics committees are an almost worldwide phenomenon (Arda 2000; Coker and McKee 2001; Goodyear-Smith *et al.* 2002; Maio 2002; Aksoy and Aksoy 2003; Kim *et al.* 2003; Hearnshaw 2004; Hyder *et al.* 2004). The common pattern of development in most countries has been to set up institutional committees on a voluntary basis, concentrating on experimental research, then to organize a more formalized national system, usually incorporating other forms of health research, and finally to create a legislative underpinning of the ethical review system, with formal regulation. Different countries are currently at different stages of development. In the USA, the 1974 National Research Act required ethical review by Institutional Review Boards (IRBs) for some forms of federally-funded research. Over time, the role of IRBs was expanded, resulting in 1991 (and updated in 2001) in a Code of Federal Regulation (45, Part 46), more usually known as the 'Common Rule' (see Box 24.7). The Common Rule provides the legal underpinning of IRB review of all federally funded research with human subjects. (Similar regulations are in place for the research funded by the US Food and Drug Administration, see Box 24.7.) In Australia, the National Health and Medical Research Council Act 1992 established the National Health and Medical Research Council (NHMRC) as a statutory body, with the Australian Human Ethics Committee (AHEC) as one of its principal committees (NHMRC 1999). In Canada, the ethical regulation of research with human subjects is governed by three Research Councils created by statute law (the Medical Research Council, the Natural Sciences and Engineering Research Council and the Social Sciences and Humanities Research Council), which issued a joint policy statement in 2003 (Tri-council Policy Statement 2003) (see Box 24.7).

In the UK, a national system of local research ethics committees (LRECs) was set up in 1991 by the Department of Health to ensure ethical review for all research projects involving National Health Service (NHS) patients (Department of Health 1991). LRECs were organized on a geographic (health authority) basis, and had independent decision-making powers, including powers to agree their own procedures, application forms and guidance to applicants. For multicentre research, involving patients in the jurisdiction of more than one LREC, the 1991 guidance suggested that LRECs should 'arrive at a voluntary arrangement under which one LREC is nominated to consider the issue on behalf of them all' (Department of Health 1991), but in practice this rarely happened. By the mid-1990s there was strong support from researchers for better arrangements to facilitate multicentre research (e.g. Middle *et al.* 1995; While 1995; Crooks *et al.* 1996), and a new system of multi-centre research ethics committees (MRECs) was set up (Department of Health 1997). Researchers carrying out studies involving fewer than five centres continued to apply to LRECs, and those with studies covering five or more centres could apply to MRECs using a standard form, with a supplementary application (on a standard form) to each relevant LREC. Even so, researchers found the process bureaucratic and slow (Lux *et al.* 2000; Tully *et al.* 2000; Lewis *et al.* 2001).

The role of ethics committees has changed since 2001 in preparation for the EU *Clinical Trials Directive* and the related move to a system of research governance (Department of Health 2001a). Following implementation of the EU *Clinical Trials Directive* in 2004, UK ethics committees now have a basis in law. Their

---

Box 24.7   Ethical regulation of research

Australia
NHMRC documents relating to ethical conduct in research:
www.health.gov.au/nhmrc/issues/researchethics.htm

Canada
Tri-council Policy Statement: Ethical Conduct for Research Involving Humans:
www.pre.ethics.gc.ca/english/policystatement/policystatement.cfm
Canadian Institutes of Health Research, ethics: www.cihr-irsc.gc.ca/e/about/2891.
shtml

UK
Central Office of Research Ethics Committees: www.corec.org.uk
New operational procedures for NHS RECs, guidance for applicants:
www.corec.org.uk/applicants/help/docs/Guidance_for_Applicants_to_RECs.pdf
Department of Health Research Governance Framework:
www.dh.gov.uk/PublicationsAndStatistics/Publications/
PublicationsPolicyAndGuidance/PublicationsPolicyAndGuidanceArticle/fs/
en?CONTENT_ID=4008777&chk=dMRd/5
The NHS R&D forum, an organisation concerned with the implementation of
research governance:
www.rdforum.nhs.uk/

USA
45 CFR 46, The Common Rule: www.hhs.gov/ohrp.humansubjects/guidance/
45cfr46.htm
The Belmont Report: www.hhs.gov/ohrp/humansubjects/guidance/belmont.htm
Regulations applying to FDA: 21 CFR 50: http://www.fda.gov/oc/ohrt/irbs/appendixb.
html
21 CFR 56: www.fda.gov/oc/ohrt/irbs/appendixc.html

---

accountability is also clearly defined: ethics committees are answerable to strategic
health authorities in England and to the Central Office of Research Ethics Committees (COREC). 'Recognized ethics committees', which are authorized to
review clinical trials, are also answerable to the UK Ethics Committee Authority
(UKECA), which comprises four ministers, one from each constituent country of
the UK, including the UK Secretary of State for Health. Finally, the UKECA is in
turn answerable to the EU, which has the power to fine the UK for any failure in
performance. The performance of ethics committees is now closely monitored to
ensure that they meet requirements (for example, the 60-day deadline for decisions).
A single, nationally standard, application form is required for all research, including
multicentre studies, and a decision is needed from only one committee (albeit with
expedited local review, termed 'site-specific assessment', as necessary). All UK
health researchers needing detailed information about how to apply for ethical
approval should therefore start with the COREC website (see Box 24.7).

The statements of principle that guide the work of research ethics committees in
the UK, USA, Canada and Australia incorporate most of the elements of the *Declaration of Helsinki* (Belmont Report 1979; NHMRC 1999; Department of Health

2003a; Tri-Council Policy Statement 2003). These statements have also been influenced by four key principles:

- *autonomy*: the obligation to respect the decision-making capacities of autonomous persons;
- *beneficence*: the obligation to provide benefits and to balance benefits against risks;
- *non-maleficence*: the obligation to avoid causing harm;
- *justice*: the obligation of fairness in the distribution of benefits and risks.

These principles have dominated biomedical ethics for the past 30 years (Beauchamp and Childress 2001) (see Box 24.8 for examples). They offer simplicity and practicality in addressing ethical problems, but they have not been without criticism (e.g. Callahan 2003; Campbell 2003; Gardiner 2003; Harris 2003). For example, the

---

Box 24.8   Extracts from the Belmont Report

Basic ethical principles

1 Respect for persons – respect for persons incorporates at least two ethical convictions: first, that individuals should be treated as autonomous agents, and second, that persons with diminished authority are entitled to protection.
2 Beneficence – persons are treated in an ethical manner not only by respecting their decisions and protecting them from harm, but also by making efforts to secure their well-being. Such treatment falls under the principle of beneficence.
3 Justice – who ought to receive the benefits of research and share its burdens? . . . For example, the selection of research subjects needs to be scrutinized in order to determine whether some classes are being systematically selected simply because of their easy availability . . . rather than for reasons directly related to the problem being studied.

Extracts from Australian *National Statement on Ethical Conduct in Research Involving Humans*
Principles of ethical conduct: integrity, respect for persons, beneficence and justice.

1.1 The guiding value for researchers is integrity, which is expressed in a commitment to the search for knowledge, to recognise principles of research conduct and in the honest and ethical conduct of research and dissemination and communication of results.
1.2 When conducting research involving humans, the guiding ethical principle for researchers is respect for persons which is expressed as regard for the welfare, rights, beliefs, perceptions, customs and cultural heritage, both individual and collective, of persons involved in research.
1.3 In research involving humans, the ethical principle of beneficence is expressed in researchers' responsibility to minimise risks of harm or discomfort to participants in research projects.
1.4 Each research project must be designed to ensure that respect for the dignity and well-being of the participants takes precedence over the expected benefits to knowledge.
1.5 The ethical value of justice requires that, within a population, there is a fair distribution of the benefits and burdens of participation in research and, for any research participant, a balance of burdens and benefits.

dominance of the principle of 'autonomy' has been criticized, although Raanan Gillon, a leading proponent of the four principles, believes this is a benefit:

> I personally am inclined to see respect for autonomy as *primus inter pares* – first among equals – among the four principles. Firstly, autonomy – by which in summary I simply mean deliberated self rule; the ability and tendency to think for oneself, to make decisions for oneself about the way one wishes to lead one's life based on that thinking, and then to enact those decisions – is what makes morality – any sort of morality – possible. For that reason alone autonomy – free will – is morally very precious and ought not merely to be respected, but its development encouraged.
>
> (Gillon 2003)

Given such views and the emphasis on experimental studies in the *Declaration of Helsinki*, it is not surprising that ethical review has tended to concentrate on the information about a study that will be given to potential participants, the way in which consent is recorded (the expectation is usually a signed consent form for each participant) and the justification and special procedures required for studies involving children, or mentally incompetent or otherwise vulnerable adults.

Ethical review works well but is not always entirely effective. For instance, despite ethical review of information sheets for clinical trials, some participants still do not fully understand the information they have been given as part of the procedure to obtain their consent for participation (Ferguson 2002; Corrigan 2003; Brown *et al.* 2004; Gammelgaard *et al.* 2004; Lizd *et al.* 2004). The close scrutiny of research involving children or mentally incapacitated or vulnerable adults means that researchers invest substantial time, effort and ingenuity in developing consent procedures and in gaining approval for their studies (Bayer and Tadd 2000; Manning 2000; Osborn and Fulford 2003; Rees and Hardy 2003; Van Staden and Kruger 2003; Glasziou and Chalmers 2004). Such review may bring benefits in the protection of patients, but it may also result in fewer evaluated interventions and services for these groups (a potential injustice).

Social science studies in health may also be disadvantaged by inflexible requirements for giving information and obtaining written consent, particularly those using qualitative methods such as participant observation or in-depth interviewing. Various authors have described, for instance, the difficulties associated with asking for signed consent, either because vulnerable or stigmatized populations may be reluctant to provide such a record of their identity or because the formal consent procedure fits poorly with the ongoing, participatory and collaborative nature of the research (Coomber 2002; Kent *et al.* 2002; Truman 2003). It is notable that Canada's Tri-Council Policy Statement (2003) is the only national policy statement on research ethics to acknowledge explicitly that studies employing social science methods may require different procedures to those used for clinical or intervention studies.

The ethical review systems in many countries have developed rapidly in the last decade. Ideas about biomedical ethics are still evolving, and even in countries where ethical guidelines have not changed, much is open to interpretation. Researchers may therefore obtain different decisions from different committees, a particular problem for multicentre and international research (Burman *et al.* 2001; Gilman *et al.* 2002; Goodyear-Smith *et al.* 2002; McWilliams *et al.* 2003; Hearnshaw 2004; Minnis 2004; Shah *et al.* 2004). It is impossible to estimate how many worthwhile studies have been prevented or delayed by ethical review and the opportunity costs of this for public health. Glasziou and Chalmers (2004) argue that ethical review is itself an unevaluated intervention: 'it is time that a more concerted effort be made to assess the likelihood of benefits, harms, and costs of different approaches to ethics review for different types of evaluation'. Legislative support for ethical review systems tends to make available some funding to train ethics committee members, but committees often have heavy workloads, they tend to be staffed by dedicated, unpaid volunteers, and they are part of a system which may not help them fulfil adequately their role of protecting research participants (Jamrozik 2000; Levine 2001; Savulescu 2001; 2002, Savulescu and Spriggs 2002). Ethical review systems will need to evolve further to address the increasing breadth and complexity of medical research.

National laws, codes and regulations

Researchers must comply with national guidance and legislation, as well as international codes, agreements and ethical review systems. Within each country, each profession has a code (or codes) that its members must comply with at all times. Professional codes and guidance vary, depending on the focus and interests of the profession (see Box 24.9 for links). As one would expect, the UK General Medical Council's guidance on good practice in research (General Medical Council 2002) is strongly influenced by the *Declaration of Helsinki*. The codes of the British Sociological Association and the Association of Social Anthropologists reflect different disciplinary inheritances, but are also strongly influenced by the ethical norms of biomedical research. Other bodies, such as the Medical Research Council, also issue guidance for research practice for their own researchers but these standards are often accepted more widely. National codes and guidance do not exist in isolation; they are regularly updated and tend to reflect changes in international codes.

In the UK there is also a new system of 'research governance' (Department of Health 2001a, 2003a), already mentioned in relation to ethics committees. Research governance codifies much existing good practice in research but further demarcates the roles and responsibilities of individuals and organizations (see Box 24.10). In the implementation of research governance by the Department of Health, the emphasis has been on reporting mechanisms, performance management and audit (Department of Health 2001b; Kerrison *et al.* 2003). This has served to increase the bureaucracy associated with research projects. For instance, UK researchers now need to seek approval from research and development departments of the hospital Trusts or the Primary Care Trusts for each research project involving NHS staff or patients in those Trusts. This process of approval is in addition to the existing system of ethical review and has the potential to be time-consuming, particularly for multicentre research (Torgerson and Dumville 2004). The requirements of research governance have also put pressures on NHS organizations; many are still in the process of capacity-building to ensure they have suitably trained staff to carry out the necessary administration, and many are still finding the best organizational arrangements for meeting the research governance requirements (Shaw *et al.* 2004).

Researchers must comply with the law at all times. This seems a simple requirement, but the law may be open to interpretation or may, on occasion, be so poorly constructed that researchers have difficulty complying with it. Two important and closely related legal issues are currently being debated in a number of countries: the use of data and the use of human tissue in research. We will focus mainly on the use of data. The central question is: 'Is it acceptable to use identifiable information about (or tissue taken from) a person for the purposes of research without their prior explicit consent?' Subject to ethical approval, this has been possible until recently. Ethical approval is in turn subject to several conditions: the data are handled by health professionals (or persons with an equivalent duty of confidentiality);

Box 24.9   UK professional codes and guidance

Association of Social Anthropologists of the UK and the Commonwealth
Ethical guidelines for good research practice: http://www.theasa.org/ethics.htm

British Psychological Society
Code of conduct, ethical principles and guidelines: http://www.bps.org.uk/about/rules5.cfm

British Sociological Association
Statement of ethical practice: http://www.britsoc.co.uk/index.php?link_id=14&area=item1

General Medical Council
Good practice in research, seeking patients' consent: the ethical considerations, and confidentiality: protecting and providing information, all available via http://www.gmc-uk.org/standards/default.htm

Medical Research Council
Good research practice, personal information in medical research, human tissue and biological samples for use in research, ethical conduct of research on the mentally incapacitated, all available via
http://www.mrc.ac.uk/index/publications/publications-ethics_and_best_practice/publications-ethics_series.htm.

Nursing and Midwifery Council
Code of professional conduct: http://www.nmc-uk.org/nmc/main/publications/$professionalConduct

Royal College of Nurses
Research ethics: RCN guidance for nurses: www.man.ac.uk/rcn/ukwide/ukethics.html

Royal College of Psychiatrists
Guidelines for researchers and for research ethics committees on psychiatric research involving human participants: http://www.rcpsych.ac.uk/publications/cr/cr82.htm

Royal Statistical Society
Code of conduct: http://www.rss.org.uk/main.asp?page=1875

Wellcome Trust
Good research practice, human participants in research:
http://www.wellcome.ac.uk/en/1/awtvispol.html

---

the identifiable information is known only to the research team and procedures for ensuring the security of information are in place; the published results do not identify individuals; and the research does not affect individuals' clinical care. Today, however, ethical approval alone would not be sufficient. The reasons why health researchers need to make use of identifiable health data are the same in any country, and examples from Canada are given in Box 24.11 (CIHR 2002).

The confusion about research with identifiable data in the UK is often attributed to the Data Protection Act 1998, but this is only partly accurate (Coleman *et al.* 2003).

Box 24.10   Research governance: roles and responsibilities

Chief investigator, investigators, other researchers
- Developing proposals that are scientifically sound and ethical.
- Seeking NHS research ethics committee approval, or independent ethical review in social care.
- Conducting research to the agreed protocol (or proposal), in accordance with legal requirements and guidance.
- Ensuring participants' welfare while in the study.
- Feeding back results of research to participants.

Research ethics committee
- Providing an independent expert opinion on whether the proposed research is ethical and respects the dignity, right, safety and well-being of participants.

Sponsor
- Taking overall responsibility for confirming that everything is ready for the research to begin, including:
- putting and keeping in place arrangements for initiation and management and funding of the study (and, for clinical trials involving medicines, applying for authorisation and making appropriate arrangements for investigational medicinal products for the trial);
- satisfying itself that the research protocol, research team and research environment have passed appropriate scientific quality assurance;
- satisfying itself the study has ethical approval before it begins;
- satisfying itself that arrangements will be kept in place for monitoring and reporting on the research, including prompt reporting of suspected serious adverse events;
- ensuring the research complies with the law.

Main funder
- Assessing the scientific quality of the research as proposed.
- Establishing the value for money of the research as proposed.
- Assessing the quality of the research environment in which the research will be undertaken, and the experience and expertise of the chief investigator, principal investigator(s) and other key researchers involved.
- Requiring that a sponsor takes on responsibility before the research begins.

Employing organization
- Promoting a quality research culture.
- Ensuring researchers understand and discharge their responsibilities.
- Ensuring the research is properly designed, and that it is well managed, monitored and reported, as agreed with the sponsor.
- Taking action if misconduct or fraud is suspected.

Care organization/responsible care professional
- Ensuring that research using their patients, service users, carers or staff meets the standard set out in the research governance framework (drawing on the ethical review and sponsor).
- Ensuring there is ethical approval for all research for which they have a duty of care.
- Retaining responsibility for research participants' care.

Box 24.11   Why do health researchers need to make secondary use of data?

1   **To study patterns of diseases in the population.** Population health or health services researchers generally need to look at whole populations, or a representative sample of individuals to address questions about geographic or temporal patterns of disease, and to develop strategies to help control and manage disease. Sometimes, all of the information needed to answer the research question is contained in databases created for other uses and the researcher does not need to individually contact the thousands of people involved to obtain any further information. The researcher does not need to know who the actual individuals are. It is information on the whole study population that is important to the researcher. However, an individual identifier is sometimes necessary to link information about the same individual across databases (e.g. data on prescriptions with data on hospital admissions) or to link information on the same individual within a given database (e.g. to identify prescriptions written to the same patient in a prescription claims database).

2   **To identify causes of disease and their impact.** The secondary use of existing data is often required to conduct studies examining the causes of disease, or to determine whether persons who are exposed to a substance are at increased risk of adverse health effects. Many epidemiological studies investigate the health effects of exposures or events that occurred in the past (e.g. exposure to asbestos among shipyard workers, or exposure of Gulf War veterans to depleted uranium).

3   **To develop and evaluate health strategies, treatments, services, programmes and policies.** Pre-existing databases are primary sources of information for monitoring and evaluating the performance of the health care system and the effectiveness of new health programmes and policies. Comprehensive databases for documenting physician visits, hospitalizations and prescription drug use are available in many provinces. Studies using this information are critical for improving the delivery of health care and ensuring that new health policies are indeed effective.

4   **To assess data quality.** Data quality is an important issue in research on populations. Research based on poor quality data is wasteful of resources and misleads policy-makers and the general public. Researchers use existing data in order to determine whether and how to refine the research method and analysis so as to draw clearer and more accurate inferences from their research results.

5   **To assemble research participants.** Existing data are also used to identify or assemble potential research participants. In these cases, individuals are identified as eligible participants are then contacted and asked whether they would agree to participate in a research study or to provide further information needed to answer a research question. Researchers may also use databases to identify potential controls or comparison populations.

The Act implements the European directive on the transfer of identifiable data (see Box 24.4), but neither the European directive nor the UK Data Protection Act was intended to block medical research. The directive codifies the conditions under which research can be done, and in other European countries its interpretation has not caused such problems; in fact Danish researchers argue that it has made epidemiological research easier (De Vet *et al.* 2003). The problem in the UK stems partly from guidance issued to the medical profession by the General Medical Council in September 2000 (General Medical Council 2000). The guidance was intended to comply with the Data Protection Act but went far beyond it, prohibiting the transfer of patient information to disease registries. As a result, many long-standing data transfer arrangements were destabilized, confusion ensued, and the General Medical Council was forced to prorogue application of its guidance to disease registries only six weeks later to avert a complete collapse of cancer registration. (The guidance was only formally updated as recently as April 2004 and, although more factually correct than before, it is still problematic – see General Medical Council 2004.) The loose wording of the Data Protection Act on 'fair processing' has also caused confusion. 'Fair processing' embodies the requirement that an individual should not be deceived or misled as to the purposes for which personal data are collected. This principle is not contentious, but in practice it has often been equated with consent, which causes difficulty. In 2002, the Information Commissioner responsible for implementation of the Data Protection Act, Elizabeth France, summed up the ongoing confusion neatly:

> I have seen a significant increase in the number of requests for assistance from individuals . . . It seems to me that there are several reasons for the increase in requests for assistance and advice. Firstly there has been an extension of the scope of Data Protection from purely automated records to many classes of manual records . . . Secondly, it is clear that many practitioners are confused between the requirements of the Data Protection Act and those of the various regulatory and representative bodies within the sector including the GMC, MRC, and BMA. To some extent the advice issued by these different bodies may reflect their different roles. To some extent it may also reflect misunderstandings of the requirements of the Act. *It is a common misconception, for instance, that the Act always requires consent of data subjects to the processing of their data.* At the same time, as private litigation increases throughout society, many health service bodies have adopted a more cautious approach to the use and disclosure of patient data, fearing that uses and disclosures of data which previously seemed unexceptional might attract action for a breach of confidence.
>
> (Information Commissioner 2002, emphasis added)

The Health and Social Care Act 2001 gave the health secretary powers to allow identifiable patient data to be used in specific circumstances without patient consent. This power was presented by government as a transitional legislative solution to difficulties with public health surveillance and medical research, required only until technical solutions around the corner rendered the use of identifiable data unnecessary. Even this approach was forcefully criticized (Anderson 2001). The Act provides temporary legislative support for health research. It does not modify the 1998 Data Protection Act in any way, but it does modify the common law on confidentiality: health professionals who comply with it are not in breach of the common law. The Patient Information Advisory Group (PIAG) was set up under Section 61 to consider applications for use of identifiable data without consent for research projects, public health surveillance and NHS functions. In practical terms, this means that any researcher who wishes to use identifiable data without consent for a research project (e.g. this includes previously unremarkable activities such as identifying a sampling frame for a survey and holding contact information for the identified individuals) must apply to the PIAG, after first obtaining ethical approval. The PIAG meets four times a year; its secretariat is provided by the Department of Health's Information Policy Unit. The PIAG's record of decisions so far has been extremely conservative. Its most recent annual report sets out the approach (see extracts in Box 24.12).

Box 24.12   Patient Information Advisory Group

Extracts from PIAG annual report, October 2003
It is our aim to ensure Section 60 [of the Health and Social Care Act 2001] is used to establish an explicit regulatory code that, whilst supporting specific activities, regulates those who gain access to patient identifiable information much more strictly than the common law has before now (p.3). In considering the merits of these applications we have determined to balance the rights of individual patients on the one hand with the potential benefits to the wider patient body and the public. In those cases where there remains an element of doubt we have always chosen to protect patient confidentiality and advise applicants to find ways of either obtaining consent to use identifiable data or working with data that has been anonymised (p.7.)

It is rarely necessary to have 100% coverage of a sample population for a research study . . . It is not sufficient for applicants to simply state that certain groups are less likely to provide consent; we seek evidence to justify such comments. Applicants must also demonstrate that the research is likely to be of particular benefit to those patients who are less likely to participate before we would consider providing Section 60 support (p.9).

How to apply for PIAG approval, and other information about PIAG
http://www.advisorybodies.doh.gov.uk/PIAG/Index.htm

The increasing use of electronic patient records over the last decade is one factor driving concerns about the confidentiality of health data. The Department of Health is planning a national system of electronic health records. It commissioned research on patients' views, consulted on a draft confidentiality strategy in 2002, and published a new code of practice on confidentiality in 2003 (see Box 24.13). The new code is conservative, largely coinciding with the PIAG's position on acceptable uses of data. Under this code, clinical audit within a single organization is considered acceptable, but Section 60 support is required for audit involving more than one organization, and for all forms of research using identifiable data by anyone other than the immediate clinical team. The code contains a bizarre distinction between acceptable uses of identifiable data for direct patient care and in other activities, such as research:

Many current uses of confidential patient information do not contribute to or support the healthcare that a patient receives. Very often, these other uses are extremely important and provide benefits to society – e.g. medical research, protecting the health of the public, health service management and financial

---

Box 24.13   Confidentiality and related issues

Australia
Draft National Health Privacy Code: www.health.gov.au/pubs/nhpcode.htm
Electronic health records project: www.health.gov.au/healthconnect/

Canada
CIHR information about privacy available via: www.cihr-irsc.gc.ca/e/about/6426.
shtml

UK
NHS Code of Practice on Confidentiality:
www.dh.gov.uk/PolicyAndGuidance/InformationPolicy/
PatientConfidentialityAndCaldicottGuardians/AccessHealthRecordsArticle/fs/
en?CONTENT_ID=4100550&chk1w6ljh
DoH-commissioned research informing Code:
www.nhsia.nhs.uk/confidentiality/pages/hw_report_1002.asp
Confidentiality issues in the NHS:
www.nhsia.nhs.uk/confidentiality/pages/default.asp
Human Tissue Bill:
www.parliam ent.the-stationery-office.co.uk/pa/cm200304/cmbills/009/2004009.htm
MRC view of Bill:
www.mrc.ac.uk/pdf-htb_views_updated_25jun04.pdf
Wellcome Trust view of Bill: www.wellcome.ac.uk/en/1/awtprerel0104n311.html
Redfern Inquiry (tissue retention): http://www.rlcinquiry.org.uk/
Regulation of Investigatory Powers Act, 2000:
Text of Act: www.hmso.gov.uk/acts/acts2000/20000023.htm
Home office information about Act: *www.homeoffice.gov.uk/crimpol/crimreduc/*
regulation/

USA
Information about HIPAA:
www.hhs.gov/ocr/hipaa/
HIPAA and database research: http://privacyruleandresearch.nih.gov/research_
repositories.asp
HIPAA and public health: www.cdc.gov/mmwr/preview/mmwrhtml/m2e411a1.htm

---

audit. However, they are not directly associated with the healthcare that patients receive and we cannot assume that patients who seek healthcare are content for their information to be used in these ways.

(Department of Health 2003b)

This position seems at variance with the Department of Health's long-established aim of evidenced-based practice. Bill Lowrance (2002), in his report on secondary uses of data in health care, cites an amusing example devised by the Confidentiality and Security Group for Scotland that shows the artificiality of this supposed divide:

Doctor: Here, this medicine will help your condition.
Patient: How do you know?

Doctor: A study of 10,000 people's experience showed that it helped 9,247 of them to get better.
Patient: Good, I'll take it. But don't let anybody know whether I get better.

Alongside the issue of consent for the use of identifiable data in research, consent for the use of tissue samples is also a looming problem in the UK. The Human Tissue Bill, which had its second reading in Parliament in January 2004, is intended to provide a comprehensive legislative framework for the taking, storage and use of all human organs and tissue (including blood, urine, hair, saliva etc.), with informed consent underpinning all activity (see Box 24.13). However, the Bill has been strongly criticized by the Wellcome Trust and Cancer Research UK (two major research charities), by the Medical Research Council and by individual clinicians and researchers. It is described as unclear, unworkable and in danger of criminalizing legitimate research activity. The Bill is a legislative response to public concern at events at Bristol Royal Infirmary and the Royal Liverpool Children's (Alder Hey) Hospital in the 1990s, where infants' organs were retained after autopsy (see Bennett 2001 and Redfern Inquiry, link in Box 24.13). However, this Bill represents such a marked shift towards a requirement for consent that Furness and Sullivan (2004) asked in a *British Medical Journal* editorial, 'Does this Bill focus so much on individual rights that the benefits to society of research and training are ignored?' They also note the potential opportunity cost of the time spent by health staff in obtaining consent, and the lack of adequate systems for holding recorded preferences:

> In Leicester, for every autopsy performed 1215 samples from living patients are examined. Across the United Kingdom, about 150 million samples are examined each year. All fall under this bill. Imagine that a paltry one minute of staff time is taken for each sample – to ask the questions, listen to the answers, record the answers, and transcribe them into a database. One hundred and fifty million minutes per year equates to 1339 full time jobs. That is the entire staff of a medium sized NHS hospital. Add another minute to provide patients with some minimal information, and another hospital is fully occupied. Another minute to answer a question, and another hospital is unavailable. The initial government statement of the financial implications of the bill ignored this cost.
> (Furness and Sullivan 2004)

Confusion about the requirements of the Data Protection Act and the various professional guidelines has caused many problems for research in the last few years in the UK. Those responsible for health data have often taken a conservative stance on potential research uses for fear of being in breach of the law. Lowrance believes that understanding about data ownership and possession has become confused:

> Data may be about a patient, for instance, but that person does not 'own' the data in the sense that they are his in some exclusive proprietary way to take away, sell, or destroy . . . data-subjects have a right to inspect data about themselves, which contributes to patient-centering of care. But although it may give the patient a photocopy or printout, or correct an error or inset an amendment at a patient's request, for a variety of medical and legal reasons no health provider or payor can relinquish possession of, or right of control over, data it has collected in providing or paying for care.
> (Lowrance 2002)

Lowrance's view contrasts sharply with the position taken by the PIAG, which has recommended Section 60 support even for administrative uses of identifiable data in NHS-wide databases, as well as for research. The special status being afforded health information is also in contrast to non-health legislation – for instance the

Regulation of Investigatory Powers Act 2000 allows the government a range of powers to access personal data without consent, including the interception of communications data such as emails and mobile phone records (see Box 24.13 for link). As a result of the new regulatory climate, health research (particularly records-based and survey research) has been blocked, hindered, or methodologically weakened by a requirement of prior consent (see Strobl *et al.* 2000; Cassell and Young 2002; Verity and Nicoll 2002; Angus *et al.* 2003; Ingelfinger and Drazen 2004; Peto *et al.* 2004; Tu *et al.* 2004). It is difficult to quantify the overall effect on research as there is no central repository of information. Failed studies tend not to reach publication, and researchers have begun to police themselves, knowing which studies are, or are not, likely to be feasible in the new climate. A recent report from the Wellcome Trust highlights the current situation as a cause for concern:

> The public must be protected from inappropriate use of personal information. However, some of the new processes around data protection and issues of consent, designed to provide public protection, create unwitting barriers to the conduct of research of clear public value. It is essential to ensure the long-term continued collection, completeness, accessibility and linkage of key data on population health such as mortality, cancer incidence, infectious disease surveillance and health service use that are required for monitoring and improving the public health. It is necessary to establish the degree to which public health research is being impeded by the current and developing regulatory framework . . . the practical aspects of the regulatory framework need to be streamlined as these processes can act as a strong cumulative disincentive to embarking on public health research.
>
> (PHS Working Group 2004)

The specificity of research participants' consent is also a major issue in the current climate, in part as a result of a misinterpretation of the Data Protection Act's fifth principle and partly due to a concern about the bounds of consent. Researchers are now being asked by ethics committees and others to destroy identifiable data on the completion of studies; ongoing research (e.g. follow-up of individuals in subsequent studies, or secondary analysis of data that includes identifiable data such as a postcode) only being allowed if there is explicit consent for further uses. Gaining consent from individuals at a later date for research that was not envisaged at the outset of the original study can be problematic (e.g. it may not be possible to contact individuals or they may not respond to a request for consent) but, as Tyrer *et al.* (2003) showed, this does not necessarily indicate an objection to the new research. The requirements of today would, if enforced in the past, have prevented some of the UK's most highly regarded and critically acclaimed studies (Doll 2001; Barker 2003).

The problems in the UK are mirrored elsewhere. In Australia, discussions about privacy and confidentiality have been central to the development of a national system of electronic records. In 2002, the Australian government published a draft National Privacy Code for consultation (see Box 24.13). The Australian code appears to give greater consideration to the public interest, and how it should be balanced with the rights of the individual. In Canada, the Personal Information Protection and Electronic Documents Act 2000 appears to have caused similar disruption to health research. The provisions of this federal Act have to be incorporated into law in each province, but differences of opinion over how to do this are reflected by two privacy commissioners:

> I would have to say I've heard an argument made and I've heard a lot of anecdotal evidence that not having the full sample somehow badly skews

epidemiological research. Not to say it is not out there, but I have not seen the persuasive evidence that this is in fact the case. I have not had somebody point to, 'The following studies that were of real importance turned out to be badly flawed because . . .', for instance.

(Privacy Commissioner for Canada cited in CIHR 2001a)

I've been persuaded that, in many, many cases, we cannot afford the bias that can be introduced through a consent requirement, at least in relation to secondary uses of existing data (for example, clinical and other data found in hospital charts). Nor does the practicality of a consent requirement respecting research using existing data leap off the page if one assumes that there exists a strong and meaningful regime for data protection. If meaningful rules exist to restrict further uses and disclosures, to protect the confidentiality and security of information, and to prohibit the use of research data or outcomes to make decisions that directly relate to data subjects – if, in other words, realistic risks of harm to individuals have been removed or sufficiently mitigated – then I suggest the price of consent is too high.

(Office of the Information and Privacy Commissioner for British Columbia 2003)

The Canadian Institutes of Health Research have argued strongly for the use of identifiable data in research and have published several documents (e.g. CIHR 2001a, 2001b, 2002) in this area (see Box 24.13).

In the USA, the Health Insurance Portability and Accountability Act (HIPAA) 1996 laid out standards for electronic transactions of health data. Congressional concerns about possible erosion of privacy led to the inclusion in the HIPAA of a mandate to protect the privacy of individuals. The Department of Health and Human Services then published a final regulation in the form of the Privacy Rule in December 2000 (see Box 24.13). This was a major change in the legal framework on the privacy of health data and has affected health research. The Privacy Rule set minimum standards for privacy protection that most 'covered entities' (i.e. health plans, health care clearing houses and health care providers) had to meet by April 2003 (National Institutes of Health 2004). Individuals may authorize the use of their data for specific research projects – a 'Privacy Rule Authorization' which lasts for six years. Research done before the introduction of the Privacy Rule suggested that substantial sample biases would ensue from the use of such authorizations (Jacobsen *et al.* 1999). Researchers can obtain a 'waiver' or 'alteration' of the need for authorization from a privacy board or institutional review board (IRB), but how much this happens in practice is unclear. Anecdotal evidence suggests that there is much confusion about the requirements of the Rule in terms of what can be considered legitimate exemptions, with no consensus of opinion among covered entities, IRBs or researchers. The concerns in the USA over the legitimate collection, storage and use of human tissue in research appear remarkably similar to those in the UK, despite the different legislative and health care environments. Levine (2001) has described the issue in relation to ethical committee approval for such research:

Institutional review boards spend seemingly endless hours trying to determine how to say to a patient, 'We want to store a sample of your blood (or other tissue removed at clinically indicated surgery) with the hope that we might be able to do some genetic studies on it sometime in the future. We don't know exactly what genetic studies we might do, but in case it turns out to be something about which the IRB feels you should be consulted, we will ask for additional informed consent'. This is difficult enough when the tissue is sampled in the course of a formal research protocol, but what about the more common cases, in which the tissue is removed by a surgeon or other physician who lacks sufficient sophistication in genetics to respond adequately to the patient's questions?

The preoccupation with the privacy and confidentiality of health data in recent years in the UK, Australia, Canada and the USA illustrates how quickly ethical norms and standards can change and the extent to which ideas about appropriate research conduct are transnational. The World Medical Association (2002b) published new guidelines on the ethical use of health databases (see Box 24.) but these reflect national debates about data rather than taking an independent lead.

Finally, it should be noted that relatively little work has been done to assess the views of the public about the uses of tissue and health data. The few available studies show that knowledge about the uses of existing health information for research is low. People do value privacy when asked about it in a research setting, but the confidentiality of health records is not a passionate concern (NHSIA, Consumers Association and *Health Which?* 2002; Willison *et al.* 2003; Adams *et al.* 2004; Robling *et al.* 2004). Studies also show that respondents consider existing uses of data to be acceptable (Richards *et al.* 2003; Holowaty *et al.* forthcoming), and that they expect public health to be protected (Jones 2003). Most studies published so far have failed to present respondents with the opportunity costs of increased privacy protection, or to have them consider the balance between individual privacy and the public interest.

Conclusions

Increased codification of research ethics over the last few decades and the introduction of research governance has led to tighter regulation of medical research. Further, the debate about access to information from medical records, without an individual's consent, for the purposes of epidemiological and health services research, has resulted in extensions to the regulatory framework. Two (related) trends can be seen as responsible for the current situation: the uncritical extension of the *Declaration of Helsinki* principles to non-experimental research; and the increased importance of individual autonomy in society, with the consequent confusion between information *owned by* individuals and information *about* individuals. Ethical regulation of medical research involving human subjects provides essential reassurance that the risk of harm for the participants has been minimized. However, the extensive regulation that is now in place represents a considerable burden to health researchers and ultimately threatens research productivity. The cost of foregone research is unquantifiable (and possibly unknowable), yet in modern health care systems, which rely on sophisticated data flows, disabling surveillance will affect the quality of health care that individuals receive. Ever-increasing scrutiny has diminishing returns and there is an urgent need for a balance to be struck between a system of effective regulation and not preventing important research and surveillance from being carried out.

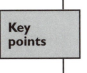

Key points

- All international guidelines relating to health research now advocate ethical review, and ethics committees are an almost worldwide phenomenon.

- Increasingly, codification of research ethics and the introduction of research governance has led to tighter regulation of medical research.

- Ethical regulation of medical research on humans provides essential reassurance that the risk of harm has been minimized for participants.

- In the UK, ethics committees now have a basis in law, their accountability is clearly defined, and their performance is closely monitored.

- The statements of principle that guide the work of research ethics committees in the UK, USA, Canada and Australia incorporate most of the elements of the *Declaration of Helsinki*.

- Ethical review has tended to concentrate on the information about a study that will be given to potential participants, the way in which consent is recorded, and the justification and special procedures required for studies involving children or mentally incompetent or otherwise vulnerable adults.

- Social science studies in health may also be disadvantaged by inflexible requirements for giving information and obtaining written consent, particularly those using qualitative methods, such as participant observation or in-depth interviewing.

- Researchers must comply with national guidance and legislation, international codes, agreements, ethical review systems, and professional codes and guidance on ethics and good research practice.

- Confusion about the requirements of the Data Protection Act, and the various professional guidelines, has caused many problems for UK research over the last few years.

- The current extensive regulatory system represents a considerable burden for researchers and threatens productivity.

Acknowledgement

We would like to thank Sara Shaw for her comments on this chapter.

References

Adams, T., Budden, M., Hoare, C. and Sanderson, H. (2004) Lessons from the central Hampshire electronic health record pilot project: issues of data protection and consent, *British Medical Journal*, 328: 871–4.

Aksoy, N. and Aksoy, S. (2003) Research ethics committees in Turkey, in S.Y. Song, Y.M. Koo and D.R.J. Macer (eds) *Bioethics in Asia in the 21st Century*. Japan: Eubios Ethics Institute.

Anderson, R. (2001) Undermining data privacy in health information, *British Medical Journal*, 322: 422–3.

Angus, V.C., Entwistle, V.A., Emslie, M.J., Walker, K.A. and Andrew, J.E. (2003) The requirement for prior consent to participate on survey response rates: a population-based survey in Grampian, *BMC Health Services Research*, www.biomedcentral.com/1472–6963/3/21.

Arda, B. (2000) Evaluation of research ethics committees in Turkey, *Journal of Medical Ethics*, 26: 459–61.

Barker, D. (2003) The midwife, the coincidence, and the hypothesis, *British Medical Journal*, 327: 1428–30.

Bastian, H. (2001) What are the effects of the fifth revision of the *Declaration of Helsinki*? Gains and losses for rights of consumer and research participants, *British Medical Journal*, 323: 1419–21.

Bayer, A. and Tadd, W. (2000) Unjustified exclusion of elderly people from studies submitted to research ethics committee for approval: descriptive study, *British Medical Journal*, 321: 922–3.

Beauchamp, T.L. and Childress, J. (2001) *Principles of Biomedical Ethics*, 5th edn. New York: Oxford University Press.

Belmont Report (1979) *Ethical Principles and Guidelines for the Protection of Human Subjects of Biomedical and Behavioral Research*. Washington: The National Commission for the Protection of Human subjects of Biomedical and Behavioral Research.

Bennett, J.R. (2001) The organ retention furore: the need for consent, *Clinical Medicine*, 1: 167–71.

Brown, R.F., Butow, P.N., Butt, D.G., Moore, A.R. and Tattersall, M.H.N. (2004) Developing ethical strategies to assist oncologists in seeking informed consent to cancer clinical trials, *Social Science and Medicine*, 58: 379–90.

Burman, W.J., Reves, R.R., Cohn, D.L. and Schooley, R.T. (2001) Breaking the camel's back: multicentre clinical trials and local institutional review boards, *Annals of Internal Medicine*, 134: 152–7.

Callahan, D. (2003) Principlism and communitarianism, *Journal of Medical Ethics*, 29: 287–91.

Campbell, A.V. (2003) The virtues (and vices) of the four principles, *Journal of Medical Ethics*, 29: 292–6.

Cassell, J. and Young, A. (2002) Why we should not seek individual informed consent for participation in health services research? *Journal of Medical Ethics*, 28: 313–17.

Cave, E. and Holm, S. (2002) New governance arrangements for research ethics committees: is facilitating research achieved at the cost of participants' interest?, *Journal of Medical Ethics*, 28: 318–21.

CIHR (2001a) *Presentation Before the Standing Committee on General Government Regarding Ontario Bill 159: An Act Respecting Personal Health Information and Related Matters*. Ottowa: Canadian Institutes of Health Research.

CIHR (2001b) *Selected International Legal Norms on the Protection of Personal Information in Health Research*. Ottawa: Canadian Institutes of Health Research.

CIHR (2002) *Secondary use of Personal Information in Health Research: Case Studies*. Ottawa: Canadian Institutes of Health Research.

CIOMS (1991) *International Guidelines for Ethical Review of Epidemiological Studies*. Geneva: Council for International Organizations of Medical Sciences.

CIOMS (2002) *International Ethical Guidelines for Biomedical Research Involving Human Subjects*. Geneva: CIOMS.

Coker, R. and McKee, M. (2001) Ethical approval for health research in central and eastern Europe: an international survey, *Clinical Medicine*, 1: 197–9.

Coleman, M.P., Evans, B.G. and Barrett, G. (2003) Confidentiality and the public interest in medical research – will we ever get it right?, *Clinical Medicine*, 3: 219–28.

Coomber, R. (2002) Signing your life away? Why research ethics committees (REC) shouldn't always require written confirmation that participants in research have been informed of the aims of a study and their rights – the case of criminal populations, *Sociological Research Online*, 7(1): wwwsocresonline.org.uk/7/1/coomber.html.

Corrigan, O. (2003) Empty ethics: the problem with informed consent, *Sociology of Health and Illness*, 25: 768–92.

Corrigan, O.P. and Williams-Jones, B. (2003) Consent is not enough – putting incompetent patients first in clinical trials, *Lancet*, 361: 2096–7.

Council of Europe (1981) *Convention for the Protection of Individuals with Regards to Automatic Processing of Personal Data* (European Treaty Series no.108). Strasbourg: Council of Europe.

Council of Europe (1997) *Convention for the Protection of Human Rights and Dignity of the Human Being with Regard to the Application of Biology and Medicine: Convention on Human Rights and Biomedicine* (European Treaty Series no.164). Oviedo: Council of Europe.

Council of Europe (2003a) *Draft Additional Protocol to the Convention of Human Rights and Biomedicine, on Biomedical Research*. Strasboug: Council of Europe, Steering Committee on Bioethics.

Council of Europe (2003b) *Draft Explanatory Report to the Draft Additional Protocol to the Convention of Human Rights and Biomedicine, on Biomedical Research*. Strasboug: Council of Europe, Steering Committee on Bioethics.

Crawley, F.P. (2004) New European clinical trials directive: is European research possible?, *British Medical Journal*, 328: 522.

Crooks, S.W., Colman, S.B. and Campbell, I.A. (1996) Costs and getting ethical approval deter doctors from participating in multicentre trials, *British Medical Journal*, 312: 1669.

De Vet, H.C.W., Dekker, J.M., van Ven, E.B. and Olsen, J. (2003) Access to data from European registries for epidemiological research: results from a survey by the International Epidemiological Association European Federation, *International Journal of Epidemiology*, 32: 1114–15.

Department of Health (1991) *Local Research Ethics Committees*. London: DoH.

Department of Health (1997) *Ethics Committee Review of Multi-centre Research: Establishment of Multi-centre Research Ethics Committees*. London: DoH.

Department of Health (2001a) *Research Governance Framework for Health and Social Care*. London: DoH.

Department of Health (2001b) *Research Governance Implementation Plan*. London: DoH.

Department of Health (2003a) *Research Governance Framework for Health and Social Care*. London: DoH.

Department of Health (2003b) *Confidentiality: NHS Code of Practice*. London: DoH.

Doll, R. (2001) What are the effects of the fifth revision of the *Declaration of Helsinki*? Research will be impeded, *British Medical Journal*, 323: 1421–22.

Edwards, S.J.L., Kirchin, S. and Huxtable, R. (2004) Research ethics committees and paternalism, *Journal of Medical Ethics*, 30: 88–91.

European Union (1995) Directive 95/46/EC of the European Parliament and of the Council of 24 October 1995 on the protection of individuals with regard to the processing of personal data and on the free movement of such data, *Official Journal of the European Communities*, L283: 31–50.

European Union (2001) Directive 2001/20/EC of the European Parliament and of the Council of 4 April 2001 on the approximation of the laws, regulations and administrative provisions of the Member States relating to the implementation of good clinic practice in the conduct of clinical Trials on medicinal products for human use, *Official Journal of the European Communities*, L121: 34–44.

Ferguson, P.R. (2002) Patients' perceptions of information provided in clinical trials, *Journal of Medical Ethics*, 28: 45–8.

Furness, P. and Sullivan, R. (2004) The human tissue bill: criminal sanctions linked to opaque legislation threaten research, *British Medical Journal*, 328: 533–4.

Gammelgaard, A., Rossel, P. and Mortensen, O.S. in collaboration with the DANAMI-2 investigators (2004) Patients' perceptions of informed consent in acute myocardial infarction research: a Danish study, *Social Science and Medicine*, 58: 2313–24.

Gardiner, P. (2003) A virtue ethics approach to moral dilemmas in medicine, *Journal of Medical Ethics*, 29: 297–302.

Gaw, A. and Mungall, M.M.B. (2004) New European clinical trials directive: implementation requires funding for effective training programmes, *British Medical Journal*, 328: 522.

General Medical Council (2000) *Confidentiality: Protecting and Providing Information*. London: GMC.

General Medical Council (2002) *Research: The Roles and Responsibilities of Doctors*. London: GMC.

General Medical Council (2004) *Confidentiality: Protecting and Providing Information*. London: GMC.

Gillon, R. (2003) Ethics needs principles – four can encompass the rest – and respect for autonomy should be 'first among equals', *Journal of Medical Ethics*, 29: 307–12.

Gilman, R.H., Aderton, C., Kosek, M., Garcia, H.H. and Evans, C.A. (2002) How many committees does it take to make a project ethical? *Lancet*, 360: 1025–6.

Glasziou, P. and Chalmers, I. (2004) Ethics review roulette: what can we learn?, *British Medical Journal*, 328: 121–2.

Goodyear-Smith, F., Lobb, B., Davies, G., Nachson, I. and Seelau, S.M. (2002) International variation in ethics committee requirements: comparison across five westernised nations, *BMC Medical Ethics*, 3: 2 (www.biomedcentral.com/1472-6939/3/2).

Guenter, D., Esparza, J. and Macklin, R. (2000) Ethical considerations in the international HIV vaccine trials: summary of a consultative process conducted by the Joint United National Programme of HIV/AIDS (UNAIDS), *Journal of Medical Ethics*, 26: 37–43.

Harris, J. (2003) In praise of unprincipled ethics, *Journal of Medical Ethics*, 29: 303–6.

Hearnshaw, H. (2004) Comparison of requirements of research ethics committees in 11

European countries for a non-invasive interventional study, *British Medical Journal*, 328: 140–1.

Hirsch, L.J. and Guess, H.A. (2001) What are the effects of the fifth revision of the *Declaration of Helsinki*? Some clauses will hinder development of new drugs and vaccines, *British Medical Journal*, 323: 1422–3.

Holowaty, E.J., Sullivan, T., Bondy, S. and Berger, E. (forthcoming) Non-consensual uses of personal health information for cancer screening and research: what does the public say?

Human, D. and Fluss, S.S. (2001) *The World Medical Association's Declaration of Helsinki: Historical and Contemporary Perspectives* (fifth draft), www.wma.net/e/ethicsunit/pdf/draft_historical_contemporary_perspectives.pdf (accessed 29 March 2004).

Hyder, A.A., Wali, S.A., Khan, A.N. *et al.* (2004) Ethical review of health research: a perspective from developing country researchers, *Journal of Medical Ethics*, 30: 68–72.

Information Commissioner (2002) *Use and Disclosure of Health Data: Guidance on the Application of the Data Protection Act 1998.* Wilmslow: Information Commission.

Ingelfinger, J.R. and Drazen, J.M. (2004) Registry research and medical privacy, *New England Journal of Medicine*, 350: 1452–53.

International Conference on Harmonization of Technical Requirements for Registration of Pharmaceuticals for Human Use (1996) *Guideline for Good Clinical Practice.* Geneva: ICH.

Jacobsen, S.J., Xia, Z., Campion, M.E. *et al.* (1999) Potential effect of authorization bias on medical record research, *Mayo Clinic Proceedings*, 74: 330–8.

Jamrozik, K. (2000) The case for a new system of oversight of research on human subjects, *Journal of Medical Ethics*, 26: 334–9.

Jones, C. (2003) The utilitarian argument for medical confidentiality: a pilot study of patients' views, *Journal of Medical Ethics*, 29: 348–52.

Kent, J., Williamson, E., Goodenough, T. and Ashcroft, R. (2002) Social science gets the ethics treatment: research governance and ethical review, *Sociological Research Online*, 7(4): wwwsocresonline.org.uk/7/4/williamson.html.

Kerrison, S., McNally, N. and Pollock, A.M. (2003) United Kingdom research governance strategy, *British Medical Journal*, 327: 553–6.

Kim, O.J., Park, B.J., Lee, S.M. *et al.* (2003) Current status of the institutional review boards in Korea: constitutional, operation and policy for protection of research participants, in S.Y. Song, Y.M. Koo and D.R.J. Macer (eds) *Bioethics in Asia in the 21st Century.* Japan: Eubios Ethics Institute.

Levine, R.J. (2001) Institutional review boards: a crisis in confidence, *Annals of Internal Medicine*, 134: 161–3.

Lewis, J.C., Tomkins, S. and Sampson, J.R. (2001) Ethical approval for research involving geographically dispersed subjects: unsuitability of the UK MREC/LREC system and relevance to uncommon genetic disorders, *Journal of Medical Ethics*, 27: 347–51.

Lidz, C.W., Appelbaum, P.S., Grisson, T. and Renaud, M. (2004) Therapeutic misconception and the appreciation of risks in clinical trials, *Social Science and Medicine*, 58: 1689–97.

Lowrance, W.W. (2002) *Learning from Experience: Privacy and the Secondary use of Data in Health Research.* London: Nuffield Trust.

Lux, A.L., Edwards, S.W. and Osborne, J.P. (2000) Responses of local research ethics committees to a study with approval from a multicentre research ethics committee, *British Medical Journal*, 320: 1182–3.

Maio, G. (2002) The cultural specifity of research ethics – why ethical debate in France is different, *Journal of Medical Ethics*, 28: 147–50.

Manning, D.J. (2000) Presumed consent in emergency neonatal research, *Journal of Medical Ethics*, 26: 249–53.

McWilliams, R., Hoover-Fong, J., Hamosh, A., Beck, S., Beaty, T. and Cutting, G. (2003) Problematic variation in local institutional review of a multicenter genetic epidemiology study, *Journal of the American Medical Association*, 290: 360–6.

Middle, C., Johnson, A., Petty, T. *et al.* (1995) Ethics approval for a national postal survey: recent experience, *British Medical Journal*, 311: 659–60.

Minnis, H.J. (2004) Ethics review in research: ethics committees are risk adverse, *British Medical Journal*, 328: 710–11.

National Institutes of Health (2004) *Research Repositories, Databases and the HIPAA Privacy Rule.* Bethesda, MD: NIH.

NHMRC (1999) *National Statement on Ethical Conduct in Research Involving Humans.* Canberra: Commonwealth of Australia.

NHSIA, Consumers Association and *Health Which?* (2002) *Share with Care! People's Views on Consent and Confidentiality of Patient Information.* London: NHS Information Authority.

Nuffield Council on Bioethics (2002) *The Ethics of Research Related to Healthcare in Developing Countries.* London: Nuffield Council on Bioethics.

OECD (2001) *OECD Guidelines on the Protection of Privacy and Transborder Flows of Personal Data.* Paris: Organization for Economic Cooperation and Development.

Office of the Information and Privacy Commissioner for British Columbia (2003) *Personal Information and Health Research: What Price Consent? What Value?* Insight Health Privacy Conference, Toronto, September.

Osborn, D.P.J. and Fulford, K.W.M. (2003) Psychiatric research: what ethical concerns do LRECs encounter? A postal survey, *Journal of Medical Ethics*, 29: 55–6.

Peto, J., Fletcher, O. and Gilham, C. (2004) Data protection, informed consent, and research, *British Medical Journal*, 328: 1029–30.

PHS Working Group (2004) *Public Health Sciences: Challenges and Opportunities.* Report of the Public Health Working Group convened by the Wellcome Trust. London: Wellcome Trust.

Pincock, S. (2004) Consent rule in EU clinical trial directive triggers concern, *Lancet*, 363: 785.

Rees, E. and Hardy, J. (2003) Novel consent process for research in dying patients unable to give consent, *British Medical Journal*, 327: 198.

Richards, M.P.M., Ponder, M., Pharoah, P. *et al.* (2003) Issues of consent and feedback in a genetic epidemiological study of women with breast cancer, *Journal of Medical Ethics*, 29: 93–6.

Robling, M.R., Hood, K., Houston, H. *et al.* (2004) Public attitudes towards the use of primary care patient record data in medical research without consent: a qualitative study, *Journal of Medical Ethics*, 30: 104–9.

Savulescu, J. (2001) Harm, ethics committees and the gene therapy death, *Journal of Medical Ethics*, 27: 148–50.

Savulescu, J. (2002) Two deaths and two lessons: is it time to review the structure and function of research ethics committees, *Journal of Medical Ethics*, 28: 1–2.

Savulescu, J. and Spriggs, M. (2002) The hexamethonium asthma study and the death of a normal volunteer in research, *Journal of Medical Ethics*, 28: 3–4.

Shah, S., Whittle, A., Wlfond, B. *et al.* (2004) How do institutional review boards apply the federal risk and benefit standards for pediatric research?, *Journal of the American Medical Association*, 291: 476–82.

Shaw, S., Macfarlane, F., Greaves, C. and Carter, Y.H. (2004) Developing research management and governance capacity in UK PCTs: a qualitative evaluation of pilot sites, *Family Practice*, 21: 92–8.

Strobl, J., Cave, E. and Walley, T. (2000) Data protection legislation: interpretation and barriers to research, *British Medical Journal*, 321: 890–2.

Tollman, S.M. (2001) What are the effects of the fifth revision of the *Declaration of Helsinki*? Fair partnerships support ethical research, *British Medical Journal*, 323: 1417–19.

Torgerson, D.J. and Dumville, J.C. (2004) Ethics review in research: research governance also delays research, *British Medical Journal*, 328: 710.

Tri-Council Policy Statement (2003) *Ethical Conduct for Research Involving Humans.* Ottawa: Medical Research Council, Natural Sciences and Engineering Research Council and Social Sciences and Humanities Research Council of Canada.

Truman, C. (2003) Ethics and the ruling relations of research production, *Sociological Research Online*, 7(4), wwwsocresonline.org.uk/8/1/truman.html.

Tu, J.V., Willison, D.J., Silver, F.L. *et al.* for the Investigators in the Registry of the Canadian Stroke Network (2004) Impracticability of informed consent in the registry of the Canadian Stroke Network, *New England Journal of Medicine*, 350: 1414–21.

Tully, J., Ninis, N., Booy, R. and Viner, R. (2000) The new system of review by multicentre research ethics committees: prospective study, *British Medical Journal*, 320: 1179–82.

Tyrer, P., Seivewright, H., Ferguson, B. and Johnson, T. (2003) 'Cold calling' in psychiatric follow up studies: is it justified?, *Journal of Medical Ethics*, 29: 238–42.

UNAIDS (2002) *Ethical Considerations in HIV Preventive Vaccine Research: UNAIDS Guidance Document.* Geneva: UNAIDS.

Van Staden, C.W. and Kruger, C. (2003) Incapacity to give informed consent owing to mental disorder, *Journal of Medical Ethics*, 29: 41–3.

Verity, C. and Nicholl, A. (2002) Consent, confidentiality, and the threat to public health surveillance, *British Medical Journal*, 324: 1210–3.

While, A.E. (1995) Ethics committees: impediments to research or guardians of ethical standards?, *British Medical Journal*, 311: 661.

Willison, D.J., Keshavjee, K., Nair, K. *et al.* for the COMPETE investigators (2003) Patient consent preferences for research uses of information in electronic medical records: interview and survey data, *British Medical Journal*, 326: 373–7.

Woods, K. (2004) Implementing the European clinical trials directive, *British Medical Journal*, 328: 240–1.

World Health Organization (1995) *Guidelines for Good Clinical Practice (GCP) for Trials of Pharmaceutical Products*, WHO Technical Report Series, no.850. Geneva: WHO.

World Medical Association (2002a) *World Medical Association Declaration of Helsinki: Ethical Principles for Medical Research involving Human Subjects.* Ferney-Voltaire: WMA.

World Medical Association (2002b) *The World Medical Association Declaration on Ethical Considerations Regarding Health Databases.* Ferney-Voltaire: WMA.

25

Training for research

Tina Ramkalawan

Introduction

There is an evident and surprising paucity of well-signposted literature relating to research training or, specifically, *health* research training.

While research itself is held in high esteem, it would seem that, until recently, little attention has been given to the challenges facing those wanting to learn *how* to do research. Historically, the research training process has not been subject to much evaluative scrutiny, and researchers have been 'trained' following a route that typically involves shadowing and working with established professional researchers. This still forms the basis of most postgraduate doctoral training today (UK Council for Graduate Education 2002).

A shortage of data prevents us from fully assessing the success of this model, although it has undoubtedly produced some excellent professional researchers. However, various government reviews (e.g. Roberts 2002; DfES 2003) have highlighted a range of concerns relating to research and the development and retention of high-quality researchers. This has also resulted in more attention being given to the process of research *training* and its outcomes.

A growth in evidence-based practice and the technology-facilitated accessibility of research information has resulted in different groups of people wanting to learn about health research for different reasons. These people include:

- those who want to critically evaluate the research;
- those who want to apply the findings to their own practice;
- those who want to do research and develop a professional research career.

The focus of this chapter is primarily for those in the third category: individuals who want to learn how to do research and are considering careers in health research. This group is potentially as diverse as health research itself. Thus, the chapter provides a preliminary consideration of some issues pertinent to research training, research conduct and research careers.

Brief overview of challenges in health research training

Training, or learning and development, is essential to becoming a health researcher. This often involves acquiring specific competencies, usually linked to a core discipline, alongside more generic or transferable skills. It also involves recognizing the need for continuous personal and professional development.

Embarking on research training involves a fair degree of organization, planning and flexibility. For example, you must determine your specific needs and objectives, identify appropriate training to meet these, finance the training, manage a research project, update and maintain knowledge and skills, and share expertise and learning. This may not always be a straightforward process.

In the UK, a variety of research courses can make the identification of appropriate and good-quality training confusing. In addition, flexibility and resourcefulness are called for when research projects do not go precisely according to plan, as is often the case. Further down the line, sharing your expertise involves learning how to communicate (and defend) your research, verbally and in writing, to a range of audiences that may include health care purchasers, providers and users as well as, more traditionally, academic peers.

In some circumstances, research learning is conducted alongside other professional responsibilities (e.g. nursing, physiotherapy, general practice). Doing research alongside clinical practice, for instance, presents its own opportunities and challenges, not least because of the potential differences in culture that can define each arena of work.

Finally, general developments and concerns about the future of scientific research in the UK are also relevant to considerations of developments in health research. In particular, these include an awareness of current potential shortcomings in research training and research career development.

Health research and health services research

There are various definitions of health and therefore of health research. Generally, a derivation of the World Health Organization's (WHO) definition is most often cited[1] (WHO 1948, 1998). As a consequence of this, health research could be broadly defined as any research that relates to the physical, mental and social well-being of individuals and populations.

> Health research is essential for improving the design of health interventions, policies and service delivery, and it accounts for the vast majority of *any* research conducted in the UK.
>
> Health services research (HSR) is a field within health research that more specifically considers the cost-effective provision of health care and related technology.

In the USA, HSR is quite clearly defined as an amalgam of the disciplines of public health, clinical medicine, economics, social survey research, systems analysis and biostatistics. It focuses on the access, delivery, outcomes and quality of health care and service. The UK shares a broadly similar definition of HSR to that of the USA, with the addition that other social sciences (e.g. sociology, psychology, anthropology) and humanities (e.g. geography) are recognized to play a larger role in the field. Consequently, a louder voice is often given to the patient experience.

The differences in health care systems between these two countries (the UK system is publicly maintained by the National Health Service – NHS; the US system is privately financed) also inevitably influence the overall research perspectives. However, changes in health care and a growth in private provision in the UK may encourage more and more areas of commonality. Certainly, health economics has become an essential component of health research and HSR in both countries, because considerations of the cost implications of health interventions and provisions are unavoidable.

Like health research, HSR is best thought of as a 'field with many disciplines'. This quality makes health research and HSR distinct from other fields, such as biomedical research. Some key differences are that:

- multidisciplinary research is essential for addressing the range of complex questions that are asked;
- the research is often conducted in context rather than in artificial situations or laboratory conditions;
- issues of public as well as of professional concern are addressed, and the research often has direct relevance to policy and to service provision.

These characteristics are important in influencing the ways in which individuals may train to do health research and be effective as health researchers. As a result, health researchers should be encouraged to adopt a multidisciplinary outlook, respect the contexts of research and the participants involved in it, and endeavour to communicate findings to policy and decision-making bodies, where appropriate.

Table 25.1 Research Councils in the UK and Key Areas of Research Funded by Each

Research Council	Abbr.	Website address	Key areas funded
Biotechnology and Biological sciences*	BBSRC	www.bbsrc.ac.uk	Agri-food; animal sciences; biochemistry and cell biology; biomolecular sciences; engineering and biological systems; genes and developmental biology; plant and microbial sciences
Council for the Central Laboratory of the Research Councils	CCLRC	www.cclrc.ac.uk	Accelerator science and technology; business and IT; central laser facility (CLF); engineering; e-science; instrumentation; particle physics; radio communications research unit (RCRU); space science and technology, radiation
Engineering and Physical Sciences Research	EPSRC	www.epsrc.ac.uk	Chemistry; engineering; information and communications technologies; infrastructure and environment; innovative manufacturing; life sciences interface; materials; mathematical sciences; physics; basic technology research
Economic and Social Research Council*	ESRC	www.esrc.ac.uk	Economic performance and development; environment and human behaviour; governance and citizenship; knowledge, communication and learning; life course, lifestyles and health; social stability and exclusion; work and organizations
Medical Research Council*	MRC	www.mrc.ac.uk	People and population studies: health services and the health of the public; neuroscience and mental health; immunology and infection; genetics, molecular structure and dynamics; cell biology, development and growth; medical physiology and disease processes
Natural Environment Research Council	NERC	www.nerc.ac.uk	Terrestrial, marine and freshwater biology; Earth, atmospheric, hydrological, oceanographic and polar sciences; Earth observation
Particle Physics and Astronomy Research Council	PPARC	www.pparc.ac.uk	Science programme; astronomy programme, e-science & grid; particle physics programme
Arts and Humanities Research Board	AHRB	www.ahrb.ac.uk	Humanities, creative and performing arts

* Research councils that provide support for health-related research in some capacity.

Sources of funding for health research and training

There are currently seven research councils in the UK and one research board (for arts and humanities). Each research council/board has its own research priority areas, which are further subdivided into specific topic areas. Within these, regularly changing research priorities are identified.

In the UK, most public funding for health research and training comes from the government's Department of Health (DoH), through its research and development programme, followed by the research councils. The DoH also has concordats with five of the research councils, primarily with the Medical Research Council (MRC),[2] which ensure collaboration in research areas of mutual interest.

Table 25.1 lists all the research councils in the UK and provides broad details of the areas that they fund. The councils that fund health research in some capacity are highlighted within the table. Table 25.2 lists some of the key western international government-funded bodies overseeing health care, delivery and/or research within their associated countries.

In addition to publicly-funded health research, a number of charities (e.g. the Wellcome Trust) and private companies (e.g. the pharmaceutical industry) finance research on specific or general health topics. Health departments in Scotland, Wales and Northern Ireland also support health and social care research and development, and other organizations provide the infrastructure that facilitates research.[3] These funders, through a variety of mechanisms and schemes, provide resources for scientific, social and educational health research in the UK. They also provide the means by which many researchers are able to undertake postgraduate and postdoctoral research training and are responsible for financing the majority of research degree (Ph.D.) students. For up-to-date information on current funding schemes, eligibility criteria and deadlines, see the relevant websites listed within Table 25.1 and at the end of this chapter.

Table 25.2   Key international health research organizations

Country	Organization
Australia	Australian Research Council (ARC) Australian Government – Department of Education, Science and Training National Health and Medical Research Council (NHMRC)
Canada	Canadian Institutes of Health Research (CIHR) Canadian Health Services Research Foundation (CHSRF)
New Zealand	Health Research Council (HRC) Ministry of Research, Science and Technology (MoRST) Foundation for Research, Science and Technology (RS&T)
UK	Department of Health – research and development programme Medical Research Council (MRC) The Wellcome Trust
USA	National Institute of Health (NIH) United States Department of Health and Human Services (HHS) Agency for Health care Research and Quality (AHRQ)

Training

Specific research training takes place at postgraduate level, with learners coming from a wide range of core disciplines to expand their research skills and further develop specific areas of expertise. The core disciplines that tend to be associated with health research are presented in Box 25.1

Box 25.1   Core disciplines studied at undergraduate/masters level commonly represented within health research

- Anthropology; medical anthropology
- Biology
- Computing; information technology
- Economics, health economics
- Epidemiology
- Geography; medical geography
- Health services research
- Mathematics; statistics
- Medical sciences; clinical medicine
- Philosophy; medical ethics
- Psychology; health psychology
- Public health
- Sociology; medical sociology

Masters and doctoral training

There are many masters-level courses that offer training in health/health-related research. It can be a minefield for potential students to navigate their way through, trying to determine which course is most appropriate and which will provide the core skills necessary for research development.

This level of choice reflects the fact that research degrees in the UK are offered by a large number of higher education establishments and institutions. In other countries, such as the Netherlands and the USA, both research and research training are concentrated in far fewer institutions. This model of research training, whereby fewer institutions are resourced to focus on research and research degrees, may also be a feature of UK higher education in the future (DfES 2003).

There are surprisingly few comprehensive resources available to facilitate the process of identifying appropriate training. However, the UK Department of Health provides a useful internet resource called RDLearning that lists health and health-related courses, with a particular emphasis on research training. It can be a useful starting point in searching for relevant postgraduate study (see www.rdlearning.org.uk). RDLearning also supports RDDirect – a telephone advisory service for all health researchers, regardless of level of experience. With an accompanying website, RDDirect provides information and advice on all aspects of the research process (see www.rddirect.org.uk). Additional research training resources can be found listed at the end of the chapter.

There is no fixed pathway to professional research. Some researchers come into research from other related careers, for example having worked in health care management or delivery. Alternatively, health researchers may have had little or no professional experience of health care prior to their research training. They may have taken a purely academic route through undergraduate and postgraduate study. These are only two examples of several possible ways into health research and are summarised in Box 25.2.

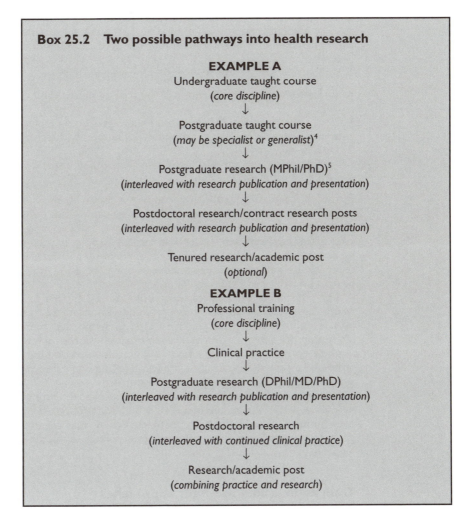

Box 25.2   Two possible pathways into health research

EXAMPLE A

Undergraduate taught course
(*core discipline*)
↓
Postgraduate taught course
(*may be specialist or generalist*)[4]
↓
Postgraduate research (MPhil/PhD)[5]
(*interleaved with research publication and presentation*)
↓
Postdoctoral research/contract research posts
(*interleaved with research publication and presentation*)
↓
Tenured research/academic post
(*optional*)

EXAMPLE B

Professional training
(*core discipline*)
↓
Clinical practice
↓
Postgraduate research (DPhil/MD/PhD)
(*interleaved with research publication and presentation*)
↓
Postdoctoral research
(*interleaved with continued clinical practice*)
↓
Research/academic post
(*combining practice and research*)

Whichever pathway is taken, some level of postgraduate study is obligatory. Most notably, if you wish to pursue a career in research, where you are ultimately designing and managing your own projects, the possession of a research doctorate (MD[6]/Ph.D./D.Phil.) is an important, if not essential, stage in your development, and demonstrates that a minimum level of competence in research has been achieved.

Situated learning

The learning acquired through doctoral research training is a classic example of *situated learning* (Lave 1988). This recognizes that studying for a Ph.D. involves more than merely being taught, but is an active, collaborative process that takes place in a fairly well-defined culture – i.e. the learning is *situated* in communities of practice (Lave and Wenger 1990).

The theory of situated learning underpins a lot of thinking concerning continued learning and professional development, which in turn increasingly informs the way we think about research training. It is, along with related theories, a useful way of viewing how individuals develop the necessary skills to become professional researchers.

Some of the key elements of situated learning are that:

• the learning occurs as a function of the activity, context and culture in which it is based;
• social interaction and collaboration are essential components of learning, which in turn help to generate 'communities of practice' with a shared culture of beliefs and a shared language;
• learners develop gradually, eventually becoming 'experts' within their community (e.g. field of research).

In studying for a Ph.D., students conduct a research project from start to finish typically over three or four years, with core guidance from one or more key supervisors. Although the student–supervisor relationship is key, most of the learning that takes place is self-directed, rather than formally taught. Experts in the field of study then examine the resulting thesis – a comprehensive and detailed critical analysis of the research – and eventually (one hopes) confer 'expert' status to the student. It can be seen how this process fulfils the criteria above.

The criteria for situated learning could also be applied to the ways in which health care professionals/practitioners acquire knowledge and skills. Thus, shifting from a culture of clinical practice to research practice can sometimes present interesting dilemmas (e.g. differences in organizational structure, methods of communication and work collaboration). Individuals who combine research with other professional activities can find themselves juggling two cultures, with each not fully appreciating the other's requirements or norms.

More practically, if you are a health care professional training to do research, you have to consider the requirements of your professional association in relation to maintaining skills and eligibility to practice. This may involve certain minimum patient contact hours or continuing professional development alongside your research.

Training in mixed methods approaches

The 'community of practice' where learning takes place can become further defined in health research by individual disciplines and the (sometimes arbitrary) barriers that can exist between them.

Core disciplines studied at undergraduate and masters level tend to introduce students to specific approaches to research. This often produces researchers with a familiarity and preference for certain methodologies over others – the most common distinction being between the use of qualitative and quantitative methods.

There is still something of a divide among researchers in identifying themselves as either quantitative *or* qualitative researchers. Ultimately, the research question and the outcomes sought will define the most appropriate methods to be used, and increasingly there is a requirement for mixed methods approaches in study design. This has encouraged greater flexibility in applying methods and learning about alternative approaches to one's own methods. To that end, it is important that quantitative researchers have a basic appreciation of qualitative methods, and that qualitative researchers have some understanding of the premise of quantitative investigation. This places students who are flexible and willing to learn about the applicability of methods from outside their core disciplines in a strong position.

Such flexibility will become progressively more important, as multi/ interdisciplinary research are explicitly recognized to be key elements of good-quality research in health and other fields (Joint Research Councils 2000; European Union Research Advisory Board 2004). Moreover, understanding a range of approaches and methodologies enables researchers to:

- communicate with a wider range of research professionals;
- critically evaluate a full range of research in determining the best project design for their work;
- appreciate the range of perspectives typically brought to and represented within health research;
- contribute more effectively to multi/interdisciplinary projects and help them to realize potential outputs.

Multidisciplinarity and interdisciplinarity in health research and training

Multidisciplinarity and interdisciplinarity are often considered to be essential in areas of health research. But although the terms are often used interchangeably, they represent different methods of collaborative work (Klein 1990).

In *multidisciplinary research*, individuals from different distinct disciplines collaborate, aiming to generate novel outputs in relation to a common goal. In order to work well, researchers need to be open to new ideas, and think and communicate outside the boundaries prescribed by their own areas of expertise. However, 'intellectually, they go home to their own discipline after work' (European Union Research Advisory Board 2004).

In *interdisciplinary research*, the process is taken a stage further. Researchers from different distinct disciplines work together to yield novel but *integrated* outputs. The aim is to synthesize different approaches and potentially create something entirely new. True interdisciplinarity is thought to be highly desirable, but difficult to achieve (Rogers *et al.* 2000).

While a lot of the research conducted in health can claim to be multidisciplinary, there is still little evidence of truly interdisciplinary work. Perhaps a lot could be done to ameliorate the challenges to interdisciplinary research by looking at the ways in which people train to do health research.

For instance, the differences between disciplines present key barriers to interdisciplinarity – differences in approaches, units of analysis, expectations, criteria and value judgements. And individual disciplines often work hard to protect the hypothetical boundaries that make them distinct. Each assumes that it has its own coherent methodologies and theories, and that its researchers share a single agreed internal language.

It is relatively easy to challenge these assumptions, and psychology presents a useful example. Psychology, as a discipline, is really an amalgam of separate sub-disciplines, each with its own conceptual framework. This spectrum of sub-disciplines is so wide that more variation can sometimes be found *within* psychology than *between* an area of psychology and another discipline entirely (e.g. biology or sociology). Nevertheless, until it is acknowledged that disciplinary boundaries are blurred, it will continue to be difficult to synthesize methods and theories.

The European Research Advisory Board emphasizes the importance of interdisciplinarity[7] in research and suggests three strategic ways in which interdisciplinary research could be facilitated. These are:

(1) A reassessment, where useful, of disciplinary demarcations.
(2) A removal of various institutional barriers to performing research.
(3) A rethinking of associated research training.

During research training, students can be encouraged to broaden their understanding of different conceptual frameworks and explore methods and approaches outside their core disciplines.

The European Research Advisory Board (2004) found anecdotal evidence that research students are very receptive to interdisciplinarity. However, maintaining this interest at postdoctoral level seemed to prove more difficult. At this level, researchers seem to revert to previous disciplinary boundaries in order to facilitate career development. Some pressure comes from the way in which organizations, from the top down, structure and categorize research. As a result, there is a perceived pressure to align oneself strongly with a core discipline that has a well-defined and established research identity.

In the USA, by contrast, interdisciplinary learning has been an active issue since the late 1890s (Rogers *et al.* 2000). There, they have begun to consider how best to embed multi/interdisciplinarity into research training, viewing it as vital for cutting-edge, innovative research. One approach taken has been to assess the added value of new multipurpose, multidisciplinary university research centres to address national scientific, technical and social problems. The NSF Integrative Graduate Education and Research Traineeship Programme (www.nsf.gov/home/crssprgm/igert) is one example. It encourages cross-departmental, cross-university *and* international collaboration through the provision of essential resources, and is perceived to be a good example of how well this approach to interdisciplinarity can work.

Competencies in health research

Research training should equip students with the core competencies necessary for research. These primarily relate to acquiring the specialized skills to design, conduct, analyse, present and publish research that makes an original contribution to the field (Quality Assurance Agency 2001).

Until recently, there has been little structured guidance on the process of studying for a Ph.D. This is now changing. In addition to learning how to actually *do* research, recommendations now suggest that research training should also contain some additional, structured elements of learning that relate to universal competencies (Metcalf *et al.* 2003). These competencies tend to focus on areas of personal and professional development and on the range of *skills*, rather than discipline-related knowledge, that research training ought to provide. These include areas such as project and time management, communication and networking skills.

The USA and other countries already provide more comprehensive guidance concerning the structure and content of research degrees, with Ph.D. programmes typically running for four years to accommodate requirements. Formal teaching is also an integrated characteristic of US doctoral training.

The Roberts Review (2002), was conducted in the UK to consider the issues pertinent to developing researchers. The review primarily concentrates on training in science, technology and engineering, but emphasizes that its findings are also relevant to health and medical research, which benefit from contributions from these disciplines. It specifically recommends that students' training should meet stringent minimum standards and '. . . *include the provision of at least two weeks' dedicated training a year, principally in transferable skills* . . .'. (4.2. Chapter 4)

In recent years, the UK Research Councils have worked together under the banner of the 'Joint Councils' to encourage greater cohesion in the training of Ph.D. students. They have identified the key skills that researchers ought to possess by the end of their training, and this provides a valuable step towards standardizing quality in research training.

To that end, the UK Research Councils provide a statement[8] of the skills training required of their research students. This is presented in Table 25.3. In identifying these competencies, the research councils were faced with a daunting task, as they had to accommodate the entire range of disciplines represented within postgraduate research. Therefore, these competencies are universal and deemed to be appropriate regardless of whether applied to research students in the arts, sciences or humanities. They highlight the generic, transferable skills which are increasingly recognized to be important to researchers' development.[9]

The joint councils are not prescriptive about the learning methods that should underpin the acquisition of these skills, but suggest that they should be developed during the course of study using a mixture of approaches. In support of this, the UK GRAD Programme, on behalf of the UK research councils, provides a number of courses and resources to facilitate this training for *all* postgraduate students. Courses and information aim to encourage a successful transition from postgraduate study to a research career. The UK GRAD website provides up-to-date information on the range of courses available and useful additional resources in this area – www.gradschools.ac.uk.

The UK is not unique in its discussions about the development and training of researchers. Debate in the USA about doctoral training raises a number of issues, some of which are consistent with those of concern in the UK. These include unease over decreasing numbers of full-time academic positions for researchers and a need for more transferable skills training. In the USA, it is also felt that the dominating emphasis on research fails to equip researchers with the skills to teach and share learning with junior colleagues.

This raises an important point about the iterative nature of research and research training. Researchers are facilitated in the process of developing their research skills by more experienced researchers. They, in turn, play an important role in supporting the training of new, less experienced research students. This emphasizes the importance of communication skills, including teaching and mentoring skills (see Table 25.3). Unfortunately, these skills are often readily neglected within the research training environment.

Research careers

Postdoctoral training

Research training does not end with the completion of a postgraduate doctoral degree; it could be argued that this is when it actually begins. Research funders and universities offer a variety of schemes targeting the most promising postdoctoral researchers. With the help of these, researchers are able to consolidate the skills acquired during their predoctoral training and better plan for career development. The schemes offer varying packages of support, but usually provide a salary and

Table 25.3   Joint councils' statement on skills required by researchers

(A) Research skills and techniques
To be able to demonstrate:
1   The ability to recognize and validate problems.
2   Original, independent and critical thinking, and the ability to develop theoretical concepts.
3   A knowledge of recent advances within one's field and in related areas.
4   An understanding of relevant research methodologies and techniques and their appropriate application within one's research field.
5   The ability to critically analyse and evaluate one's findings and those of others.
6   An ability to summarize, document, report and reflect on progress.

(B) Research environment

To be able to:
1   Show a broad understanding of the context, at the national and international level, in which research takes place.
2   Demonstrate awareness of issues relating to the rights of other researchers, of research subjects, and of others who may be affected by the research, e.g. confidentiality, ethical issues, attribution, copyright, malpractice, ownership of data and the requirements of the Data Protection Act.
3   Demonstrate appreciation of standards of good research practice in their institution and/or discipline.
4   Understand relevant health and safety issues and demonstrate responsible working practices.
5   Understand the processes for funding and evaluation of research.
6   Justify the principles and experimental techniques used in one's own research.
7   Understand the process of academic or commercial exploitation of research results.

(C) Research management

To be able to:
1   Apply effective project management through the setting of research goals, intermediate milestones and prioritization of activities.
2   Design and execute systems for the acquisition and collation of information through the effective use of appropriate resources and equipment.
3   Identify and access appropriate bibliographical resources, archives and other sources of relevant information.
4   Use information technology appropriately for database management, recording and presenting information.

(D) Personal effectiveness

To be able to:
1   Demonstrate a willingness and ability to learn and acquire knowledge.
2   Be creative, innovative and original in one's approach to research.
3   Demonstrate flexibility and open-mindedness.
4   Demonstrate self-awareness and the ability to identify own training needs.
5   Demonstrate self-discipline, motivation and thoroughness.
6   Recognize boundaries and draw upon/use sources of support as appropriate.
7   Show initiative, work independently and be self-reliant.

(E) Communication skills

To be able to:
1   Write clearly and in a style appropriate to purpose, e.g. progress reports, published documents, thesis.
2   Construct coherent arguments and articulate ideas clearly to a range of audiences, formally and informally through a variety of techniques.
3   Constructively defend research outcomes at seminars and viva examinations.
4   Contribute to promoting the public understanding of one's research field.
5   Effectively support the learning of others when involved in teaching, mentoring or demonstrating activities.

(F) Networking and teamworking

To be able to:
1 Develop and maintain cooperative networks and working relationships with supervisors, colleagues and peers, within the institution and the wider research community.
2 Understand one's behaviours and impact on others when working in and contributing to the success of formal and informal teams.
3 Listen, give and receive feedback and respond perceptively to others.

(G) Career management

To be able to:
1 Appreciate the need for and show commitment to continued professional development.
2 Take ownership for and manage one's career progression, set realistic and achievable career goals, and identify and develop ways to improve employability.
3 Demonstrate an insight into the transferable nature of research skills to other work environments and the range of career opportunities within and outside academia.
4 Present one's skills, personal attributes and experiences through effective CVs, applications and interviews.

Source: www.grad.ac.uk/3_2_1.jsp

resources for training and travel (e.g. see www.mrc.ac.uk for details of postdoctoral schemes offered by the UK MRC; see individual websites at the end of this chapter for details of schemes provided by other funders).

A variety of European and international awards are also available (e.g. www.cordis.lu/en). Furthermore, several postdoctoral award schemes actively encourage researchers to gain experience in a department/institution different to the one they are currently in. Periods of postdoctoral research in other national and international institutions can provide valuable opportunities for personal and professional growth.

Within health research, schemes are often organized to provide awards for clinical and non-clinical researchers. In so doing, institutions/awarders attempt to recognize the different opportunities and pressures that may confront researchers from clinical backgrounds (e.g. medicine). Clinical researchers are often ineligible to apply for schemes designed for non-clinical researchers and vice versa, so eligibility criteria should always be checked carefully when considering applying for an award.

Contract research staff and career researchers

General patterns of employment suggest that individuals will seek to change careers a number of times in their lifetime, and researchers are no exception (European Union Research Advisory Board 2002). Some professional researchers aim for the top of their field, wanting to seek funding for their research and manage their own teams as principle investigators. They might be referred to as 'career researchers'. Others will aim to fill one of the essential roles within research project teams that enable the research to be conducted. The nature of fixed-term funding for projects often results in these researchers being employed for the duration of the funded project, and hence they are often referred to as 'contract research staff'.

This is not a clear-cut distinction and in reality there is often a lot of overlap between the two roles. Career researchers often work for years as contract research staff before securing an established research or academic post, while there are many examples of principal investigators who are regularly employed on fixed-term contracts.

Not all professional researchers aspire to becoming principal investigators, but health research would be impossible without the contribution made by all types of researcher at all levels. Health research relies heavily on input from a large number of contract research staff.

The current predominance of fixed-term contracts in research has presented a number of challenges for contract research staff and for continuity and quality in health research. Contract research staff are often faced with having to regularly search and apply for new posts, and frequently need to relocate to maximize opportunities. In the long-term, this leads to numerous frustrations, not least a lack of security for the individuals involved. Research then suffers, as experienced researchers choose to leave to pursue other careers that offer better salaries and greater stability.

Recently, government reviews have recognized these dilemmas for researchers and it has been proposed that mechanisms be instituted to minimize the disincentives to working in research and to facilitate research careers (DTI 1997–2002; Roberts 2002). The Roberts Review, for example, identifies several problems for postdoctoral researchers, such as:

- increasingly uncompetitive salaries in relation to other industries and resultant poor recruitment and retention of permanent academic staff;
- unsatisfactory training in the (generic) skills required in an academic career or in business research.

Consequently, the Roberts Review makes a number of recommendations for increasing capacity in scientific research, which are pertinent to health research. It recommends the provision of higher salaries for postdoctoral researchers, fewer fixed-term contracts and a wider availability of additional (transferable) skills training. Mechanisms have been put in place to facilitate a reduction in fixed-term contracts. But, generally, how quickly these recommendations can be realized, and whether or not they are sufficient to stem a flow of researchers out of research (and out of UK-based public research) remains to be seen.

Alternatively, academic/higher education institutions also offer postdoctoral researchers a variety of fellowship schemes and, more commonly, lectureship posts. Lectureships will require researchers to contribute to teaching and administration alongside their research activity. This can put additional pressure on time, and there is an active debate about the growing divide between research and teaching within institutions. This has impacted on the number of researchers applying for academic lectureships and there is evidence that professional researchers are increasingly showing preference for positions that enable them to focus on research at the exclusion of teaching responsibilities (HEFCE 2004a). Adopting the models of research and research training found in other countries (e.g. the Netherlands, Germany, USA), where research activity is concentrated in fewer specialist institutions, has been presented as one possible solution (HEFCE 2004a, 2004c).

Conclusions

This chapter has aimed to provide a brief overview of some of the issues pertinent to training for health research. Some of these relate to the fact that health research is a broad field with many disciplines and a preponderance of multidisciplinary research.

At masters' level, the provision of health-related training has increased over the years, and prospective students in some areas are confronted with a variety of courses to choose from. Better signposting would facilitate the process of identifying appropriate training and, although there are some helpful resources, the options are by no means exhaustive.

A review of professional health care training is currently being conducted by the Quality Assurance Agency for Higher Education (QAA).[10] Although this review concentrates on *professional* health care training funded by the DoH, and excludes research degrees, it may include some taught postgraduate courses of relevance to new health researchers, particularly those from professional health care backgrounds.

The process of studying for a doctoral research degree was considered within one theoretical learning framework, namely that of situated learning. This lends itself to an understanding of how students are trained within an overarching research culture. However, within this, disciplines and sub-disciplines can be protective of the boundaries that define their approaches to research, and these can present barriers to multidisciplinarity and interdisciplinarity.

As a result, it is suggested that, alongside their core expertise, Ph.D. students in health research should be encouraged to learn something about different approaches and methodologies to their own. Generic transferable skills are also important and have been identified by the Joint Research Councils as valuable learning outcomes. As a result, an element of structured teaching in these areas is now often integrated into Ph.D. programmes, and nationally-run courses and workshops provide further options.

It is also important that health researchers develop good communication skills and learn to communicate research findings to a variety of audiences. Health research often has indirect or direct implications for health care and delivery. As a result, it is necessary to think about the need to present to policy- and decision-makers, health care practitioners and users, as well as a variety of interest groups and researchers.

Finally, considering broader developments in research may help to inform your training/research choices and plans. Over recent years, research training in general has been informed by a number of reports (e.g. Roberts 2002; Metcalf *et al.* 2003; European Union Research Advisory Board 2004; HEFCE 2004b). Many of the issues raised are relevant to health research. Amongst them are recommendations relating to:

- developments in UK and European research funding;
- the structure of research and the provision of research training;
- the training needs and skills requirements of research students;
- the removal of various barriers to research career development.

These reports reflect a general commitment to UK research and the development and support of UK researchers. They will most definitely shape training and careers within the research environments of the future.

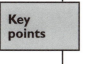

Key points

- People want to learn about health research in order to critically evaluate the research, to apply the findings to their own practice, and/or to do research and develop a professional research career.

- Training in health research involves acquiring specific competencies, usually linked to a core discipline, alongside more generic or transferable skills. It also involves recognizing the need for continuous personal and professional learning and development.

- There is no fixed pathway to professional research. Some individuals come into health research from health-related careers, and others may have had little or no professional experience of health care prior to their research training.

- The learning acquired through doctoral research training is a classic example of situated learning, which recognizes that studying for a Ph.D. is also an active collaborative process that takes place in a well-defined culture.

- Core disciples studied at postgraduate level tend to introduce students to specific approaches to research, leading to methodological preferences.

- Increasingly there is a requirement for mixed methods approaches in study design, requiring greater flexibility in applying methods.

- In multidisciplinary research, people from different disciples collaborate, aiming to generate novel outputs in relation to a common goal.

- In interdisciplinary research, the process is taken a stage further: researchers from different disciplines work together to yield novel but integrated outputs; this approach has a longer tradition in the USA.

- Research training should equip students with the core competencies necessary for research, specifically the skills to design, conduct, analyse, present and publish research that makes an original contribution to the field.

- Research training does not end with the completion of a postgraduate degree; it could be argued that this is when it begins.

Notes

1 Health: a dynamic state of complete physical, mental, spiritual and social well-being and not merely the absence of disease or infirmity (WHO 1998).
2 At the time of writing, each of the four UK health departments has concordats with the MRC, EPSR, BBSRC, NERC and ESRC. These agreements set out the aims and principles for collaboration between the health departments and each council to ensure effective development, funding, management, dissemination and exploitation of publicly-funded research of mutual interest.
3 These include: the Department for Education and Skills (DfES), through the Higher Education Funding Council for England (HEFCE); the Department of Trade and Industry (DTI), through their Office of Science and Technology.
4 A specialist course includes courses such as health economics or medical statistics, which focus on a particular discipline and approach; a generalist course may be health services research or health research methods, which provide a more general overview of various disciplines, methods and approaches.
5 Research degrees (e.g. Ph.D.) are not essential for all research posts, although some level of postgraduate training is usual (e.g. masters level). It is also common for undergraduates with good first degrees to go straight to research doctoral training. A first or upper second class degree in an appropriate subject is the minimum requirement stipulated by research councils for Ph.D. studentships.
6 The MD is currently the only 'professional doctorate' available in the UK. This is defined as: 'a programme of advanced study and research which, while satisfying the university criteria for the award of a Doctorate, is designed to meet the specific needs of a professional group external to the University, and which develops the capability of individuals to work within a professional context' (UK Council for Graduate Education 2002). It has been criticized for the varying standards applied to its assessment and award.
7 The Board uses the term *interdisciplinary* to cover both multidisciplinary and interdisciplinary approaches.
8 Joint Statement of the Research Councils'/AHRB Skills Training Requirements for Research Students, developed with the UK research councils, Arts and Humanities Research Board, UK HEIs and the UK GRAD Programme.
9 It is important to note that the research councils/AHRB emphasize that these generic

skills should not detract from the key element of development – i.e. training in research skills and techniques; making an original contribution to knowledge; publishing research.
10 QAA review of health care programmes (2003–6) is commissioned by the DoH in partnership with the Nursing and Midwifery Council, Health Professions Council and the Workforce Development Confederations/Strategic Health Authorities.

Resources

Agency for Health care Research and Quality (AHRQ): www.ahrq.gov/fund/training/trainix.htm
Australian Government, Department of Education, Science and Training, Research Training Scheme Guidelines for 2004: www.dest.gov.au/highered/research/rts.htm
Australian Research Council: www.arc.gov.au/arc_home/default.htm
Canadian health services research foundation: www.chsrf.ca/home_e.php
Cipolla, R. (1995) *Guidelines on PhD Research and Supervision*, http://mi.eng.cam.ac.uk/~cipolla/phdguide.html
Dept of Health Research and Development: www.dh.gov.uk/PolicyAndGuidance/ResearchAndDevelopment/fs/en
For more detailed discussion on the topic of situated learning and learning styles: http://tip.psychology.org/lave.html
Foundation for Research, Science and Technology (RS&T): www.frst.govt.nz
Free online database for researchers' CVs, for access by potential employers: www.cvs.ac.uk
Higher Education Funding Council for England (HEFCE): www.hefce.ac.uk
Information for UK organizations on the EUs Sixth Framework Programme, a source of support for leading-edge research and technological development: http://fp6uk.ost.gov.uk
King's Fund: www.kingsfund.org.uk
Medical Research Council (MRC) (UK): www.mrc.ac.uk
Ministry of Research Science and Technology, NZ: www.morst.govt.nz/default.asp?CHANNEL=Channels&PAGE=Home
NHS University (NHSU) – aims to provide learning and development opportunities to NHS and social sector employees: www.nhsu..nhs.uk
NSF Integrative Graduate Education and Research Traineeship Programme (the IGERT Programme) – a collaborative multidisciplinary Ph.D. education and training programme in the US: www.nsf.gov/home/crssprgm/igert.
Office of Science and Technology: www.ost.gov.uk/index_v4.htm
Quality Assurance Agency for Higher Education: www.qaa.ac.uk
Research Councils UK Postgraduate Training Group (PTG): www.gradschools.ac.uk
Research councils UK: www.rcuk.ac.uk
Research training opportunities offered by NIH: http://grants1.nih.gov/training/
The European Research Advisory Board (EURAB) – provides advice on the design and implementation of EU research policy: http://europa.eu.int/comm/research/eurab/index_en.html
UK Council for Graduate Education: www.ukcge.ac.uk
UK Department of Health (DoH): www.dh.gov.uk
UK Graduate Careers website: www.prospects.ac.uk
United States Department of Health and Human Services: www.hhs.gov/
Wellcome Trust: www.wellcome.ac.uk
Guidance on research and research training
Higher Education & Research Opportunities in the UK (HERO): www.hero.ac.uk
Postgraduate research opportunities: www.jobs.ac.uk
Prospects – postgraduate study information, education and courses: www.prospects.ac.uk
RDDirect: www.rddirect.org.uk
RDLearning: www.rdlearning.org.uk
Research and Development Information (UK): www.rdinfo.org.uk
UK Universities directory of postgraduate training courses: www.postgraduateprospects.co.uk

References

DfES (Department for Education and Skills) (2003) *The Future of Higher Education*. London: The Stationery Office.

DTI (Department of Trade and Industry) (1997–2002) *Final Report of the Research Careers Initiative*: London: DTI Publications.

European Union Research Advisory Board (2002) *Some Issues Affecting the Future of University Research in the EU. Final Report*. http://europa.eu.int.

European Union Research Advisory Board (2004) *Interdisciplinarity in Research. Final Report*. http://europa.eu.int.

HEFCE (Higher Education Funding Council for England) (2004a) *Higher Education in the United Kingdom*. Bristol: HEFCE.

HEFCE (Higher Education Funding Council for England) (2004b) *HEFCE Strategic Plan 2003–08*. Bristol: HEFCE.

HEFCE (Higher Education Funding Council for England) (2004c) *Improving Standards in Postgraduate Research Degree Programmes: Statement on Progress*. Bristol: HEFCE.

Joint Research Councils (2000) *Promoting Interdisciplinary Research & Training – Report of the Joint Research Council Visits to 13 UK Universities*.

Klein, J. (1990) *Interdisciplinarity: History, Theory and Practice*. Detroit, MI: Wayne State University Press.

Lave, J. (1988) *Cognition in Practice: Mind, Mathematics and Culture in Everyday Life*. Cambridge: Cambridge University Press.

Lave, J. and Wenger, E. (1990) *Situated Learning: Legitimate Peripheral Situated Learning*. Cambridge: Cambridge University Press.

Metcalfe, J., Thompson, Q. and Green, H. (2003) *Improving Standards in Postgraduate Research Degree Programmes: A Report to the Higher Education Funding Councils of England, Scotland and Wales*. Bristol: HEFCE.

Quality Assurance Agency (QAA) (2001) *The Framework for Higher Education Qualifications in England, Wales and Northern Ireland*. Gloucester: QAA.

Roberts, G. (2002) *SET for Success: The Supply of People with Science, Technology, Engineering and Mathematics Skills*. The report of Sir Gareth Roberts' Review, 15 April 2002. London: HM Treasury.

Rogers, Y., Scaife, M. and Rizzo, A. (2000) *Isn't Multidisciplinarity Enough? When do we Really Need Interdisciplinarity?* www-sv.cict.fr/coctos/pjs/interdisciplinarity/Interpaper Rogers.html.

UK Council for Graduate Education (2002) *Professional Doctorates*. Staffordshire: UKCGE.

WHO (World Health Organization) (1948) Preamble to the *Constitution of the World Health Organization* as adopted by the International Health Conference, New York, 19–22 June 1946. Geneva: World Health Organization.

WHO (World Health Organization) (1998) *101st session of the WHO Executive Board*. Geneva: World Health Organization.

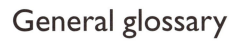

General glossary

acquiescence response set ('yes-saying') respondents will more frequently endorse a statement than disagree with its opposite.

atomistic fallacies assume that the results of individual studies apply between areas.

attrition loss of sample members over time in longitudinal and experimental research with post-tests.

Bayesian approach starts with a **prior belief** (expressed as a probability distribution) about the likely values of the parameters, and then uses the observed data to modify this belief.

bias deviation in one direction of the observed value from the true value of the construct being measured (as opposed to random error).

blind concealing the assignment of people to experimental or control group in experiments. Concealment can be from the people or from both the people and the person carrying out the intervention, e.g. treating doctor ('double blind').

case a single unit in a study (e.g. a person or setting, such as a clinic, hospital).

case–control study people who have the outcome of interest (e.g. disease) and a control group of individuals without the disease are selected for investigation; the proportions with the exposure of interest in each group are then compared.

case–parent trio design cases and their parents are genotyped, but the parents themselves are not the controls, instead hypothetical pseudo-siblings are constructed using the other three genotypes, which could have been transmitted from the parents to the case, but were not.

case–sibling study discordant sibling pairs used as controls.

case study a research method which focuses on the circumstances, dynamics and complexity of a single case, or a small number of cases.

causal hypothesis a statement that predicteds that one phenomenon will be the result of one or more other phenomena that precede it in time.

causal relationships observed changes (the 'effect') in one variable are due to earlier changes in another.

central limit theorem the sampling distribution approaches normality as the number of samples taken increases.

central tendency (a) Mean: the arithmetic mean, or average, is a measure of central tendency in a population or sample. The mean is defined as the sum of the scores divided by the total number of cases involved. (b) Median: this is the middle value of the observations when listed in ascending order; it bisects the observations (i.e. the point below which 50 per cent of the observations fall). (c) Mode: a measure of central tendency based on the most common value in the distribution (i.e. the value of X with the highest frequency).

clinical case series clinicians often collect a series of cases that they have seen in the course of their clinics or ward work. Such case series are sometimes used as a source of descriptive data.

clinical trial an experiment where the participants are patients.

closed question the question is followed by predetermined response choices into which the respondent's reply is placed.

cluster a sample unit which consists of a group of elements.

cluster sampling probability sampling involving the selection of groupings (clusters) and selecting the sample units from the clusters.

coding the assignation of (usually numerical) codes to each category of each variable.

cohort the population has a common experience or characteristic which defines the sampling (i.e. all born in the same year).

concept an abstraction representing an object or phenomenon.

confidence interval a confidence interval calculated from a sample is interpreted as a range of values which contains the true population value with the probability specified.

confounding factors an extraneous factor (a factor *other* than the variables under study), *not controlled for*, distorts the results. An extraneous factor only confounds when it is related to dependent variables and to the independent variables under investigation. It makes them appear connected when their association is, in fact, spurious.

conjoint analysis a generic term used to describe a range of methods for eliciting preferences by asking people to rate, rank or choose between carefully constructed scenarios that differ in the level of important characteristics (cues). Responses represent people's rank ordering of preferences, in response to systematic, factorial manipulation of independent variables, and are analysed using regression techniques to establish the relative importance of each cue and the trade-offs that people make between cues.

content analysis the systematic analysis of observations obtained from records, documents and field notes.

control group the group in the experimental research that is not exposed to the independent variable (intervention).

control variable a variable used to test the possibility that an empirically observed relationship between an independent and dependent variable is spurious.

convenience sample a sample that is fortuitously gathered or found in one place, setting or source.

cost–benefit analysis assignation of a monetary value to the benefits of a programme, and making comparisons with the monetary costs of the programme for an assessment of efficiency.

cost–consequence analysis uses a mixture of relevant clinically based measures, such as survival, symptom-free days, as well as patient-based measures relating to symptoms and/or quality of life.

cost–effectiveness analysis comparison of different programmes producing the same type of non-monetary benefit in relation to their monetary costs for an assessment of efficiency.

cost minimization compares the cost of achieving the same outcome.

cost–utility analysis relates the project's cost to a measure of its usefulness or outcome (utility).

crisis theory the individual strives towards homeostasis and equilibrium, and therefore crises are self-limiting as people work towards achieving stability.

critical appraisal a discipline for increasing the effectiveness of reading, by providing a comprehensive checklist for examining the quality of a research report.

critical incident approach uses interviews to investigate the factors, reasoning and processes involved in recent, memorable situations.

cross-section at one point in time.

cross-sectional study describes the frequency (or level) of a particular attribute in a defined population, or sample, *at one point in time*.

decision analysis a systematic quantitative approach for assessing the relative value of one or more different decision options.

deduction a theoretical or mental process of reasoning by which the investigator starts off with an idea, and develops a theory and hypothesis from it; then phenomena are assessed in order to determine whether the theory is consistent with the observations.

dependent variable(s) the variable(s) the investigator wishes to explain – the dependent variable is the expected outcome of the independent variable.

discrete choice modelling a method of measuring stated preferences, whereby respondents are asked to make a series of pairwise choices between scenarios which differ in the levels of important characteristics.

dispersion a summary of a spread of cases in a figure (measures include quartiles, percentiles, deciles, standard deviations and the range).

ecological fallacy assumes that the average characteristics of *populations*, and the results of ecological studies, are applicable to *individuals* within the population. Relationships between variables are estimated at one level of analysis (eg. the clinics) and then wrongly extrapolated to another (e.g. the individual patients).

ecological study the unit of observation and analysis is a group rather than an individual.

effect size a numerical index of the magnitude of an observed association.

emic perspective individuals' interpretations of their behaviour, customs or beliefs.

empirical based on observation.

empiricism a philosophical approach that the only valid form of knowledge is that which is gathered by use of the senses; explanations should be based on actual observations, rather than theoretical statements.

ethnography the study of people in their natural settings; a descriptive account of social life and culture in a defined social system, based on qualitative methods (e.g. detailed observations, unstructured interviews, analysis of documents). This method is used by anthropologists.

ethnomethodology a method for the study of a cultural group, and more specifically meaning *the methods of the people*; the study of how people use social interaction to make sense of situations (to create their 'reality') (*see also* phenomenology, interpretive approach, symbolic interactionism).

etic perspective investigators' interpretations of research participants' behaviour, customs or beliefs.

experiment a scientific method used to establish cause and effect relationships between the independent and dependent variables. At its most basic, the experiment is a situation in which the independent (experimental) variable is fixed by manipulation by the investigator or by natural occurrence. The *true* experimental method involves the random allocation of participants to experimental and control groups. Ideally, participants are assessed before and after the manipulation of the independent variable in order to measure its effects on the dependent variable.

experimental group the group that is exposed to the independent variable (intervention) in experimental research.

field research research which takes place in a natural setting.

focus groups a research method of interviewing people while they are interacting in small groups.

framing bias the way in which information is presented can affect people's perceptions of it.

frequentist framework for statistical inference assumes that there is a true (fixed) population value for the parameter that we are trying to estimate.

frequency distribution the number of observations of each of the values within a variable.

functionalism theory based on interrelationships within the social system as a whole; how they operate and change, and their social consequences for individuals, sub-systems and societies.

grounded theory the investigator develops conceptual categories from the data and then makes new observations to develop these categories. Hypotheses are derived directly from the data.

health behaviour an activity undertaken by a person for the purpose of preventing disease or detecting it at an asymptomatic stage.

health outcome in the context of health services, outcomes relate to the effect of service interventions on individuals' previous health status, in relation to the aims of the intervention; in the broader context of health and illness, outcome can simply be defined in relation to the individual's goals and priorities.

health service needs need for effective services.

health status, subjective or perceived an individual's experience of mental, physical and social functioning and well-being.

heuristics use of short cuts in decision-making to simplify the process, known as rules of thumb (classic heuristics are characterized as intuitive processes similar to perception).

hierarchical data data on different levels or layers (e.g. area, household, individual member of household).

hypothesis a tentative solution to a research question, expressed in the form of a prediction about the relationship between the dependent and independent variables.

hypothetico-deductive method beginning with a theory and, in a deductive way, deriving testable hypotheses from it, the hypotheses are then tested by gathering and analysing data and the theory is supported or refuted (*see* deduction).

idiographic research which studies individuals, and which attempts to understand people or social situations in relation to their unique characteristics, without attempting to make generalizations.

incidence cases (e.g. of disease) which first occur in a population in a defined period of time.

incremental costs the extra costs of moving from one service to another.

independent variable(s) the explanatory or predictor variable(s) – the variable hypothesized to explain the dependent variable(s).

indicator measurement tool used for monitoring and evaluation.

individualistic or reductionist fallacy inferences about groups are wrongly drawn from data about individuals.

induction begins with the observation and measurement of phenomena and then develops ideas and general theories about the universe of interest.

inferential statistics these enable the researcher to make inferences about the characteristics of the population of interest on the basis of observations made on a sample of that population.

information acquisition patterns the order and combination in which information is searched in the process of making a judgement or decision.

information bias misclassification of, for example, people's responses due to error or bias.

interaction the direction and/or magnitude of the association between two variables depends on the value of one or more other variables.

interdisciplinary research researchers from different distinct disciplines work together to yield novel but *integrated* outputs. The aim is to synthesize different approaches and potentially create something entirely new.

interpretive approach the theoretical perspective that social scientists must include the meaning that social actors give to events and behaviour; symbolic interactionists and ethnomethodologists hold interpretive perspectives and subscribe to the philosophy of phenomenology.

interval data the data points (classes) are ordered and the size of the difference between the points is specified, but the zero point and unit of measurement are arbitrary (e.g. temperature – the zero point differs on the two scales commonly used).

intervening variable the independent variable affects the dependent variable through another (intervening) variable. This is also referred to as indirect causation.

interventional (experimental) study the investigator tests whether modifying or changing something about the study participants alters the development or course of the outcome.

interview a research method which involves a trained interviewer asking questions and recording respondents' replies. Interview questions can be structured (printed on a questionnaire with set question wording and pre-coded response categories), semi-structured (mostly open-ended questions, i.e. with no pre-coded response categories) or unstructured and in-depth (listed topics about which interviewers probe respondents for their views and experiences).

judgement analysis models the influence of case information on judgement or decision-making.

leading question question phrased in a way which leads the respondent to believe that a certain reply is expected.

lens model/framework a model of judges' or decision-makers' use of information in terms of its usefulness.

lens model equation a regression-based equation expressing a judge's accuracy in terms of models of the criterion being judged and the judgement, and the match between these.

level of measurement categorization of measuring instruments, and their resulting data, into four types: nominal, ordinal, interval, ratio.

longitudinal at more than one point in time.

marginal cost(s) the extra cost(s) of producing one extra unit of output.

mathematical health care evaluation model an analytic methodology that accounts for events over time and across populations, based on primary or secondary data, to estimate the effects of an intervention on valued health consequences and costs.

Mendelian randomization investigates genetic variant-disease associations that are not generally susceptible to the reverse causation or confounding which may distort interpretations of conventional observational studies.

meta-analysis the systematic process whereby a single quantitative measure of effect is derived from the combination of effects from a number of separate studies.

missing data information that is not available for a particular case (e.g. person) for which other information is available (e.g. owing to item non-response).

mixed methods combined qualitative and quantitative designs: the use of qualitative and quantitative techniques in parallel or sequentially.

model a description of some system intended to predict what happens if certain actions are taken.

moderating variable the variable that determines the effect of one variable on another.

multidisciplinary research researchers from different distinct disciplines collaborate, aiming to generate novel outputs in relation to a common goal.

multivariate statistics analysis of three or more variables simultaneously; for example, they can explain the association of two variables after adjusting for one or more others (e.g. multiple and logistic regression analysis, factor analysis).

naturalistic decision-making approach uses methods which aim to study decision-making in as natural or realistic settings as possible.

naturalistic research descriptive research in natural, unmanipulated, social settings using less obtrusive, qualitative methods.

need includes felt need (want), expressed need (demand), normative need (experts' definitions which can change over time in response to knowledge) and comparative need (comparisons with others and considerations of equity).

nominal data the classes are mutually exclusive, but have no intrinsic order or value (e.g. classification of capitals: Berlin, London, Milan, Paris, Stockholm).

nomothetics the science of general laws; a belief in general laws that influence behaviour or personality traits; aims to generalize research findings.

normal distribution a mathematically defined curve which is an ideal or a theoretical distribution that occurs frequently in real life, especially in sampling. The normal distribution is a symmetrical, bell-shaped curve, rising smoothly from a small number of cases at both extremes to a large number of cases in the middle; and the average (mean) corresponds to the peak of the distribution; it is enveloped by a curve and equation.

null hypothesis a statement that there is no relationship between the dependent and independent variables.

observation (in social science) a research method in which the investigator systematically watches, listens to and records the phenomenon of interest.

observational studies (in epidemiology) involve the investigator collecting data on factors (**exposures**) associated with the occurrence or progression of the outcome of interest, without attempting to alter the exposure status of subjects.

operationalize the development of proxy measures which enable phenomena to be observed empirically (i.e. measured).

opportunity cost the value of the best alternative use of a programme's resources (i.e. the value forgone by the investment in the programme).

ordinal data classes which can be placed in rank order (e.g. bigger than, preferred to, higher than) but in which the amount by which one class is bigger than/preferred is not specified (e.g. behaviour and attitudes: much more, more, about the same, less, much less; strongly agree, agree, neither agree nor disagree, disagree, strongly disagree; social class I professional, II semi-professional, III non-manual, III manual, IV semi-skilled, V unskilled).

P value P is the symbol of the probability associated with the outcome of a test of a null hypothesis (i.e. the probability that an observed inferential statistic occurred by chance, as in $P < 0.05$); p (small p) is used for proportions. Statistical tests exist which, in appropriate study designs and samples, can test for the probability of observing the values obtained.

paradigm a set of ideas (hypotheses) about the phenomena under inquiry.

paradigm shift this occurs if, over time, evidence accumulates which refutes, or is incompatible with, the paradigm, and thus the old paradigm is replaced by a new one.

participant observation a research method in which the investigator takes part in (i.e. has a 'role' in) the social phenomenon of interest.

patient/client-based assessment measure an instrument which aims to measure individuals' perceptions of their condition, and/or its effects on their lives, and changes in this/ these following an intervention.

pattern recognition combinations of information matching those stored in long-term memory are associated (apparently automatically) with a particular judgement, hypothesis or action, as if the pattern of cues is recognized. Used mostly in relation to visual information (e.g. when evaluating dermatology slides, X-rays, etc.).

performance indicator a quantitative measure incorporating dimensions of efficiency and equity.

perspective a way of interpreting empirical phenomena.

phenomenological sociology is based on the concept of the social construction of reality through the social interaction of people (social actors), who use symbols to interpret each other and assign meanings to perceptions and experiences (*see also* ethnomethodology, interpretive approach, symbolic interactionism).

phenomenology the philosophical belief that, unlike matter, humans have a consciousness. They interpret and experience the world in terms of meanings and actively construct an individual social reality.

positivism aims to discover laws using quantitative methods and emphasizes *positive facts*. It assumes that human behaviour is a reaction to (i.e. determined by) external stimuli and that it is possible to observe and measure social phenomena using the principles of the natural scientist, and to establish a reliable and valid body of knowledge about its operation based on empiricism and the hypothetico-deductive method.

power calculation a measure of how likely the study is to produce a statistically significant result for a difference between groups of a given magnitude (i.e. the ability to detect a true difference).

precision the ability of a measure to detect small changes in an attribute.

preference methods (stated) elicit people's preferences for alternative goods or services; conjoint analysis and discrete choice modelling are two methods of measuring and analysing stated preferences.

preference (stated) discrete choice modelling (in contrast to conjoint analysis) is based on random utility theory: an individual's utility consists of a systematic and random component (the random component implies that the investigator can only predict the *probability* that a person will choose a particular alternative).

prevalence the number of instances of a phenomenon in a specified population at a designated time.

prevalence ratio the number of cases (e.g. of disease) in a population at one point in time, expressed as a ratio of the population's size.

process tracing a general term that characterizes a variety of methods developed to track the reasoning process as it unfolds over time, leading to a decision.

prospective study collection of data over the forward passage of time (future).

psychometric validation the process by which an instrument is assessed for reliability and validity by mounting a series of defined tests on the population group for whom the instrument is intended.

purposive sample a sample in which respondents, subjects or settings are deliberately chosen to reflect some features or characteristics of interest.

qualitative research social research which is carried out in the field (natural settings) and analysed largely in non-statistical ways.

quality of life in relation to health (health-related quality of life) the *perceived effects* of disease and treatment on different areas of life; not simply about states and feelings of healthiness or wellness (which come within definitions of perceived health status).

quantitative research the measurement and analysis of observations in a numerical way.

quota sample sampling technique which takes account of characteristics of the wider population, making sure that their distribution is replicated in the composition of the study sample.

random error the errors in the study (usually from the sampling) randomly vary and sum to zero over enough cases; random error results in an estimate being *equally* likely to be above or below the true value.

random sampling this gives each of the units in the target population a calculable and non-zero probability of being selected.

randomization assignment at random of people to experimental and control groups in experiments.

randomized controlled trial a planned and rigorously controlled experiment, which compares the outcomes of a group receiving an intervention with those observed in a comparable group receiving a control intervention.

range a measure of dispersion which is based on the lowest and highest values observed.

ratio data scores are assigned on a scale with equal intervals and a true zero point.

reactive (Hawthorne) effect a guinea-pig effect (awareness of being studied). If people feel they are being tested they may feel the need to create a good impression, or if the study stimulates new interest in the topic under investigation then the results will be distorted.

recognition primed decision-making with experience people acquire a large repertoire of patterns or schemata which enable them to recognize and immediately categorize new situations as familiar or not.

reductionism the view that the phenomenon of interest can be explained within the lowest level of investigation (e.g. in biology, the cellular or chemical level). In sociology, this is known as atomism, which argues that the social system is no more than a collection of individuals, and in order to understand the social system we simply need to understand individuals.

reductionist fallacy inferences about groups are wrongly drawn from data about individuals.

regression to the mean an extreme measurement on a variable of interest which contains a degree of random error; on subsequent measurements, this value will tend to return to normal. The implication is that if a group of patients with a severe disease rating at a particular point in time have been selected for study, they may improve in the short term, independently of any intervention, simply because of the random variation inherent in the disease.

relative risk the incidence rate for the condition in the population exposed to a phenomenon divided by the incidence rate in the non-exposed population.

relativism no single system of knowledge or beliefs (or 'social facts') exists; it is dependent on context (i.e. culture).

reliability the extent to which the measure is consistent and minimizes random error (its repeatability).

research design this refers to the strategy of the research – how the sampling is conducted, whether a descriptive or experimental design is selected, whether control groups are needed, what variables need to be operationalized and measured, what analyses will be conducted.

research methods or techniques these are the methods of data collection – interview, telephone, postal surveys, diaries and analyses of documents, observational methods and so on. They are also the instruments to be used.

response bias the non-responders differ from responders in relation to the variable of interest.

response rate the number and percentage of people who respond positively to the invitation to take part in the study.

response shift the process whereby internal standards and values are changed.

responsiveness a measure of the association between the *change* in the observed score and the change in the true value of the construct (*see also* sensitivity).

retrospective study collection of data over past time (looking backwards).

reverse causation the causal direction of the observed association is opposite to that hypothesized. Experiments deal with reverse causation by the manipulation of the experimental (independent) variable, measuring the dependent variable before and after this manipulation.

sample a sub-set of a population.

sampling techniques used to obtain a sub-set of a population without the expense of conducting a census (gathering of information from *all* members of a population).

sampling distribution the distribution of means of all possible different samples of *n* observations that can be obtained from this population. It has a mean equal to the population mean. It is a normal distribution (assuming the sample size is large enough).

sampling error any sample is just one of an almost infinite number that might have been selected, all of which can produce slightly different estimates. Sampling error is the probability that any one sample is not completely representative of the population from which it was drawn.

sampling frame a list of the sampling units from which the sample can be drawn.

scaling the assignation of numbers to responses (e.g. relating to attitudes, beliefs, perceptions) following a specified method and set of associated rules.

script activation scripts (abstract patterns of information describing the features seen [e.g. in an illness], and the order in which they are seen) are stored in long-term memory. They are activated (possibly unconsciously) when combinations of information, approximating the abstract forms, are perceived.

selection bias systematic differences between those selected and not selected for study; thus, study members are biased and not representative of the target population.

sensitivity ability of the actual gradations in the scale's scores to reflect any changes adequately; probability of correctly identifying affected person ('case').

sensitivity analysis a method for making plausible assumptions about the margins of error in the results, and assessing whether they affect the implications of the results. The margins of error can be calculated using the confidence intervals of the results or they can be guessed.

simple random sample a probability sampling method that gives each sampling unit an equal chance of being selected in the sample.

skewed distribution a distribution in which more observations fall on one side of the mean than the other.

snowball sample starting with an initial contact, the researcher asks this contact for referrals to other respondents who may be able to contribute to the research topic.

social theory an explanation of something and can just be an answer to 'what', 'when' or 'why' questions; also refers to more developed bodies of structured knowledge that may have developed over time.

specificity a measure of the probability of correctly identifying a non-affected person (i.e. 'non-case') with the measure.

spurious association an observed association between the dependent and independent variables which is false (spurious) because the association is caused by a third extraneous variable which intervenes. If the latter is controlled the observed association disappears.

standard deviation this is the most common measure of dispersion. It is based on the difference of values from the mean value (the spread of individual results round a mean value); it is the square root of the arithmetic mean of the squared deviations from the mean.

standard error this is a measure of the uncertainty in a sample statistic; the standard deviation of the sampling distribution is called the standard error. It is related to the population variation. The standard error of a mean is the standard deviation of the population divided by the square root of the sample size. The formula is given in standard statistical texts.

standardized mortality rate deaths e.g. per 1000 of the population standardized for age.

standardized mortality ratio compares the standard mortality rate for the standard (whole) population with that of particular regions or groups (index population), and expresses this as a ratio.

statistical significance significance at the 0.05 per cent level means that five times in 100 the results could have occurred by chance, i.e. if the test was performed 100 times, on five occasions significant results will occur by chance.

structural approaches in clinical decision-making statistical analyses of the relationship between judgements or decisions made, and information about the clinician, client or setting.

survey a method of collecting information from a sample of the population of interest (known as a sample survey).

survivor bias the most severely affected cases die earlier than other cases.

symbolic interactionism perspective concerned with the meanings of phenomena to individuals, and how these meanings are produced in social exchanges. Focuses on the details of interactions between individuals, rather than the wider social system, and in particular the use of symbols in communications and in the creation of a sense of self and a sense of social reality (*see also* phenomenology, ethnomethodology, interpretive approach).

systematic error the errors in the study result in an estimate being more likely to be *either* above or below the true value, depending upon the nature of the systematic error in any particular case.

systematic random sampling a sample in which every *k*th case is selected from the population (*n*) (with a random starting point).

systematic research the process of research should be based on an agreed set of rules and processes which are rigorously adhered to, and against which the research can be evaluated.

systematic review methodical and deliberate survey and assessment of a body of evidence relating to a particular health issue; it is prepared with a systematic approach to minimizing study biases and random errors.

theory a set of logically interrelated propositions and their implications.

theoretical framework the conceptual underpinning of a research study. This may be based on an emergent theory or a specific conceptual model.

think aloud the concurrent verbalization of thoughts as they pass through a respondent's consciousness. A process-tracing technique aiming to externalize the contents of working memory during problem-solving/decision-making.

triangulation the use of three or more different research methods (i.e. multiple methods) to investigate the phenomenon of interest.

Type I error (or alpha error) the error of rejecting a true null hypothesis.

Type II error (or beta error) the failure to reject (i.e. acceptance of) a null hypothesis when it is actually false.

unidimensional the items comprising a measurement scale form a single dimension that reflects one concept.

utility of a health state a cardinal measure of the strength of an individual's preference for particular health outcomes when faced with uncertainty.

validity, ecological the realism of the research results in real life settings, i.e. outside the artificial research setting.

validity, external the extent to which the research findings can be generalized to the wider population of interest and applied to different settings.

validity, internal the extent to which the instrument is really measuring what it purports to measure.

variable an indicator assumed to represent the underlying construct or concept, produced by the operationalization of the latter.

Index

Note on using this index: (i) common terms are indexed in alphabetical order; (ii) specialist terms, with specialized and relevant uses of common terms, are indexed within specialist subject headings.

RESEARCH METHODS IN HEALTH
INVESTIGATING HEALTH AND HEALTH SERVICES

Ann Bowling

Praise for the first edition of *Research Methods in Health*:

> . . . a brilliantly clear documentation of different philosophies, approaches and methods of research about health and services. Laid out in an accessible and manageable way, it covers an enormous amount of material without sacrificing thoroughness . . . I would recommend it to a broad readership.
>
> *MIDIRS Midwifery Digest*

> . . . This major research textbook is as good as an introduction to the field as you are likely to find.
>
> *The International Journal of Social Psychiatry*

> . . . an easy to read book with excellent background information on the theory and practice of research. A summary of main points, key terms and recommended reading follows each chapter and there is a useful glossary of terms at the end of the book for quick reference . . . I particularly liked the checklists when undertaking literature reviews and writing research proposals.
>
> *British Journal of Health Care Management*

This new edition of Ann Bowling's well-known and highly respected text has been thoroughly revised and updated to reflect key methodological developments in health research. It is a comprehensive, easy to read guide to the range of methods used to study and evaluate health and health services. It describes the concepts and methods used by the main disciplines involved in health research, including: demography, epidemiology, health economics, psychology and sociology.

The research methods described cover the assessment of health needs, morbidity and mortality trends and rates, costing health services, sampling for survey research, cross-sectional and longitudinal survey design, experimental methods and techniques of group assignment, questionnaire design, interviewing techniques, coding and analysis of quantitative data, methods and analysis of qualitative observational studies, and types of unstructured interviewing.

With new material on topics such as cluster randomization, utility analyses, patients' preferences, and perception of risk, the text is aimed at students and researchers of health and health services. It has also been designed for health professionals and policy makers who have responsibility for applying research findings in practice, and who need to know how to judge the value of that research.

Contents
Part one: Investigating health services and health: the scope of research – Part two: The philosophy, theory and practice of research – Part three: Quantitative research: sampling and research methods – Part four: The tools of quantitative research – Part five: Qualitative and combined research methods, and their analysis – Index.

512pp   0 335 20643 3 (Paperback)   0 335 20644 1 (Hardback)

MEASURING DISEASE
A REVIEW OF DISEASE SPECIFIC QUALITY OF LIFE MEASUREMENT SCALES
Second Edition

Ann Bowling

Praise for the first edition:

> . . . text that is remarkably detailed and comprehensive in its coverage of a range of quality of life measures . . . Bowling's book provides an important step towards the development of measures of quality of life that are both sensitive and rigorous.
>
> *Journal of Epidemiology & Community Health*

> . . . a most useful and comprehensive addition to the literature . . . The book is readable, well referenced and up to date. I recommend any group that wishes to attempt to measure health outcomes to consider adding this book to their resource list.
>
> *Australian Health Review*

> . . . this book gives an in-depth and comprehensive insight in health-related quality of life scales . . . a most valuable guide in helping the reader search for the scale with the best psychometric properties. Furthermore, this book will contribute highly to the improvement of disease-specific measurement of quality of life and to the comparability of measurement results.
>
> *Journal of Health Psychology*

This is a thoroughly updated and revised edition of *Measuring Disease*. It supplements the author's previous work *Measuring Health* (2nd edition). In assessing the outcome of disease and treatments, measurement scales must be relevant to their specific effects, necessitating the use of disease specific questionnaires. There is now considerable interest in measures which are multi-dimensional, and which are more sensitive than generic measures to specific disease and treatment effects. This book reviews disease specific measures of quality of life and, where relevant, popularly used symptom and single dimension scales. It is intended as a source book for researchers, medical and health care practitioners who are involved in the measurement of the outcome of health services.

Contents
Preface – List of Abbreviations – Health-related quality of life: conceptual meaning, use and measurement – Cancers – Psychiatric conditions and psychological morbidity – Respiratory conditions – Neurological conditions – Rheumatological conditions – Cardiovascular diseases – Other disease- and condition-specific scales – Appendix: a selection of useful scale distributors and addresses – References – Index.

420pp   0 335 20641 7 (Paperback)

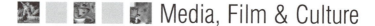
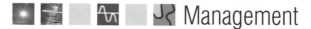
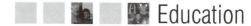
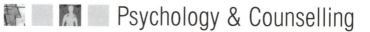
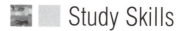
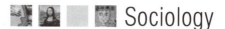
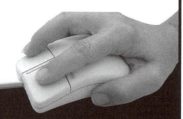
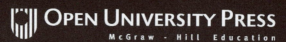